Great Ormond Street
Handbook of Paediatrics

The product of a world centre of excellence in teaching and medical and surgical practice, this new edition of a bestseller has been revised throughout for easier quick reference. Building on the range of expertise showcased in the previous editions, this text incorporates updated material and new figures to helpfully illustrate clinical features and epidemiology. This compact volume offers expert knowledge useful for trainees and professional clinicians in other disciplines.

- Offers unparalleled range of expertise in a compact volume
- Provides both paediatricians in training and practice and professionals in many other disciplines with expert knowledge
- Combines the advantages of a colour atlas with those of a short textbook covering clinical features, epidemiology, investigations, and differential diagnosis

T0386166

Great Ormond Street Handbook Series

Great Ormond Street Handbook of Congenital Ear Deformities
An Illustrated Surgical Guide
Neil W Bulstrode & Ahmed Salah Mazeed

Great Ormond Street Handbook of Paediatric Vascular Anomalies
An Illustrated Guide to Clinical Management
Neil W Bulstrode, Alex Barnacle, Maanasa Polubothu

Great Ormond Street Handbook of Paediatrics
An Illustrated Guide, Third Edition
Stephen D Marks, Simon Blackburn, Stephan Strobel

For more information about this series, please visit: https://www.routledge.com/Great-Ormond-Street-Handbook-Series/book-series/GOSH

Great Ormond Street Handbook of Paediatrics

An Illustrated Guide

Third Edition

Edited by

Stephen D Marks, MD MSc MRCP DCH FRCPCH
Simon Blackburn, MEd FRCS(paed.surg) FFST
Stephan Strobel, MD, PhD, MRCP(Hon), FRCP, FRCPCH

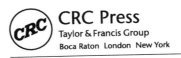
CRC Press
Taylor & Francis Group
Boca Raton London New York

CRC Press is an imprint of the
Taylor & Francis Group, an **informa** business

Designed cover image: Shutterstock 397786159. Bibiz1

Third edition published 2025
by CRC Press
2385 NW Executive Center Drive, Suite 320, Boca Raton FL 33431

and by CRC Press
4 Park Square, Milton Park, Abingdon, Oxon, OX14 4RN

CRC Press is an imprint of Taylor & Francis Group, LLC

© 2025 Taylor & Francis Group, LLC

Second edition published by CRC Press 2016

Library of Congress Cataloging-in-Publication Data
Names: Strobel, Stephan editor | Blackburn, Simon, 1979- editor | Marks, Stephen D editor
Title: Great Ormond Street handbook of paediatrics / edited by Stephen D Marks, Simon Blackburn and Stephan Strobel.
Other titles: Handbook of paediatrics
Description: Third edition. | Boca Raton, FL : CRC Press, 2025. | Includes bibliographical references and index.
Identifiers: LCCN 2024014422 (print) | LCCN 2024014423 (ebook) | ISBN 9781032006871 paperback | ISBN 9781032006918 hardback | ISBN 9781003175186 ebook
Subjects: MESH: Pediatrics | Child Health | Adolescent Health | Handbook | LCGFT: Handbooks and manuals
Classification: LCC RJ45 .G76 2025 (print) | LCC RJ45 (ebook) | NLM WS 39 | DDC 618.92–dc23/eng
LC record available at https://lccn.loc.gov/2024014422
LC ebook record available at https://lccn.loc.gov/2024014423

ISBN: 9781032006918 (hbk)
ISBN: 9781032006871 (pbk)
ISBN: 9781003175186 (ebk)

DOI: 10.1201/9781003175186

Typeset in Palatino
by Deanta Global Publishing Services, Chennai, India

Contents

Foreword

It is a great privilege to write the Foreword for the third edition of the *Great Ormond Street Handbook of Paediatrics* after my predecessors, Sir Cyril Chantler and Tessa Blackstone. Surgical, medical and genetic techniques have hugely advanced since this handbook was first published in 2007 where it has been the winner of the 2007 Royal Society of Medicine & Society of Authors Book Awards. It is wonderful to see that the authors and the three editors, who are experts in their fields, have thoroughly revised the contents of this important handbook. The text is both concise and clear and the images are of the highest quality, made possible through the excellent work undertaken by the hospital's Department of Medical Illustration. It is refreshing to see an up-to-date textbook containing such high quality figures covering a wider range of conditions which makes it easier on the eye of the reader!

The hospital was the first children's hospital in the United Kingdom and was founded by Dr Charles West, opening in 1852 with just ten beds. Although still situated in Great Ormond Street, the hospital and healthcare has completely changed over the last 170 years, now with over 300 consultants who form part of the experienced multidisciplinary teams that work together to provide the best care for children and their families. Great Ormond Street Hospital for Children NHS Foundation Trust (GOSH) is an international centre of excellence in child healthcare and the largest paediatric centre in the United Kingdom. GOSH is an acute specialist paediatric hospital with over 60 clinical specialties and subspecialties, with a mission to provide world-class care to children and young people with rare, complex and difficult-to-treat conditions, yet the authors cover all common and rare medical and surgical conditions of childhood. Patients receive first class care, including advanced therapy medicinal products and gene therapies, in our research hospital which links closely with our academic partners, University College London Great Ormond Street Institute of Child Health and the National Institute for Health and Social Care Research (NIHR) Great Ormond Street Hospital Biomedical Research Centre. We have state of the art laboratory and research facilities at GOSH and UCL now with the Zayed Centre for Research into Rare Disease in Children, which has opened since the second edition of this handbook.

I am sure that this handbook will be an invaluable resource and superb reference book for all those who provide healthcare for children and young people, including doctors from general practitioners to general paediatricians, specialists and trainees as well as medical students, paediatric nurses and members of the multidisciplinary teams.

I would like to thank all the contributors as well as the three editors who are passionate about medical education and have spent so much time editing the book, which I am sure will be read not just in the United Kingdom, but also internationally. Like the previous editions, I do hope that it will be translated into other languages and of use to those in low and middle income countries.

Ellen Schroder
Chair
Great Ormond Street Hospital
for Children NHS Foundation Trust

About the Editors

Stephen D Marks, MD MSc MRCP DCH FRCPCH is a Consultant Paediatric Nephrologist and clinical lead for renal transplantation at Great Ormond Street Hospital for Children NHS Foundation Trust (GOSH). He is Professor of Paediatric Nephrology and Transplantation at University College London Great Ormond Street Institute of Child Health and Director of the NIHR GOSH Clinical Research Facility.

Simon Blackburn MEd FRCS(paed.surg) FFST is a Consultant Neonatal and Paediatric Surgeon at Great Ormond Street Hospital where he is also Co-Director of Education and of the Learning Academy.

Stephan Strobel, MD, PhD, MRCP(Hon), FRCP, FRCPCH, is an Emeritus Professor of Paediatrics and Clinical Immunology, University of Plymouth and Honorary Professor of Paediatrics and Clinical Immunology, University College London Institute of Child Health and Great Ormond Street Hospital for Children NHS Foundation Trust, UK.

Contributors

Nele Alders
Institute of Tropical Medicine
Antwerp, Belgium

Anoushka Alwis
Consultant Paediatric Neurologist, General
Neurology, Headache and Neurovascular
Service
Great Ormond Street Hospital for Children
NHS Foundation Trust, London, UK

Angela Barnicoat
Former Consultant in Clinical Genetics, Great
Ormond Street Hospital for Children NHS
Foundation Trust, London, UK

Jack Bartram
Consultant Paediatric Haematologist, Great
Ormond Street Hospital for Children NHS
Foundation Trust, London, UK

Richard Bowman
Consultant Paediatric Ophthalmologist, Great
Ormond Street Hospital for Children NHS
Foundation Trust, London, UK

Paul Brogan
Professor of Vasculitis and Honorary
Consultant Paediatric Rheumatologist, Great
Ormond Street Hospital for Children NHS
Foundation Trust, London, UK

Alex Broomfield
Consultant, Metabolic Unit, Great Ormond
Street Hospital for Children NHS Foundation
Trust, London, UK

Rossa Brugha
Respiratory Consultant, Great Ormond Street
Hospital for Children NHS Foundation Trust,
London, UK

Neil Bulstrode
Consultant Plastic Surgeon, Great Ormond
Street Hospital for Children NHS Foundation
Trust, London, UK

Michelle Carr
Consultant Fetal and Paediatric Cardiologist,
Great Ormond Street Hospital for Children
NHS Foundation Trust, London, UK

Abraham Cherian
Consultant Paediatric Urologist, Great Ormond
Street Hospital for Children NHS Foundation
Trust, London, UK

Tanzina Chowdhury
Consultant Paediatric Oncologist, Great
Ormond Street Hospital for Children NHS
Foundation Trust, London, UK

Samantha Cooray
Department of Paediatrics, Women and
Children's Services, Homerton Healthcare NHS
Foundation Trust, London, UK

Paula Coyle
Consultant Paediatric Otolaryngologist,
University College London Hospital, London,
UK

Mehul T Dattani
Consultant in Paediatric Endocrinology,
Great Ormond Street Hospital for Children,
NHS Foundation Trust, London, UK

David Dunaway
Consultant Craniofacial Surgeon, Great
Ormond Street Hospital for Children NHS
Foundation Trust, London, UK

Deborah M Eastwood
Consultant Paediatric Orthopaedic Surgeon,
Great Ormond Street Hospital for Children
and Royal National Orthopaedic Hospital NHS
Foundation Trusts, London, UK

Simon Eccles
Consultant Craniofacial and Plastic Surgeon,
Great Ormond Street Hospital for Children
NHS Foundation Trust, London, UK

Noelle Enright
Consultant Paediatric Neurologist, Great
Ormond Street Hospital for Children NHS
Foundation Trust, London, UK

Ru-Xin Foong
Consultant in Paediatric Allergy, Evelina
Children's Hospital, Guy's and St Thomas'
Hospitals NHS Foundation Trust, London, UK

Adam T Fox
Consultant in Paediatric Allergy, Guy's and St
Thomas' NHS Foundation Trust, London, UK

Edward Gaynor
Consultant Paediatric Gastroenterologist and
Lead, Gastrointestinal Allergy, Great Ormond
Street Hospital for Children NHS Foundation
Trust, London, UK
Chair of Quality Standards, British Society of
Paediatric Gastroenterology, Hepatology and
Nutrition, UK

Sara Ghorashian
Consultant Paediatric Haematologisy and
Honorary Senior Lecturer, Great Ormond
Street Hospital for Children NHS Foundation
Trust, London, UK

Sri Gore
Consultant Ophthalmologist and Oculoplastic
Surgeon, Great Ormond Street Hospital for
Children NHS Foundation Trust, London, UK

Adriaan Grobbelaar
Department of Plastic Surgery, Great Ormond
Street Hospital
Department of Plastic and Hand Surgery,
University of Bern, Switzerland
Professor, UCL Department of Surgery and
Interventional Sciences

Stephanie Grünewald
Consultant, Metabolic Unit, Great Ormond
Street Hospital for Children NHS Foundation
Trust, London, UK

Darren Hargrave
Clinical Paediatric Oncologist, Great Ormond
Street Hospital for Children NHS Foundation
Trust, London, UK

Robert H Henderson
Consultant, Great Ormond Street Hospital for
Children NHS Foundation Trust, London, UK

Susan Hill
Gastroenterology Consultant, Specialist in
Nutrition and Intestinal Insufficiency, Great
Ormond Street Hospital for Children, NHS
Foundation Trust
Honorary Senior Lecturer, UCL Institute of
Child Health, London, UK

David Inwald
Consultant in Paediatric Intensive Care,
Addenbrooke's Hospital, Cambridge University
Hospitals NHS Foundation Trust, Cambridge

Winnie Ip
Consultant Immunologist, Great Ormond
Street Hospital for Children NHS Foundation
Trust, London, UK

Christopher Jephson
Consultant Paediatric Otolaryngologist, Great
Ormond Street Hospital for Children NHS
Foundation Trust, London, UK

Loshan Kangesu
Consultant Plastic Surgeon, Great Ormond
Street Hospital for Children NHS Foundation
Trust, London, UK

Jonathan Leckenby, MD, PhD
Honorary Consultant Plastic Surgeon, Great
Ormond Street Hospital, London
Assistant Professor, Departments of Surgery
and
Neuroscience, University of Rochester Medical
Center, Rochester, New York, USA

Keith Lindley
Consultant Paediatric Gastroenterologist, Great
Ormond Street Hospital for Children NHS
Foundation Trust, London, UK

Florian Moenkemeyer
Consultant in Paediatric Cardiology, Great
Ormond Street Hospital for Children NHS
Foundation Trust, London, UK

Paul Morris
Consultant Plastic Surgeon, Great Ormond
Street Hospital for Children NHS Foundation
Trust, London, UK

Dhanya Mullassery
Consultant Neonatal and Paediatric Surgeon,
Great Ormond Street Hospital for Children
NHS Foundation Trust, London, UK

Ken Nischal
Professor and Director, Paediatric
Ophthalmology, Strabismus and Adult Motility,
Children's Hospital of Pittsburgh, UPMC
School of Medicine of Pittsburgh, University of
Pittsburgh, Philadelphia, USA

Juling Ong
Consultant Paediatric Plastic Surgeon, Great
Ormond Street Hospital, London, UK

Philip Ostrowski
Consultant in Clinical Genetics and Genomic
Medicine, Great Ormond Street Hospital for
Children NHS Foundation Trust, London, UK

Nandinee Patel
Consultant in Paediatric Allergy, St Mary's
Hospital, Imperial College Healthcare NHS
Trust
Honorary Senior Clinical Lecturer, Imperial
College London, London, UK

Justin Penner
Department of Infectious Diseases, Great
Ormond Street Hospital, London, UK

Catherine Peters
Consultant Paediatric Endocrinologist, Great
Ormond Street Hospital for Children NHS
Foundation Trust, London, UK

Mark Peters
Professor of Paediatric Intensive Care,
University College London Great Ormond St
Institute of Child Health and Great Ormond
Street Hospital for Children NHS Foundation
Trust, London, UK

Clarissa Pilkington
Consultant Paediatric and Adolescent
Rheumatologist, Great Ormond Street Hospital
for Children NHS Foundation Trust, London, UK

Maanasa Polubothu
Consultant Paediatric Dermatologist, Great
Ormond Street Hospital for Children NHS
Foundation Trust, London, UK

Michael Quail
Consultant Paediatric Cardiologist,
Great Ormond Street Hospital for Children
NHS Foundation Trust, London, UK

Liam Reilly
Paediatric Immunology, Infectious Diseases
& Allergy, Great North Children's Hospital,
Newcastle upon Tyne Hospitals NHS
Foundation Trust, UK

Patricia Rorison
Consultant Cleft & Plastic Surgeon, Great
Ormond Street, London. UK

Sohaib R. Rufai
NIHR Academic Clinical Lecturer in
Ophthalmology, University of Leicester
Ulverscroft Eye Unit, UK

Amir Sadri
Consultant Plastic Surgeon, Great Ormond
Street Hospital & The Royal London Hospital,
London, UK

Richard Scott
Consultant and Honorary Senior Lecturer
in Clinical Genetics, Great Ormond Street
Hospital for Children NHS Foundation Trust,
London, UK

Delane Shingadia
Department of Infectious Diseases, Great
Ormond Street Hospital, London, UK

Keith Sibson
Haemophilia Consultant, Great Ormond Street
Hospital for Children NHS Foundation Trust,
London, UK

Branavan Sivakumar
Consultant Hand, Plastic and Reconstructive
Surgeon, Great Ormond Street Hospital
for Children and Royal Free Hospital NHS
Foundation Trusts, London, UK

Olga Slater
Consultant Paediatric Oncologist, Great
Ormond Street Hospital for Children NHS
Foundation Trust, London, UK

Naima Smeulders
Consultant Paediatric Urologist, Great Ormond
Street Hospital for Children NHS Foundation
Trust, London, UK

Gillian Smith
Consultant Plastic and Reconstructive Surgeon,
Great Ormond Street Hospital for Children
NHS Foundation Trust, London, UK

Helen Spencer
Consultant Respiratory Paediatrician, Great
Ormond Street Hospital, London, UK

Alison Steele
Honorary Consultant, Great Ormond Street
Hospital for Children NHS Foundation Trust,
London, UK

Andrew Turnbull
Consultant Respiratory Paediatrician, Great
Ormond Street Hospital, NHS Foundation
Trust, London, UK

Anna Uwagboe
Consultant Paediatrician, Watford General
Hospital and the Lighthouse, Camden, UK

Ajay Vora
Consultant Paediatric Haematologist, Great
Ormond Street Hospital for Children NHS
Foundation Trust, London, UK

Emma Wakeling
Consultant in Clinical Genetics, North East
Thames Regional Genetic Service, Great
Ormond Street Hospital for Children NHS
Foundation Trust, London, UK

Austen Worth
Paediatric Immunology, Great Ormond Street
Hospital for Children NHS Foundation Trust,
UK
Associate Professor, University College
London, UK

Mildrid Yeo
Paediatric Genetics and Metabolic Consultant,
Paediatric Genetics Department, KK Women's
and Children's Hospital, Singapore

1 Emergency Medicine

David Inwald and Mark Peters

INTRODUCTION

A simple, structured approach to an acutely ill child has been the focus of the initiatives of Advanced Paediatric Life Support (APLS) and European Paediatric Advanced Life Support (EPALS) courses.

The advantages of this structured approach are clear: clinical problems are addressed in order of urgency and the chances of significant omissions are reduced. In all acutely ill children the airway (A), breathing (B) and circulation (C) should be assessed (and supported if inadequate) before a more detailed assessment is undertaken.

This chapter will outline the emergency management of the most common conditions requiring treatment in paediatric practice. In contrast to the APLS/EPLS approach we include some details of ongoing care. This does not mean to distract from the vital importance of the initial assessment and resuscitation. All readers involved in the care of acutely unwell children are encouraged to train in APLS/EPALS.

AIRWAY OBSTRUCTION

See also the chapter 'Respiratory Medicine'.

Stridor is an inspiratory noise related to obstruction of the extrathoracic airway. Dynamic intrathoracic airway obstruction can also result in expiratory stridor in conditions such as bronchomalacia or tracheomalacia. Obstruction of the extrathoracic airway is most commonly due to acute conditions, such as viral laryngotracheitis, bacterial tracheitis, foreign body aspiration and other conditions such as quinsy, retropharyngeal abscess, epiglottitis, inhalation of hot gases and angioneurotic oedema. Airway obstruction can also occur as a result of chronic lesions such as subglottic or tracheal stenosis, vascular ring, airway haemangiomata and polyps. These may present in the context of an intercurrent viral infection which may make airway obstruction worse.

Immediate Assessment and Management

Initial assessment should include rapid physical examination of the airway, breathing and circulation, with particular attention to the work of breathing (i.e. respiratory rate, recession, use of accessory muscles) and pulse oximetry. Cyanosis, distress, exhaustion or oxygen saturations of < 92% in air are all signs of severe obstruction and possible impending collapse. Children with these signs may require urgent intubation and ventilation. Intubation may be difficult and senior anaesthetic help should be summoned. Children with milder obstruction may require more specific management (see below). The presence of a high fever in a toxic-looking child should raise the possibility of bacterial tracheitis or epiglottitis. If the child is stable, a brief history should be taken with regard to recent coryzal illness (suggestive of viral tracheitis), foreign body aspiration and *Haemophilus* influenza immunisation.

Investigations

Radiological investigations are not routinely required. Lateral neck x-rays are rarely helpful. Imaging, which may include a chest radiograph and CT neck and thorax, should only be performed when the child is stable. Laboratory investigations need only be performed if intravenous access is required.

Further Management
Bacterial Tracheitis and Viral Tracheitis (Croup)

Children with mild or moderately severe viral tracheitis who do not require immediate intubation should be commenced on enteral or intravenous dexamethasone. However, children with bacterial tracheitis or severe viral tracheitis occasionally require intubation (Figures 1.1 and 1.2). A senior anaesthetist should be called as the child may require inhalational anaesthesia. Paralysing agents should be used with care in this setting as when muscle tone is lost the airway may completely obstruct. While waiting for help, nebulised adrenaline can be helpful in reducing airway oedema. Children with suspected bacterial tracheitis may be septic and require volume resuscitation prior to intubation. They should have blood cultures sent and antibiotics to cover *Staphylococcus* and

DOI: 10.1201/9781003175186-1

1

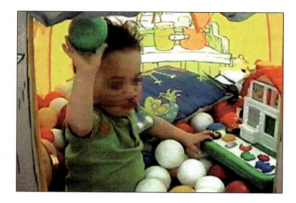

Figure 1.1 A two-year-old child with viral tracheitis intubated in the ICU. As the lungs are unaffected he does not require mechanical ventilation. A humidification device is attached to the end of the tube to prevent secretions drying in the airway.

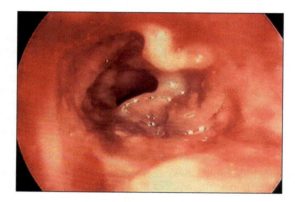

Figure 1.2 Bacterial tracheitis in an 18-month-old child who presented with a high pyrexia, shock and stridor.

Streptococcus infections should be commenced. There is a risk of early tube obstruction with pus and debris in children with tracheitis.

Foreign Body

Aspiration of a foreign body may result in an asymptomatic child or cardiorespiratory collapse. Clearly, partial or complete obstruction at the level of the larynx or trachea may require urgent resuscitation. Again, senior anaesthetic help should be summoned. It may be possible to remove the foreign body at laryngoscopy using some Magill's forceps. If not, an urgent tracheostomy may be required as a temporising measure. A foreign body further down the airway may cause partial or complete obstruction of one or more major bronchi. A chest radiograph may demonstrate areas of hyperinflation or collapse, depending on the degree of airway obstruction (Figures 1.3a and 1.3b). If in any doubt, inspiratory and expiratory films and the radiographic appearance of the pulmonary vascular tree will help to determine which lung is abnormal. These children need to be referred to a specialist centre where rigid bronchoscopy can be performed to remove the foreign body (Figure 1.4).

Other

Epiglottitis has become extremely rare since the introduction of *Haemophilus* influenza immunisation (Figure 1.5). If it is suspected, however, senior anaesthetic, ENT and paediatric advice should be sought. The airway should be secured, by tracheostomy if necessary. Antibiotic therapy with cover for *Haemophilus* infection should be commenced. Quinsy (peritonsillar abscess) will require

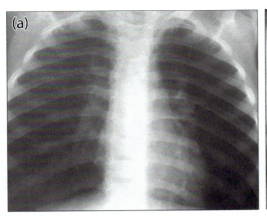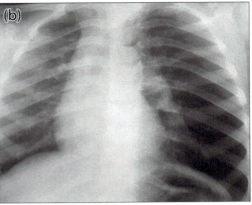

Figure 1.3a, b Inspiratory (a) and expiratory (b) chest radiographs in a 4-year-old child with an inhaled peanut in the left main bronchus. Though foreign bodies usually cause occlusion of the entire airway lumen and distal collapse, in this case the peanut is causing a ball-valve effect and the left lung does not deflate on expiration

incision and drainage, sometimes with a period of airway support while post-operative oedema settles. Anatomical lesions such as airway haemangiomata, vascular rings and tracheal stenosis may require specific surgical management (Figures 1.6, 1.7 and 1.8).

ANAPHYLAXIS

Anaphylaxis is a potentially life-threatening allergic reaction (Figure 1.9). Symptoms are usually sudden. They may include airway, breathing and circulation problems and skin or mucosal changes, although these may be absent in up to 20% of cases.

Anaphylaxis is a Type I hypersensitivity reaction triggered by crosslinking of IgE on mast cells. It occurs when enough antigen enters the systemic circulation to activate circulating basophils and tissue mast cells. This results in the release of inflammatory mediators, particularly histamine, prostaglandins and leukotrienes. These mediators cause massive peripheral vasodilation (cardio-respiratory arrest, shock), increased vascular permeability (angio-oedema, airway obstruction and urticaria), intense contraction of non-vascular smooth muscle (bronchoconstriction), abdominal pain, nausea, vomiting and tachycardia. Anaphylaxis may be due to drugs, insect stings, foods, plants, chemicals or latex.

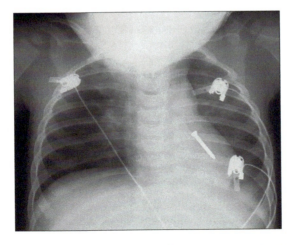

Figure 1.4 Nail in the left main bronchus. This will require removal with a rigid bronchoscope. Physiotherapy and flexible bronchoscopy are contraindicated, as both may cause the foreign body to slip further down the airway

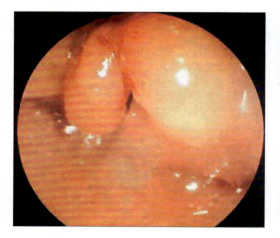

Figure 1.5 Acute inflammation of the epiglottis due to viral infection. The child required intubation

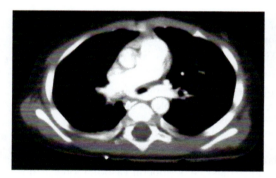

Figure 1.6 Left pulmonary artery vascular sling demonstrated by contrast CT scanning. The child presented with stridor.

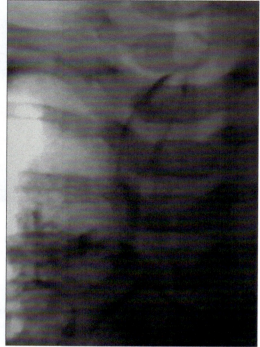

Figure 1.7 Congenital tracheal stenosis demonstrated by contrast bronchography. Surgical management was required.

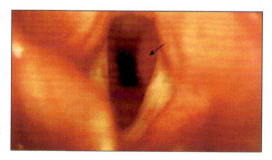

Figure 1.8 An airway haemangioma in a six-month-old child who presented with stridor. These lesions often present during viral lower respiratory tract infections when they are unmasked by additional airway swelling. The clue to the diagnosis may be the presence of haemangiomas elsewhere.

Recognition

Clinical assessment should include rapid physical examination, with attention to airway, breathing and circulation, measurement of peak expiratory flow rate (PEFR) in older children able to perform the technique and pulse oximetry. Children should be examined for generalised oedema, angio-oedema, erythematous rash and urticaria and a history taken for substance exposure (with particular reference to drugs or foodstuffs).

Immediate Management

Patients should be treated lying flat, with legs elevated if possible, with high-flow oxygen if $SpO_2 < 95\%$. If stridor is present, airway angio-oedema is likely and senior anaesthetic assistance should be summoned. Intramuscular adrenaline should be administered as soon as possible in anaphylactic shock. Adrenaline doses may be repeated at five-minute intervals. Intravenous adrenaline may be used if anaphylaxis is refractory, e.g. after two doses of intramuscular adrenaline. Hypotension in anaphylaxis is due to vasodilatation and capillary leak and intravenous fluid will be necessary to restore circulation. Bronchospasm, if present, may respond to adrenaline and corticosteroids. If mechanical ventilation is necessary, a

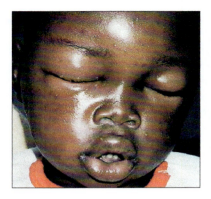

Figure 1.9 Severe anaphylaxis in an 11-month-old baby caused by bee stings with oedematous eyelids and lips, wheeze and shock.

slow rate and long expiratory time should be used to allow full expiration to occur. Refractory bronchospasm should be treated as severe asthma (see also the chapter 'Respiratory Medicine').

Antihistamines are now considered a third-line intervention and should not be used during initial emergency treatment. Non-sedating oral antihistamines, in preference to chlorphenamine, may be given following initial stabilisation, especially in patients with persisting skin symptoms. Steroids are no longer advised in the absence of bronchospasm.

Follow Up

The causative allergen may be identified by taking a careful history. However, all patients should be referred to a specialist clinic for allergy assessment.

Management primarily consists of avoidance. However, patients should also be instructed to carry an emergency management or action plan and to wear a warning bracelet or necklace. Patients or parents of children at risk of anaphylactic reactions should carry injectable adrenaline at all times and know how to use it in an emergency.

ASTHMA

See also the chapter 'Respiratory Medicine'.

Asthma is a chronic disease characterised by reversible airflow obstruction, with recurrent bouts of wheezing and breathlessness. However, all that wheezes is not asthma and important differential diagnoses of acute severe asthma include foreign body aspiration and bronchiolitis. Asthma has increased in prevalence over recent years and now affects 10 to 20% of children in the United Kingdom. Acute exacerbations of asthma represent 10 to 15% of all acute medical admissions in children. About 20 children and about 1400 adults die in the United Kingdom every year due to acute severe asthma. Common factors leading to acute exacerbations include viral respiratory infections, irritants, exercise, and allergens.

Recognition

Clinical assessment should include rapid physical examination, with attention to airway, breathing and circulation, measurement of peak expiratory flow rate (PEFR), in children old enough to manage it, and pulse oximetry. Routine blood gas analysis is not recommended as arterial puncture is painful and may cause acute decompensation. Clinical assessment is more useful. Very severe tachypnoea is unusual in severe asthma and may suggest another diagnosis or toxic effects of bronchodilators. Work of breathing is a useful indicator.

Immediate Management

Hospital management of acute severe or life-threatening asthma should be with high-flow oxygen, nebulised salbutamol and ipratropium bromide, and oral or intravenous corticosteroids. Salbutamol and ipratropium bromide can safely be given continuously until improvement has occurred, when the dose frequency can be reduced. Consider adding magnesium sulphate to each nebuliser in the first hour in children with a short duration of acute severe asthma symptoms presenting with SpO_2 < 92%. Oxygen should be given before, during and after administration of inhaled bronchodilators, to avoid hypoxaemia. Intravenous salbutamol and/or magnesium sulphate may be considered if the patient does not respond to first-line therapy. Aminophylline may be used in severe or life-threatening asthma unresponsive to maximal doses of bronchodilators and corticosteroids. Salbutamol and or aminophylline toxicity (tachypnoea, tachycardia, low pCO_2 and lactic acidosis) are not uncommon and may be confused with unresponsive asthma especially if these are seen after an initial improvement.

If life-threatening features are present, senior help and an experienced anaesthetist should be summoned. In the meantime, the airway should be maintained, oxygen should be administered by a rebreathing mask and intravenous access secured for administration of corticosteroids and bronchodilators. Intravenous bronchodilators should be given with cardiac monitoring, as they can cause arrhythmias.

Investigations

A chest radiograph should be obtained after initial stabilisation in any child with features of severe or life-threatening asthma, or with a first episode of wheezing, to exclude a foreign body, pneumothorax and mucus plugging (Figures 1.10 and 1.11). Routine chest radiographs in all cases of acute asthma are not necessary.

Indications for Ventilatory Support

- Patients who are tired (falling work of breathing or respiratory rate with increasing pCO_2).

- Those with a reduced conscious level.

- Those who continue to deteriorate despite maximal therapy.

Blood gas analysis is not a substitute for clinical assessment and the focus should remain on the clinical state of the patient.

Intubation

The patient should be pre-oxygenated and 10 to 20 mls/kg fluid bolus given electively. Patients with acute severe asthma are often volume depleted and vasodilated. Ketamine (which has some bronchodilator activity) is a useful induction agent.

Ventilation Strategies

High airway resistance may lead to a prolonged expiratory phase during artificial ventilation, and slow ventilation rates may be required (10 to 15 breaths per minute). Blood gases should not be normalised and high $PaCO_2$ values may be tolerated without harm ('permissive hypercapnia') provided the pH remains > 7.1 in the absence of other organ failure. Some PEEP is necessary to counteract intrinsic PEEP. Neuromuscular paralysis should be discontinued as soon as possible as the combination of corticosteroids and paralysing agents is associated with an increased risk of critical illness neuropathy.

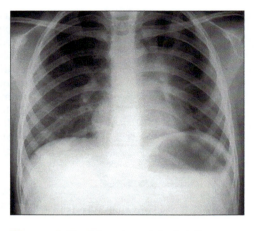

Figure 1.10 Plugging of the left lingular bronchus in acute severe asthma in an eight-year-old girl. The left heart border is indistinct but the left diaphragm is clearly seen.

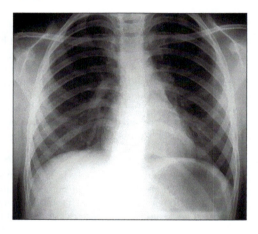

Figure 1.11 The plug seen in in Figure 1.10 was expectorated after bronchodilators were given.

While Ventilated

Key in the management of asthma is generous humidification and physiotherapy to mobilise secretions and mucus plugs. Drug treatment may include continued neuromuscular paralysis, ketamine by continuous infusion (for both sedative and bronchodilator effect), intravenous bronchodilators, corticosteroids and antibiotics. Weaning from mechanical ventilation can be difficult. Any child requiring PICU admission for acute severe asthma should be referred to a paediatric respiratory specialist for outpatient follow-up on hospital discharge.

BRONCHIOLITIS

See also the chapter 'Respiratory Medicine'.

Bronchiolitis is a clinical syndrome of infancy characterised by respiratory distress with both crepitations and wheezes on auscultation. It is often preceded by a coryzal illness and usually has a viral aetiology: respiratory syncytial virus (RSV), influenza, parainfluenza and adenovirus are common. Secondary bacterial infection is rare. Small airway obstruction leading to hyperinflation is typical, although many severe cases also have localised or diffuse atelectasis (Figure 1.12).

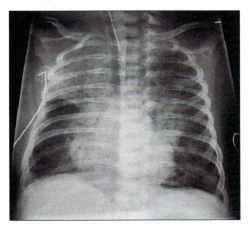

Figure 1.12 Respiratory syncytial virus infection with features of acute respiratory distress syndrome, showing generalised air space shadowing in addition to areas of collapse and hyperinflation.

Recognition

Clinical assessment should include rapid physical examination, with attention to airway, breathing, circulation and pulse oximetry. In very sick infants, capillary or venous blood gases can help to guide treatment. However, clinical assessment is still more important than blood gas analysis.

Immediate Management

Low flow oxygen via nasal cannula should be given to maintain saturations > 90%. Humidified high-flow nasal cannula oxygen and CPAP may also be of benefit, although definitive trials are awaited. Intravenous fluids may be given as bolus to maintain intravascular volume then maintenance if the child is unable to feed. Beware hyponatraemia from reduced free-water clearance due to SIADH. Nasogastric feeding may be preferred in the acute phase. Bronchodilators, including nebulised adrenaline, do not shorten the length of admission or alter the outcome. Antibiotics, antivirals and corticosteroids are generally not of benefit.

Investigations

If severely unwell, alternative diagnoses such as pneumonia and empyema should be considered. This group of infants will require a chest radiograph. Further investigations should include a nasopharyngeal aspirate for viral immunofluorescence. Underlying conditions such as lung, cardiac or neurological disease, or immunodeficiency, should be considered in infants with severe or persistent symptoms.

Indications for Ventilatory Support

Assisted ventilation is required in a small proportion of infants, who often fall into one of the high-risk groups. Ventilatory support may be required in infants who are tired, who have a reduced conscious level or who continue to deteriorate with worsening respiratory failure with progressive hypoxaemia or hypercarbia. As with asthma, blood gas analysis is not a substitute for clinical assessment and the focus should remain on the clinical state of the patient.

Intubation

Ventilation is rarely required and is often accompanied by a transient worsening of gas exchange.

Ventilation Strategies

If ventilation is necessary, a low tidal volume lung protective strategy can be adopted with tidal volumes of 4 to 7 mls/kg, PIP < 30, low respiratory rate, and permissive hypercapnia, SpO$_2$ target of 88–92%, allowing the pH to go down to 7.2. Moderate PEEP (6–8) typically helps to counteract intrinsic PEEP.

While Ventilated

There is no proven treatment for bronchiolitis other than good supportive care. Extracorporeal membrane oxygenation (ECMO) has been used in very severely affected infants with excellent results.

CARDIAC EMERGENCIES

Cardiac emergencies in childhood are rare. Cyanosis in the neonatal period, pulmonary oedema, cardiogenic shock and arrhythmia are the common modes of presentation of previously undiagnosed disease.

CYANOSIS

Cyanosis in a newborn infant or baby should raise suspicion of a right to left shunt due to congenital heart disease (Figure 1.13a and 1.13b) but in a newborn can also be due to persistent pulmonary

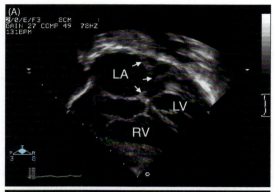

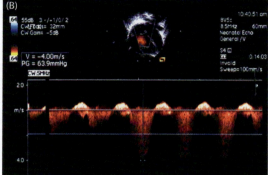

Figure 1.13 Echocardiography showing cor triatriatum with pulmonary hypertension. Figure (A) shows the abnormal left atrium (LA) obstructing flow into the left ventricle (LV); (B) shows the tricuspid regurgitant jet with a pressure gradient of 64 mmHg, indicating systemic right ventricle (RV) pressure due to pulmonary hypertension. The child was a 5-month-old baby who presented with respiratory failure, cyanosis and failure to thrive.

hypertension of the newborn or respiratory causes. It is possible, although now extremely rare, for children in later life with congenital left to right shunts to develop pulmonary hypertension and for the shunt to reverse, causing cyanosis. This situation is known as Eisenmenger's syndrome but is now very rare in high-income countries.

Any newborn child with persistent cyanosis which cannot be explained by a respiratory cause should be presumed to have a cardiac lesion. Prostaglandin E2 should be commenced to maintain ductal patency and the infant referred to a paediatric cardiology centre for further investigation and management. Prostaglandin E2 may cause apnoea and transfer may require the airway to be secured with an endotracheal tube.

CARDIOGENIC PULMONARY OEDEMA

Pulmonary oedema may occur in conditions associated with elevated left atrial pressure (e.g. mitral stenosis (Figure 1.14)) or in the context of a left to right shunt with pulmonary overflow (e.g. ventricular septal defect (Figure 1.15)). If cardiac output is preserved the clinical presentation may be as respiratory failure with or without a history of feeding difficulties and failure to thrive. The presence of viral or bacterial respiratory pathogens may further confuse the picture. A murmur or hepatic enlargement may give a clue to a cardiac diagnosis, as may the presence of cardiomegaly or pulmonary oedema on the chest radiograph. Echocardiography will be necessary to make an anatomical diagnosis.

Children should be treated for 'Acute Lung Injury/ARDS' with the caveat that high concentration inspired oxygen and normocapnea should be avoided to reduce pulmonary blood flow if a left to right shunt is present. Diuretics may be useful. Failure to wean from mechanical ventilation after any associated infection has resolved may be an indication for transfer to a cardiac centre for surgical repair.

CARDIOGENIC SHOCK

Cardiogenic shock can occur in the newborn period, most commonly when the duct closes in duct-dependent lesions with left heart obstruction, for example, hypoplastic left heart syndrome, coarctation of the aorta or critical aortic stenosis. An aberrant left coronary artery can have a similar presentation, usually a few weeks later (Figure 1.16). Cardiogenic shock may also occur secondary to acquired disease at any time, the most common of which in childhood is viral myocarditis or dilated cardiomyopathy (Figure 1.17).

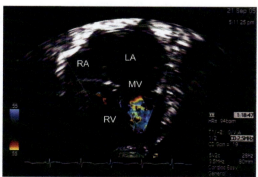

Figure 1.14 Echocardiography showing congenital mitral stenosis. Note the enlarged left atrium.

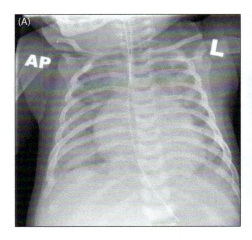 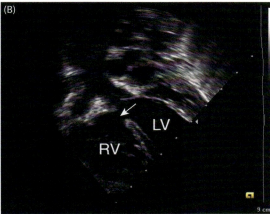

Figure 1.15 Chest radiograph (A) showing cardiomegaly and pulmonary oedema in a 4-month-old with a large ventricular septal defect (B). The presentation was with respiratory failure in association with viral infection.

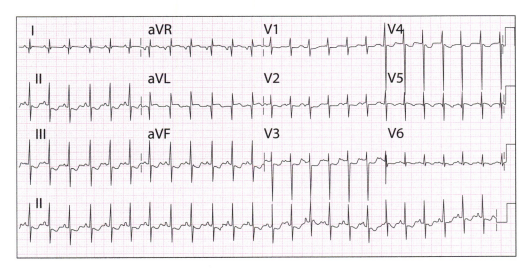

Figure 1.16 12-lead electrocardiograph of a 6-week-old infant with anomalous origin of the left coronary artery from the pulmonary artery (ALCAPA). The infant presented with poor feeding, lethargy and tachypnoea. Q waves are present in lead I and aVL, ST segment elevation in aVL and ST segment depression in II, III, and aVF and the anterior chest leads consistent with a full-thickness anterior infarct.

However, myocardial dysfunction with or without coronary occlusion can occur in Kawasaki disease shock syndrome (see the chapters 'Infectious Diseases' and 'Rheumatology') (Figures 1.18 and 1.19) or in Paediatric Inflammatory Multisystem Syndrome Temporally Associated with SARS-CoV-2 (PIMS-TS), which may occur a few weeks after acute infection with SARS-CoV-2. Specialist advice should be sought when managing children with these conditions.

Arrhythmias, particularly supraventricular tachycardia, may also present as cardiogenic shock in infancy (Figure 1.20).

Infants presenting with cardiogenic shock in the newborn period should be presumed to have duct-dependent circulation until proven otherwise and prostaglandin E2 should be commenced to maintain the systemic circulation. The differential diagnosis includes sepsis, and infants should be commenced on broad-spectrum intravenous antibiotics after blood cultures have been taken. An enlarged liver is often a clue to a cardiac diagnosis. Electrocardiography and cardiac troponin are useful investigations. These infants are often profoundly acidotic and may require airway support,

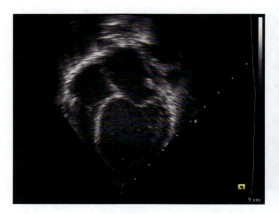

Figure 1.17 Echocardiography showing severe left ventricular dilatation in an 8-month-old with cardiomyopathy due to Vitamin D deficiency.

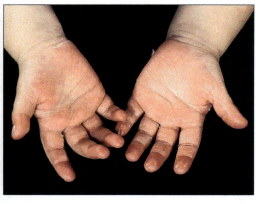

Figure 1.18 Desquamation of the hands in a 4-year old with Kawasaki disease.

mechanical ventilation, fluids, bicarbonate and inotropes to maintain cardiac output. Older, previously well children presenting with cardiogenic shock will require similar management but without attention to the possibility of duct-dependent circulation. Transfer to a paediatric cardiac centre should be arranged for ongoing care.

ARRHYTHMIAS

The commonest arrhythmias in the newborn period are congenital complete heart block (often secondary to maternal systemic lupus erythematosus (SLE) and transplacental carriage of anti-Ro and/or anti-La antibodies) or supraventricular tachycardia due to an aberrant conduction pathway such as in Wolff–Parkinson–White syndrome. In later life, supraventricular tachycardia is also the

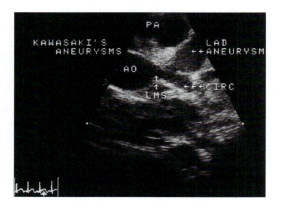

Figure 1.19 Echocardiography showing left anterior descending coronary artery aneurysm in Kawasaki disease. Short axis view shown. Key: AO – aorta; LMS – left main stem; LAD – left anterior descending; CIRC – circumflex; PA – pulmonary artery. (Courtesy of Dr Robert Yates.)

commonest arrhythmia. Supraventricular tachycardia usually presents as cardiogenic shock in a young baby (see above) or as palpitations or syncope in an older child. Ventricular arrhythmias are extremely rare in childhood and may be due to cardiac (e.g. anomalous coronary artery, long QT syndrome, other channelopathy) or non-cardiac causes, (e.g. poisoning, hyperkalaemia or acidosis).

ACUTE ENCEPHALOPATHIC ILLNESS

CONVULSIVE STATUS EPILEPTICUS

Convulsive status epilepticus (CSE) is defined as a convulsive seizure that continues for longer than five minutes, or convulsive seizures that occur one after the other with no recovery between. CSE in childhood is a life-threatening condition with a serious risk of neurological sequelae. Although the outcome from an episode of CSE is mainly determined by its cause, duration is also important. In addition, the longer the duration of the episode, the more difficult it is to terminate.

Between 0.4 and 0.8% of children experience an episode of CSE before the age of 15 years; 12% of first seizures in childhood are CSE which carries a mortality rate of approximately 4%. Neurological sequelae of CSE, such as epilepsy, motor deficits, learning difficulties, and behaviour problems, are rare but occur in a small minority of children.

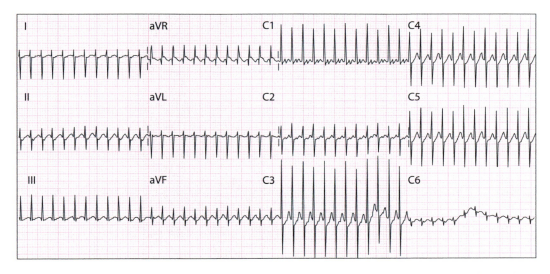

Figure 1.20 12-lead electrocardiograph showing AV re-entry tachycardia in a 6-month-old baby with an accessory AV pathway. The ventricular rate is about 200–250, P waves are absent and the QRS complexes are narrow with normal morphology.

Recognition

Initial assessment and resuscitation should address airway, breathing and circulation (A, B, C). High-flow oxygen should be administered if hypoxaemic and the blood glucose level measured by stick testing. A brief history and clinical examination should be undertaken.

Immediate Management of CSE

If intravenous access is available, lorazepam should be given. Lorazepam is equally or more effective than diazepam and causes less respiratory depression. Lorazepam also has a longer duration of anti-seizure effect (12–24 hours) than diazepam (15–30 minutes). If after ten minutes the convulsion has not stopped or another convulsion has begun, a second dose of lorazepam should be given, assuming intravenous access is established. An alternative to lorazepam is buccal midazolam followed by rectal diazepam.

If seizure activity continues for a further ten minutes and in the unlikely event that intravenous access is still not possible, an intraosseous needle should be inserted. Continuing convulsive activity indicates a longer-acting intravenous anticonvulsant is required. Recent trials have shown that levetiracetam has similar efficacy to the well-established recommendations of phenytoin or phenobarbitone and may have a preferable side effect profile. Heart rate, ECG and blood pressure monitoring during infusion are recommended, particularly as intravenous phenytoin can cause arrhythmias.

OTHER ENCEPHALOPATHIC ILLNESS

Children presenting with non-convulsive acute encephalopathies may present with reduced conscious level, psychosis or confusion. These children may also be in non-convulsive status epilepticus. Structural and non-structural causes should be considered, including space-occupying lesions, meningoencephalitis, autoimmune disease such as acute demyelinating encephalomyelitis (ADEM) (Figure 1.21), anti-NMDA receptor antibody encephalitis, stroke, metabolic disorders and trauma including non-accidental injury.

Investigations

If seizure activity is present, once it has ceased, a full examination including examination of the central nervous system and fundoscopy should be performed. Presentation with non-convulsive encephalopathy, new onset seizures, focal seizures or residual focal neurology suggest a structural cause and neuroimaging will be required. Fundoscopy may reveal retinal haemorrhages suggestive of non-accidental injury (see the chapter 'Child Protection'). Children with no previous history of

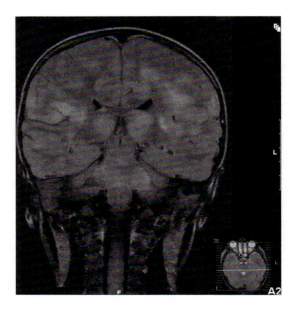

Figure 1.21 T2 weighted MRI scan in an 8-year-old child with acute disseminated encephalo-myelitis, showing multiple areas of increased signal in the white matter. The child presented in convulsive status epilepticus.

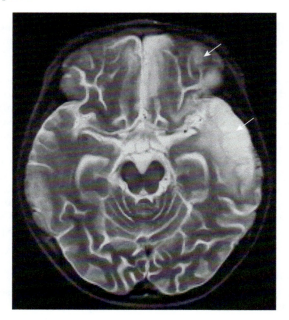

Figure 1.22 T2-weighted magnetic resonance image in transverse section of a two-year-old with intractable seizures due to herpes simplex encephalitis. Increased signal, representing oedema, is seen in the left prefrontal and temporal lobes.

a seizure disorder who remain encephalopathic should be presumed to have an infective aetiology until proven otherwise, particularly if a fever is present, and given aciclovir, a cephalosporin and a macrolide to cover for the common causes of infective encephalopathy (Figures 1.22, 1.23, 1.24).

Blood should be sent for a full blood count, urea and electrolytes, anticonvulsant, calcium, magnesium and blood glucose levels. Consideration should be given, particularly in infants, to sending metabolic investigations including lactate and serum ammonia, acylcarnitine blood spots and

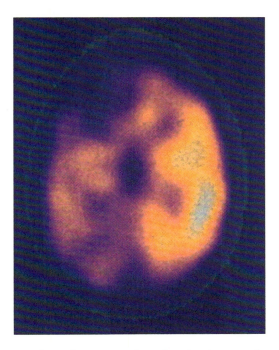

Figure 1.23 Perfusion scan from the same patient showing increased uptake in the same area.

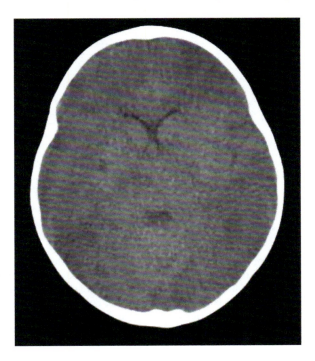

Figure 1.24 Generalised cerebral oedema with infarction in a child with pneumococcal meningoencephalitis.

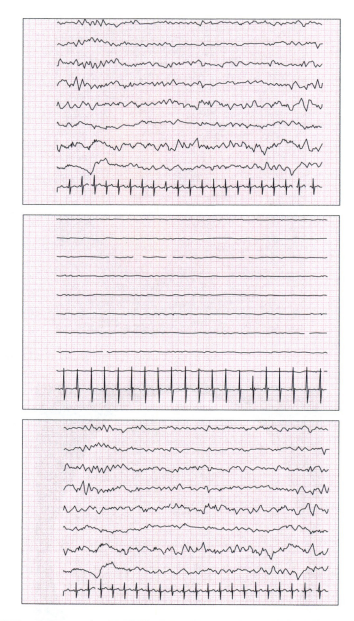

Figure 1.25 EEGs of a 5-month-old child with a history of neonatal seizures responding to phenobarbitone presented with increasingly severe and prolonged seizures with tonic–clonic and myoclonic elements. Top: During status epilepticus, high amplitude (note the change in calibration) repetitive sharp waves are seen continuously. Middle: Following an injection of pyridoxine the EEG activity disappears, returning after eight to nine hours. Bottom: An interictal EEG shows age-appropriate activity. The child had pyridoxine-dependent seizures and was maintained fit-free on regular pyridoxine after the diagnosis was made. (Courtesy of Dr Stuart Boyd.)

plasma amino acids and urine organic acids. Appropriate specimens should also be sent for bacterial, viral and mycoplasma culture, serology and PCR. Lumbar puncture should be avoided until it is clear that intracranial pressure is not raised. Further investigation when the child is stable may include neuroimaging and neurophysiological investigation (Figure 1.25 – three panels).

Indications for Ventilatory Support

If after intravenous levetiracetam, phenytoin or phenobarbitone, the child remains in CSE, or the airway is not protected because of reduced conscious level, then rapid sequence induction of anaesthesia should be performed using thiopentone or propofol. If neuromuscular paralysis is used, this should be short-acting so as not to mask clinical signs of seizure. Once ventilated, standard neuroprotective measures should be instituted including good oxygenation, avoidance of hyper or hypocapnia, maintenance of blood pressure, normothermia and adequate sedation. Mannitol or 3% saline should be considered if clinical signs of raised ICP develop.

For children under 3 years of age with a prior history of chronic, active epilepsy who present with an episode of established CSE, specialist advice should be sought. Some infants may respond to intravenous pyridoxine if the seizures are pyridoxine-dependent or pyridoxine-responsive, or to biotin, in cases of biotinidase deficiency.

Once ventilated, the child will need to be transferred to a paediatric intensive care unit (PICU). Advice on ongoing management should be sought from a paediatric neurologist.

DIABETIC KETOACIDOSIS

See also the chapter 'Endocrinology'.

Diabetic ketoacidosis (DKA) is the common presentation of insulin-dependent diabetes mellitus (IDDM) in childhood. The primary cause is insufficient endogenous or therapeutic insulin to allow adequate cellular uptake of glucose and inhibition of ketogenesis. This decompensation is frequently precipitated by an infective illness. The main clinical picture is of dehydration resulting from hyperglycaemia-induced osmotic diuresis, and a profound metabolic acidosis (with an increased anion gap) from the accumulation of acidic ketone bodies.

Initial Assessment and Resuscitation

As with all acutely ill children the initial assessment of a child with DKA focuses on airway, breathing and circulation. Altered conscious level on presentation is an important poor prognostic factor and should trigger the early involvement of senior help. Children in DKA will be tachypnoeic as they attempt to compensate for metabolic acidosis by reducing $PaCO_2$. A low pH (< 7.0) or low $PaCO_2$ (< 2.5 kPa) indicate severe disease with a high risk of cerebral oedema. In the rare cases that require artificial ventilation for exhaustion or shock, the initial target $PaCO_2$ must be similar to the value that the patient was achieving. This will prevent worsening of acidosis and cerebral oedema. The heart rate, blood pressure and peripheral perfusion must be regularly assessed. It is now recommended that all patients are given a 10 mls/kg fluid bolus on presentation; those in shock should be given a 20 mls/kg fluid bolus and then reassessed. The possibility of infection must be considered. Newer recommendations for more aggressive fluid resuscitation are not universally accepted. The baseline risk of cerebral oedema should be balanced against the typically much lower risks of shock in DKA.

Indications for referral to PICU include pH < 7.1, shock, depressed sensorium and children < two years. Any significant reduction in conscious level should prompt discussion with anaesthetic and/or paediatric intensive care unit staff. Cerebral oedema in DKA is unpredictable but has been associated with a low $PaCO_2$ on presentation, rapid changes in osmolarity and the use of bicarbonate. Treatment of cerebral oedema is essentially supportive as with raised intra-cranial pressure after traumatic brain injury (see below). Control of $PaCO_2$, support of the circulation and avoiding low plasma osmolarity, along with osmolar therapy for acute treatment, are the main strategies. There is no evidence to support invasive intra-cranial pressure monitoring.

Initial Investigations

These should include glucose, urea and electrolytes, bicarbonate, creatinine, plasma osmolality, liver and bone profile, FBC, electrolytes, arterial blood gas, urinalysis (for ketonuria and glycosuria) and partial septic screen (e.g. MSU, blood cultures). Hourly blood glucose levels should be performed. Urea and electrolytes, including phosphate, should be checked regularly.

Further Management

Rehydration should be slow over 48 hours with regular checks of serum electrolytes and osmolality. A urinary catheter should be placed in the presence of oliguria or reduced conscious level.

An insulin infusion should not be commenced until intravenous fluids have been running for at least one to two hours as there is some evidence that cerebral oedema is more likely if insulin is started early. Once started, the insulin infusion should continue until resolution of ketoacidosis. To prevent a precipitous drop in plasma glucose, glucose should be added to the intravenous fluid when plasma glucose falls to 14 mmol/l. Potassium replacement therapy should be started immediately in the maintenance fluid. Bicarbonate administration should be avoided. Anticoagulation should be considered in older children particularly those with femoral central venous lines. A nasogastric tube should be considered in all cases with any reduction in conscious level or if there is a history of vomiting.

PAEDIATRIC ACUTE RESPIRATORY DISTRESS SYNDROME (PARDS)

PARDS is the term used to describe the pulmonary response to a broad range of injuries occurring either directly to the lung or as the consequence of injury or inflammation at other sites in the body (Figure 1.26). It is characterised by Type 1 (hypoxaemic) respiratory failure not explained by cardiac failure or fluid overload and imaging findings of new infiltrates consistent with acute pulmonary parenchymal disease within seven days of a known clinical insult. Diagnostic criteria were developed for the syndrome in 2015 by the Paediatric Acute Lung Injury Consensus Conference.

Common causes of PARDS
- Sepsis
- Infective pneumonia
- Trauma
- Aspiration/near drowning
- Burns/inhalational injury
- Massive blood transfusion
- Transfusion-related acute lung injury

Pathogenesis

PARDS is classically characterised by widespread airway collapse, surfactant deficiency and reduced lung compliance. It is an inflammatory disorder with three phases: an exudative phase, a proliferative phase and a fibrotic phase. Many studies of adult ARDS show that survivors return to normal lung function, with complete resolution of pulmonary fibrosis.

Initial Assessment

Assessment of the child with respiratory failure follows the standard ABC approach, with an emphasis on the work of breathing and on the effects of hypoxaemia on other organ systems, particularly the heart and brain. Once an initial assessment of severity has been made and supportive

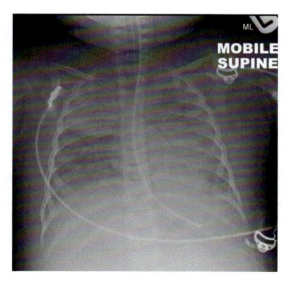

Figure 1.26 Severe ARDS in a 5-year-old with H1N1 influenza. The child did not survive.

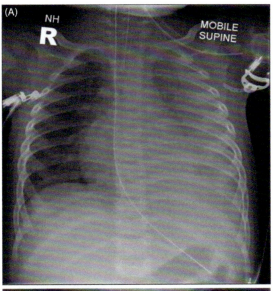

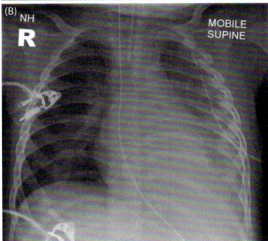

Figure 1.27 Empyema due to left lower lobe pneumococcal pneumonia in an 8 month old before (a) and after (b) drainage. The child was ventilated, treated with antibiotics and intrapleural urokinase and made a full recovery.

measures instituted, appropriate investigations should be arranged to determine the underlying cause so that specific therapy may be commenced. For example, infection requires appropriate antibiotic therapy and empyema, if present, should be drained (Figures 1.27a and 1.27b).

Supportive Therapy

Supportive therapy ranges from oxygen by face mask, to non-invasive ventilation, endotracheal intubation and mechanical ventilation, prone positioning, inhaled nitric oxide (iNO) and extra-corporeal membrane oxygenation (ECMO). Non-invasive ventilation refers to ventilatory support without endotracheal intubation. This includes continuous positive airway pressure (CPAP) or biphasic positive airways pressure (BiPAP) via face mask or nasal mask. Mechanical ventilation should be considered in any child who is tiring due to excessive work of breathing, or who has cardiovascular compromise or a reduced conscious level due to respiratory failure. While worsening hypoxaemia or worsening hypercarbia may confirm the imminent need for ventilation, as always, blood gas analysis is not a substitute for clinical assessment.

Ventilatory Support

The goals of treating patients with PARDS are to maintain adequate gas exchange while avoiding ventilator induced lung injury, and to give time to treat the underlying cause of the condition.

Oxygenation

High concentration inspired oxygen should be avoided to limit the risk of direct cellular toxicity and to avoid reabsorption atelectasis. SaO_2 targets of 88 to 92 have been shown to improve outcomes. Positive end expiratory pressure (PEEP) may improve oxygenation by encouraging movement of fluid from the alveolar to the interstitial space, recruiting collapsed alveoli, increasing in functional residual capacity and preventing cyclical alveolar collapse. A long inspiratory time may also improve lung recruitment.

Lung Protective Ventilation

Traditional mechanical ventilation, using high tidal volumes and low PEEP, is likely to induce lung injury in patients. However, a 'lung protective strategy', optimizing PEEP, using a tidal volume of < 6 mls/kg, permissive hypercapnia, and pressure-limited ventilation has been shown to improve outcome.

High-Frequency Oscillatory Ventilation (HFOV)

Although there are no trial data to support the use of HFOV, in PICU it is still often used for patients with PARDS. It delivers small tidal volumes (typically 2 mls/kg) and may prevent 'atelectotrauma', keep the lungs open, improve alveolar recruitment and ventilation/perfusion matching.

PARDS Due to SARS-CoV-2

In critically ill adults COVID-19 pneumonitis has been shown to respond to corticosteroids, antivirals and anti-interleukin 6 antibodies. These may be considered in some paediatric cases; advice should be sought from a specialist in infectious diseases.

SEPSIS

The definition of in children has recently been updated to 'an infection with a life-threatening organ dysfunction'. Respiratory, cardiovascular, neurological and coagulation dysfunction are incorporated in the operational definition of the 'Phoenix Score 2024'. Any cardiovascular dysfunction can be described in the context of infection can be described as septic shock.

The characteristic pattern of worsening cardiovascular, respiratory and subsequently other organ system dysfunction is termed 'multiple organ failure'. While the most extreme cases of severe sepsis are seen with gram-negative infections (classically *Neisseria meningitidis*) (Figures 1.28 and 1.29) the same pattern can be seen in response to many organisms including viruses and fungi.

Initial Assessment and Resuscitation

The immediate care of a child with suspected septic shock follows the principles of A, B, C (airway, breathing and circulation) followed by specific therapy for the probable causative organism. Depressed conscious level (GCS ≤ 8), poor airway reflexes, tachypnoea and requirement for supplemental oxygen indicate an impending need for assisted ventilation. Such signs will usually be accompanied by significant shock and hence induction of anaesthesia presents a significant risk. This can be minimised by volume replacement, pre-oxygenation, and selection of a cardiostable anaesthetic agent. An adrenaline bolus should be prepared and available. Optimal drugs for induction include ketamine and/or fentanyl. Myocardial depressive agents

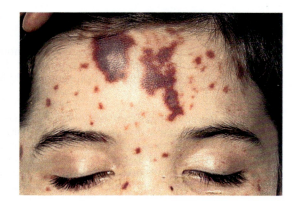

Figure 1.28 Rash of meningococcal disease with purpura and petechiae.

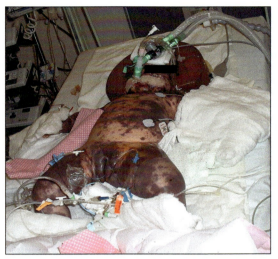

Figure 1.29 Infant with meningococcal sepsis in multiorgan failure.

such as thiopentone, midazolam or propofol are not good choices in children with septic shock. Intubation should be performed by the most experienced staff available. Children with meningococcal disease should be orally intubated unless a coagulopathy has been excluded.

If the child is in shock, peripheral (or central) venous access should not be attempted for more than 90 seconds. Initial resuscitation via an anterior tibial intraosseous needle is easy and effective. Cardiovascular decompensation should be immediately treated with 10 mls/kg of intravenous fluid (ideally balanced crystalloid) which can be safely repeated while management is continuing. Inotropes, if required, may be safely delivered peripherally before central venous access is obtained. Intubation should be considered after administration of 40 to 60 mls/kg due to the likelihood of evolving pulmonary oedema due to capillary leak.

Investigations

These should include full blood count, clotting screen (including fibrinogen and D-dimers or fibrin degradation products to look for evidence of disseminated intravascular coagulopathy), urea and electrolytes, calcium, magnesium, phosphate, liver function tests, blood and urine for culture and rapid antigen screening and/or bacterial or viral PCR where available. Lumbar puncture should not be performed in children with coagulopathy or with a reduced conscious level.

Further Management
Antibiotics

Appropriate antibiotic therapy should be commenced as soon as possible, ideally after taking blood and urine for culture. The only exception to this is in meningococcal disease, where the primary care provider may have already administered parenteral benzylpenicillin.

Circulatory Support

In children and infants with shock, 10 to 20 mls/kg fluid boluses should be used, with careful reassessment after each bolus to enable early identification of signs and symptoms of fluid overload (hepatomegaly, bilateral basal lung crackles and jugular venous distention). The use of fresh frozen plasma (FFP) or packed cells as volume should be considered to correct coagulopathy and to maintain haematocrit. In the presence of persistent hypotension inotropic support should be initiated. Noradrenaline or adrenaline should be used as first-line vasoactive drugs. Dopamine is no longer recommended but can be used if adrenaline and noradrenaline are not available.

Coagulopathy

Profound coagulopathies should be treated with FFP. Low fibrinogen concentrations suggest DIC and can be replaced with cryoprecipitate. Low platelet counts in the absence of clinical bleeding should not be supplemented. Specialist haematology advice should be sought if necessary.

Other

Children with severe sepsis may develop multiorgan failure and require multiple supportive treatments including ventilation, inotropes, renal support and even ECMO. These should be continued while specific measures are taken to treat the infection, including antibiotic therapy and surgical source control if necessary. Some children with severe infection develop limb compartment syndrome in the acute phase or skin and limb necrosis and gangrene in the recovery phase. These may require specialist management including plastic, orthopaedic and vascular surgery.

TRAUMA

TRAUMATIC BRAIN INJURY

Head injury is the major cause of death in children after infancy. The majority of cases in this age group are the result of blunt trauma, with road traffic collisions and falls responsible for most. In infancy, most serious head injuries are non-accidental (see the chapter 'Child Protection') (Figure 1.30). Penetrating injuries are rare in the UK. The majority of head injuries seen in emergency departments are minor. The probability of a serious injury is increased by a violent mechanism of injury (e.g. pedestrian versus car, fall from a height), reduced conscious level – either on history or still present on examination, focal neurological signs and penetrating injury (Figures 1.31, 1.32, 1.33). A combination of these factors makes a serious injury very likely.

Initial Assessment and Resuscitation

The initial assessment and management of the severely injured child follows the routine of <C> catastrophic haemorrhage, A airway (and cervical spine), B breathing and C circulation. Catastrophic haemorrhage should be controlled by compression or surgery as appropriate. Direct airway trauma is rare but loss of the airway due to reduced conscious level and absent cough and gag reflexes are common. The conscious level must be assessed and any concern about the ability to protect the airway should be managed with intubation and ventilation to avoid hypoxaemia or hypercarbia. All children with serious head injuries should be considered to have sustained a cervical spine injury (because of the relatively high risk of ligamentous injury in childhood). Local guidance for imaging should be followed.

Retinal haemorrhages are more common in non-accidental than accidental head injury (Figure 1.34). If there is uncertainty about mechanism, formal ophthalmological assessment with retinal photography should be undertaken as soon as possible.

Hypoventilation raises arterial carbon dioxide levels leading to cerebral vasodilatation and increased intracranial pressure (ICP). The aim of respiratory support in severe head injury is to avoid hypercarbia and maintain $PaCO_2$ in the normal range. Lower levels are detrimental and may contribute to cerebral ischaemia via excessive cerebral vasoconstriction. Hypotension must be avoided in order to maintain cerebral perfusion. Fluid resuscitation may be required, but in cases with severe cerebral oedema, inotrope or vasopressor treatment may be essential to maintain cerebral perfusion pressure (CPP). A child who has been ventilated with a severe head injury must

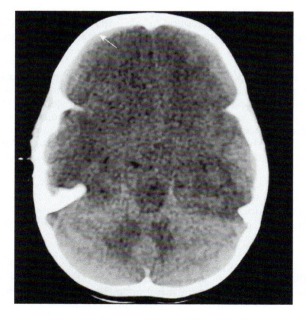

Figure 1.30 Severe non-accidental injury in a 2-year-old child. There is a right subdural haematoma and severe cerebral oedema and infarction.

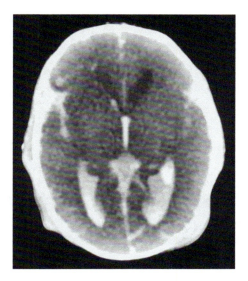

Figure 1.31 Traumatic brain injury with intraventricular and subarachnoid blood. Generalized cerebral oedema is also present.

receive both sedation and analgesia to assist in the control of raised ICP.

Management after Initial Stabilisation

Primary brain injury occurs on impact. The care of the child with head injury is aimed at avoiding secondary brain injury. This can be summarised as providing a 'well-perfused and well-oxygenated brain'. Three principal mechanisms lead to the generation of secondary brain injuries: hypoxaemia, reduced cerebral perfusion and metabolic disturbances (e.g. hypoglycaemia, hyponatraemia). Raised ICP may occur due to a rapidly expanding intracranial haematoma or acute hydrocephalus resulting in a decrease in cerebral perfusion – a neurosurgical emergency. However, raised ICP is more commonly the result of diffuse cerebral oedema in children. In this scenario, the circulation must be supported to maintain cerebral blood flow.

Although there is consensus on the ongoing intensive care management of children with head injuries, there is a very limited evidence base on which to support current practice. Treatments commonly employed include head up 30° tilt, midline head position, sedation, analgesia and intracranial pressure monitoring with circulation support (fluid and vasopressors) to maintain cerebral perfusion pressure. Mannitol or 3% saline may be useful to decrease ICP prior to emergency neurosurgical intervention. Some centres use phenytoin or levetiracetam as post-traumatic seizure prophylaxis. Hyperventilation can be harmful as it reduces cerebral perfusion and is not recommended. Hypothermia and corticosteroids are not of benefit.

THE CHILD WITH MULTIPLE INJURIES

Few paediatricians will be regularly involved with the resuscitation of children with multiple injuries. Such cases must be approached in a structured way (<C>, A, B, C – see above), in order to identify and treat life-threatening injuries. Focused abdominal sonography in trauma (FAST) scanning is generally no longer recommended as it may delay definitive imaging

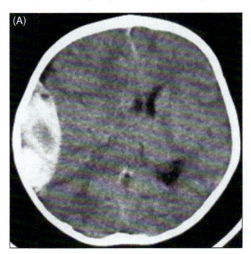
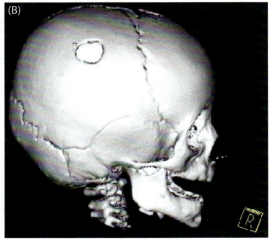

Figure 1.32 CT scan (a) showing right sided acute extradural haemorrhage with mass effect in a 7 month old who rolled off a changing mat onto a hard floor. The baby required a craniotomy (b) and made a full recovery.

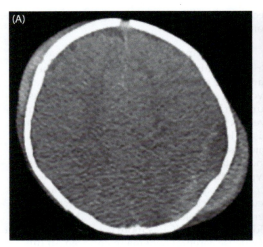 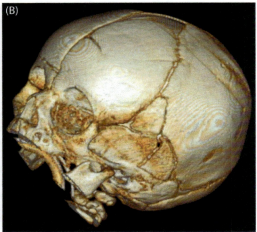

Figure 1.33 CT scan (a) showing left sided acute subdural haemorrhage with cerebral oedema in a 3 month old who was dropped to the floor and sustained multiple skull fractures (b). The haemorrhage was drained and the child made a full recovery after a period of neurointensive care.

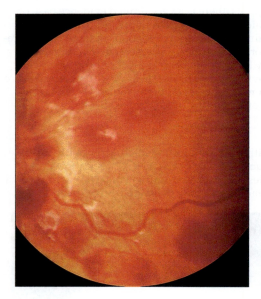

Figure 1.34 Multiple domed subhyaloid retinal haemorrhages in a case of non-accidental injury caused by shaking. The white spots in the centre of the haemorrhages are light reflexes. Fundoscopy should be performed in all infants presenting with significant head injuries.

(Figures 1.35, 1.36, 1.37). The care of a child with multiple injuries can be best achieved in large centres with all the relevant specialities available onsite (eg. anaesthesia/ICU, radiology, orthopaedics, neurology, general, cardiothoracic, maxillofacial and plastic surgery).

Initial Assessment and Resuscitation

This is identical to that already described for the child with a head injury. As before, the patient should be considered to have a cervical spine injury until they are awake and able to demonstrate normal neurology in the absence of neck pain and with appropriate imaging, if necessary. Airway assessment must include an assessment of the airway reflexes and conscious level as well as the effects of any direct trauma or foreign body.

Haemorrhagic shock is the main threat to the circulation in multiple trauma. The priority is early control of haemorrhage and fluid resuscitation, ideally with a combination of packed cells, FFP and platelets. Secure intravenous or intra-osseous access will be required (ideally away from the site of obvious injuries) and fluid resuscitation of 5 to 10 mls/kg should be given, repeated as necessary, until haemorrhage control is achieved. Acute tension pneumo- or haemo-pneumothorax may require emergency aspiration and drainage. Cardiac injuries should be considered and treated if present. Blood samples for full blood count, coagulation screen, blood group and cross-matching should be taken as early as possible. Resuscitation must continue while sites of potential blood loss are assessed and treated.

Management after Initial Stabilisation

After immediately life-threatening <C>ABC problems have been addressed, a careful examination to detail all injuries must be undertaken, including log-rolling to examine the back and

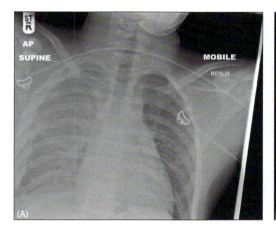
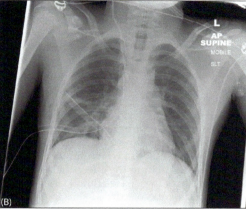

Figure 1.35 Right sided haemothorax in association with cardiac tamponade in a 15 year old after penetrating thoracic injury before (a) and after (b) thoracotomy.

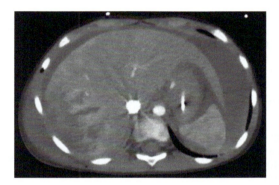

Figure 1.36 Liver maceration with intraperitoneal blood in a 3 year old with blunt abdominal and thoracic trauma. The child made a full recovery with non-operative management.

Figure 1.37 Intraperitoneal air due to perforation of a viscus, infarction of the left kidney and pancreatic haemorrhage and intraperitoneal blood in a 7 year old after a crush injury to the abdomen. Laparotomy is mandatory in the context of perforation.

thoraco-lumbar spine. It is at this stage that imaging appropriate to the injuries (e.g. CT cervical-spine, head, thorax and abdomen) should be performed if haemodynamic stability can be obtained. If stability cannot be achieved, 'damage control' surgery by appropriate surgical teams may be required prior to imaging. The purpose of 'damage control' surgery is to mitigate any immediately life-threatening injuries and to regain physiological stability rather than to provide definitive treatment for all injuries. The management of non-immediately life-threatening injuries may be deferred.

Blood loss from fractures (especially to the pelvis or femora) is easily underestimated and may require early fixation. Hepatic, renal, splenic and other vascular injuries are all sites of potentially lethal haemorrhage though many such injuries, particularly those caused by blunt trauma can be managed without surgical intervention in children. Some will, however, require interventional radiology or surgery.

BURNS

The initial management of a child with severe burns can be summarised as 'forget about the burn'. The priorities remain airway, breathing and circulation. If the mechanism of burn is unclear or there is co-existent trauma then cervical spine precautions must be observed. Analgesia must also be addressed urgently.

General Approach to the Child with Burns

Reduced conscious level and airway obstruction from facial or inhalational burn injury are the major causes of airway obstruction in burns. A child with facial or airway burns should be assessed for early intubation because of the high risk of swelling tissue (Figure 1.38).

Smoke inhalation or reduced chest wall movement from circumferential burns must be considered. High-flow oxygen should be administered to cases in which smoke inhalation is possible (to limit the effects of carbon monoxide poisoning). Large fluid losses will occur through areas of burned skin in proportion to the area affected. Complex formulae exist for calculating fluid replacement required but this should not confuse the initial management. Immediate circulation support should be as for shock from any cause with 10 mls/kg fluid boluses. If shock is present, it should not be ascribed to fluid losses through the burn without considering the possibility of associated fractures or other injuries.

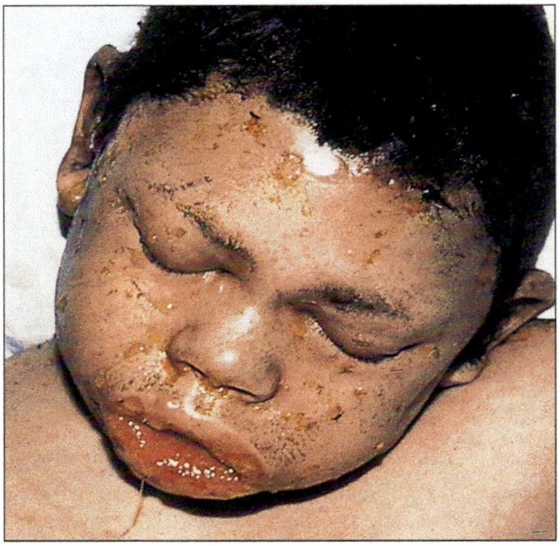

After the initial resuscitation, ongoing care including fluid management should be undertaken in combination with the specialised burns centre and/or paediatric intensive care unit.

Figure 1.38 Facial oedema with eyelid and lip swelling caused by a flash burn. Swelling occurs up to 24 hours after the injury and the airway must be secured with an endotracheal tube.

POISONING

Suspected poisoning in children results in 40,000 visits to Accident and Emergency departments in England and Wales every year and 15 to 20 deaths. Poisoning may occur accidentally in a young child or toddler, intentionally in teenagers or deliberately in some cases of child abuse and fabricated and induced illness (see the chapter 'Child Protection').

Recognition and Assessment

Primary assessment should be directed to airway patency, adequacy of breathing and circulation and neurological status. Acidotic breathing is seen in salicylate or ethylene glycol poisoning. QRS prolongation and ventricular tachycardia may be seen in tricyclic antidepressant poisoning. A depressed conscious level suggests poisoning with opiates, sedatives, antihistamines or hypoglycaemic agents. Small pupils suggest opiate poisoning but large pupils suggest amphetamines, atropine or tricyclic poisoning. Convulsions are associated with many drugs, particularly tricyclic antidepressants.

Immediate Management

Airway patency should be maintained, with intubation if necessary. Children with cardiorespiratory failure or a decreased conscious level should receive high-flow oxygen through a face mask with a reservoir if the airway is patent. Shock should be treated with fluid boluses rather than inotropes as inotropes can cause arrhythmia in combination with some toxins. Cardiac dysrhythmias caused by poisons need specific treatment, which should be discussed with a Poisons Centre. Hypoglycaemia should be treated with 2 mls/kg intravenous 10% dextrose and convulsions treated with diazepam, midazolam or lorazepam. Naloxone should be given if the pupils are very constricted or there is a history of opiate poisoning.

Investigations

When intravenous access is obtained, blood should be sent for a full blood count, urea and electrolytes, paracetamol and salicylate levels, toxicology, and blood glucose. Urine specimens can be sent for toxicological analysis. Monitoring should include ECG, blood pressure, pulse oximetry, core temperature, blood glucose and sometimes blood gases.

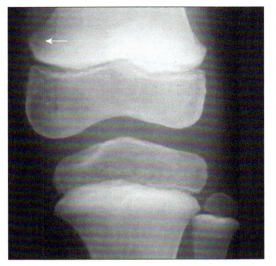

Figure 1.39 Lead poisoning causing a dense metaphyseal line at the growing ends of long bones. Chelation can be affected with dimercaprol, edetate calcium disodium and 2,3 dimercaptosuccinic acid. Management should be undertaken in conjunction with the local poisons unit.

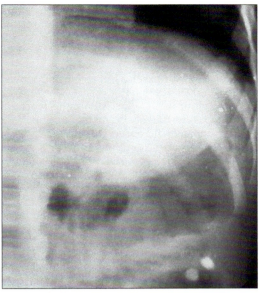

Figure 1.40 Multiple dense opacities seen in stomach and left flank in a 2-year-old boy who had ingested his mother's iron tablets. He was treated with desferrioxamine and made a full recovery.

Further Management
Gut Decontamination

Activated charcoal can be given as a single dose (50 grams for children over 12 years, 1 g/kg body-weight for a child up to 12 years) up to one hour after ingestion of a toxin. Beyond this time adsorption is reduced. Gastric lavage is rarely required as benefit rarely outweighs risk; advice should be sought from a specialist toxicologist, particularly following ingestion of iron or lithium, which are not adsorbed to activated charcoal. Whole gut irrigation is rarely required.

Paracetamol Poisoning

N-acetyl cysteine should be given as soon as possible after a large overdose of paracetamol or if levels are toxic four hours after ingestion. In cases which are not straightforward, advice should be taken from a specialist toxicologist and from a liver transplant unit.

Other

Management for other poisons should be guided by advice from a specialist toxicologist and may include chelating agents, antidotes and active elimination techniques such as haemofiltration (Figures 1.39 and 1.40).

REFERENCES
- Pediatric Acute Lung Injury Consensus Conference Group. Pediatric acute respiratory distress syndrome: Consensus recommendations from the Pediatric Acute Lung Injury Consensus Conference. *Pediatr Crit Care Med.* 2015;16:428–439.
- Weiss SL, et al. Executive summary: Surviving sepsis campaign international guidelines for the management of septic shock and sepsis-associated organ dysfunction in children. *Pediatr Crit Care Med.* 2020;21:186–195.
- BSPED interim guideline for the management of children and young people under the age of 18 years with Diabetic Ketoacidosis, 2020. https://www.bsped.org.uk/media/1798/bsped-dka -guideline-2020.pdf, accessed 1st June 2021.

- Kochanek PM, et al. Guidelines for the management of pediatric severe traumatic brain injury, third edition: Update of the brain trauma foundation fuidelines. *Pediatr Crit Care Med.* March 2019;20(3S):S1–S82.
- Hodgetts TJ, Mahoney PF, et al. ABC to <C>ABC: Redefining the military trauma paradigm. *Emerg Med J.* 2006;23:745–746.
- Mahoney PF, Russell RJ, et al. Novel haemostatic techniques in military medicine. *J R Army Med Corps.* 2005;151:139–141.
- NICE clinical guideline: Meningitis (bacterial) and meningococcal septicaemia in under 16s: Recognition, diagnosis and management. Clinical guideline [CG102]. Published: 23 June 2010. Last updated: 01 February 2015. https://www.nice.org.uk/guidance/cg102, accessed 1st June 2021.
- Advanced Life Support Group (ALSG). *Advanced Paediatric Life Support: A Practical Approach to Emergencies*, 6th Edition. Wiley; 2016.
- British guideline on the management of asthma. A national clinical guideline. First published 2003. Revised edition published July 2019. https://www.brit-thoracic.org.uk/quality-improvement/guidelines/asthma/, accessed 1st June 2021.
- Bronchiolitis in children: Diagnosis and management. NICE guideline [NG9]. Published: 01 June 2015. https://www.nice.org.uk/guidance/ng9, accessed 1st June 2021.
- NICE clinical guideline: Epilepsies: Diagnosis and management. Clinical guideline [CG137]. Published: 11 January 2012 Last updated: 12 May 2021. https://www.nice.org.uk/guidance/cg137, accessed 1st June 2021.
- NICE clinical guideline: Fever in under 5s: Assessment and initial management. Clinical guideline [CG160]. Published: 22 May 2013. https://www.nice.org.uk/guidance/cg160, accessed 1st June 2021.

2 Child Protection

Alison Steele and Anna Uwagboe

INTRODUCTION

Child maltreatment exists in all cultures across the world. There is international agreement that child maltreatment is wrong, requiring active prevention and intervention by governments. This has been enshrined in Article 19 of The United Nations Convention of the Rights of the Child (UNCRC) that states:

> *all children have a right to protection from all forms of physical and mental violence, injury or abuse, neglect and maltreatment or exploitation, including sexual abuse while in the care of parent(s), legal guardians or another person who has the care of the child.*

A child is anyone under the age of 18 years as defined by the UN Convention on the Rights of the Child and this is enshrined in British law. In this chapter the terms 'child' and 'young person' are used interchangeably depending on the context.

Currently 196 countries are party to the UNCRC and once a country has ratified the treaty they are bound to its terms by international law.

The Global Status Report on Preventing Violence Against Children 2020 found that, in 2017, around 40,000 children were murdered worldwide. This report details the fragmented and limited progress made by governments across the world to end violence against children following the recommendations of the UN Secretary General's report in 2006.

The report also addresses the impact of our changing climate, social exclusion, deprivation caused by the world economic crisis and mass migration. It emphasises that the greatest effects of violence against children are in the early years because it can result in irreversible detrimental effects on child development and well-being.

In the United Kingdom, a series of high-profile child deaths have shaped attitudes and legislature towards child protection. Legislation reinforces the responsibilities of persons and organisations that work with children and/or adults with parenting responsibilities within the United Kingdom to safeguard the children under their care.

The prevalence of child maltreatment within the United Kingdom is difficult to determine accurately because it is normally hidden from view. The Crime Survey for England and Wales in March 2019 estimated that one in five adults aged 18 to 74 years (8.5 million people) had experienced at least one form of maltreatment in childhood.

SAFEGUARDING AND CHILD PROTECTION SYSTEMS WITHIN THE UNITED KINGDOM

Safeguarding is the process of ensuring children have healthy happy lives and reach their full potential. Child protection is a process that occurs when professionals act on concerns that parents or carers may be significantly harming their children.

All nations in the United Kingdom have multi-agency guidance which should be referred to but there are two fundamental underlying principles which are:

- Safeguarding is everyone's responsibility.
- There must be a child-centred approach.

Early intervention and help are pivotal in supporting families to prevent child maltreatment. Much of the work that health professionals undertake with children and families is aimed at providing this support. They work closely with families and professionals in hospitals, community health, social services and education in a 'team around the child' approach.

Some families need intensive support which includes social services. This support involves a child and family assessment by a social worker and the formulation of a Child in Need plan (CIN plan). This approach falls under Section 17 of the Children Act. CIN plans are made with the family's consent. Children who have a CIN plan are those with complex disabilities who require coordinated multidisciplinary support and those with complex psychosocial needs who are not yet at the threshold for child protection interventions.

DOI: 10.1201/9781003175186-2

The Children Act 1989 describes the duty of local authorities to intervene in family life. In cases of suspected maltreatment, this does not require parental consent. The threshold for this type of intervention is when maltreatment is likely to or has occurred. The legal term for this is 'significant harm'. Harm is defined in the Children Act as 'ill-treatment or the impairment of health or development including, for example, impairment suffered from seeing or hearing the ill-treatment of another'.

The common assessment framework (CAF) is a tool which offers a way of assessing which children may be more vulnerable and what support can be offered. Vulnerability to maltreatment will be elicited in full history taking.

THE ROLE OF HEALTH PROFESSIONALS

Health professionals have an increasingly important role including:

- Working collaboratively with other professionals to provide families with support.
- Advocating for the child's voice to be heard.
- Recognising and referring children at risk of significant harm.
- Providing a chronology of significant events with explanations of the medical findings.
- Contributing to enquiries about a child and family.
- Appropriate information sharing.
- Participating in the child protection processes including attending strategy meetings and child protection conferences.
- Playing a part in delivery of the Child Protection Plan (CPP).
- Providing therapeutic help to maltreated children.
- Writing reports for child protection conferences and court.
- Appearing as a witness when called in either family or criminal court.

CASE STUDY: DANIEL PELKA

Daniel was killed by his mother and stepfather in March 2012 when he was 4 years old. Although Daniel died some years ago, the lessons learned continue to be relevant today.

In the six months prior to his death, Daniel was subject to physical maltreatment, emotional abuse and neglect. There were multiple indicators to suggest Daniel was maltreated prior to his death and several opportunities for professionals to intervene. The police were called to the family home on many occasions for reports of domestic abuse. Daniel's mother had a history of alcoholism and her pattern of behaviour did not change despite multiple interventions by professionals.

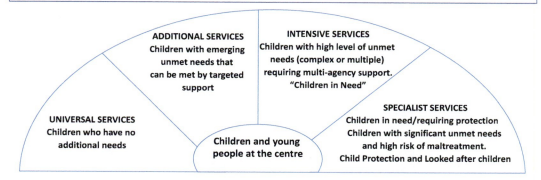

Figure 2.1 The windscreen representing the continuum of need. A child's smooth transition through this continuum is supported by appropriate information sharing while keeping the child's welfare at the centre of all interventions provided by services.

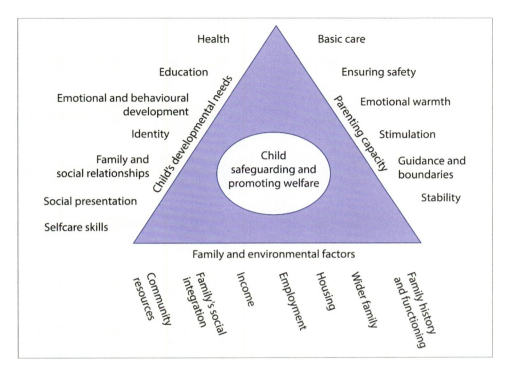

Figure 2.2 Common assessment framework triangle. (From https://www.gov.uk/government/ uploads/system/uploads/attachment_data/file/190604/DFES-04320-2006-ChildAbuse.pdf, with permission under the Open Government Licence.)

Daniel was brought to ED in early 2011 by his stepfather with a spiral fracture in his left arm that had occurred the day before. Examining doctors noticed multiple bruises on his arm and abdomen. The injury was explained by him jumping off a couch and although abuse was suspected, the medical evidence was inconclusive. His mother and stepfather mislead professionals using Daniel's sister older sister to explain his injuries as accidental. Social care referrals were made but they ultimately did not identify a need for ongoing intervention.

Daniel started school in September 2011 and staff at the school noticed he was always hungry and would sometimes scavenge from the bins. Daniel was also noted to have multiple bruises and unexplained marks seen by different members of school staff, but these were not recorded or linked to his starvation. Daniel was seen by a paediatrician in February 2012 when his weight loss and behaviour regarding food was linked to a medical condition. The paediatrician was unaware of the bruises noted by school staff and three weeks after this review Daniel died. He had a significant head injury as well as 40 other injuries and was very emaciated.

Daniel's growth chart clearly demonstrated his faltering growth.

Although professionals were largely unaware of the extent of maltreatment that Daniel suffered, this may have been uncovered if there was greater information sharing, more child-focused interventions by professionals and a consideration that abuse might be a differential when assessing Daniel's presentation.

PAEDIATRIC ASSESSMENT OF A CHILD WITH SUSPICION OF MALTREATMENT
General Approach

It is important to assess the child in a rigorous way irrespective of whether there is an allegation of maltreatment, an unexplained injury, or the incidental discovery of maltreatment during any medical consultation. The only difference from the diagnostic process in any other disorder is that when maltreatment is diagnosed or suspected the management occurs within a multi-agency

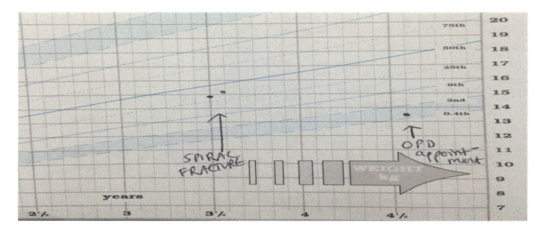

Figure 2.3 Case study – serious case review on the Daniel Pelka.

context of assessment and planning for the child. Many maltreated children will have co-existing medical problems.

There should be a system in place in each locality to triage child protection referrals and to determine where they need to be assessed by a health professional. The options may be within a community paediatric clinic, at hospital or in a sexual abuse referral centre.

Consent

Ideally, every child should be seen with a parent, unless this is not considered to be in the best interests of the child. You must obtain consent from someone with parental responsibility or from the child if they are Gillick competent. It is also very important that the child understands and agrees to the assessment, taking into account their developmental stage.

Documentation

It is vital to document findings fully as any consultation can be subject to legal scrutiny. The notes should be clear, precise, contemporaneous, and signed.

Body maps should be used with detailed descriptions and explanations for any lesion seen.

Photographs should be taken with consent on approved devices in line with national and local policy. Important statements made by the child/parents should be recorded verbatim. Facts need to be distinguished from clinical opinion. Additional care should be taken in documenting time, place and people present as well as who provided the history, including the child.

History Taking

Ideally a parent/carer will be present and able to provide details of the pregnancy, birth, neonatal period and past medical history. It is important to explore potential differential diagnoses of medical conditions that could account for all or part of the presentation.

Clinicians should try to speak to the child alone. Risk factors and vulnerabilities for maltreatment should be noted in the history.

Unmet health needs such as outstanding immunisations or dental caries should be established.

Examination

A thorough general physical examination should be conducted, to include height, weight and head circumference plotted on growth charts. The whole body should be examined including hair, nails, mouth, teeth, ears, nose, head, skin and hidden areas, e.g. behind ears, between toes.

The child's demeanour, response to carer, play, attention and behaviour should be recorded during the examination as well as whether or not the child was able to co-operate. If the examination is incomplete, it should be explained why this is.

Ensure the child has a clear explanation of the process and with their agreement, it is important to examine their buttocks and external genitalia. If sexual abuse is suspected, a more detailed examination of the ano-genital area should be undertaken by an expert.

Investigations

Investigations are directed by the presentation to ensure that all injuries are detected, and medical conditions are ascertained. The RCPCH Companion which is updated regularly details guidance on investigations.

Diagnosis/Opinion

An opinion on whether the assessment supports a diagnosis of child maltreatment is vital because it will guide social services and the police with the next steps.

If there is uncertainty this should be acknowledged.

Management

This includes the clear communication of the opinion verbally and in writing to the child's family, social services and the police as appropriate. The immediate safety of the child and any siblings should be considered. It is important that the plan also addresses any unmet health needs. Health professionals should ensure appropriate follow-up and/or referrals are arranged, timely reports compiled, and child protection meetings are attended.

TYPES OF MALTREATMENT AND NEGLECT

The commonly used categories of maltreatment in the United Kingdom are physical abuse, emotional abuse, sexual abuse and neglect. These categories can overlap.

Child maltreatment should be part of the differential in any child presenting to health services.

Physical Maltreatment

This is a form of maltreatment which may involve hitting, shaking, throwing, poisoning, burning/scalding, drowning, suffocating, or otherwise causing physical harm to a child. Fabricated or induced illness can be a form of physical maltreatment.

It is important to remember that a maltreated child can have a normal physical examination.

Where physical signs are present, certain characteristics in the history should alert you to suspicion of child maltreatment. These include:

- Inconsistent or changing story.

- Unclear mechanism of injury.

- Delay in presentation.

- Abnormal interaction between child and carer.

- Abnormal behaviour of parents/caregivers.

- Unexplained injuries in a non-ambulant child is always suspicious for maltreatment.

Bruising

Bruising is a very common finding in children. Accidental bruising is strongly related to the mobility of the child. The majority of school-aged children will have bruising at any given time with accidental bruising tending to be over bony prominences and on the front of the body, often corresponding to sites that are bumped in falls. Other accidental bruising may occur when younger children are pulling to stand and bump their head.

The distribution of accidental bruising varies with the developmental age of the child; crawling babies typically injure their chin, nose, and forehead while older children have bruises to their knees and shins. It is very unusual for pre-mobile children to sustain bruises accidentally and therefore bruises in this age group should raise significant concerns about the possibility of maltreatment.

Bruising on soft parts of the body like the buttocks, genitalia, cheeks, is rarely seen in non-abused children, even in those who have bleeding disorders. Abusive bruising can occur anywhere but are most commonly found on soft tissue areas. Multiple bruises or bruises in clusters are suspicious. Bruises inflicted with significant force may have

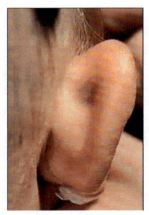

Figure 2.4 Bruising to the pinna suggestive of pinching.

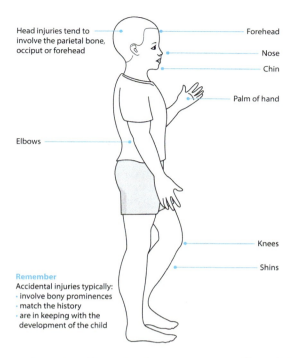

Head injuries tend to involve the parietal bone, occiput or forehead

Forehead

Nose

Chin

Palm of hand

Elbows

Knees

Shins

Remember
Accidental injuries typically:
- involve bony prominences
- match the history
- are in keeping with the development of the child

Figure 2.5 Typical sites of accidental injuries. (With permission, Harris J, Sidebotham P, Welbury R *et al. Child Protection and the Dental Team: an introduction to safeguarding children in dental practice.* COPDEND: Sheffield, 2006: www.cpdt.org.uk.)

surrounding petechiae and this finding is strongly correlated with maltreatment. Inflicted bruises may bear the imprint of a hand or implement, which can be correlated with allegations.

Ageing of Bruises

Evidence suggests that bruises cannot be aged from clinical assessment.

Burns and Scalds

Burns are a common cause of emergency presentations in children and can be associated with maltreatment of all types, particularly neglect. The most common type of intentional burn is a forced immersion scald injury.

The distribution of intentional scalds (burns from hot liquids) is likely to involve the lower limbs, be bilateral and be in the posterior part of the body (buttocks). These scalds typically have clear margins and a symmetrical distribution. They may show a 'glove and stocking' distribution or skin sparing in buttock creases (the 'hole in doughnut' effect). Features that should increase suspicion include co-existent unrelated injuries and a history of previous maltreatment or current vulnerability. The history about the cause of the scald may be inconsistent with the findings, for example a history of a scald from flowing water when the examination findings indicate immersion.

Intentional burns are more commonly reported on the back, shoulders, or buttocks. These often have sharp demarcated edges which may show the imprint of whatever was used to inflict the burn for example, cigarettes, irons, hair straighteners. Intentional cigarette burns cause symmetrical round, well-demarcated burns of uniform thickness.

Accidental burns are more commonly from flowing water, splashes or spills. They are characteristically asymmetrical, of differing depths and more likely to involve the head, neck, trunk and upper extremities e.g. a small child grabbing a cup containing a hot drink from a raised surface. These burns may indicate a lack of supervision.

It is important to also consider conditions that may mimics burns such as staphylococcal infections, e.g. impetigo, staphylococcal scalded syndrome.

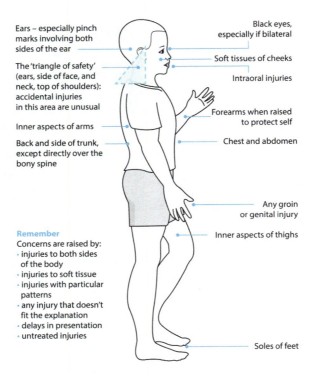

Ears – especially pinch marks involving both sides of the ear

The 'triangle of safety' (ears, side of face, and neck, top of shoulders): accidental injuries in this area are unusual

Inner aspects of arms

Back and side of trunk, except directly over the bony spine

Black eyes, especially if bilateral

Soft tissues of cheeks

Intraoral injuries

Forearms when raised to protect self

Chest and abdomen

Any groin or genital injury

Inner aspects of thighs

Soles of feet

Remember
Concerns are raised by:
· injuries to both sides of the body
· injuries to soft tissue
· injuries with particular patterns
· any injury that doesn't fit the explanation
· delays in presentation
· untreated injuries

Figure 2.6 Typical sites of inflicted injuries. (With permission, Harris J, Sidebotham P, Welbury R *et al. Child Protection and the Dental Team: an introduction to safeguarding children in dental practice.* COPDEND: Sheffield, 2006: www.cpdt.org.uk.)

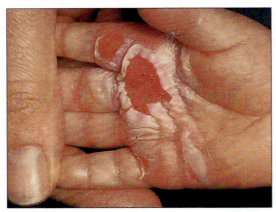

Figure 2.7 Contact burn on palm from touching hot object.

Fractures

Fractures may present with pain, swelling and bruising, but some fractures caused by maltreatment may be clinically silent or a loss of function may be the only indicator in a younger child.

As with other injuries, the characteristics of a fracture alone cannot be used to distinguish between accidental and inflicted injury.

In general, there is an inverse correlation between the age of a child and the probability of a fracture being the result of maltreatment. The greatest risk of maltreatment causing a fracture is in those aged less than 4 months of age.

Investigations, which may include a full skeletal survey, should be considered to detect any occult injuries in a child under 2 years with an injury thought to be inflicted or with a sibling who has an inflicted injury. These investigations should be in keeping with current national guidance.

In a child with a fracture, it is important to exclude any predisposing skeletal disorder such as osteogenesis imperfecta or osteopenia of prematurity. It is important to still consider the possibility of inflicted injuries in children with known pathologies.

Ageing of Fractures

Serial images may help in dating fractures, as may a radionuclide scan. Evidence suggests that dating of fractures is an inexact science and can be confounded by further injuries or immobilisation. Always seek advice from a paediatric radiologist.

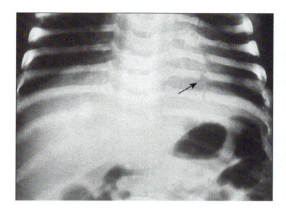

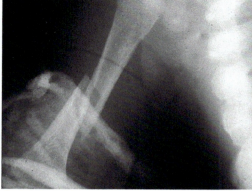

Figure 2.8 Posterior rib fractures.

Figure 2.9 Fracture of the humeral shaft.

Types of Fractures

Rib Fractures – Multiple rib fractures and posterior rib fractures are more likely to be inflicted than accidental or due to underlying pathology. CPR (cardiopulmonary resuscitation) is unlikely to cause rib fractures. Posterior rib fractures in a child who has been resuscitated on a firm surface are inconsistent with the biomechanics of CPR.

Femoral Fractures – In children less than a year old a spiral fracture is the most common type of inflicted femoral fracture.

Humeral fractures – A spiral or oblique fracture of the humerus may result from an applied twisting force and is therefore highly suspicious for maltreatment, in children less than 5 years.

Metaphyseal Fractures – These fractures are also known as corner fractures or bucket handle fractures and occur at the growing plate which is at the end of each long bone. These are more commonly seen in inflicted injury and occur when there is a shearing/whiplash force to the limbs. They are often occult and so not detected easily on imaging unless specifically looked for.

Skull Fractures – The commonest skull fracture is that of a single, linear, hairline parietal fracture which may occur either accidentally or as a result of an inflicted injury. Skull fractures are more frequent in accidental trauma than in inflicted injury but multiple, depressed, growing, bilateral fractures or those crossing suture lines are more common in inflicted injury.

Skull fractures need an appropriate history of a significant incident, usually of a fall from several feet onto a firm or hard surface, to account for them. Fractures resulting from accidental domestic falls rarely result in intracranial injuries. Skull fractures do not heal by developing callus and cannot be dated from radiographic appearances.

Other Types of Physical Injury

Head injury is the most common cause of death in maltreated children, as well as having serious long-term consequences in children who survive. 'Shaken baby syndrome', described in the 1960s, is characterised by intracranial and intraocular bleeding often resulting in long-term brain damage.

Intracranial injury can be caused by impact, shaking or a combination of both. Presentations can vary from visible injuries such as soft tissue swelling or bruising to the head as well as non-visible injuries to the brain which present with impaired consciousness, apnoea, seizures or irritability. In the baby with an open fontanelle the signs may be less obvious, and a parent/carer may only report poor feeding or excessive crying.

Distinguishing inflicted from non-inflicted brain injury remains a challenge, but the recent RCPCH systematic review provides the best framework to assess this probability. Retinal haemorrhages together with apnoeas in children under 3 years of age, strongly correlate with inflicted head trauma. Other co-existing features that increase the suspicion of maltreatment include seizures, rib and long bone fractures.

The combination of encephalopathy, subdural haemorrhages and retinal haemorrhages is suggestive of an episode of shaking. It may also include an impact injury which could be against a hard or soft surface. The damage to the brain appears related to its rapid acceleration and deceleration during shaking/impact.

It is increasingly being recognised that spinal injuries can occur in association with inflicted head trauma. These injuries are often occult and need to be specifically sought.

Neuroimaging should be undertaken in any infant with encephalopathic features, focal neurological signs or haemorrhagic retinopathy. It is also important to consider in infants presenting with ALTE/BRUE (apparent life-threatening event/brief resolved unexplained events). The Royal College of Radiologists guidelines on the radiological investigation of suspected physical abuse in children provide good guidance on imaging modalities.

Visceral Injuries – They are difficult to detect and need to be considered if there are other serious/significant injuries. They are detected by specific imaging and blood markers of liver and pancreatic damage.

Bites and Oral Injuries – An adult human bite mark is always an inflicted injury and is therefore highly suspicious for maltreatment.

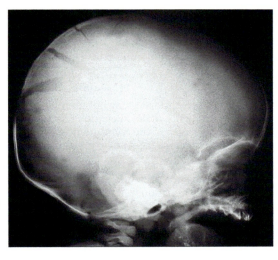

Figure 2.10 Branched skull fracture emanating from the occipital bone.

Bites can be swabbed for DNA and it can be helpful to refer to a forensic odontologist who may be able to help distinguish between child bites, adult bites and animal bites.

Ear Nose, Throat and Oral Injuries – Epistaxis is a rare presentation in children aged less than 2 years and warrants investigation as it is associated with asphyxiation.

A torn frenum of the upper or lower lip in isolation is not diagnostic of inflicted injury but needs to be assessed in the context of history and social concerns.

FABRICATED OR INDUCED ILLNESS (FII)

Induction of illness in a child by a parent is very rare, fabrication of symptoms is less rare, and it is often the actions of doctors in response to inaccurate parental reporting that causes much of the harm. FII (previously known as Munchausen's Syndrome-by-proxy) can be motivated either by erroneous beliefs or be the result of deliberate manipulation. The child can come to harm both physically and emotionally when the parent fabricates symptoms.

Perplexing presentations are clinical situations where there are concerns that FII might be the reason why the child's presentation, reported symptoms, and lack of response to prescribed treatment is puzzling. However, at this stage FII has yet to be established. In these situations, it is important to consider FII as a differential diagnosis and act in accordance with national guidance.

Management of these children and families can be challenging and it is important to avoid multiple referrals and best to have one paediatrician working closely with the general practitioner. Thorough history taking is paramount and it may be appropriate to perform some baseline investigations to exclude common causes of reported symptoms. In general, the approach should be one of transparency and reassurance while trying to avoid iatrogenic harm with unnecessary investigations; there will often be improvement following reassurance that a medical cause is not present and only a minority will need consideration of child protection proceedings.

SEXUAL ABUSE

Sexual abuse involves forcing or enticing a child or young person to take part in sexual activities, not necessarily involving physical contact, whether or not the child is aware of what is happening. Sexual abuse also includes non-contact activities, such as involving children in the production or viewing of sexual images/sexual activities, encouraging children to behave in sexually inappropriate ways or grooming a child in preparation for abuse. Increasingly grooming is occurring online and sexual abuse via the internet has become a major problem.

A child under 13 is not legally capable of consenting to sexual activity, but a degree of discretion is allowed so as not to stigmatise peer with peer activity. It is however imperative to ascertain whether there is sexual exploitation involving a power differential, age difference or lack of agreement.

Incidence

Although sexual abuse accounts for a minority of Child Protection Plans in the United Kingdom, it is often unrecognised and therefore frequently missed.

Presentation

Sexually abused children may not manifest any signs or symptoms. They may not make allegations for fear of not being believed or because of the consequences.

Child sexual abuse (CSA) may present in a variety of ways.

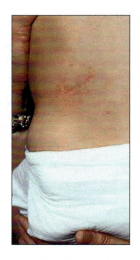

Figure 2.11 Bite marks on the back of an 8-month-old girl.

1. Allegation: This may be in the acute period when forensic samples may be gathered, but more commonly the child will allege non-recent abuse.

2. Physical symptoms: A wide range of physical symptoms may be linked to CSA, these include: constipation, dysuria, recurrent urinary tract infections, abnormal vaginal/penile discharge, recurrent ano-genital itching/discomfort, rectal fissures and bleeding (distinguish vaginal from rectal). A benign medical cause may often explain the symptoms, but sexual abuse should always be considered.

3. Emotional/behavioural: Sudden changes in behaviour maybe an indicator of sexual abuse but are often very non-specific. It is always important to ask the child if there is anything worrying them or if there is anyone making them feel uncomfortable. Other non-specific symptoms include:

   - Sleep disturbance or nightmares
   - Anxiety, depression, withdrawal
   - Aggression, attention seeking and/or poor concentration
   - Sexualised behaviour
   - Functional symptoms – recurrent headaches, abdominal pain
   - New onset soiling and wetting
   - Self-harm
   - Suicidal ideation
   - Running away
   - Risk taking behaviour
   - Eating disorders

Achieving Best Evidence (ABE) Interview

Following an allegation, the child is interviewed by a trained professional in a purpose-built suite with audio-visual recording facilities. This is used as evidence in court.

Assessment

All acute medical needs for children presenting following sexual abuse should be addressed by emergency and paediatric departments.

The United Kingdom has Sexual Assault Referral Centres (SARCs) that provide specialised forensic examinations, medical care, support, and follow up. The forensic sampling time frame is < 72 hours for children under 13 years and seven days for children over 13 years old. Children presenting acutely, within the forensic timeframe, should have intimate body swabs taken (semen, saliva, hair and other substances) and their clothing obtained for forensic analysis by expert laboratories.

In cases of non-recent assault an appropriate referral should be made to local specialist children health services for assessment.

The ano-genital examination should be done by a specialist using a colposcope for photo documentation. Acute genital, anal or oral injury can result in a variety of physical signs but most children alleging sexual abuse have normal physical findings.

This assessment is a specialised child protection assessment which includes addressing the child's health, safeguarding and forensic needs.

It is always important to consider the need for post coital contraception, pregnancy screening, hepatitis B and HIV prophylaxis, STI screening and treatment.

EMOTIONAL MALTREATMENT

This is the persistent maltreatment of a child causing severe adverse effects on the child's emotional development. All types of child maltreatment involve the child sustaining emotional damage but this type of maltreatment can occur in isolation.

Emotional maltreatment can involve active abuse or emotional unavailability or neglect. Both emotional abuse and neglect refer to relationships, rather than single events and are defined as persistent, non-physical harmful interactions with a child by a caregiver.

It is the impact on the child and their functioning that demonstrates the negative effects of these interactions.

In addition to emotional unavailability, unresponsiveness and neglect, the following negative interactions may be involved:

- Negative attributions or beliefs about the child

- Developmentally inappropriate interactions with the child

- Failure to recognise the child's individuality

- Failure to promote the child's social adaptations

The impact of these interactions varies but may include the following:

Infants: Feeding difficulties, crying, poor sleep, delayed development, and unresponsiveness.

Toddler/Pre-school: Head banging, rocking, clingy and developmental delay especially language and social skills.

School age: wetting, soiling, poor performance, antisocial behaviour, feeling worthless, unloved, inadequate, frightened, or corrupted.

Adolescents: low self-esteem, depression, self-harm, substance misuse, eating disorders, oppositional, aggressive, and delinquent behaviour.

Growth problems and behavioural signs such as 'frozen watchfulness' may indicate emotional maltreatment. It is important to consider emotional maltreatment as a differential diagnosis when assessing other presentations such as ADHD and autistic spectrum condition.

It is important to observe and record contemporaneously concerns about parent – child interactions and the impact they may be having on the child and take appropriate action.

Neglect

Neglect is the persistent failure of the parent to meet the child's basic needs. Unlike the other forms of maltreatment, it is the result of omission rather than deliberate acts. Although a single incident of neglect may result in significant damage, in general neglect is about an overall life experience.

It is important that professionals address issues of neglect in a supportive fashion. Poverty and deprivation undoubtedly negatively impact children, but these are issues that society has to address, and should be differentiated from parental acts of omission. Neglect can occur in any socioeconomic class but is more often recognised in association with deprivation.

Neglect is harmful and can be life-threatening, it needs to be taken as seriously as the other types of maltreatment.

Neglect can have both physical and emotional components. A helpful framework for categorising neglect is described in RCPCH Child protection companion and includes:

- Emotional neglect

- Abandonment

- Medical neglect

- Nutritional neglect

- Educational neglect

- Physical neglect
- Failure to provide supervision and guidance

Early recognition and intervention is important to prevent this type of harm which can have life-long consequences and become an intergenerational issue.

ADOLESCENCE

Many adolescents are maltreated or at risk of maltreatment, but this may well not be recognised. Challenging behaviour in adolescence is often not linked to their early childhood experiences or current maltreatment issue and they are often labelled as difficult. Each patient should be considered as an individual with experiences, medical needs, and rights appropriate to their age and stage of development. When assessing an adolescent patient it is usually appropriate to speak to them alone without a parent or carer present and to undertake a HEADSS (Home Education/Employment, Eating, Activities, Drugs, Sexuality, Suicide/Depression and Safety) diagnostic checklist.

VULNERABILITY AND RESILIENCE

There are recognised factors that impact the likelihood of maltreatment occurring. However, none of these factors have a causal link and there will be families who provide excellent parenting despite very difficult circumstances. It is therefore helpful to assess the risks, vulnerability, and resilience factors in a non-judgemental fashion.

Adverse childhood experiences (ACEs) are traumatic events occurring in childhood that can be detrimental to a child's long-term health, emotional and social developmental outcome. These ACEs include child maltreatment, growing up in a family where there is a history of domestic abuse, parental mental health difficulties, alcohol, or drug abuse, witnessing inhumane treatment, community disruption, poverty, discrimination, parental conflict and other factors influenced by the wider society. Analysis of serious case reviews of serious or fatal child maltreatment have shown that ACEs, in particular the trio of violence within the family home, parental mental health difficulties and drug abuse are prevalent.

It is important to note that children who have significant ACE's are not irreparably damaged and with appropriate interventions, permanent harm can be prevented.

As well as factors that make children vulnerable to maltreatment, there are other factors that make children more resilient to the effects of maltreatment. A strong relationship with an adult who values them, a variety of personality characteristics and a high cognitive ability are a few examples.

CASE STUDY: OXFORD SERIOUS CASE REVIEW

In 2013 several members of a gang were convicted of charges relating to child sexual exploitation (CSE) over a period of eight years in Oxford. The perpetrators had targeted as many as 50 vulnerable children with affection, alcohol and drugs while isolating them from caregivers. The children were then subjected to physical maltreatment and sexual abuse while being trafficked across the United Kingdom.

These children, most of whom were under local authority care, often did not understand they were being exploited. The investigation into this case identified that some professionals working with the children failed to recognise that grooming and sexual exploitation was taking place. The children were frequently missing from home and had behavioural changes as a result of the abuse which professionals looking after them often viewed as 'difficult girls making bad choices'. There was also poor understanding by professionals around consent and CSE.

This case highlighted the need for CSE training among professionals and importance of keeping children at the heart of the issue by recognising their vulnerability instead of viewing them as 'challenging individuals' who are difficult to manage. It also demonstrated the impact of a lack of information sharing between agencies and a heavy reliance on the victims to support criminal investigations/proceedings.

CONTEXTUAL SAFEGUARDING

Contextual safeguarding is an approach to understanding and responding to children's experiences of harm outside their families. This concept recognises that the relationships that young people form in their neighbourhoods, in school and online may result in maltreatment. The following list briefly describes some contextual safeguarding issues:

Self-Harm

Self-harm is widespread in adolescence and may indicate maltreatment. Bullying particularly online is commonly associated with self-harm. Self-harm includes a spectrum of presentations which include cutting, medication overdose, chemical and heat burns.

Bullying

Bullying can take many forms. Children who are bullied may show a range of symptoms and, at worst, may present to health services following physical assault or self-harm.

Digital Harm

Children and young people increasingly report adverse experiences online. It is often vulnerable children who are affected by maltreatment online. It is always worth asking specifically about cyberbullying, misinformation via social media groups as well as potential grooming and exploitation online.

Gangs and Criminal Exploitation

Gang culture which is often associated with children being exploited to assist gangs in criminal behaviour. Young people can be recruited by gangs to facilitate the transport of drugs and contraband between cities and rural locations. This is often called 'county lines' activity. The young people involved become very vulnerable, often recruit their peers and present with injuries and challenging behaviour.

Sexual Exploitation

Sexual exploitation in the United Kingdom and elsewhere remains a largely hidden problem. Child sexual exploitation is a form of child sexual abuse. It occurs where an individual or group takes advantage of an imbalance of power to coerce, manipulate or deceive a child or young person into sexual activity in exchange for something the victim needs or wants, and/or for the financial advantage or increased status of the perpetrator or facilitator.

A victim may have been sexually exploited even if they perceive the activity to be consensual. Child sexual exploitation can also occur online and doesn't need to involve physical contact. Many children are unaware that maltreatment is taking place.

Sexual exploitation of a child may start with a grooming period where the abuser forms a relationship with the child, often supplying them with drugs and alcohol prior to the sexual abuse starting. Suspicions that a child is being sexually exploited include relationships with older men, behavioural changes, going missing and self-harm.

Honour Based Violence and Forced Marriage

Honour based violence is a term used to define violence committed within the context of the extended family which is motivated by a perceived need to improve standing within the community which is assumed to have been lost due to the behaviour of the victim. Common triggers are refusing an arranged marriage, having a relationship outside the approved group, homosexual relationships, reporting domestic abuse and attempting divorce with associated custody of children. It is important to believe young people who report they are at risk of this form of maltreatment and work with them alongside social services and the police to ensure their safety.

Forced marriage is when a person faces physical, social and emotional pressure to marry an individual not of their choosing. This can sometimes occur during visits abroad to countries outside the United Kingdom. There is a specific government Forced Marriage Unit which can help and advice to individuals or professionals including supporting legal action to help protect the individual.

Female Genital Mutilation (FGM)

FGM is a cultural practice involving cutting or removal of parts of the female genitals practiced on millions of women worldwide. It is prevalent in areas of sub-Saharan Africa, Arab states as well as parts of Asia, Eastern Europe and Latin America.

There are four main types of FGM which range from piercing/pricking the female genitalia through to removal of all of the labia and clitoris with narrowing of the vaginal opening.

FGM is often performed by traditional circumcisers or cutters who do not have any medical training, although in some countries it is done by a medical professional.

There are no health benefits to FGM and it can cause serious short and long-term health problems.

Women and children who have undergone FGM require support and treatment. FGM is often an isolated issue and not connected to other forms of child maltreatment but further evaluation of the risks of FGM within the family should be explored.

In October 2015 it became a mandatory duty for all health professionals in England and Wales to report known cases of FGM in under 18-year-olds to the police. Known cases are defined as a child disclosing FGM or concerns arising from examination findings.

Modern Slavery and Trafficking

Children can be trafficked within, into and out of the United Kingdom. This occurs against their will and is usually for the purposes of criminal and sexual exploitation or forced labour. These children would have experienced multiple types of adversity and can have complex presentations. It is important that these groups are not criminalised when they are involved in criminal activities. The Modern Human Slavery and Trafficking Unit in the UK combat this issue and can be contacted for advice and support.

Refugees and Unaccompanied Asylum Seekers

Refugees have multiple health needs and inevitably have experienced adversity and trauma. This situation is currently compounded by the restrictions to universal healthcare within the United Kingdom for this group of children and their families. Child migrants to the United Kingdom who are unaccompanied are the responsibility of the state.

WHAT TO DO WHEN YOU SUSPECT MALTREATMENT

This depends on the professional's level of experience and seniority, but if maltreatment is suspected then safeguarding children procedures must be followed.

Occasionally immediate action is required which can be discussed with organisation's specialist safeguarding teams or out of hours with senior managers. It is an individual's professional responsibility to ensure that appropriate action has been taken and to escalate any remaining concerns to the safeguarding team, if necessary. Referrals to social services will always require written information, but some teams may take an initial referral via telephone in an emergency.

If the child is in immediate danger, it is best to telephone the police as they are the only agency who can act immediately to ensure a child's welfare.

What Happens Next?

If social services assess that a child has been subject to significant harm, they will carry out a child protection investigation which is called a Section 47 enquiry. This enquiry may be undertaken by social services alone or jointly with the police who may be investigating a potential crime against a child. The decisions made about Section 47 enquiries take place at a strategy meeting led by social services. If social services assess that significant harm is likely, they will call an initial Child Protection Conference. This Conference is attended by the family and professionals who also provide written reports.

Professionals at the Conference are asked their opinion on whether the child is likely to suffer or has suffered significant harm. If this is the case a Child Protection Plan is formulated which will include the need for further assessment and intervention to protect the child or children involved. Although unborn children have no legal rights, they can have a CPP which becomes active following their birth. A core group which includes key professionals and the family, meet at regular intervals between review child protection conferences, to implement the objectives of the CPP.

It is hoped that the CPP will work and that in due course children can be stepped down to a CIN plan and ultimately from social work involvement. Families do not have to consent to CPPs. Information sharing is vital when a child is on a CPP as it indicates a high level of concern about the welfare of a child. It is important that throughout the process the child's views are sought and seriously considered.

Where there are immediate or ongoing serious concerns about the welfare of a child the local authority will apply to the family court to obtain parental responsibility for the child.

Parental responsibility encompasses all the rights and duties of parents towards their children. The issue of who has parental responsibility for children can be quite complex.

Birth mothers and fathers named on the birth certificate have parental responsibility unless the child has been adopted. There are other court orders that can grant parental responsibilities to other parties such as relatives.

When the local authority gains parental responsibility through the family court their responsibility is overriding and they can place the child in an alternative home to ensure their well-being. Children placed outside the family home by a local authority are termed 'looked after children'. There are looked after children health teams who oversee their health.

In parallel with family court processes whose priority is the welfare of children, the police may investigate any potential crime against the child. There may be a prosecution of any potential perpetrators of crime in the criminal courts. Although the evidence produced in both family and criminal court is of comparable quality, the threshold for a judge in family court to grant a legal order is that the concern has been proved 'on the balance of probabilities'. In a criminal court however, the prosecution must prove (usually to a jury) the defendant's guilt beyond reasonable doubt. In the criminal process the focus is on the perpetrator, although achieving a criminal conviction can also protect children from the convicted individual.

CONCLUSION

It is important that all health professionals are aware of the part they play in the child protection system, which is mandated by their professional bodies. Child safeguarding is everyone's business and requires health professionals to share information appropriately. Health professionals' aim is to support families in caring for their children, but when concern arises about maltreatment it is their duty recognise this and respond appropriately.

RESOURCES

- The Global status report on preventing violence against children 2020
- RCPCH Child Protection Evidence – Systematic reviews
- Child Protection Companion – RCPCH
- Working Together to Safeguard Children (Department for Education) – 2018
- National Guidance for Child Protection in Scotland (Scottish Government, 2021, updated 2023)
- Social Services and Well-Being (Wales) Act 2014
- Co-Operating to Safeguard Children and Young People in Northern Ireland (Department of Health, 2017)
- Perplexing Presentations/Fabricated or Induced Illness in Children RCPCH guidance 2021

3 Infectious Diseases

Nele Alders, Justin Penner and Delane Shingadia

The current spread of infectious diseases and multi-resistant organisms are a worldwide problem that has a greater impact on low-income countries.

BACTERIA

NEONATAL MENINGITIS

Incidence

Rates of culture-proven meningitis in developed countries, including the United Kingdom, is estimated to be approximately 0.3/1000 live births. Incidence and aetiology of neonatal meningitis has changed significantly in the past two decades as a result of universal vaccination programmes. Low birth weight infants (< 2500 g), prematurity, traumatic delivery, premature rupture of membranes, chorioamnionitis and/or maternal peripartum infection are all risk factors for development of meningitis in the neonatal period.

Aetiology/Pathogenesis

The most common organisms to cause neonatal meningitis include: group B streptococcus (> 50%), *E. coli* (20%), and rarely listeria monocytogenes (5–10%). Vertical transmission during delivery is the most common source of infection. Neonates are at greatest risk of meningitis secondary to the continuing development of humoral and cellular immunity and phagocytic migration. Complement pathway inefficiency further predisposes to infections with encapsulated bacteria.

Clinical Presentation

Clinical signs and symptoms of neonatal meningitis are non-specific, often leading to late diagnosis and poorer outcomes. Fever or hypothermia may be the only presenting sign. Other signs and symptoms may include: irritability, poor feeding, abnormal heart rate or respiratory impairment, poor peripheral perfusion, apnoea, feeding intolerance, hypotonia and diarrhoea. Seizures, bulging fontanelle and focal neurological findings are late signs which impart poor prognosis. Nuchal rigidity is not commonly appreciated in neonates diagnosed with meningitis.

Diagnosis

When suspicion of neonatal meningitis presents, blood cultures, urine cultures, and a lumbar puncture are required for bacteriologic confirmation. Microscopy and culture of cerebrospinal fluid is the gold standard for isolation of the causative bacterial agent. Molecular diagnostics, such as polymerase chain reaction (PCR), may be useful in neonates who have already been treated with antibiotics at the time of lumbar puncture. Cell count (elevated > 20), low glucose, and high protein in the CSF supports a diagnosis of meningitis. Cranial imaging with or without spinal imaging (ultrasound and/or MRI) is often undertaken to assess for the presence of bacterial collections, especially in cases with persistent fever or focal neurologic signs.

Treatment

Use of broad-spectrum antibiotics, most typically a third-generation cephalosporin in combination with an aminoglycoside provides empiric coverage for both gram-negative bacterial and group B streptococcus aetiologies in the neonatal period. The addition of aminopenicillin provides additional coverage for listeria. Once a pathogen is isolated, targeted antibiotic therapy can be instituted. Meningitis caused by gram-negative bacteria and listeria are treated with a total of three weeks of antimicrobial coverage whereas cases caused by group B streptococcus require two to three weeks of treatment. Cerebral abscesses require longer treatment with up to six weeks of antibiotics and occasionally surgical intervention.

MENINGOCOCCAL INFECTIONS

Incidence

In 2018/2019 in England and Wales there were 525 cases of confirmed invasive meningococcal infections, a substantial decline since peak infections of 2595 in 1999/2000. Infants remain the most

DOI: 10.1201/9781003175186-3

commonly affected age group. The disease tends to be sporadic but more prominent in winter months. Occasional small outbreaks occur in the United Kingdom.

Aetiology/Pathogenesis

Neisseria meningitis is a gram-negative diplococcus bacterium. Thirteen serogroups are recognised by their different capsular polysaccharide antigen. Most disease is caused by serogroups A, B, C, Y and W-135. In the United Kingdom, due to the introduction of the group C conjugate vaccine in 1999, serogroup B strains are now responsible for the majority of cases of meningococcemia, although a shift in strain prevalence due to widespread vaccination against the B strain is also increasingly evident.

Asymptomatic carriage of meningococci in the upper respiratory tract may occur in 5–15% of the population. Humans are the only natural hosts. Transmission of meningococcus occurs from person to person via respiratory droplet spread. In some individuals, meningococci are able to invade the circulation (also the meninges), with the resultant release of bacterial products, including endotoxin, thereby initiating an inflammatory process. The end result is vascular endothelial damage that results in capillary leak syndrome (responsible for severe hypovolemia), and intravascular thrombosis with subsequent vascular occlusion and extensive organ damage.

Clinical Presentation

Meningococcal disease most commonly presents as bacterial meningitis (15% of cases), septicaemia (25% of cases) or as a combination of both (60% of cases). Meningococcaemia usually manifests as an abrupt onset of fever, malaise and a characteristic petechial rash (Figure 3.1) that may initially be maculopapular. In its most devastating form, large ecchymotic areas develop (purpura fulminans) (Figure 3.2), with disseminated intravascular coagulation (DIC), shock and coma, which can lead to a rapidly fatal outcome, despite appropriate therapy. The presentation of

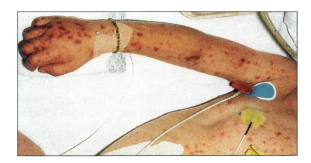

Figure 3.1   Meningococcal infections demonstrating petechial rash.

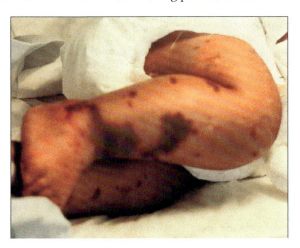

Figure 3.2   Meningococcal infection with disseminated intravascular coagulation.

meningococcal meningitis is much the same as other forms of meningitis with fever, headache, vomiting, and neck stiffness. Complications of invasive meningococcal disease include arthritis, pericarditis, endophthalmitis, and pneumonia. Widespread necrosis may require amputations and reconstructive surgery.

Diagnosis

Due to the rapidity of disease development, clinical diagnosis is paramount. Blood and/or CSF cultures may be positive; blood cultures tend to be positive in 50% of cases, whilst CSF cultures are positive in 70%. Whole blood PCR test for N. meningitidis should also be obtained. This is a very sensitive test, especially in cases where prior antibiotics have been given.

Treatment

Early recognition, initiation of antibiotic therapy (intramuscular or IV benzylpenicillin 1200 mg for children > 10 years of age, 600 mg for those aged from 1 to 9 years, and 300 mg for those younger than 1 year) and prompt referral to hospital is essential for a good outcome. In-patient treatment consists of initial empiric therapy with IV cefotaxime or ceftriaxone, until confirmation of the aetiology of the invasive disease. These antibiotics can be continued for the full course of treatment (5–7 days). Patients should be admitted to the Paediatric Intensive Care Unit (PICU), and elective ventilation may be required for severely ill patients. Hypovolaemic shock, manifested by cold peripheries, poor capillary refill, tachycardia and oliguria should be corrected promptly with boluses of IV fluid (colloids or crystalloids). Treatment of raised intracranial pressure and correction of DIC and maintenance of circulation are also priorities.

TUBERCULOSIS

Incidence

There has been a dramatic resurgence of tuberculosis (TB) worldwide. In low-income countries, this increase is strongly associated with poverty, homelessness, and urban overcrowding, including the AIDS epidemic. The breakdown in TB control programmes, multiple drug resistences and the increase in the number of individuals from areas of high endemicity have also contributed. The United Kingdom is designated as a low incidence country (< 40/100,000) with an estimated rate per 100,000 in 2019 of 8/100,000, although specific regions have rates that approach or exceed the cut-off of endemicity. A total of 5500 cases were reported in the United Kingdom in 2019 of which 169 cases were in children < 15 years old. Among these 52.4% had only extra-pulmonary disease, the most common site being lymph node disease (19.3% intrathoracic nodes; 13.3% extrathoracic nodes).

Aetiology/Pathogenesis

Mycobacterium tuberculosis, an acid-fast bacillus, is the major cause of human TB. Transmission occurs via inhalation of airborne particles, usually from an adult with sputum smear-positive pulmonary TB (cavitary TB). The inhaled organisms multiply in alveolar macrophages and spread via lymphatics to regional lymph nodes. The primary complex (Ghon) consists of local disease at the portal of entry and the involved regional lymph nodes. Some tubercle bacilli can spread via the bloodstream to establish metastatic infection in the lungs, reticuloendothelial system and various other organs. After six to eight weeks, cell-mediated immunity develops (skin test conversion), and is usually followed by progressive healing of infected foci. In a small proportion of patients, symptomatic disease will develop at the time of primary infection. In general, complications in children occur within 6 to 12 months after initial infection.

Clinical Presentation

Most children infected with *M. tuberculosis* are asymptomatic. Patients may present with radiographic abnormalities consistent with hilar or mediastinal lymphadenopathy, cervical adenitis, pulmonary involvement (atelectasis, consolidation, pleural effusion) (Figures 3.3 and 3.4), miliary (Figure 3.5) or CNS disease. Later manifestations may include: bone and joint, renal, and cutaneous disease. The classic symptoms of TB, fever, night sweats, and loss of weight are rare in young children.

Diagnosis

Definitive diagnosis is made via the identification and isolation of *M. tuberculosis* from early morning gastric aspirates or from other normally sterile body fluids (CSF, pleural fluid, urine, sputum). Recovery of organisms may take up to ten weeks by conventional solid media culture methods;

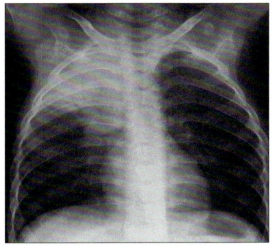

Figure 3.3 Tuberculosis: pulmonary involvement.

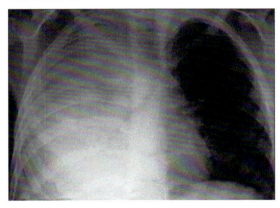

Figure 3.4 Tuberculosis with right pleural effusion.

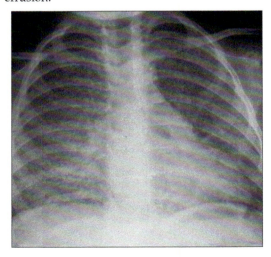

Figure 3.5 Miliary TB.

using the BACTEC radiometric liquid system this can be reduced to two weeks. Newer more rapid methods of diagnosis, including PCR and the use of DNA probes such as GeneXpert, have become available. A positive tuberculin skin test (Mantoux reaction > 5 mm induration) is suggestive of either infection in an asymptomatic individual, or disease in a symptomatic patient. Interferon-gamma release assays (IGRAs) are also increasingly used and measure interferon-gamma production from T-lymphocytes in response to stimulation from antigens that are fairly specific for *M. tuberculosis* complex. Thus they have been mainly introduced as an adjunct to or in lieu of tuberculin skin tests (TST), particularly in the context of false-positive TST due to BCG or non-tuberculous mycobacteria.

Treatment

It is important to differentiate between infection and disease. Asymptomatic tuberculin-positive cases with normal chest x-rays (infection) are treated with isoniazid (INH) 10 mg/kg and rifampicin 15 mg/kg (for three months) or INH monotherapy for six months (chemoprophylaxis). Pulmonary disease, including TB adenitis, requires short-course chemotherapy which consists of a two-month course of INH (10 mg/kg), rifampicin (15 mg/kg), pyrazinamide (35 mg/kg), and ethambutol (20 mg/kg), followed by INH and rifampicin for a further four months. Miliary TB and TB meningitis are treated for a total of 12 months (two months with four drugs, ten months with two drugs). For all treatment protocols, modifications should be made based on drug susceptibility. A weaning course of adjunctive steroids (six weeks) should be used in cases of CNS disease, pericardial, laryngeal, or endobronchial disease. When multidrug resistant (MDR-TB), extensively drug resistant (XDR-TB) or rifampicin resistant TB (RR-TB) is isolated or when the index case is known or suspected to have resistant disease, an individualised combination of drugs should be used based on the WHO groupings (A–C) of antimycobacterial drugs. Longer courses, typically a minimum of 12 to 18 months are required for resistant TB disease. Fixed-dose combination tablets are preferred in order to minimise pill burden and to improve compliance.

NON-TUBERCULOUS MYCOBACTERIAL INFECTIONS
Incidence

More than 120 species of non-tuberculous mycobacterial (NTM) infections have been implicated in human disease. There is a marked variation of disease incidence in different geographical regions. In resource rich countries, NTMs are more common than infection due to *M. tuberculosis*. In resource limited countries, chronic cervical adenitis is mostly secondary to *M. tuberculosis*.

Aetiology/Pathogenesis

Non-tuberculous mycobacteria are acid-fast bacilli (AFB) and are classified as rapidly growing species (e.g. *Mycobacterium fortuitum*, *Mycobacterium abscessus*, *Mycobacterium chelonae*) or slowly growing species (e.g. *Mycobacterium avium* complex (MAC), *Mycobacterium marinum*, and *Mycobacterium kansasii*).

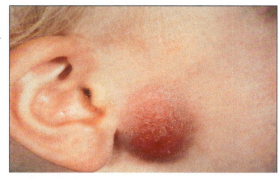

Figure 3.6   Lymphadenitis.

The predominant NTM disease in children is cervical lymphadenitis due to MAC. The organisms are ubiquitous and are found in soil, food, and water. Transmission results from environmental acquisition by inhalation or ingestion (lymphadenitis and pulmonary diseases) or direct contact (cutaneous and soft tissue diseases) from a contaminated source.

Clinical Presentation

NTM causes four main clinical syndromes in children: lymphadenopathy, skin and soft tissue infection (Figure 3.6), pulmonary disease (predominantly in children with underlying pulmonary conditions, e.g. cystic fibrosis), and disseminated disease (predominantly in immune-compromised children). The most common presentation is the development of chronic localised lymphadenopathy. Affected nodes tend to be in the anterior cervical chain and submandibular area (less commonly preauricular, postauricular and submental lymph nodes). The affected nodes are usually unilateral, firm, painless, and may be fixed to underlying tissues. They often develop an overlying, superficial, dark reddish or purplish hue (Figure 3.6). The natural history is for fluctuance to develop with eventual chronic discharging sinus formation and scarring. Occasional low-grade fever may be present but other constitutional symptoms are rare.

Diagnosis

Isolation and identification of non-tuberculous AFB by culture or PCR from specimens taken from sites such as blood, sputum, bronchial lavage, CSF, bone marrow, lymph node aspirate or other sterile body sites is required for a definitive diagnosis. A positive Mantoux test of (> 5 mm of induration) is suggestive of NTM in a child with a negative chest x-ray and negative family history of TB. Cases of disseminated disease should be evaluated for primary or secondary immunodeficiency, including neutrophil function deficiencies.

Treatment

Complete surgical excision of the involved lymph nodes is the definitive treatment for non-tuberculous lymphadenitis. If this is not possible, a period of antimycobacterial therapy may be necessary (up to six months usually). Pending results of sensitivity testing, a regimen of clarithromycin 15 mg/kg/day and rifampicin 15–20 mg/kg/day, with or without ethambutol 15 mg/kg/day, is often used.

Management of cutaneous disease and disease at other sites may also require both antimicrobial therapy and surgical debridement. Triple or quadruple antimycobacterial therapy to which the isolate is susceptible (macrolide, rifampicin, ethambutol, quinolone +/– amikacin) is generally indicated for disseminated disease in immunocompromised patients. Some species like *M. abscessus* and *M. chelonae* may be more resistant to standard first-line treatment and require more complex and prolonged treatment.

LYME DISEASE

Incidence

In England and Wales, Lyme disease is the most common vector-borne human infection. Although it remains rare, rates have increased since reporting began in 1986. In 2017 there were 1579 cases identified (incidence of 2.7/100,000 population). The cases reported were most commonly in the summer and early autumn.

Aetiology/Pathogenesis

Lyme disease is caused by the spirochete *Borrelia burgdorferi*. Transmission typically occurs from tick vectors (*Ixodes* species in Northern Europe). Tick bites usually need to be longer than 24 hours for human infection to occur. The incubation period is 3 to 20 days with a median of 12 days. Only tick bites from *Borrelia burgdorferi* infected carriers cause Lyme disease.

Clinical Presentation

The clinical presentations of *Lyme borreliosis* vary widely and are often divided into different stages, namely early localised, early disseminated, and late disease. Early localised disease has a distinctive targetoid rash called erythema migrans (EM) occurring at the inoculum site with a slow expansion over weeks with central clearing (Figure 3.7). Other features that may accompany the rash include: fever, malaise, headache, neck stiffness, myalgia, and arthralgia. Early disseminated disease is characterised by multiple erythematous skin lesions and can be accompanied by: cranial nerve palsies, lymphocytic meningitis, myocarditis, and conjunctivitis. Late disease is characterised by neurological involvement and commonly by pauciarticular relapsing arthritis.

Diagnosis

Serological testing is the most useful diagnostic test, although these tests may be negative in the first few weeks of infection.

In the United Kingdom, the Lyme Borreliosis Unit of Public Health England uses a two-stage diagnostic approach, the first being an enzyme immune assay (EIA) screen followed by an immunoblot or western blot to confirm antibodies. Early localised disease is a clinical diagnosis as the typical EM rash occurs prior to seroconversion.

Treatment

Early localised disease, carditis, and focal disease affecting cranial or peripheral nerves is treated with doxycycline (> 12 years) or amoxicillin (< 12 years) orally for 21 days. Azithromycin for 17

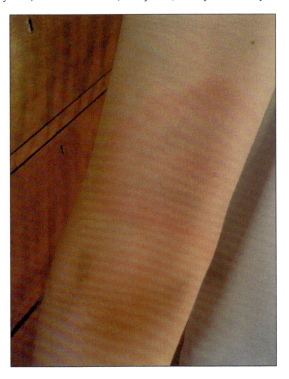

Figure 3.7 Lyme disease with erythema migrans rash.

days can be used where there is a definite history of penicillin allergy except in cases of Lyme carditis due to the risk of QT prolongation. IV ceftriaxone is recommended for CNS involvement and myocardial involvement with haemodynamic instability for 21 days duration. Treatment with doxycycline/amoxicillin is extended to 28 days in the setting of Lyme arthritis. If symptoms persist after an appropriate antibiotic course a second course can be considered in rare circumstances. Prolonged and repeated antibiotic courses beyond a second treatment is not recommended. A Jarish–Herxheimer reaction (a transient clinical phenomenon that occurs in patients infected by spirochetes who undergo antibiotic treatment) can occur after treatment especially in cases with high spirochaete burden.

STAPHYLOCOCCAL TOXIC SHOCK SYNDROME

Incidence

Although first described in children in the United States in 1978, most cases of staphylococcal toxic shock syndrome (TSS) occurred in young menstruating women using tampons in the following decades. The incidence of TSS declined sharply after the withdrawal of highly absorbent tampon brands. In the United Kingdom, non-menstrual TSS is now more common than menstrual TSS. Children < 16 years of age accounted for 39% of TSS cases, most caused by burns and skin and soft tissue infections.

Aetiology/Pathogenesis

The most common aetiologic agent is toxic shock syndrome toxin-1 (TSST-1) producing strains of *S. aureus*. Often *S. aureus* is merely a coloniser of a body site and does not cause focal infection, however, the toxin produced has superantigen properties and is able to cause widespread activation of the immune system with consequent endothelial damage. This results in multi-system organ damage secondary to capillary leak syndrome, loss of intravascular volume and tone, and interstitial oedema and occasionally death.

Clinical Presentation

An acute febrile illness characterised by the onset of a diffuse macular rash, mucositis (Figure 3.8), myalgia, gastrointestinal symptoms, hypotension can lead to multi-organ system dysfunction including renal failure. Desquamation of the trunk (Figure 3.9) begins after seven days, followed by palmoplantar desquamation.

Diagnosis

Diagnosis is based on established clinical criteria. Laboratory abnormalities usually include anaemia, clotting derangements, thrombocytopenia, elevated creatinine phosphokinase (CPK), and in some patients evidence of liver and/or kidney injury. Isolates of *S. aureus* (from superficial and sterile sites) should be examined for their ability to produce TSST-1.

There is a broad differential diagnoses which includes invasive group A streptococcal toxic shock, drug reaction, Kawasaki disease, enteric fever, dengue, leptospirosis and septic shock due to other pathogens (e.g. gram-negatives).

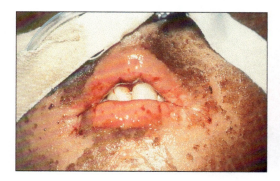

Figure 3.8 Staphylococcal toxic shock syndrome with mucositis.

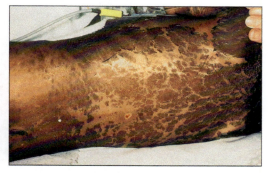

Figure 3.9 Staphylococcal toxic shock syndrome with flaky desquamation of the trunk.

Treatment

Supportive management of multi-system organ failure is key alongside antibiotic therapy with an antistaphylococcal agent whilst eradicating the source of toxin production (removal of any foreign body and/or irrigation of wound). The addition of clindamycin may be useful given its antitoxin properties. IV immunoglobulin should be considered in severely ill patients.

SYPHILIS

Incidence

Syphilis infections rose by 20% from 2016 compared with 2017. Increased rates (3.8/100,000) of syphilis infection have been seen in women of childbearing age (20–24 years). Recent Public Health England data show increases in congenital syphilis with 21 cases diagnosed between 2010 and 2017. Reports from incident investigations suggest a more widespread infection. Syphilis infections continue to rise, highlighting the importance in recognition of congenital syphilis. A rise in atypical cases in neonates born to mothers with negative first-trimester screening infected during pregnancy requires additional vigilance.

Aetiology/Pathogenesis

Syphilis is caused by the bacterial spirochaete *Treponema pallidum* sp. pallidum. Haematogenous dissemination of the spirochaete can cause multi-organ dysfunction with the most severe of cases seeding the CNS. Infection can lay dormant causing symptoms later in childhood if not promptly recognised and treated in the neonatal period.

Clinical Presentation

Heightened suspicion is essential as approximately two-thirds of infants with congenital syphilis are asymptomatic at birth. Signs and symptoms of early congenital syphilis include: rash, blistering or peeling skin lesions, lymphadenopathy, hepatosplenomegaly, jaundice, osteochondritis, funisitis, haemorrhagic rhinitis, failure to thrive and ophthalmological abnormalities. Late signs of missed congenital syphilis in children include: gummatous skin lesions, saddle nose, craniofacial and long bone abnormalities, sensorineural hearing loss, and dental anomalies among others.

Diagnosis

Serological evaluation should include treponemal IgM enzyme immunoassay (EIA) in conjunction with a paired quantitative non-treponemal test and Treponema pallidum particle agglutination assay (TPPA) of the infant and mother. Assays for IgG (i.e. TPPA or rapid plasma reagin) in the infant can be positive as a result of passive transfer (to a maximum of 18 months of age) whether or not the infant is infected. Direct molecular testing with PCR or dark field microscopy of skin lesions, nasopharyngeal aspirates, and/or placenta may assist diagnosis. A comprehensive set of diagnostic investigations including: standard haematological, renal and liver biochemistry, a lumbar puncture with CSF syphilis serology, ophthalmology and audiology evaluations, and radiographs of long bones (as clinically indicated) should be completed.

Treatment

Recommended treatment for neonatal congenital syphilis is benzyl penicillin 30 mg/kg IV 12 hourly for the first seven days of life then eight hourly for three additional days for a total of ten days.

VIRUSES

ENTEROVIRUSES

Incidence

The true incidence of enteroviral infections is largely unknown as most infections are subclinical or diagnosed clinically. Larger scale outbreaks of respiratory illness (e.g. EV-D68), acute haemorrhagic conjunctivitis (EV-D70 and CV-A24v), and hand-foot-and-mouth disease are common. Infections are typically seasonal with increased infection rates in the spring and early summer.

Aetiology/Pathogenesis

Enteroviruses are single-stranded RNA viruses of the picornaviridae family. This group of viruses includes polioviruses, coxsackieviruses A and B, echoviruses, and other serotypes of the enterovirus family (68–71, 73–91, 100–101). Enteroviruses are transmitted by direct contact with respiratory secretions and stool or contaminated water sources. Infections may also be transmitted vertically from mother to foetus causing congenital enterovirus syndrome.

Clinical Presentation

Rarely, severe foetal anomalies have been attributed to congenitally acquired enterovirus infection although the majority of cases are asymptomatic. Suspicion for congenital enterovirus syndrome should be raised in the setting of unexplained severe pneumonitis, carditis, neurological manifestations, sepsis and stillbirth, particularly in the context of concurrent unexplained maternal illness. The spectrum of childhood disease includes: meningoencephalitis, flaccid paralysis, rash, hand-foot-and-mouth disease, conjunctivitis, myopericarditis and wheeze.

Diagnosis

Clinical diagnosis is common. Isolation of virus by PCR in blood, respiratory secretions, throat/nasopharyngeal swabs, stool, or CSF by RT-PCR is confirmatory. Paired maternal samples and sampling of placental tissue can help support a diagnosis of vertically acquired enterovirus.

Treatment

Supportive treatment is paramount. Severe cases of congenital enterovirus and in those with primary immunodeficiencies (i.e. X-linked agammaglobulinemia) can be considered for treatment with IVIG.

HIV INFECTION AND AIDS

Aetiology/Pathogenesis

HIV disease is secondary to infection with a human RNA retrovirus (usually HIV-1, less commonly HIV-2), trophic for CD4 T-lymphocytes. Transmission is via one of three routes:

- Perinatal infection (antenatal, peri-partum or via breastfeeding).
- Transfusion of infected blood products or via contaminated needles.
- Sexual transmission.

HIV is able to integrate into the host's genome through the action of its reverse transcriptase enzyme. The eventual consequences of infection are a gradual CD4 T-cell depletion and a resultant cell-mediated immunodeficiency. The occurrence of a major opportunistic infection or cancer defines a diagnosis of AIDS.

Incidence

The UNAIDS 2019 report states that 9.38 million people worldwide are living with HIV (1.8 million children), the majority in sub-Saharan Africa. According to the Collaborative HIV Paediatric Study (CHIPS), in 2020 a total of 2210 children were reported to be living with HIV in the United Kingdom. Major progress has been made in the United Kingdom, as elsewhere, in reducing the rate of vertical transmission of HIV. When interventions were virtually non-existent, the vertical transmission rate among diagnosed women was 25.6%. However, the overall transmission rate from diagnosed women who receive combination antiretroviral therapy (ART) with an undetectable viral load is very low (0.27% in 2012–2014).

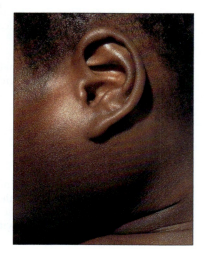

Clinical Presentation

Infants surviving the first 6 to 12 months of life receiving no antiretroviral treatment are often asymptomatic for the first few years of childhood. Generalised lymphadenopathy, hepatosplenomegaly, failure to thrive, parotitis, (Figure 3.10) and lymphocytic interstitial pneumonitis (LIP) are often seen in combination when children become symptomatic. Approximately 25% of children present in the first year with

Figure 3.10 Parotitis in HIV infection.

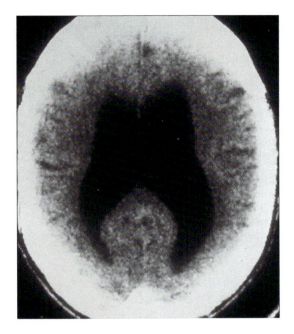

Figure 3.11   HIV encephalitis.

an AIDS-defining illness. AIDS-defining conditions observed in children include: *Pneumocystis jirovecii* pneumonia (PJP), recurrent bacterial infections, failure to thrive, HIV encephalitis (Figure 3.11), CMV retinitis (Figure 3.12), LIP, pulmonary/oesophageal candidiasis, cryptosporidiosis, chronic herpes simplex virus (HSV), Kaposi sarcoma, and MAC infection. With widespread antenatal HIV testing of pregnant women, and administration of early antiretroviral therapy for infected infants, infants and children on combination ART now rarely develop opportunistic infections or symptomatic disease.

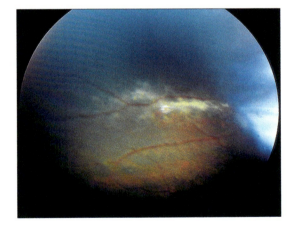

Figure 3.12   CMV retinitis.

Diagnosis

A confirmed positive HIV antibody test (ELISA) is diagnostic of HIV infection in children over 18 months. In younger infants, because placentally transmitted antibody may persist for up to 18 months, the diagnosis is usually made with a positive plasma HIV RNA or DNA PCR test. Infants are considered infected if the initial sample is confirmed by a second virological test performed on a separate specimen taken more than four weeks after birth. Other laboratory findings may show low CD4 cells (both absolute percentage and total number), lymphopenia, hypergammaglobulinemia and thrombocytopenia.

WHO guidelines recommend that all patients living with HIV should be commenced on ART regardless of clinical, immunological, or virological status. There are now more than 30 medications in six drug classes available to treat HIV. Unfortunately not all are licensed for children or have paediatric formulations available.

A typical ART regimen usually consists of two nucleoside reverse transcriptase inhibitors (NRTI), in addition to a third agent: an integrase inhibitor, nonnucleoside reverse transcriptase inhibitor (NNRTIs) or a boosted protease inhibitor (PI). This combination will need to be changed, if or when there is evidence of therapy failure, medication intolerance or when regimen simplification is desired. Prophylaxis with daily co-trimoxazole is important in the prevention of PJP in the neonatal period and at older ages if the CD4 count falls below 350 cells/mm^3. All immunisations are indicated in this group of patients, except BCG (if CD4 < 25%), which may be considered for asymptomatic children in those countries with high incidence of TB or where community/household transmission risk is high.

It is essential that infected children and their families receive comprehensive care that addresses both the medical and psychosocial aspects of this disease. This is best done by a multidisciplinary team that includes: an adult physician, a paediatrician, psychologist, social worker, HIV counsellor, physiotherapist, pharmacist and a dietician.

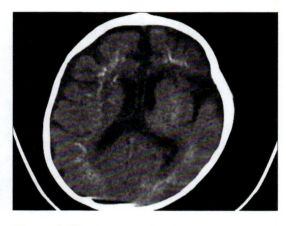

Figure 3.13 Congenital CMV with intracellular calcification.

CONGENITAL CYTOMEGALOVIRUS

Incidence

CMV is a ubiquitous virus that only infects humans. Transmission occurs horizontally (by direct person-to-person contact through secretions), vertically (from mother to child before, during or after birth) and via blood products from infected donors. Approximately 1% of all live-born infants are infected in utero and excrete CMV at birth, making this the most common congenital viral infection.

Aetiology/Pathogenesis

CMV is a double-stranded DNA virus (*Herpesviridae* family) that causes primary infection followed by latency established in cells of myeloid lineage. Seropositivity increases with age and in populations from lower socioeconomic status. Congenital infection is thought to be transmitted from maternal blood via the placenta and is 40 times more common following primary infection in the mother during pregnancy than in those who have serological evidence of previous CMV infection.

Clinical Presentation

Congenital CMV infection is asymptomatic in the majority of babies at birth; however, 10% will have features evident at birth (so-called symptomatic congenital CMV infection) that include: intrauterine growth restriction, jaundice, purpura, hepatosplenomegaly, microcephaly, intracerebral calcifications (Figure 3.13) and retinitis. Sensorineural hearing loss is the most common sequelae of congenital infection, occurring more often in those infants with symptomatic infection. Hearing loss may be present at birth or occur later, in the first years of life. Developmental delay may also occur. In contrast to congenital infection, postnatally acquired infection (usually acquired through breast milk) is not associated with clinical illness except in preterm or immunocompromised infants where systemic infections can occur.

Diagnosis

CMV infection is diagnosed by PCR or by serology. Serology is of limited use in those under 1 year of age, due to passive maternal antibody transfer, but may be useful in older children. CMV IgM measurements may indicate primary infection but are only positive in approximately 70% of congenitally infected infants. Identification of CMV from samples obtained within the first three weeks of life (PCR of bloods, saliva and urine) usually indicate congenitally acquired infection. Dried blood spots (Guthrie card) taken shortly after birth may be used retrospectively to confirm the presence of congenital CMV using PCR, although sensitivity typically ranges between 30 and 70%. Examination for end-organ dysfunction in congenitally acquired CMV, i.e. thrombocytopaenia, hepatic dysfunction, ophthalmology and audiology examinations for chorioretinitis and sensorineural hearing loss, and neuroimaging (for neuronal migration deficits, calcifications, and neuronal inflammatory changes) are essential in the classification of symptomatic congenital CMV.

Treatment

Data in neonates with symptomatic congenital CMV disease involving the central nervous system suggest possible benefit of six weeks of IV ganciclovir for protecting against hearing loss and potentially in decreasing developmental impairment at 1 to 2 years of age. Six months of oral valganciclovir in symptomatic neonates has also been shown to modestly improve hearing and developmental outcomes in the long term, although a direct comparative study with IV ganciclovir has so far not been conducted. Antiviral therapy is not recommended routinely in asymptomatic neonates and young infants because of possible drug toxicities, particularly neutropenia. Trial evidence for anti-viral treatment beyond the neonatal period suggests no benefit.

INFECTIOUS MONONUCLEOSIS

Incidence

Infection with Epstein-Barr Virus (EBV) usually occurs early in life, more than 90% become infected. Acute primary EBV infection is typically subclinical and is not synonymous with infectious mononucleosis (IM), unless characteristic clinical findings are present. The incidence of IM is highest in the adolescent age group (15–24 years). The virus is excreted in saliva and spread by direct contact (i.e. kissing, sharing of water bottles, etc.).

Aetiology/Pathogenesis

EBV is a herpes virus that has special affinity for B-lymphocytes. Initial infection takes place in pharyngeal epithelial cells followed by spread to B-lymphocytes. In acute stages of IM, the number of infected circulating B-cells may be as high as 20%. Proliferation of EBV is regulated by natural killer cells and T-cytotoxic suppressor cells. Atypical lymphocytes represent T-lymphocytes responding to infected B-cells.

Clinical Presentation

Typical manifestations of IM include: fever, exudative pharyngitis (Figure 3.14), lymphadenopathy, hepatosplenomegaly and atypical lymphocytosis. Complications include: upper-airway obstruction, thrombocytopenia, jaundice, and CNS pathology (aseptic meningitis, encephalitis, Guillain–Barré syndrome). EBV is associated with post-transplant lymphoproliferative disease (PTLD). Patients with mutations causing primary immune disorders (e.g. X-linked lymphoproliferative disease) might be unable to control EBV infection and can develop overwhelming infection. Burkitt B-cell lymphoma, Hodgkin lymphoma and nasopharyngeal carcinoma are associated with EBV infection.

Diagnosis

Laboratory diagnosis is typically made using serologic tests: non-specific tests such as mono-spot or the Paul–Bunnell test (heterophile antibody tests), and/or more specific tests identifying antibodies against various viral components of EBV (VCA, EA [D&R], EBNA). Acute infection is characterised by the presence of IgM against VCA. Quantitative PCR is routinely used in transplant recipients to detect those patients who have EBV reactivation to prevent PTLD. Non-specific laboratory changes include an absolute lymphocytosis (> 10% atypical lymphocytes) often with neutropenia, and raised liver enzymes.

Treatment

IM is a self-limited disease, hence treatment is supportive. Steroids have been shown to be beneficial in upper-airway obstruction due to tonsillar hypertrophy and adenopathy. Aciclovir has activity against EBV, but clinical

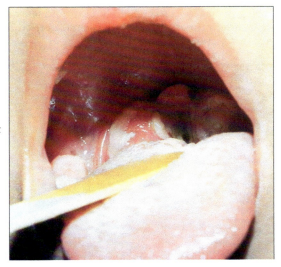

Figure 3.14 Exudative pharyngitis in infectious mononucleosis.

trials have not shown any clear benefit. Specific monoclonal antibodies (anti-CD20) such as rituximab have been shown to be beneficial in selective groups of patients.

MEASLES

Incidence

Prior to universal immunisation programmes measles was common in childhood, with epidemics occurring every 2 to 3 years. More than 90% of individuals had symptomatic infection by the age of 10 years. Until the late 1990s, measles was responsible for just under 1 million deaths worldwide, mainly in resource-poor countries. Since then, due to upscaling of global immunisation programmes, the death rate from measles has decreased substantially. Nevertheless, recent decreases in vaccination rates have resulted in periodic outbreaks worldwide.

Aetiology/Pathogenesis

Measles is caused by the measles virus, an RNA virus of the genus Morbillivirus, of the Paramyxoviridae family. It is transmitted by droplet infection, with the virus replicating initially in the respiratory tract. During the prodromal period, and for a short time after the rash appears, it is found in nasopharyngeal secretions, blood, and urine. Patients are infectious from four days before the rash appears, until four days after its appearance. The incubation period generally is 8 to 12 days from exposure to the onset of symptoms.

Clinical Presentation

Measles begins with a prodromal period of three to five days, characterised by: a fever, cough, runny nose and conjunctivitis. Koplik's spots (greyish white dots) (Figure 3.15) appear on the buccal mucosa opposite the upper and lower premolar teeth some 24 to 48 hours before the onset of rash. These are a pathognomonic exanthem of measles and may persist up to two to three days after the rash has appeared. The characteristic rash usually appears around the fourth day, as the fever peaks, and spreads in a cephalocaudal distribution (Figure 3.16).

Diagnosis

Diagnosis is typically clinical. Salivary tests for detecting the presence of antimeasles IgM antibodies and/or PCR are available for confirmatory diagnosis. Serologic tests (ELISA) are also used to detect IgG and IgM antibodies. A nasopharyngeal aspirate can also be used to confirm the diagnosis by performing immunofluorescence testing for the presence of measles antigen.

Complications

Complications include: otitis media, pneumonia, laryngotracheitis and encephalitis. These may occur as a result of the primary viral illness or due to secondary bacterial infection. Subacute sclerosing panencephalitis (SSPE) is a rare and late complication of measles infection, occurring many years after primary infection. It is characterised by the onset of gradual intellectual deterioration, ataxia, and seizures.

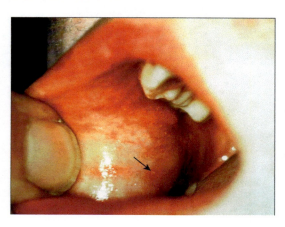

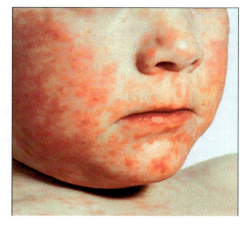

Figure 3.15 Koplik's spots present on the buccal mucosa.

Figure 3.16 Measles exanthem – a blanching maculopapular eruption.

Treatment

No specific treatment is indicated for measles, and treatment is supportive. Vitamin A should be given to children who are malnourished, immunodeficient, or known to be vitamin A deficient.

Prognosis and Prevention

Mortality is around 1:1000 and is greatest in infants and adults. Prevention is through routine immunisation with MMR. In outbreaks and/or in countries where measles remains endemic, the first dose of vaccine can be given at nine months. Early doses require boosting after 12 months, due to possible lower efficacy in infants < 1 year of age.

VARICELLA (CHICKEN POX)

Incidence

Chicken pox is a highly contagious disease with an estimated 90% of susceptible household contacts developing the disease after exposure.

Aetiology/Pathogenesis

The *Varicella zoster* virus (VZV) is a herpes virus with an incubation period of approximately 14 days (ranging between 10 and 21 days). Transmission occurs by direct contact or via airborne spread from respiratory secretions. Virus replication occurs in regional cervical lymph nodes following infection of conjunctivae and/or mucosa of the nasopharynx. A primary viraemia ensues in four to six days, with viral replication occurring in the liver, spleen and other organs. A secondary viraemia occurs at ten days, with spread of virus to the skin and subsequent appearance of rash. Children are infectious one to two days before the rash appears until crusting of the lesions. Exposure to VZV in the antenatal period can also cause serious consequences to the developing fetus and neonate. Congenital varicella syndrome results from exposure in the first 20 weeks of pregnancy and remains rare with an estimated incidence of 1–2% after maternal exposure. Disseminated neonatal infection can occur in infants born to non-immune mothers who contract VZV infection in the week before, or up to a week after delivery.

Clinical Presentation

Varicella is generally a benign illness characterised by the appearance of a maculopapular vesicular rash, fever, malaise and anorexia. The rash, often accompanied by fever, may be pruritic and usually crusts over in five days. It progresses in a centripetal distribution, with lesions at all stages (macules, papules, vesicles, crusts) present simultaneously (Figure 3.17). In the immunocompromised patient, varicella can be life-threatening with a mortality of 7%.

Congenital varicella syndrome classically presents with skin scarring, limb defects and ophthalmologic abnormalities whereas neonatal varicella can present with disseminated disease and overwhelming viral sepsis.

Diagnosis

The most reliable serological tests to detect specific VZV IgM and IgG are the fluorescent antibody to membrane antigen test (FAMA) and the ELISA assay. Direct PCR testing of skin lesions or body fluids (blood, CSF) is the most commonly used diagnostic test.

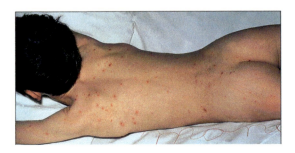

Figure 3.17   Characteristic lesions of varicella (chicken pox).

Treatment

Simple measures are sufficient for most patients, i.e. fluids, antipyretics and topical lotions. Oral aciclovir is not recommended routinely for treatment of uncomplicated chickenpox in otherwise healthy children. It may be considered for the older child (> 12 years), or for those patients taking short courses of steroids. Infection in the immunocompromised host, CNS, orbital, or severe/disseminated disease should be treated with IV aciclovir 500 mg/m^2 per dose, three times daily, for seven to ten days. Children with varicella should not receive salicylates because of the risk of Reye syndrome.

Prognosis

Complications develop in 5% of normal children, the most common being secondary bacterial infection. Other complications include pneumonitis (Figure 3.18), glomerulonephritis, hepatitis, encephalitis and orchitis (Figure 3.19). Severe complications, requiring hospital admission, are rarer and include: sepsis, necrotising fasciitis, encephalitis, and pneumonia. In untreated immunocompromised children, one-third of patients will develop disseminated disease. Varicella is responsible for 20 to 30 deaths per year in the United Kingdom.

Prevention

Strict isolation of cases is necessary if patients are admitted to hospital. Incubation period extends from 24 to 48 hours before, until five days after the appearance of the rash. Consideration of varicella zoster immunoglobulin should be given to susceptible individuals (particularly pregnant women > 20 weeks gestation, neonates, and immunocompromised children) in contact with

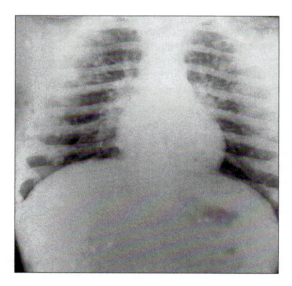

Figure 3.18   Pneumonitis in varicella (chicken pox).

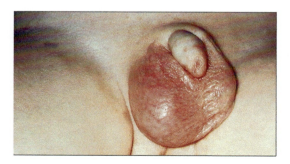

Figure 3.19   Orchitis in varicella (chicken pox).

chickenpox. A live-attenuated varicella vaccine is available which protects approximately 98% of children and 75% of adolescents and adults.

HERPES ZOSTER (SHINGLES)

Incidence

Herpes zoster infection is less common in children than in adults. It is a more common event in the immunosuppressed patient, especially after bone marrow transplantation (BMT). There is an association between the early development of chickenpox and the appearance of zoster later in childhood.

Aetiology/Pathogenesis

Shingles occur as a result of reactivation of latent VZV in the dorsal root ganglia after primary infection with chicken pox. When cell-mediated immunity to VZV declines (e.g. onset of immunodeficiency, old age), the virus can begin replicating in the ganglia and is transported along the axon to the sensory nerve endings in the skin, replicating locally to produce the characteristic vesicular lesions.

Clinical Presentation

The eruptive phase of herpes zoster infection in children starts with the appearance of grouped red papules, which are dermatomal in distribution. These rapidly progress to vesicles, pustules, and scab formation in around 5 to 10 days. The lesions may be accompanied by pain, fever and malaise. The most commonly affected dermatomes tend to be the thoracolumbar (Figure 3.21)

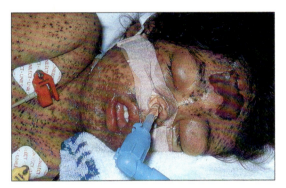

Figure 3.20   Varicella (chicken pox) in an immunocompromised patient.

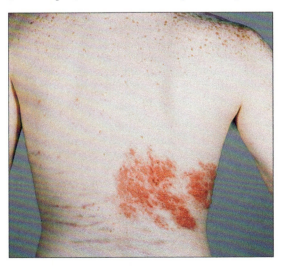

Figure 3.21   Thoracolumbar infection in herpes zoster (shingles).

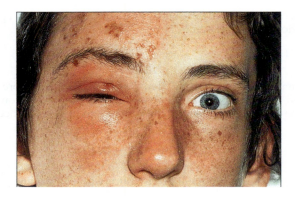

Figure 3.22   Ophthalmic infection in herpes zoster (shingles).

and trigeminal, especially the ophthalmic division (Figure 3.22). The rash is typically present for about seven days. Immunocompromised children may present with prolonged, multi-dermatomal lesions, and disseminated disease.

Diagnosis
Diagnosis is typically clinical but PCR testing of skin lesions is a commonly used adjunct test.

Treatment
Immunocompromised children with zoster should receive IV aciclovir 500 mg/m^2/dose, three times daily, for seven to ten days. Healthy children with uncomplicated zoster do not require systemic antiviral therapy.

Prognosis
The risk of postherpetic neuralgia is rare in children.
   Immunocompromised children may develop unusual or relapsing cutaneous lesions.

Prevention
A live attenuated varicella vaccine may be protective in some groups of immunosuppressed children.

KAWASAKI DISEASE
(See also the chapters 'Emergency Medicine and Rheumatology').

Incidence
The disease is most prevalent in Japan, where epidemics occur frequently. In the United Kingdom there is an estimated incidence of 15 per million children, which is probably an underestimate. About 80% of affected patients are under 4 years of age. There is little evidence for person-to-person transmission, although siblings of index cases have been affected as have some contacts of index cases.

Aetiology/Pathogenesis
Clinical features suggest an infectious aetiology, however, a microbial agent has not been conclusively identified. Current evidence suggests that the disease is the result of superantigen activity (i.e. a toxin with superantigen properties is able to cause widespread activation of the immune system, huge cytokine release and consequent initiation of generalised inflammatory changes and vasculitis). The pathological lesion in Kawasaki disease is thus a vasculitis affecting small arteries throughout the body with a predilection for the coronary vessels. Medial disruption and formation of coronary artery aneurysms (CAA) may occur.

Clinical Presentation
Kawasaki disease is an acute febrile illness of unknown aetiology, affecting predominantly infants and young children. It is a leading cause of acquired heart disease in children. It is

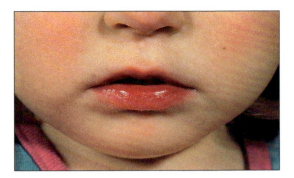

Figure 3.23 Mucositis in Kawasaki disease.

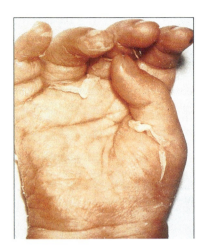

Figure 3.24 Desquamation of the hand.

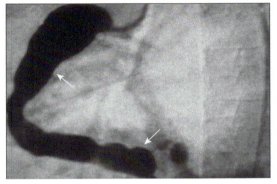

Figure 3.25 Cardiac involvement with coronary arteritis and aneurysm formation.

characterised by a prolonged remittent fever, mucositis and skin rash.

Diagnosis

The diagnosis is based on the presence of five of six principal clinical criteria (mentioned above), without other explanation for the illness. Laboratory investigations are non-specific with evidence of a widespread severe inflammatory process.

Treatment

A single high dose of IVIG (2 g/kg) given over 1 to 12 hours, within the first ten days of the illness, along with the initiation of high-dose aspirin therapy (100 mg/kg/d in four divided doses) is the mainstay of treatment. Once the fever has subsided (or on the 14th day) the aspirin is reduced to 3–5 mg/kg once daily as antiplatelet therapy and continued for two to three months. ECHOcardiography is obtained at diagnosis, one week into the illness and at four to six weeks after the start of the illness. If CAA are detected, dipyridamole may be added to the aspirin therapy and continued long term.

Prognosis

In patients not receiving high-dose immunoglobulin within the first ten days of the illness, the incidence of CAA is 15–30%. In treated patients the incidence is less than 5%. Regression of CAA may occur in around 50% of patients over a one to two year period. Sudden death from coronary thrombosis and myocardial infarction may occur in untreated patients.

NEONATAL HERPES SIMPLEX VIRUS

Incidence

Herpes simplex virus (HSV) infection of the neonate can be acquired during the intrauterine, intrapartum, or postnatal period. The majority of neonatal HSV infections are due to HSV-2 (75%). More than 85% of cases occur after vaginal exposure during delivery.

Aetiology/Pathogenesis

Following direct exposure to the virus at delivery, the newborn may develop localised disease on the skin, eye or mouth (45%), central nervous system (30%), or disseminated disease (25%). A higher incidence of neonatal herpes has been documented in babies born to mothers with primary infection (25–50%) as compared with recurrent genital herpes infection (2%).

Clinical Presentation

The hallmark of infection is a vesicular eruption (clusters of vesicles on an erythematous base) on the skin (Figure 3.26). Presentation is usually within the first two to four weeks of life. Central nervous system disease often presents with meningoencephalitis and/or seizures. Disseminated infection may present with severe liver dysfunction, DIC and or pneumonitis, mimicking sepsis or a metabolic disorder.

Diagnosis

HSV is most commonly isolated from neonatal skin or mucous membranes, blood or CSF by PCR or immunofluorescence.

Treatment

Aciclovir, 60 mg/kg/d in three divided doses, intravenously for 14 days (21 days for encephalitis or disseminated disease) is recommended. Disease may reoccur after discontinuation of therapy. Long-term oral suppressive therapy in neonates (Aciclovir) for 6–12 months has recently been shown to be effective in preventing relapse. Neonates with ocular involvement (keratoconjunctivitis) should also receive topical antiviral treatment (3% vidarabine).

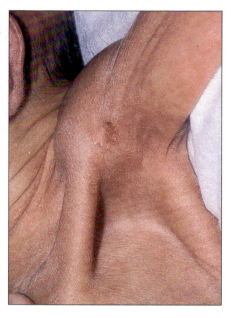

Figure 3.26 Neonatal herpes simplex virus infection. Vesicular eruption.

SARS-COV-2

Incidence

Severe acute respiratory syndrome coronavirus 2 (SARS-CoV-2), a novel zoonotic coronavirus causing severe respiratory symptoms in adults (coronavirus disease 2019 [COVID-19]), was first identified in China in December 2019. The first cases of COVID-19 in the United Kingdom were identified on 29 January 2020 with the World Health Organisation (WHO) subsequently declaring COVID-19 a pandemic on 11 March 2020. Children represent a small proportion of the total number of confirmed COVID-19 cases, with older adults and those with underlying co-morbidities particularly affected.

Aetiology/Pathogenesis

SARS-CoV-2 is the virus that causes COVID-19 and the post-viral phenomenon in children called paediatric inflammatory multi-system syndrome temporally associated with SARS-CoV-2 (PIMS-TS). SARS-CoV-2 is a single-stranded RNA virus belonging to the β-coronavirus family. It mainly enters human cells by binding to the angiotensin converting enzyme 2 (ACE-2), which is broadly expressed in vascular endothelium, respiratory epithelium, alveolar monocytes and macrophages. The virus primarily spreads between people through close contact and via respiratory droplets with airborne transmission. The upper respiratory tissue is initially infected, but later in the disease process replication in the lower respiratory tract may generate secondary viraemia. An extensive attack against target organs that express ACE-2 can ensue, such as heart, kidney, gastrointestinal tract, and the greater endovascular system.

Clinical Presentation

The majority of children with reported acute SARS-CoV-2 infections are asymptomatic or have mild disease. Clinical features in symptomatic children are typically mild compared to adults. The most common presenting features are: cough, fever, upper respiratory tract symptoms, loss of smell, myalgia, sore throat, lethargy, diarrhoea, vomiting and skin rash.

In April 2020 paediatricians in the United Kingdom first described a new clinical presentation in children which appeared to be a delayed immune response to SARS-CoV-2, resembling Kawasaki disease and toxic shock. This emerging post-viral phenomenon was named PIMS-TS or multisystem inflammatory syndrome in children (MIS-C). Children with PIMS-TS present with persistent high-grade fever, high inflammatory markers, and often hypotension evolving to shock.

Other common symptoms include: abdominal pain, vomiting, diarrhoea, maculopapular rash, conjunctivitis, enlarged lymph nodes, swollen hands and feet, myocardial dysfunction, coronary abnormalities, pericarditis, valvulitis, encephalitis, acute kidney injury, and a procoagulable state. Admission to intensive care may be necessary. In most cases make a full recovery with appropriate management.

Diagnosis

Polymerase chain reaction (PCR) tests detect viral SARS-CoV-2 RNA in the upper respiratory tract. SARS-CoV-2 antibody is not recommended to diagnose acute infection but can be used to detect previous infection or vaccination and is often used as an adjunct for diagnosis of PIMS-TS. Chest x-rays and CT scans are often normal in children, however, some children with more severe disease have bilateral pneumonia with ground glass opacities. In children with PIMS-TS, lymphocytopaenia, neutrophilia, elevated CRP, ferritin, D-dimers, fibrinogen, and LDH is often seen. Deranged liver transaminases and raised creatinine also is frequently observed.

Treatment

Supportive care is the cornerstone of treatment of both COVID-19 and PIMS-TS. Children with severe respiratory infection or PIMS-TS require hospital admission. Children may need oxygen, fluid and electrolyte support, empiric antibiotics, and thromboprophylaxis can be considered. Despite a lack of evidence from controlled paediatric trials, remdesivir, tocilizumab, and glucocorticoids (dexamethasone) have been used in paediatric patients with severe COVID-19 in line with adult RCT evidence. Trials to determine optimal treatment for PIMS-TS are ongoing. Immunoglobulins and steroids, and in refractory cases biologics such as tocilizumab and anakinra have been used. New antiviral drugs include molnupiravir and ritonavir.

PROTOZOA/FUNGI/TROPICAL DISEASES/MISCELLANEOUS

CONGENITAL TOXOPLASMOSIS

Incidence

The incidence of maternal toxoplasmosis in the United Kingdom is thought to be around 1:500 pregnancies. The transmission rate to the foetus is approximately 40%. A higher risk of congenital infection being associated with the latter stages of pregnancy although severe symptomatic foetal disease is more commonly acquired in the first trimester. Most infants with congenital toxoplasmosis (CTx) are asymptomatic at birth (90%). The British Paediatric Surveillance Unit estimates that about 14 infants per year are born in the United Kingdom with severe symptomatic CTx.

Aetiology/Pathogenesis

Toxoplasma gondii is an intracellular coccidian parasite with a worldwide distribution. Members of the cat family are the definitive hosts. Humans acquire the disease by consumption of poorly cooked meat or ingestion of oocysts from soil or contaminated food. When the disease is acquired in pregnancy, transplacental transmission of the parasite may occur with potentially serious sequelae for the foetus.

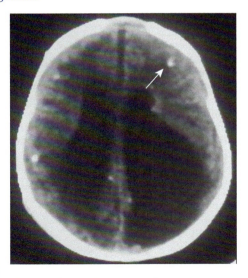

Clinical Presentation

Clinical manifestations include the 'classic triad' of: hydrocephalus, intracranial calcification (Figure 3.27) and chorioretinitis. Other non-specific features that may be seen include: jaundice, hepatosplenomegaly, thrombocytopenia, maculopapular rash, macrocephaly, lymphadenopathy, microphthalmia and seizures.

Diagnosis

A diagnosis of CTx can be made by detection of specific Toxoplasma IgM or IgA (ELISA/ISAGA), elevated dye test titres, persistence of specific IgG antibodies

Figure 3.27 Intracerebral calcification.

beyond 12 months (passively transmitted antibodies usually disappear by this time in an uninfected child), isolation of the parasite by mouse inoculation, or molecular detection by PCR (blood, CSF, amniotic fluid). Other ancillary investigations include CT/MRI brain, CSF (pleocytosis and high protein), placental examination, and ophthalmologic and audiology examinations.

Treatment

It is recommended that all infants with CTx be treated irrespective of clinical findings. Therapy should be for a total of 12 months with a combination of pyrimethamine and sulfadiazine. Steroids are given for chorioretinitis or severe CNS disease.

CRYPTOSPORIDIOSIS
INCIDENCE

Disease prevalence is higher in less developed countries (with the highest incidence in young children aged 6–24 months). There are approximately 4000–5000 reported cases per year in the United Kingdom. Symptoms appear after an incubation period of 2 to 14 days. Person-to-person transmission is most common, although animal-to-human (farm livestock) and waterborne outbreaks occur.

Aetiology/Pathogenesis

Cryptosporidium species are intracellular coccidian protozoan parasites that invade the epithelial lining of the intestinal and respiratory tracts. Following ingestion of oocysts, excystation occurs with the release of sporozoites that attach to intestinal epithelial cells, forming parasitiphorous vacuoles (Figure 3.28). An asexual intestinal cycle leads to reinfection of enterocytes and a sexual intestinal phase produces oocysts that are excreted in the stools. *C. parvum* and *C. hominis* are the primary species that infect humans.

Clinical Presentation

Infection in immunocompetent individuals results in a self-limited diarrhoeal illness (average of ten days), associated with low-grade fever, anorexia, abdominal pain and weight loss. The infection in immunocompromised patients, especially those with defective cellular immunity, is characterised by chronic profuse watery diarrhoea, malabsorption, extreme weight loss and, in some cases, death. Disseminated disease (pulmonary, biliary tract) may also be seen in this population.

Diagnosis

Definitive diagnosis is made by microscopic identification of oocysts in stool specimens stained with a modified acid-fast technique, by stool PCR, or by identification of the organism in jejunal tissue obtained at biopsy. At least three separate stool specimens should be examined before considering the test to be negative.

Treatment

Immune competent hosts typically recover spontaneously with supportive therapy consisting of adequate fluid replacement. To date, there is no fully effective therapeutic agent against *Cryptosporidium* spp. Paramomycin, azithromycin, nitazoxanide and hyperimmune bovine colostrum have all been used with limited success. The FDA has approved a three day course of nitazoxanide for treatment of all people 1 year of age and older with cryptosporidium diarrhoea. However, this is usually reserved for severe disease or for immunocompromised individuals. Other combination therapies include azithromycin and paromomycin with or without nitazoxanide.

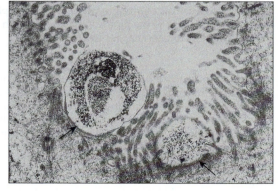

CYSTICERCOSIS
(NEUROCYSTICERCOSIS)
Incidence

Cysticercosis is endemic in rural areas of Latin America, South East Asia, and Africa. Prevalence is high in areas with poor sanitation

Figure 3.28 Appearance of parasitiphorous vacuoles at biopsy in cryptosporidiosis.

and where swine are fed animal feed. Autopsy studies in some areas show that up to 3.5% of the population have cysticercosis.

Aetiology/Pathogenesis

The disease is caused by infection with the larval stage (cysticerci) of the pork tapeworm, Taenia solium (Figure 3.29). It is acquired by ingesting eggs of the pork tapeworm that are shed in the faeces of human carriers (the adult tapeworm is acquired via eating inadequately cooked pork). Autoinfection is also a recognised route of infection. Between 24 to 72 hours after the eggs are ingested, larvae hatch and penetrate the small intestinal wall and then migrate haematogenously to sites throughout the body. Symptoms appear when a granulomatous reaction eventually ensues around dead or dying cysts.

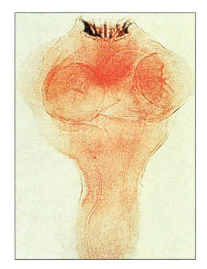

Figure 3.29   Taenia solium (cysticercosis).

Clinical Presentation

Symptoms depend on the location, size and number of cysticerci. Any tissue can be affected, the most common being brain, subcutaneous tissue, muscle, and eye. Painless lumps under the skin are characteristic of subcutaneous cysticerci. Involvement of the CNS (neurocysticercosis) presents with new-onset seizures in more than half of affected patients, four to eight years after infection. Other neurological symptoms include: transient hemiplegia, obstructive hydrocephalus, and meningitis.

Diagnosis

Neurocysticercosis is diagnosed with a CT scan of the head (Figure 3.30) showing multiple enhancing and non-enhancing cysts that later become calcified. The enzyme-linked immunotransfer blot detects antibodies to Taenia solium.

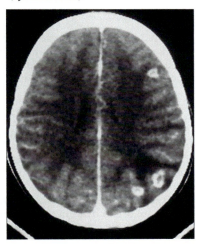

Figure 3.30   Appearance of the head (CT scan) in cysticercosis.

Treatment

Cysticidal therapy is beneficial in those children with multiple cysts, viable cysts, or symptomatic disease. The two drugs used for this indication are albendazole (15 mg/kg/d in two divided doses for four weeks) and praziquantel (50 mg/kg/d in three divided doses for two to four weeks). Albendazole is preferred over praziquantel because of fewer drug interactions, e.g. with anticonvulsants. Dexamethasone is given during the first week of treatment to reduce the inflammatory reaction induced by the dying larvae. Anticonvulsants may also be required.

MALARIA

Incidence

According to the WHO, in 2023 there were 249 million new cases of malaria worldwide(mainly in Africa), with around 625,000 deaths. Children under the age of 5 years are the most vulnerable group and account for 67% of malaria deaths. Their numbers are declining. In the United Kingdom, approximately 1600 cases of imported malaria are seen each year, with 10–15% occurring in children. Developments of malaria vaccines have yielded promising protective results.

Aetiology/Pathogenesis

Malaria is caused by invasion of erythrocytes by one of the species of intracellular protozoa of the genus *Plasmodium*. Those species infecting humans are: *P. falciparum* (Figure 3.31), *P. vivax*, *P. ovale*, *P. malariae* and *P. knowlesi*. Transmission of the parasite is usually through the bite of an infected

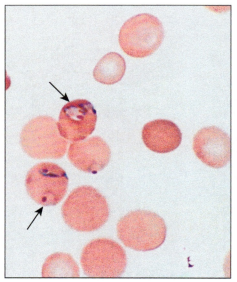

Figure 3.31 *Plasmodium falciparum.*

female Anopheles mosquito. Severe complications seen in *P. falciparum* malaria are the result of the high parasitaemia, followed by sequestration of parasitised red blood cells in deep vascular beds (including the cerebral vasculature). Vascular occlusion subsequently occurs with resultant tissue anoxia and the development of clinical symptoms, including a diffuse encephalopathy in cerebral malaria.

Clinical Presentation

Symptoms tend to be paroxysmal with high fever, chills, sweating and headaches, and jaundice and anaemia, as a result of haemolysis. Hepatosplenomegaly may be found on physical examination. P falciparum tends to cause the most severe disease, ranging from cerebral malaria (Figure 3.32), renal failure, shock, pulmonary oedema, hypoglycaemia, and haemoglobinuria ('blackwater fever').

Diagnosis

A thick smear, stained by Giemsa, identifies the presence of malarial parasites in the peripheral blood and a thin smear identifies the malarial species causing disease, as well as parasite count (reported as percentage of red blood cells infected). Rapid diagnostic tests (RDT), which detect parasite antigens in the blood, are often used in non-hospital settings in low-income countries or as an additional rapid screening test in some laboratories in middle to high-income countries. The presence of thrombocytopenia is also suggestive of malaria.

Treatment

All children with malaria due to *P. falciparum* require admission to hospital for at least 24 hours.

Uncomplicated malaria without evidence of vital organ dysfunction and low parasitemia can be started on oral therapy. Artemisinin-based combination therapy is the first choice of treatment; if this is not available atovaquone-proguanil, mefloquine and quinine-based regimens can be considered. Resistance profiles of the country where transmission occurred should be taken into account.

In cases of severe *P. falciparum* malaria with high levels of parasitemia (> 2%) and/or signs of significant organ dysfunction, IV artesunate should be started. If this is not available, IV quinine dihydrochloride can be given but should be co-administered with doxycycline, tetracycline or clindamycin. For other strains of malaria, chloroquine is the drug of choice, and hydroxychloroquine is a second-line alternative. In case of infection with *P. vivax* and *P. ovale* presumptive anti-relapse therapy (by eradicating hypnozoite forms that remain dormant in the liver) with

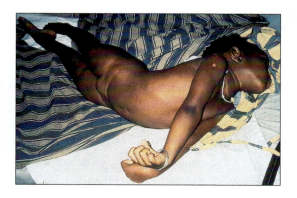

Figure 3.32 Cerebral malaria.

primaquine should be administered. This must be avoided or given with caution under expert supervision in patients with glucose-6-phosphate dehydrogenase deficiency (G6PD) in whom it may cause severe haemolysis.

SCHISTOSOMIASIS (URINARY)

Incidence

Schistosomiasis is endemic in Africa, the Middle East, Asia and South America. The presence of the specific snail host and the inappropriate disposal of human excreta in the environment are essential in maintaining the widespread distribution of the disease. Worldwide, approximately 200 million people are infected with the five major species of schistosomes.

Aetiology/Pathogenesis

Acute schistosoma infection typically presents with fever and rash known as Katayama fever. *Schistosoma haematobium* is a blood fluke (trematode) that inhabits the venous plexuses of the urinary bladder. The retained eggs cause an inflammatory reaction with the formation of multiple granulomas and eventual fibrotic lesions, leading to obstructive uropathy. The expelled eggs hatch in fresh water and the liberated miracidiae penetrate the body of the snail intermediate host. Cercariae are eventually released that penetrate the skin of human swimmers, and then migrate to the lung and liver and finally to the venous plexus of the bladder. The remaining common human schistosome species (*Schistosoma mansoni, japonicum, intercalatum, megonki*) reside in the adult form in the mesenteric plexus. Eggs are shed in the stool as opposed to the urine.

Clinical Presentation

The early manifestations in children infected with *S. haematobium* are frequency, dysuria and terminal haematuria. Symptoms of obstructive uropathy (straining, dribbling, incomplete emptying of the bladder and urgency) occur in advanced infection. End-stage disease results in hydronephrosis (Figure 3.33) and uraemia. Obstruction of the mesenteric plexus in the remainder of the *Schistosoma* species results in hepatosplenomegaly. CNS involvement is occasionally seen.

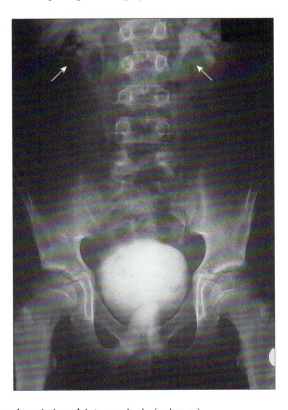

Figure 3.33 Hydronephrosis in schistosomiasis (urinary).

Diagnosis

Microscopic examination of centrifuged urine demonstrates the characteristic *S. haematobium* eggs with the lateral spine (Figure 3.35). Egg excretion in urine often peaks between noon and 2 pm. Biopsy of the bladder mucosa may be necessary if urine tests are negative. Non-haematobium species eggs can be seen on microscopy of stool. Serological tests (ELISA, RIA) to detect schistosomal antibodies are available.

Treatment

Praziquantel is the treatment of choice although paediatric-friendly formulations are lacking. Some authorities recommend this to be repeated after two weeks.

VISCERAL LEISHMANIASIS (KALA-AZAR)

Incidence

90% of visceral leishmaniasis (VL) cases occur in India, Bangladesh, Nepal, Sudan, Ethiopia and Brazil. In Europe, VL may occur along the Mediterranean coast of southern Europe. Cases of VL occurring in non-endemic areas usually arise as a result of travel to endemic areas.

Aetiology/Pathogenesis

VL is a zoonosis caused by Leishmania species (*L. donovani*, *L. infantum* and *L. chagasi*), which are intracellular protozoan parasites. They are transmitted through the bite of the female phlebotomine sandfly. The incubation period for VL typically ranges from two to six months.

Clinical Presentation

Following inoculation through the bite of an infected phlebotomine sandfly, parasites spread throughout the mononuclear macrophage system to the spleen, liver, and bone marrow. The typical presenting features include: fever, anorexia, failure to thrive, hepatosplenomegaly, lymphadenopathy, and pancytopenia. Untreated VL is often fatal. Reactivation of latent VL may also occur in those who become immunocompromised, including people with HIV or those undergoing transplantation.

Diagnosis

Definitive diagnosis is made by demonstration of the parasite in the spleen or bone marrow (Figure 3.35). Splenic aspiration has the highest sensitivity but is a high-risk procedure. Lymph node aspiration is used in some parts of the world for rapid identification of parasites. Serological testing is also used, but false positives can occur due to other infectious diseases such as trypanosomiasis.

Treatment

First-line treatment for VL is liposomal amphotericin B for a total of ten days duration although shorter courses and lower doses are being studied in high-prevalent, resource-limited settings.

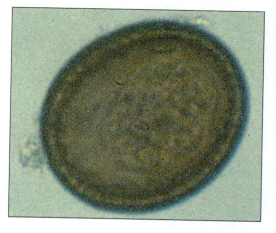

Figure 3.34 Characteristic *S. haemotobium* egg, with lateral spine.

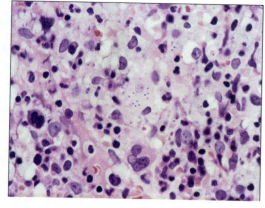

Figure 3.35 Visceral leishmaniasis. Bone marrow showing intracellular Leishmania organisms (amastigotes).

Sodium stibolgluconate is an alternative treatment although it carries a high risk of toxicity, particularly cardiac. Recent concerns about antimonial resistance in India and Nepal mean that these drugs will be less effective in South Asia. Recently, oral miltefosine for 28 days has been shown to have similar efficacy to liposomal amphotericin and has the advantage of not requiring IV therapy.

INVASIVE *ASPERGILLOSIS*

Incidence

Aspergillus species are ubiquitous saprophytic moulds present in the environment. The major risk factor for developing invasive *Aspergillus* infection is a quantitative or qualitative deficiency of neutrophil granulocytes such as those occurring in children with haematologic malignancies, primary immunodeficiencies (e.g. chronic granulomatous disease) and haematopoietic stem-cell or solid organ transplantations. The incidence among these patients is 0.4% (range: 0.1–30%). Aspergillus species are second only to *Candida* species in the frequency of opportunistic mycoses. Outbreaks of disease have been reported on cancer and transplant units that are in close proximity to construction sites.

Aetiology/Pathogenesis

Infection with the organism is usually initiated by inhalation of airborne spores. In the immuno-compromised host, *Aspergillus* tends to invade blood vessels resulting in infarction, necrosis, and haematogeneously disseminated disease. *A. fumigatus* and *A. flavus* are the most common species causing invasive *Aspergillus* in children and neonates.

Clinical Presentation

The most common clinical presentation is pulmonary aspergillosis. These patients present with persistent fever that does not respond to antibiotics, abnormal chest x-ray or CT (often with new infiltrates appearing) (Figure 3.36), cough, haemoptysis and/or pleuritic chest pain. Other clinical syndromes indicative of disseminated disease include: cutaneous disease (Figure 3.37), spinal osteomyelitis, central nervous system infection, (Figure 3.38) and renal tract involvement.

Diagnosis

Definitive diagnosis requires histopathological evidence of *Aspergillus hyphae* in tissue, as well as isolation of an *Aspergillus* species in culture. Histopathological stains reveal dichotomously branched and septate hyphae. Testing of serum biomarkers such as Galactomannan (GM) antigen or beta-D-glucan assays of blood and other biological fluids may be helpful in diagnosing invasive *Aspergillus*. GM is a polysaccharide released from *Aspergillus* during active growth and is a relatively specific marker for IA in the right clinical context, in contrast to beta-D-Glucan which can be positive in the setting of various invasive fungal infections.

Treatment

General management principles for IA include prompt initiation of antifungal therapy, control of predisposing conditions, reduction of immunosuppressive therapy, and surgical intervention.

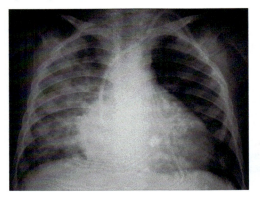 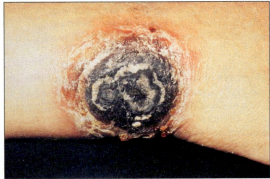

Figure 3.36   Invasive *Aspergillosis*, chest x-ray.   **Figure 3.37**   Invasive *Aspergillosis*, skin lesion.

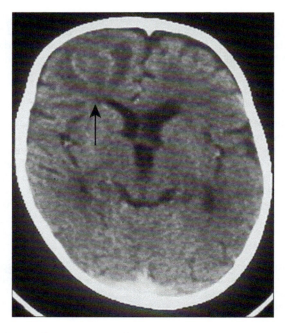

Figure 3.38 *Invasive Aspergillosis,* cerebral abscess.

Primary treatment for proven or probable IA is intravenous voriconazole (patients ≥ two years) with therapeutic drug monitoring and liposomal amphotericin B. Secondary options include combinations with echinocandins (caspofungin, micafungin) and/or alternative azoles (posaconazole, isavuconazole). The duration of treatment is often a minimum of 6 to 12 weeks but will depend on clinical response, degree of immune suppression and recovery of neutropenia.

NEONATAL SYSTEMIC CANDIDIASIS
Incidence

Candida has emerged as an important cause of neonatal infections and is associated with significant morbidity and mortality, especially in extremely low and very low birth weight

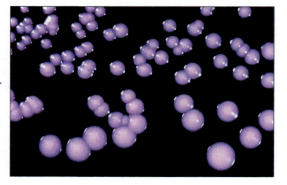

Figure 3.39 Neonatal systemic candidiasis showing typical colonies of *Candida* spp.

infants. The incidence of invasive candidiasis in neonates depends on the gestational age and the weight (< 5% for infants born at ≥ 28 weeks; up to 10–20% for 23 to 24 weeks).

Aetiology/Pathogenesis

Members of the genus *Candida* are ubiquitous, and form a heterogenous group of single-cell eukaryotic, dimorphic organisms, which grow as yeast cells (Figure 3.39).

Most *Candida* infections are nosocomially acquired. *Candida* colonise the gastrointestinal tract and disseminated infection results from translocation across the gastrointestinal epithelia. *Candida albicans* is the most frequent species in neonates, but *C. parapsilosis, C. tropicalis, C. glabrata* are all increasingly recognised. The main risk factors for systemic candidiasis are prematurity and low birth weight, prolonged use of indwelling intravascular catheters, the administration of multiple courses of broad-spectrum antibiotics, use of total parenteral nutrition (TPN), abdominal surgery, necrotising enterocolitis (NEC), antacids and endotracheal intubation.

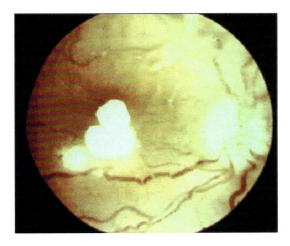

Figure 3.40 *Candida* endophthalmitis in neonatal systemic candidiasis.

Clinical Presentation

Although individual organ system involvement (e.g. UTI, meningitis) can occur, infection occurs much more often as a result of disseminated Candida infection from haematogenous spread. Catheter-related infections and disseminated candidiasis, usually involving the kidney, heart, eyes and CNS are the clinical syndromes most often seen. The incidence of catheter-related infections increase if the catheter has been in place for more than seven days. Neonates exhibit non-specific signs of sepsis (feeding intolerance, apnoea, hyperglycaemia and temperature instability).

Diagnosis

Diagnosis of candidiasis is made by isolation of the fungus from blood, which are positive in 80% of infected neonates. As fungal cultures require a minimum of one to four days of incubation, if clinical suspicion is high, appropriate antifungal treatment should be started awaiting results. Polymerase chain reaction (PCR) tests to detect fungal ribosomal DNA (18S) in blood samples can be used in conjunction with cultures if available as a diagnostic adjunct.

The suspicion or diagnosis of *Candida* infection should prompt investigations for multi-system involvement from dissemination. A thorough work-up including: culture of blood, urine and cerebrospinal fluid, ultrasound of liver spleen, kidney and cranium, ophthalmic exam and an echocardiogramme should be performed. Renal candidiasis may be manifested by the presence of 'fungal balls' in kidney; Candidal endophalmitis (Figure 3.40) is also the result of haematogenous spread of *Candida* spp. to the eye.

Treatment

Primary treatment for neonatal invasive *Candida* is amphotericin B or fluconazole. Alternatively, echinocandins can be considered for non-renal disease although data in neonates is limited. Provided no organ involvement or underlying immunological deficit, the duration of therapy is 14 days after sterile blood cultures. Disseminated disease requires four to six weeks of treatment. Removal or replacement of intravenous and urinary catheters and/or implanted prosthetic devices should be strongly considered. Surgical removal of the foci may be necessary in specific circumstances.

REFERENCES

- Ku LC, Boggess KA, Cohen-Wolkowiez M. Bacterial meningitis in infants. *Clin Perinatol.* 2015;42(1):29–viii.
- Hovmand N, Collatz Christensen H, Fogt Lundbo L, et al. Nonspecific symptoms dominate at first contact to emergency healthcare services among cases with invasive meningococcal disease. *BMC Fam Pract.* 2021:1–8.
- Haworth CS, Banks J, Capstick T, et al. British Thoracic Society guidelines for the management of non-tuberculous mycobacterial pulmonary disease (NTM-PD). *Thorax.* 2017;72:ii1–ii64.

- Egi M, Ogura E, Yatabe T, et al. The Japanese clinical practice guidelines for management of sepsis and septic shock 2020 (J-SSCG 2020) acute medicine & surgery. *J Intensive Care*. 2021:1–170.
- Cherry J, Demmler-Harrison GJ, Kaplan SL, Steinbach WJ, Hotez PJ. *Human Immunodeficiency Virus and Immunodeficiency Syndrome*. 8th ed. 2018.
- Kimberlin DW, Jester PM, Sánchez PJ, et al. Valganciclovir for symptomatic congenital cytomegalovirus disease. *N Engl J Med*. 2015 Mar 5;372(10):933–943.
- Swann OV, Holden KA, Turtle L, et al. Clinical characteristics of children and young people admitted to hospital with covid-19 in United Kingdom: Prospective multicentre observational cohort study. *BMJ*. 2020 Aug 27;370:m3249. doi:10.1136/bmj.m3249.
- Warris A, Lehrnbecher T, Roilides E, et al. ESCMID-ECMM guideline: Diagnosis and management of invasive aspergillosis in neonates and children. *Clin Microbiol Infect*. 2019 Sep;25(9):1096–1113.
- Green Book: Infectious Diseases and Vaccinations https://assets.publishing.service.gov.uk/government/uploads/system/uploads/attachment_data/file/206232/Green-Book-updated-070513.pdf (Accessed 20th January 2022).

4 Respiratory Medicine

Rossa Brugha, Andrew Turnbull and Helen Spencer

CYSTIC FIBROSIS

Incidence

The incidence of cystic fibrosis (CF) is approximately 1 in 2500 in Caucasians with a wide variation in other groups. Carriers are healthy individuals with a population frequency of 1 in 20–25 in the United Kingdom.

Aetiology and Genetics

Cystic fibrosis (CF) is an autosomal recessive disease caused by variants in the *cystic fibrosis transmembrane regulating* (CFTR) gene on the long arm of chromosome 7. The most common variant in Caucasians is p.Phe508del, accounting for some 70% of variants seen in Northern Europeans. Over 1500 variants are described, a number of which appear specific to ethnic groups.

CFTR codes for the CFTR protein. This controls a chloride channel on the cell surface with associated effects on some sodium transport channels which, when abnormal, results in viscid, sticky secretions in the airways, sinuses, liver and pancreas. Absence of the vas deferens in males leads to decreased fertility in many cases. Cystic fibrosis-related diabetes occurs mainly in adolescents and adults and low bone density can be an issue. The liver may be affected leading to portal hypertension, splenomegaly and cirrhosis.

Clinical Presentation

Neonatal screening for CF is routine for newborn babies in the United Kingdom. Prior to this, the most common presentations of CF were recurrent chest infections, failure to thrive and steatorrhoea. Children presenting with these features should be investigated for CF as children may be missed on screening (or born in countries without a newborn screening programme). Other modes of presentation include neonatal bowel obstruction due to meconium ileus in about 10–15% of cases (Figure 4.1).

Family members can be screened for CF or carrier status if a diagnosis is made in a family. Some babies are picked up on screening but subsequently do not meet the diagnostic criteria for CF; in the United Kingdom these children are termed 'screen positive, indeterminate diagnosis' and this is a challenging area for parents and clinicians. As they get older, depending on genotype (e.g. R117H, D1152H) these children may show a decrease in CFTR function and go on to fulfil criteria for 'classical CF'. Nasal polyposis, pancreatitis, periportal cirrhosis, bronchiectasis and male infertility are features of a late diagnosis, which may occur in adulthood in those with milder phenotypes.

Diagnosis

The diagnosis of CF is by identification of two CF disease-causing variants, which is possible with extended gene testing in nearly all cases. Elevated sweat chloride (> 60 mmol/L) is the key diagnostic criteria, particularly in those with typical clinical features in whom two recognised disease-causing variants are not identified. Children may present with signs of pancreatic insufficiency even before screening results are available. Pancreatic insufficiency is confirmed by low levels of faecal elastase (< 15 mcg/g). Chest disease is highly variable in severity. Early changes can be identified on specialist lung function testing at 3 months of age. A pattern of recurrent lower respiratory tract infections, obstruction by viscous mucus and heightened inflammatory response leads to a destructive process to the airways and may result in bronchiectasis (Figure 4.2) with finger clubbing (Figure 4.3). Common organisms cultured from the secretions include *Staphylococcus aureus*, *Haemophilus influenzae* and *Pseudomonas aeruginosa*, *Aspergillus*, non-tuberculous *Mycobacteria*, *Burkholderia* complex and *Stenotrophomonas*.

Treatment

Treatment is multifaceted including specific molecules that correct cytoplasmic misfolding of the CFTR protein ('correctors' e.g. tezacaftor, elexacaftor) and molecules that increase the probability of the CFTR channel opening on the epithelial surface ('potentiators', e.g. ivacaftor). Data from Phase 3 trials shows that these molecules increase lung function and body mass index. Access

DOI: 10.1201/9781003175186-4

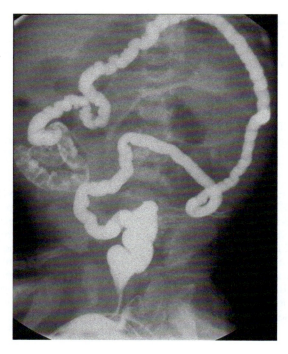

Figure 4.1 Meconium ileus in cystic fibrosis. Contrast study showing micro-colon and typical filling defects in the terminal ileum.

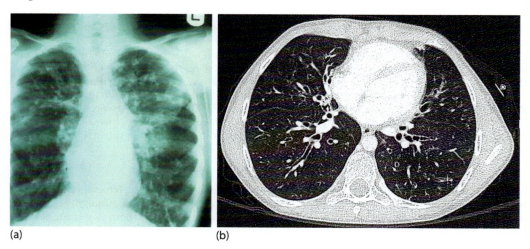

(a)   (b)

Figure 4.2 (A) Chest x-ray and (B) CT scan of advanced cystic fibrosis lung disease. There is severe overinflation, generalised bronchial wall thickening, cystic destruction and bilateral bronchiectasis.

to these medications depends on age and genotype and currently around 10–15% of patients are ineligible.

The key approaches to preventing deteriorations are good nutrition and aggressive early treatment of respiratory infections. Retention of sticky infected secretions in the chest results in repeated cycles of infection and inflammation, which damages lung tissue. The principles are therefore to make secretions less sticky (with mucolytic nebulisers), less infected (with antibiotics) and out of the chest (via daily chest physiotherapy).

As age increases there may be persistent symptoms of cough, chronic sputum production and wheeze related to the development of long-term airway damage and bronchiectasis. The major

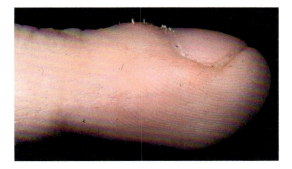

Figure 4.3   Finger clubbing.

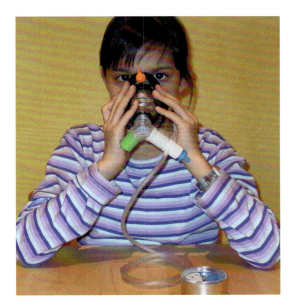

Figure 4.4   A child using a PEP mask to assist with sputum clearance.

pathogen that increases in prevalence with age is *Pseudomonas aeruginosa*. When initial infection occurs it should be treated with oral ciprofloxacin and inhaled colomycin or tobramycin in an attempt to achieve eradication. Prophylactic inhaled colomycin or tobramycin may be needed long term. Intensive two-week courses of IV antibiotics are often necessary to control *Pseudomonas*-related lung infection. *Burkholderia cepacia* is another important organism, usually multi-resistant, which can cause severe and even fatal lung disease in a small but important number of cases. Non-tuberculous mycobacteria are an important disease-causing pathogen in CF.

Cross-infection between patients is best prevented by separation and avoidance of physical contact. Treatment of the chest requires physiotherapy by a number of techniques in many cases on a daily basis (Figure 4.4).

Mucolytic agents such as nebulised 7% hypertonic sodium chloride and DNase may also be of significant benefit in children with CF who have reduced lung function and significant cough and sputum production.

Pancreatic insufficiency is seen in over 80% of CF cases and requires supplementation with pancreatic enzymes. Given in sufficient amounts a normal or energy-rich diet is well tolerated. The exact dose of daily enzymes is individualised by the CF dietician. Most children will receive additional vitamin supplementation with careful monitoring of vitamin A, E and D levels at an annual review.

Other important bowel-related problems include distal intestinal obstruction syndrome (DIOS) which requires treatment with lactulose, oral acetylcysteine, gastrograffin or a macrogol (Klean prep) depending on severity. Intestinal obstruction can occur due to DIOS or secondary to adhesions from previous surgery or stricture formation. CF-related diabetes is seen in children and increasingly in adolescents. Assessment of glucose metabolism is part of the annual review of all older children with CF. Liver dysfunction leading to hepatic cirrhosis is another problem seen in 10–15% of children, especially in adolescence. This can lead to splenomegaly, portal hypertension, oesophageal varices and haematemesis. The use of ursodeoxycholic acid may be helpful in slowing the progress of hepatic disease over time. Liver transplantation is useful in those with end-stage disease.

Prognosis

Long-term survival in cystic fibrosis is increasing steadily; the impact of the new modulators on long-term survival is unknown but predicted to significantly increase lifespans.

CHRONIC LUNG DISEASE OF PREMATURITY

Chronic lung disease (CLD) of prematurity, also referred to as bronchopulmonary dysplasia (BPD) is the primary respiratory complication that develops as a consequence of mechanical ventilation and oxygen supplementation for acute respiratory distress after premature birth.

Incidence

The risk of CLD of prematurity is inversely proportional to gestational age and birth weight. Incidence data vary according to the definitions of CLD used, with estimates ranging from one-third to two-thirds of survivors born before 28 weeks of gestation.

Aetiology/Pathogenesis

CLD of prematurity represents the response of the lungs to acute injury during a critical period of lung growth. Complex interactions between several adverse stimuli, such as inflammation, hyperoxia, mechanical ventilation and infection in the immature lungs contribute to CLD of prematurity.

BPD was first described in the 1960s in premature neonates with severe respiratory distress syndrome (RDS), who had been exposed to aggressive mechanical ventilation and high concentrations of inspired oxygen. This 'old' form of BPD was seen in the pre-surfactant era and characterised by extensive inflammatory and fibrotic changes in the airways and lung parenchyma. It has largely been replaced since the 1990s (the post-surfactant era), by a new form of the condition that occurs in more immature infants (< 32 weeks gestation averaging < 1000g in birth weight), with less severe RDS and less obvious iatrogenic injury. The 'new' BPD, now referred to as CLD of prematurity, is mainly a developmental disorder in which the immature lung fails to reach its full structural complexity, developing fewer, larger alveoli with a global reduction in the surface available for gas exchange. The airways are somewhat spared, and inflammation is usually less prominent than in the 'old' BPD.

Clinical Presentation

Recurrent wheezing and frequent viral respiratory tract infections requiring hospital admission in the early years of life are very common in infants born before 33 weeks of gestation. In addition, recurrent or persistent respiratory exacerbations may be due to structural lesions such as tracheo-bronchomalacia or subglottic stenosis, or chronic aspiration from gastro-oesophageal reflux or swallow dysfunction. Chronic cough and wheeze may persist to school age. Symptoms resembling asthma with spirometric evidence of airflow limitation are often labelled as asthma. Although there is some overlap of symptoms, the causal mechanisms, risk factors, therapeutic response and natural history are different. Clinical improvement is usually seen over time and symptoms progressively subside.

Diagnosis

The diagnosis of BPD is currently based on the need for supplemental oxygen for at least 28 days after birth, and its severity is graded according to the respiratory support required at near-term gestation (36 weeks postmenstrual age) (Table 4.1). However, prematurity *per se* may to some extent result in long-term respiratory symptoms and lung function abnormalities irrespective of the duration of oxygen dependence in the neonatal period.

Table 4.1: Diagnostic Criteria for Establishing CLD of Prematurity According to Gestational Age

Gestation	Less than 32 weeks	More than 32 weeks
Time of assessment	36 weeks postmenstrual age	> 28 days but < 56 days postnatal age
Mild CLD of prematurity	Breathing room air at 36 weeks postmenstrual age	Breathing room air by 56 days postnatal age
Moderate CLD of prematurity	Need for < 30% O_2 at 36 weeks postmenstrual age	Need for < 30% O_2 to 56 days postnatal age
Severe CLD of prematurity	Need for > 30% O_2 ± PPV or CPAP at 36 weeks postmenstrual age	Need for > 30% O_2 ± PPV or CPAP at 56 days postnatal age

CPAP – continuous positive airway pressure; PPV – positive pressure ventilation

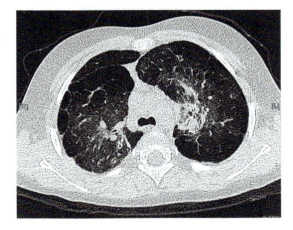

Figure 4.5 A CT scan of a child with chronic lung disease of prematurity showing extensive changes with fibrosis, air trapping, areas of collapse and bronchial wall thickening in the perihilar regions.

The investigative work-up in a premature infant who is oxygen or ventilator dependent includes CT chest with contrast to evaluate extent of lung disease and assess the pulmonary vasculature (Figure 4.5), gastro-oesophageal reflux workup and assessment of swallow, bronchoscopy and bronchogram for tracheobronchomalacia (Figure 4.6), and echocardiography for features suggestive of pulmonary hypertension.

Treatment

- Oxygen supplementation for hypoxaemia (SpO_2 < 92%).

- Ventilatory support: some infants with established severe CLD of prematurity cannot be weaned from positive pressure support or high inspired oxygen concentrations and require long-term ventilatory assistance. In many cases this can be achieved non-invasively with continuous positive airway pressure (CPAP) or intermittent positive pressure ventilation (IPPV) delivered for a proportion (≤ 16 h) of the day and usually during sleep only. For the small proportion of infants with chronic hypoventilation and/or severe tracheobronchomalacia and hypercarbia, tracheostomy with prolonged invasive ventilation may be appropriate.

- Pharmacological treatment includes treatment with diuretics, bronchodilators, inhaled or systemic corticosteroids and anti-reflux medication.

Prognosis

Although most children with CLD of prematurity show gradual symptomatic improvement with growth, they have reduced respiratory reserve with substantive obstructive lung disease that persists into adulthood.

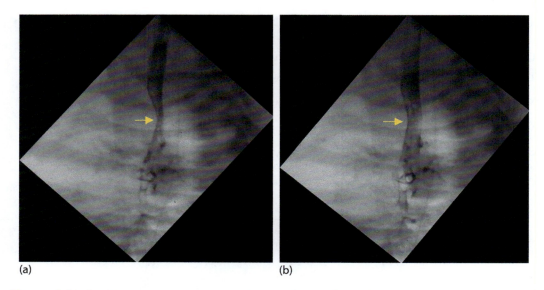

(a)　　　　　　　　　　　　　　　　　　(b)

Figure 4.6a, b   A contrast tracheogram of a premature infant with recurrent apnoea and cyanosis demonstrating significant tracheal malacia (a), which distends to normal dimensions following a continuous positive pressure of 10 cm of water during the contrast study (b).

PRESCHOOL WHEEZE

Incidence

Wheezing in the preschool years is extremely common, approximately one in three children will have at least one episode of wheeze prior to their third birthday, and by 6 years of age this figure increases to one in two children.

Aetiology/Pathogenesis

Wheeze in preschool children is mostly associated with viral upper respiratory tract infections, which can recur frequently, and is not usually associated with underlying airway inflammation, at least between episodes. Spontaneous resolution of wheezing occurs in many children by school age, while some will exhibit persisting symptoms and these children are at risk of developing asthma by mid-childhood. Allergic sensitisation before age 3 years, respiratory syncytial virus (RSV) and rhinovirus-associated wheezing illnesses in the early years, genetic predisposition, poor pulmonary function, exposure to cigarette smoke and traffic-derived air pollution, recurrent and severe episodes of wheeze in the first three years of life and parental history of asthma or atopy are all described as risk factors for persistence of wheezing from preschool to school age.

Clinical Presentation

Efforts to characterise wheeze phenotypes based on the pattern or duration of symptoms (+/– atopic status) have demonstrated significant variability in evolution and persistence of symptoms but have not corresponded with distinct differences in underlying pathophysiology or response to treatment. It appears that frequency and severity of wheezing episodes are better predictors of long-term outcomes.

Diagnosis

Diagnosis is based on history and clinical examination, although examination findings may be normal between wheeze episodes. Wheeze reported by parents can easily be confused with other respiratory noises (stridor, noisy breathing) favouring alternative diagnoses. Physician-diagnosed wheeze is a reliable indicator of lower airway obstruction.

Differential Diagnosis

Although most cases of recurrent wheeze in the preschool years are triggered by viral illness, the differential diagnosis is broad and several conditions should be considered in children with atypical presentations:

- Laryngotracheomalacia
- Foreign body in the airway
- Chronic aspiration from gastro-oesophageal reflux or swallow dysfunction
- Vascular ring or congenital tracheal stenosis
- Congenital lung lesions
- Tracheo-oesophageal fistula
- Cystic fibrosis
  - Primary ciliary dyskinesia
  - Immune deficiency

Acute Treatment

Treatment of acute wheezing episodes is with an inhaled short-acting beta$_2$-agonist (SABA) such as salbutamol, delivered by metered-dose inhaler through a spacer with a mask (children < 3 years) or mouthpiece. Oral corticosteroids have not been shown to be beneficial in preschool children with wheeze who can be managed at home, and are therefore only recommended for children with severe wheezing episodes requiring hospital admission and frequent SABA and/or supplemental oxygen or respiratory support.

Maintenance Treatment

Non-pharmacological approaches to maintenance treatment in children with preschool wheeze include avoidance of adverse exposures (environmental tobacco smoke, aeroallergens in those who are sensitised, air pollution), education on correct medication delivery, and understanding of the steps to follow during an acute episode, according to a wheeze action plan.

In children with frequent and/or severe episodes of wheeze, particularly those requiring hospitalisation, a trial of pharmacological treatment is justified. The strongest evidence favours a trial of daily low-dose inhaled corticosteroids (ICS), with recent data suggesting a greater likelihood of response in children with raised blood eosinophils or evidence of allergic sensitisation. Montelukast, a leukotriene receptor antagonist (LTRA), used intermittently at the onset of symptoms or continuously, can be trialled as an alternative or add-on therapeutic option, although the evidence of benefit is weaker than for ICS. Any treatment should be initiated as a trial (typically for two to three months) with regular reassessment of response.

Prognosis

The overall natural history of preschool wheeze is favourable, with resolution of symptoms in the majority of children by school age. Frequent and severe episodes and presence of atopy are associated with persistence of symptoms, along with a host of associated risk factors. Inhaled corticosteroids do not prevent disease progression when used as maintenance treatment, but they do have some effect on symptom control and exacerbations.

ASTHMA

Asthma is characterised by chronic airway inflammation, variable airflow limitation and bronchial hyper-responsiveness. Rather than being a single disease, the symptoms and signs of asthma represent a final common endpoint related to several biological, immunological and physiological mechanisms that produce multiple phenotypes, which further interact with genetic and environmental factors to produce variability in disease severity and expression.

Incidence

Asthma is the most common chronic disease in children, with a prevalence of 5–20% in high-income countries and a lower, but rising, prevalence in many low-income and middle-income countries. Consistently higher prevalence is reported in urban compared with rural children, which may be accounted for by a potential protective effect of microbial exposure in rural environments.

Aetiology/Pathogenesis

A number of risk factors are recognised for the development of asthma. These include frequent wheezing during the first three years of life, parental history of asthma, history of eczema, allergic rhinitis, wheezing with triggers other than colds, blood eosinophilia of ≥ 4%, allergic sensitisation to aeroallergens and/or foods. Other factors that may contribute to the risk of developing asthma are exposure to tobacco smoke, air pollution, frequent antibiotic use in infancy, obesity and genetic susceptibility.

Asthma is characterised by airway inflammation, of which the predominant subtype is eosinophilic and associated with allergic sensitisation to environmental aeroallergens. Respiratory viral infections, particularly human rhinovirus, are the key trigger for acute asthma attacks and may also be important in the pathogenesis of asthma, although the mechanisms of this are incompletely understood. Patients may have airway remodelling, which includes reticular basement membrane thickening, epithelial fragility, airway smooth muscle hypertrophy and hyperplasia, extracellular matrix deposition and mucous-secreting gland hypertrophy. The onset and course of airway inflammatory changes and remodelling in children of all ages is not fully characterised, but several studies show that by 6 years of age, children with persistent asthma symptoms demonstrate poor lung function, airway inflammation and remodelling, which is typical of adult asthma.

Clinical Presentation

The probability of asthma is high in a child who presents with frequent or recurrent wheeze, cough, difficulty breathing and chest tightness. Symptoms can occur in response to, or are worse after, exercise or other triggers such as exposure to pets, cold or damp air, or with emotions or laughter. Symptoms can be worse at night and early morning in some children. When symptomatic, widespread wheeze is heard on auscultation and there is improvement in symptoms and lung function in response to bronchodilator administration.

Diagnosis

- The diagnosis of asthma is a clinical one, based on the presence of characteristic symptoms (wheeze, dyspnoea, chest tightness, and cough) that vary in time and intensity, supported by evidence of variable airflow limitation or airway inflammation

- Variable airflow limitation may be demonstrated by spirometry with bronchodilator reversibility (Figure 4.8), excessive variability in twice-daily peak expiratory flow rate (PEFR), or by positive exercise or bronchial challenge test. A CXR during an acute presentation may demonstrate hyperinflation with air trapping (Figure 4.7).

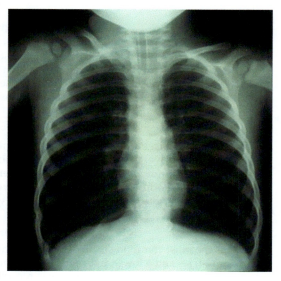

- Raised fractional exhaled nitric oxide (FeNO) is a marker of eosinophilic airway inflammation and may provide support for a diagnosis of asthma.

- In children with a high probability of asthma, it is reasonable to proceed to a trial of treatment and reserve further investigations to those with poor/no response.

- In children with a low probability of asthma, other conditions should be considered and further investigations planned accordingly (Table 4.2).

Treatment

The aims of asthma management are to achieve control of symptoms, reduce risks of future attacks and attenuated lung function growth

Figure 4.7 Severe overinflation with air trapping in asthma.

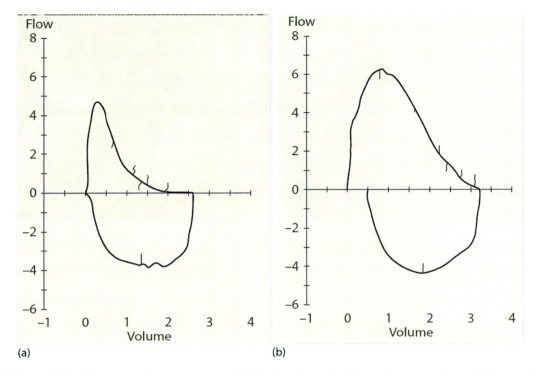

Figure 4.8a, b Flow volume loops of a child before bronchodilator showing a classical 'scooped out' appearance of the expiratory loop (a) and after bronchodilator (b). There is improvement in the peak expiratory flow and FEV1.

Table 4.2: Differential Diagnosis of Asthma in Children

Vascular rings
Gastro-oesophageal reflux
Swallow dysfunction and aspiration
Congenital heart disease with congestive cardiac failure
Inducible laryngeal obstruction or dysfunctional breathing
Cystic fibrosis
Non-CF bronchiectasis
Inhaled foreign body (Figure **4.9**)
Tracheobronchomalacia
Hypersensitivity pneumonitis
Airway compression by mediastinal lymph nodes

and minimise treatment-associated adverse effects. Control of asthma according to the British Thoracic Society (BTS)/Scottish Intercollegiate Guidelines Network (SIGN) guidelines for the management of asthma is defined as:

■ No daytime symptoms or nighttime awakening due to asthma.

■ No need for rescue medication.

■ No asthma attacks.

■ No limitations on activity including exercise.

■ Normal spirometric lung function.

 • Minimal side effects from medication.

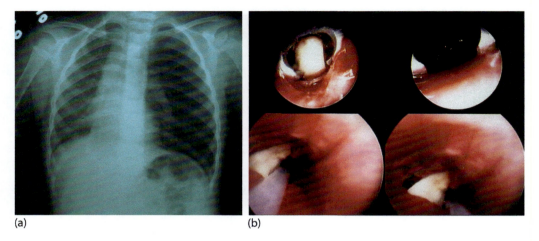

(a) (b)

Figure 4.9a, b   A child presenting with acute wheezing and unilateral overinflation on chest x-ray (a) shows on rigid bronchoscopy (b) to have inhaled a peanut into the left main bronchus leading to a ball valve overinflation.

Acute Treatment

See also the chapter 'Emergency Medicine'.

Maintenance Treatment

Non-Pharmacological Treatment

Children and young people with asthma and their parents/carers should be supported in self-management with the use of personalised asthma action plans, along with education and regular review of medication adherence and inhaler technique, and avoidance of exacerbating factors.

Pharmacological Treatment

Evidence-based recommendations for asthma treatment are outlined in the BTS/SIGN guidelines and the Global Initiative for Asthma (GINA) report, and follow a stepwise approach, with up- or down-titration of therapy to achieve control. Treatment recommendations differ for younger (5–12 years old for BTS/SIGN, 6–11 years old for GINA) and older children. At all steps short-acting β_2 agonists (SABA) are the recommended treatment for immediate relief of symptoms, according to a personalised asthma action plan. Recent changes in recommendations include earlier use of ICS and ICS-long acting β_2 agonist (LABA) combinations depending on age. A stepwise approach for maintenance therapy is outlined below:

Step 1: First-line controller options for younger children are either a monitored trial of regular twice-daily low-dose ICS via spacer device, or low-dose ICS taken whenever SABA is taken. The dose of ICS should be titrated to the lowest dose at which effective asthma control is achieved, as administration of ICS ≥ 400 µg/d of beclometasone (BDP) or equivalent may be associated with systemic side effects, such as growth failure and adrenal suppression. For older children (≥ 12 years) first-line controller options are either regular twice-daily ICS or as-needed low-dose ICS-formoterol.

Step 2: For children (all ages) with symptoms or SABA use ≥ three times/week, or with night waking ≥ one night/week, or an asthma attack in the last year, regular twice-daily ICS via a spacer is recommended. The dose of ICS should be titrated to the lowest effective dose.

Step 3: If symptom control is suboptimal at a dose of 400 µg/day of BDP or equivalent, a combination of ICS–LABA should be considered as first add-on therapy. Alternatives include increasing ICS to medium dose, or adding a leukotriene receptor antagonist (LTRA).

Step 4: If there is a response to addition of LABA, but optimal symptom control is not achieved then increasing ICS to a maximum of 800 µg/day of BDP and/or adding LTRA should be considered along with a specialist referral.

Step 5: The small minority of children not responding to step 4 therapy should be managed in a specialist paediatric asthma service, and should be carefully evaluated to ensure the diagnosis is correct, to identify comorbidities and/or persistent exacerbating factors, and to ensure the correct medication is being prescribed and taken. High-dose ICS–LABA +/– LTRA +/– tiotropium may be appropriate, along with evaluation of inflammatory phenotype for consideration of biologic therapies, such as the anti-IgE monoclonal antibody omalizumab.

Prognosis

Several studies show that ICS controls symptoms and maintains lung function in the majority of children with asthma, but is not disease-modifying.

BRONCHIOLITIS

Bronchiolitis is a clinically diagnosed acute viral respiratory infection, characterised by cough, tachypnoea and/or chest recessions, with wheeze or crackles on auscultation. In European countries the definition of bronchiolitis is limited to infants < 12 months of age whereas in North America the definition extends to children with viral lower respiratory tract infections with wheeze up to 24 months of age.

Incidence

It is estimated that around 33% of all infants will develop bronchiolitis (from all viruses) in their first year of life, with the peak incidence at 3–6 months of age. Of these children, 70% are infected with RSV and 22% develop symptomatic disease. It is a seasonal illness occurring between late autumn and early spring, when respiratory viruses are widespread in the community.

Aetiology/Pathogenesis

Bronchiolitis is primarily caused by viral infections, particularly RSV, which accounts for around 75% of cases. Other viruses, such as rhinovirus, influenza, parainfluenza, adenovirus and human metapneumovirus are also implicated.

The viral infection starts in the upper respiratory tract and spreads to the lower airways in a few days, resulting in inflammation of the bronchiolar epithelium, with peribronchial infiltration of white blood cells and oedema of the submucosa and adventitia. Plugs of sloughed, necrotic epithelium and fibrin in the airways cause significant small airway obstruction resulting in hyperinflation, air trapping, atelectasis and ventilation/perfusion mismatch leading to hypoxemia.

Clinical Presentation

Infants characteristically present with rhinorrhoea, followed within one to two days by onset of a dry wheezy cough, tachypnoea and chest wall recessions. The infant may be irritable and refusing feeds. On auscultation prolonged expiratory phase, high-pitched expiratory wheeze and fine inspiratory crackles may be heard. Apnoea can be the presenting feature, especially in the very young and in premature infants.

Most infants tend to deteriorate clinically in the first 72–96 hours of the illness, before gradual symptom improvement. Children with other comorbidities such as, prematurity, CLD of prematurity and congenital heart disease are at increased risk of severe RSV disease.

Diagnosis

- There is no role for any diagnostic tests in the routine management of bronchiolitis in the community.

- In the hospital setting, detection of the causative virus is helpful in reducing nosocomial spread by cohorting patients.

- Chest radiograph, although non-specific, typically shows bilateral hyperinflation with patchy areas of peribronchial infiltrates, collapse or consolidation (Figure 4.10). These should not be routinely requested.

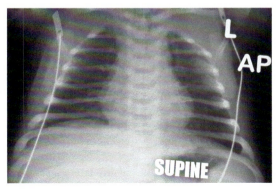

Figure 4.10 A child with severe bronchiolitis showing areas of hyperinflation and peribronchial thickening.

Differential Diagnosis

- Pulmonary causes:
  - Preschool wheezing disorders
  - Pneumonia
  - Congenital lung disease
  - CF
  - Inhaled foreign body
  - Childhood interstitial lung disease
- Non-pulmonary causes:
  - Congenital heart disease
  - Sepsis
  - Severe metabolic acidosis
- Primary immunodeficiency with opportunistic infection

Treatment

Most children with bronchiolitis are managed at home, with careful observation and adequate fluid administration. Children with moderate to severe respiratory distress should be hospitalised, with a low threshold for hospitalisation in those with other comorbidities.

Antivirals such as nebulised ribavirin are not recommended. There is no role for systemic or inhaled corticosteroids or leukotriene receptor antagonists, or for nebulised hypertonic saline or nebulised adrenaline. The mainstay of treatment is supportive therapy:

- Oxygen supplementation for hypoxaemia: recent UK trial data support a permissive hypoxaemia target of $SpO_2 \geq 90\%$.

- Maintain fluid balance: consider nasogastric feeding in infants who cannot maintain oral intake.

- Inhaled or nebulised bronchodilators are not routinely recommended,

- The use of nasal CPAP can be helpful in those who have significant respiratory failure.

- Prophylactic therapy: palivizumab is a humanised monoclonal RSV antibody that does not prevent infection but is used for prophylaxis against severe RSV bronchiolitis. It is given intramuscularly during the RSV season. It is recommended in high-risk groups, such as children with chronic lung disease on supplemental O_2, infants under 6 months of age with significant congenital heart disease and children under 2 years of age with severe congenital immune deficiency. A newer monoclonal antibody for RSV (nirsevimab) which is a single dose injection has also been introduced in some countries. Recently, RSV vaccines have been developed which can be given to mothers during pregnancy and have been shown to reduce severe RSV bronchiolitis in infants.

Prognosis

Acute bronchiolitis can be associated with later respiratory morbidity, the mechanisms of which are poorly understood. It is controversial whether there is prior genetic or environmental susceptibility to respiratory morbidity, or whether the bronchiolitis illness is the primary insult to the growing lung.

PNEUMONIA

Incidence

Pneumonia is a leading killer of children in developing countries, causing an estimated 1.9 million deaths globally in children under the age of 5 years. The European incidence of community-acquired pneumonia is approximately 33/10,000 in children aged 0–5 years and 14.5/10,000 in children aged 0–16 years.

Aetiology

Pneumonia usually begins as nasopharyngeal infection followed by spread into the lower respiratory tract. The source of the infection can be community acquired or nosocomial. Bacteria, viruses, atypical organisms and fungi can all cause pneumonia. Respiratory viruses appear to be responsible for approximately 40% of cases of community-acquired pneumonia in children who are hospitalised, particularly in those under 2 years of age, whereas *Streptococcus pneumoniae* is responsible for 27–44% of community-acquired pneumonia. Table 4.3 lists causative organisms according to age.

Clinical Presentation

Typical presenting features include fever, cough, tachypnoea, breathlessness or difficulty in breathing, chest wall recessions and hypoxia in severe infections. Crackles heard on auscultation increases the likelihood of a diagnosis of pneumonia. Wheeze in young children suggests a viral aetiology and in older subjects the possibility of *Mycoplasma pneumoniae* infection. *Mycoplasma* infections in older children are associated with headache and myalgia and *Chlamydia trachomatis* infections in neonates are associated with sticky eyes.

In terms of severity, the WHO recommends hospital admission in children with chest wall recessions. In a developed world setting, the BTS guidelines regarding admission to hospital are shown in Table 4.4.

Diagnosis

Radiological findings are accepted as the gold standard for defining pneumonia, but chest radiographs are not routinely indicated in children suspected of having pneumonia. The BTS guidelines suggest that a chest radiograph be considered in a child < 5 years old, with a fever > 39°C of unknown origin and without features typical of bronchiolitis (**Figures** 4.11–4.13). Microbiological investigations are not generally recommended for those being managed in the community, but blood cultures should be performed in hospitalised children.

Differential Diagnosis

There are few conditions that encompass all of fever, cough, breathlessness and unilateral chest signs on auscultation, as many mimics of pneumonia will give bilateral chest signs. A few key conditions should be considered when taking the history and considering initial investigations:

Table 4.3: Organisms Causing Pneumonia According to Age

Neonates
Common organism: Group B streptococci, gram-negative enteric bacteria, CMV, *Ureaplasma urealyticum, Listeria monocytogenes, Chlamydia trachomatis*
Less common: *Streptococcus pneumoniae*, Group D *Streptococcus*, anaerobes
Infants
Common organisms: RSV, coronaviruses, parainfluenza viruses, influenza viruses, adenovirus, metapneumovirus, *Streptococcus pneumoniae, Haemophilus influenzae, Mycoplasma pneumoniae, Mycobacterium tuberculosis*
Less common: *Bordetella pertussis, Pneumocystis jirovecii*
Preschool children
Common organisms: RSV, coronaviruses, parainfluenza viruses, influenza viruses, adenovirus, metapneumovirus, *Streptococcus pneumoniae, Haemophilus influenzae, Mycoplasma pneumoniae, Mycobacterium tuberculosis*
Less common: *Chlamydia pneumoniae*
School age
Common organisms: *Mycoplasma pneumoniae, Chlamydia pneumoniae, Streptococcus pneumonia, Mycobacterium tuberculosis*, respiratory viruses

Table 4.4: British Thoracic Society Guidelines – Factors Indicating Need for Admission of a Child with Pneumonia

Temperature > 38.5°C

Oxygen saturations ≤ 92%

Respiratory rate > 70/min in infants or > 50/min in older children

Nasal flaring, intermittent apnoea, grunting

Moderate to severe chest wall recessions

Infant not feeding or signs of dehydration in older children

Tachycardia

Capillary refill time ≥ 2 seconds

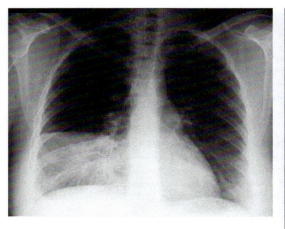

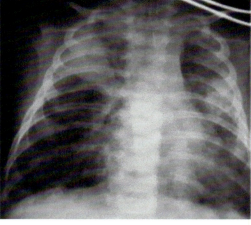

Figure 4.11 X-ray of a patient with a dense right middle lobe pneumonia secondary to a pneumococcal pneumonia, showing obliteration of the right cardiac border but preservation of the right diaphragmatic shadow.

Figure 4.12 A child with bordetella pertussis showing diffuse patchy changes in both lung fields and segmental atelectasis of the right upper lobe.

- Cardiac failure, e.g. secondary to a large VSD in an infant

- Nephrotic syndrome with hypoalbuminaemia and pulmonary oedema

- Acute cholecystitis

- Diaphragmatic palsy

- Appendicitis with hypoventilation of the lung bases

- Sickle chest crisis

- Inhaled foreign body

- Acute leukaemia with anaemia

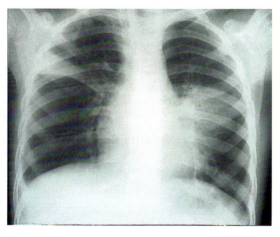

When pulmonary tuberculosis is suspected, consecutive early morning, pre-prandial, pre-ambulatory gastric washings are indicated and are more sensitive than bronchoalveolar lavage (BAL). Measuring acute phase reactants are not of any clinical utility.

Figure 4.13 A child with a *Mycoplasma pneumoniae* showing diffuse changes predominantly affecting the lingula with segmental collapse of the right upper lobe.

Treatment

Treatment can be divided according to whether the child is treated in the community or admitted to hospital.

In the community:

- In low and middle income countries oral co-trimoxazole and amoxicillin are found to be effective.

- In high income countries children are usually treated with amoxicillin with or without clavulanic acid or with a macrolide when mycoplasma infection is suspected.

In the hospital:

- Supportive:

  - Oxygen supplementation for hypoxaemia ($SpO_2 < 92\%$)

- IV fluids if the child is dehydrated
- Antipyretics and analgesics

■ Specific:

- Oral amoxicillin with or without clavulanic acid are the antibiotics of choice, and a macrolide may be added when mycoplasma infection is suspected. IV antibiotics are indicated only if the child is unable to tolerate oral antibiotics. Optimal duration of treatment is unknown but most recommend 5–7 days.

Prognosis

The great majority of children make a complete recovery. Very few go on to develop acute complications such as pleural empyema. Long-term complications such as bronchiectasis are more likely to occur where there is an underlying abnormality including recurrent aspiration, immune deficiency or malnutrition.

EMPYEMA

In respiratory medicine an empyema is a collection of pus in the pleural space, which in children usually occurs as a complication of bacterial pneumonia caused most commonly by *Streptococcus pneumoniae* and *Staphylococcus aureus*.

Aetiology/Pathogenesis

The incidence of childhood empyema is increasing worldwide, affecting about 3.3 per 100,000 children and nearly 1 in 150 children hospitalised with pneumonia progress to empyema. The pleural space normally contains about 0.3 ml/kg body weight of pleural fluid. Pneumonia can cause pleural inflammation and the resulting increased vascular permeability allows migration of inflammatory cells into the pleural space. This can progress to an empyema following bacterial invasion across an inflamed epithelium.

Clinical Presentation

Children commonly present with pneumonia symptoms, such as fever, cough, breathlessness, exercise intolerance, poor appetite, abdominal pain and malaise. They may have pleuritic chest pain and lie on the affected side to splint the involved side or sit with a curved spine. On examination, a pleural collection is suggested by decreased chest expansion, dull note on percussion and reduced or absent breath sounds on the affected side. Some children may be hypoxic due to ventilation–perfusion mismatch.

Diagnosis

Blood tests include haemoglobin, acute phase reactants such as total white cell and neutrophil counts and C reactive protein.

Pleural collection is evident on a chest radiograph (Figure 4.14). An ultrasound scan of the chest will confirm the presence of a pleural fluid collection (Figure 4.15), which may be septated with fibrous bands. The ultrasound can also guide chest drain insertion with the sonographer marking the optimum drainage site. CT of the chest is not routinely indicated for the diagnosis of empyema. Pleural fluid should be sent for gram stain, bacterial culture and may be sent for 16s PCR to identify the causative organism.

Treatment

■ Supportive:

- Oxygen supplementation for hypoxaemia ($SpO_2 < 92\%$).

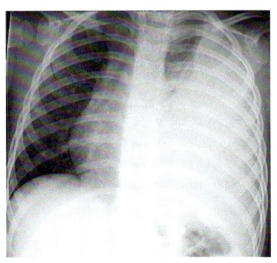

Figure 4.14 Chest radiograph showing a large left-sided pleural effusion with obliteration of the costophrenic angle.

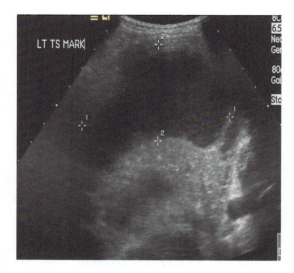

Figure 4.15 Chest ultrasound on patient in Figure 4.14 showing the presence of pleural fluid (between markers).

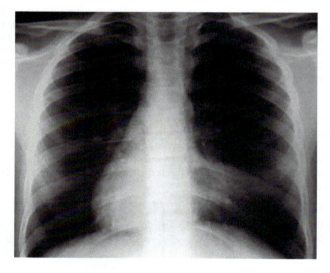

Figure 4.16 Bronchiectasis associated with primary ciliary dyskinesia showing a chest x-ray with situs inversus and consolidation in the left hemithorax (anatomical right lung).

- IV fluids if the child is dehydrated.
- Antipyretics and analgesics.

■ IV antibiotics (start with a broad-spectrum empirical cover against *S. pneumonia, S. pyogenes and S. aureus*). Further antibiotic management should be rationalised according to microbiological results.

■ Specific treatment:

- The primary treatment of choice is chest drain insertion with instillation of intrapleural urokinase twice a day for three days. Urokinase acts as a fibrinolytic to break down the fibrous septae in the empyema, allowing fluid to drain. Recombinant tissue plasminogen activator (t-PA, alteplase) may be used if urokinase is unavailable. Chest drain is removed when there is minimal discharge (40–60 ml/24 h).

- Surgical opinion for video-assisted thoracoscopic debridement is indicated as rescue therapy if there is poor or no clinical and radiological response to the primary approach.

Therapeutic response is monitored by how the child is clinically (fevers, oxygen requirement, and appetite), blood tests measuring acute phase reactants and a chest radiograph performed after completion of the urokinase course. Patients can be discharged from hospital if they remain afebrile for 24 hours after chest drain removal. Oral antibiotics are continued for one to two weeks post discharge.

Prognosis
The majority of affected children are previously healthy and make a complete recovery. Most chest radiographs are abnormal at discharge but return to normal between three and six months.

BRONCHIECTASIS
Bronchiectasis describes chronic dilatation and suppuration of the bronchi and bronchioles; 'ectasia' is dilation or distension of a hollow organ. It is not a diagnosis, and the cause for bronchiectasis should be sought; it is commonly referred to in paediatrics as 'non-CF bronchiectasis' to differentiate this group from the well phenotyped group with bronchiectasis secondary to CF.

Incidence
The incidence of non-CF bronchiectasis has decreased markedly in developed countries with improved immunisation programmes, improved hygiene and nutrition, reduced housing density and (for some) improved access to medical care. However, non-CF bronchiectasis remains common among disadvantaged groups in affluent countries, with a reported incidence of 15–20 per 1000 children among Alaskan Upiks and Indigenous Australians. While non-CF bronchiectasis remains common in the developing world, it is difficult to estimate the prevalence due to presumed under-reporting/diagnosis.

Aetiology/Pathogenesis
Non-CF bronchiectasis results from a variety of airway injury and predisposing conditions that lead to recurrent or persistent airway infection, inflammation and injury (Table 4.5). Studies report

Table 4.5: Causes of Non-CF Bronchiectasis in Children

1 Impaired immunity
- Primary immunodeficiency disorders (SCID, CVID, Hyper IgE)
- Ectodermal dysplasia
- Ataxia telangiectasia
- Bloom syndrome
- DNA ligase I defect
- Secondary immunodeficiency (HIV infection, immunosuppressive treatment)

2 Altered pulmonary host defence
- Primary ciliary dyskinesia (**Figure 4.16**)
- Impaired mucociliary clearance

3 Airway injury caused by infections
- Pulmonary tuberculosis
- Severe measles bronchopneumonia
- Pertussis

4 Airway injury caused by recurrent aspiration pneumonitis
- Gastro-oesophageal reflux disease
- Swallow dysfunction with aspiration (as seen in neurodevelopmental disorders)
- Tracheo-oesophageal fistula

5 Syndromes associated with bronchiectasis
- Young syndrome
- Yellow nail lymphoedema syndrome
- Marfan syndrome
- Usher syndrome
- Mounier-Kuhn syndrome
- Williams–Campbell syndrome
- Ehlers–Danlos syndrome

6 Others
- Retained foreign body in the airways
- Autoimmune diseases
- Allergic bronchopulmonary aspergillosis

an unidentified cause in 25–48% of all children with non-CF bronchiectasis. The severity and distribution of bronchiectasis is heterogeneous and varies according to aetiology and host response.

Mucous clearance in bronchiectasis is affected by a combination of factors, such as airflow limitation, abnormal quality and quantity of mucous production and bacterial elements that cause ciliary slowing, dyskinesia and mucous stasis. This leads to a vicious cycle of decreased mucociliary clearance, increased bacterial colonisation, biofilm formation and persistent infection.

Clinical Presentation

Children usually present with chronic or recurrent cough with sputum production. Some children may present with wheeze, shortness of breath and failure to thrive. On clinical examination digital clubbing may be present and persistent crackles with or without wheeze may be heard on auscultation.

Diagnosis

- A baseline chest x-ray should be performed in patients with symptoms of bronchiectasis, but mild cases of bronchiectasis may not be evident.

- Computed tomography (CT) scan of the lungs is the gold standard to establish the presence of bronchiectasis (Figures 4.17 and 4.18) and should be performed in all patients when there is a clinical suspicion.

If bronchiectasis is confirmed on CT, further investigations should be performed to establish cause and severity of disease. A stepwise prioritisation of investigations is suggested depending on the clinical features of the individual patient.

- Lung function (spirometry) should be assessed in all children old enough (usually age 5 years and above) to perform the tests.

- Sputum or cough swabs for microbiology.

- Immunoglobulins, vaccine responses and lymphocyte subsets to screen for immunodeficiency.

- Sweat test and genetics for CF.

- Gastrointestinal investigations such as 24-hour pH study, impedance study and upper gastrointestinal barium studies to rule out gastro-oesophageal reflux, and video fluoroscopy to rule out swallow dysfunction and aspiration.

- Nasal NO as a screening test and ciliary investigations to rule out primary ciliary dyskinesia, particularly in those patients who present with associated symptoms of rhinitis and sinusitis.

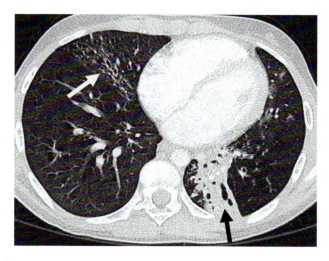

Figure 4.17 CT chest in 13-year-old female with common variable immunodeficiency. There is bronchiectasis with mucus plugging in the right middle lobe (white arrow). There is (chronic) collapse with bronchial dilatation of the left lower lobe, clearly seen on CT scan (black arrow).

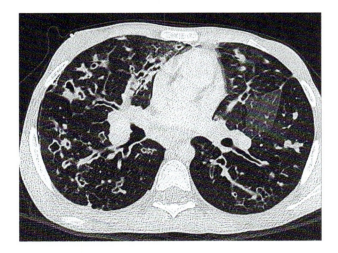

Figure 4.18   CT chest showing severe established bronchiectasis of unknown cause.

- Flexible bronchoscopy when a single lobe is affected, and in some patients with frequent infections where a pathogen is not identified.

- Consideration of microlaryngobronchoscopy (MLB) or tube oesophagram to assess for trachea-oesophageal fistula or laryngeal cleft

Treatment

The goal is to prevent disease progression, reduce infective exacerbations and maintain or improve pulmonary function. This is achieved by:

- Identification and treatment of underlying conditions, such as primary immunodeficiency, gastro-oesophageal reflux disease.

- Early recognition and treatment of acute infective exacerbations with antibiotics.

- Prophylactic antibiotics to suppress microbial load.

- Regular chest physiotherapy with airway clearance techniques.

- Immunisation: pneumococcal vaccine and annual influenza vaccine is recommended.

- Some children with airflow limitation and bronchodilator response on spirometry may benefit from a trial of inhaled corticosteroids.

- In localised bronchiectasis not responding to medical treatment, surgical removal of damaged segments or lobes may be considered to avoid 'spill-over' infection of other lobes of the lung.

Prognosis

Non-CF bronchiectasis in children is potentially reversible and disease progression is preventable with early diagnosis and appropriate treatment.

INTERSTITIAL LUNG DISEASE

Childhood interstitial lung disease (chILD) is a spectrum of a heterogeneous group of rare lung diseases resulting from varied pathogenic processes that include genetic factors, associated systemic diseases and pathological inflammatory responses to stimuli. It is not a single disease or diagnosis, chILD is an 'umbrella term' encompassing what are likely to be many, poorly understood disease process with a common end point of impaired gas diffusion across an abnormal alveolar-capillary interface, typically due to inflammation or fibrosis in the interstitium.

Incidence

This is an extremely rare condition, with an estimated prevalence of 3.6 cases per million children.

Aetiology/Pathogenesis

Within the spectrum of childhood ILD, conditions of known aetiology (such as hypersensitivity pneumonitis, storage disorders, connective tissue disorders [Figure 4.19], pulmonary vasculitides, surfactant dysfunction mutations [Figures 4.20 and 4.21]), and conditions of unknown aetiology (such as desquamative interstitial pneumonia, lymphoid interstitial pneumonia, non-specific interstitial pneumonia and pulmonary alveolar proteinosis, among several others) have been described. Some chILDs are unique to infants, such as diffuse developmental disorders (where the lung tissue is incorrectly formed, e.g. acinar dysplasia, congenital alveolar dysplasia, alveolar-capillary dysplasia) and specific conditions of undefined aetiology, such as neuroendocrine cell hyperplasia of infancy and pulmonary interstitial glycogenosis (postulated to be dysregulation of the systems involved in normal fetal maturation of the lung). In older children and adolescents, it may be that repeated alveolar injury or inflammation results in increased myofibroblast action resulting in lung fibrosis.

Clinical Presentation

There is a high incidence of prematurity (28%) and neonatal onset of symptoms and a family history of lung disease (34%). Common presenting features are tachypnoea, dyspnoea, cough and wheeze, exercise intolerance, failure to thrive and frequent respiratory infections. On physical examination, tachypnoea and chest wall retractions are seen, and fine crackles are commonly heard. In severe cases hypoxemia, clubbing and signs of pulmonary hypertension may be present.

Diagnosis

Diagnosis is made by a combination of history and clinical examination, lung function, chest x-ray and chest CT appearances, and lung biopsy where indicated. An individualised systematic approach is essential in the evaluation of childhood ILD due to the extensive differential diagnosis.

Treatment

Supportive:

Oxygen supplementation for hypoxaemia ($SpO_2 < 92\%$)

Adequate nutrition

Annual influenza vaccination

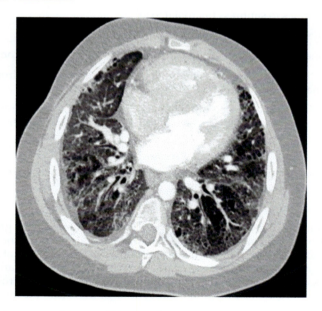

Figure 4.19 CT chest in an 11-year-old boy with systemic lupus erythematosus, showing extensive interstitial lung disease. Diffuse ground-glass attenuation, cystic changes and diffuse fibrosis with some honeycombing is seen.

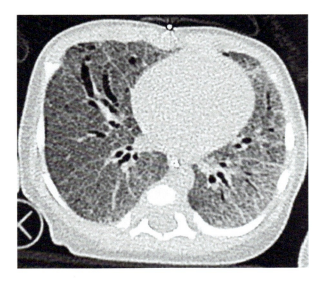

Figure 4.20 CT chest in a neonate with ABCA3 deficiency showing widespread interlobular septal thickening and diffuse hazy ground glass opacification. There are proximally dilated bronchi in both lungs, particularly prominent in the right middle lobe with scattered small subpleural lucencies in the right lung, suggesting subpleural cystic change, probably due to barotrauma.

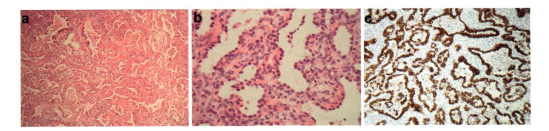

Figure 4.21 Lung histopathology of patient from Figure 4.20. There is marked thickening of the interstitium, Type 2 pneumocyte hyperplasia and accumulation of macrophages without evidence of inflammatory infiltrates (A and B – H&E stains). The lung structure is simplified and immunostaining for cytokeratin (C) confirms Type 2 pneumocyte hyperplasia. Surfactant protein gene analysis confirmed ABCA3 deficiency.

Treatment of chILD is determined by the underlying diagnosis. If an associated diagnosis is not found then treatment depends on disease severity and includes high doses of intravenous or oral steroids, hydroxychloroquine (or other immunomodulatory drugs including mycophenolate mofetil, cyclophosphamide, azathioprine), and azithromycin.

Prognosis
The clinical course is extremely variable from complete resolution without treatment in conditions such as neuroendocrine hyperplasia of infancy, to resolution or remission on treatment for some forms of desquamative interstitial pneumonitis, to progression and early death in some forms of surfactant protein deficiency.

PNEUMOTHORAX
Incidence and Aetiology
A pneumothorax is air in the pleural space, outside the lung and internal to the chest wall. This can occur either due to rupture of the lung surface, or by external puncture of the thoracic wall. The incidence is reported as 23 cases per 100,000 of population per year. A pneumothorax may

occur for a variety of reasons, shown in Table 4.6. Spontaneous pneumothorax is not uncommon in adolescent males even in the absence of other underlying lung pathology. In other cases, there may be intrinsic pulmonary anomalies such as congenital cysts or connective tissue disorders (e.g. Ehlers–Danlos or Marfan syndrome). Some cases are familial.

Clinical Presentation

There may be a sudden onset of chest pain in association with breathlessness and cyanosis. Physical examination may reveal decreased air entry and hyper-resonance to percussion on the affected side. If the air is under tension this is an emergency situation requiring immediate treatment, there will be mediastinal or even tracheal shift to the opposite side, which compresses blood flow in major vessels. The condition may be associated with air leak elsewhere such as surgical emphysema onto the chest wall, abdomen, into the neck or down the arm.

Diagnosis

Chest x-ray will show the pneumothorax (Figure 4.22) and any associated air leaking elsewhere such as into the mediastinum or subcutaneous tissue. Pleural sliding is absent on lung ultrasound, but chest x-ray is the gold standard for diagnosis.

Table 4.6: Causes of Pneumothorax

• Spontaneous	Idiopathic
	Familial, e.g. Ehlers–Danlos syndrome
	Congenital subpleural blebs/cysts
• Trauma	Penetrating or blunt chest injury
• Foreign body aspiration	
• Asthma	
• Cystic fibrosis	
• Iatrogenic	Intubation, Positive pressure ventilation, Venous cannulation, Bronchoscopy (increased risk with biopsy via bronchoscope)
• Pneumonia	Bacterial, Viral
• Rare diseases	Histiocytosis, Congenital lobar emphysema, Congenital cystic malformation
• Toxic inhalation	

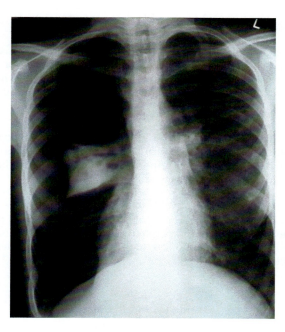

Figure 4.22   The x-ray of a child with a large right-sided pneumothorax resulting in complete collapse of the right lung.

Treatment

Treatment of pneumothorax is either conservative (if symptoms are minimal can watch and wait until it resolves), or active (remove the air from the pleural cavity by chest tube drainage). In those with minor symptoms, spontaneous recovery usually occurs and is in theory assisted by the administration of oxygen. Otherwise a chest tube should be inserted under local or general anaesthesia. Needle aspiration alone is associated with a high recurrence rate and younger patients won't tolerate this painful procedure; as a general anaesthetic will be required definitive treatment (a chest drain) is indicated. The drain should be placed under a water seal so that air does not leak back into the pleural cavity. If the chest drain shows continuous bubbling this is an indication that there is a broncho-pleural fistula and other interventions such as interventional radiology bronchoscopic glue, surgical correction or pleurodesis may be required. Thoracoscopic intervention can be particularly helpful in this situation.

CONGENITAL THORACIC MALFORMATIONS

These are congenital abnormalities of lung growth that occur in the first trimester, during early fetal lung development. There is a spectrum of abnormalities, and hybrid lesions occur. Although individually rare, the incidence has increased over the last two decades following the advent of high-resolution antenatal ultrasound examination of the fetal lung. This has resulted in difficult clinical decisions especially related to the entirely asymptomatic child with a small lesion. Congenital thoracic malformations encompass:

- Bronchogenic cyst
- Congenital lobar overinflation (CLO)/congenital large hyperlucent lobe (CLHL)/congenital segmental overinflation (CSO)
- Congenital pulmonary airway malformation (CPAM)
- Bronchopulmonary sequestration (BPS)

Management of these malformations is concentrated in specialist centres, and as uncertainty exists about their prognosis there is controversy about their management. Babies identified with CTMs on routine antenatal ultrasound should be referred to a respiratory paediatrician working within an MDT consisting of experienced radiologists, histopathologists and thoracic surgeons.

LUNG TRANSPLANTATION

Introduction

Lung transplantation is a treatment option for those with end-stage parenchymal or vascular lung disease (Tables 4.7 and 4.8). Bilateral sequential lung transplantation is now the commonest procedure undertaken. Heart–lung transplants are becoming increasingly rare, not only because of the shortage of donors available but also because of increased recognition that right heart recovery is possible in patients with severe idiopathic pulmonary arterial hypertension. Heart–lung transplant is required if there is significant left ventricular dysfunction or an uncorrectable heart defect along with pulmonary hypertension. Single lung transplantation is usually only considered in adult patients with non-suppurative lung disease. Living lobar donation (receiving two lower lobes from two living donors) is considered in few centres.

Although survival has improved over the years, lung transplants do not offer a cure as patients receive high-level immunosuppression to prevent graft rejection, with the concomitant risks (opportunistic infections and certain cancers). However, most patients will have rapid and sustained improvement in quality of life after transplantation.

Treatment

After transplantation, patients are usually maintained on three immunosuppressive medications life-long, which include prednisolone, a calcineurin inhibitor such as tacrolimus or ciclosporin, and a cell cycle inhibitor such as mycophenolate mofetil (MMF) or azathioprine. Prophylaxis against *Pneumocystis jirovecii*, CMV and fungal infection are required.

Complications

Complications following lung transplantation are common. A delicate balance is required in avoiding under-immunosuppression risking rejection and over-immunosuppression, which may

Table 4.7: Indication for Lung Transplantation Assessment

Cystic fibrosis	$FEV_1 < 30\%$ or Rapidly declining FEV_1 Acute exacerbation requiring ICU Recurrent pneumothorax Recurrent haemoptysis not controlled with embolisation Oxygen dependent Hypercapnea Desaturation < 90%with exercise Poor quality of life
Pulmonary arterial hypertension	NYHA Functional class III or IV, Commencement of IV vasodilator therapy, Declining haemodynamics/ECHO, six min walk test < 350 metres Syncope Haemoptysis
Surfactant protein deficiencies	Surfactant protein B deficiency – at diagnosis Surfactant protein C, ABCA3 deficiency have a more variable course – refer when evidence of interstitial lung disease and clinical deterioration
Pulmonary veno-occlusive disease and pulmonary capillary haemangiomatosis	At diagnosis
Other interstitial lung disease	Progressive clinical decline and decrease in lung function despite medical therapy
Obliterative bronchiolitis	Progressive clinical decline and decrease in lung function despite medical therapy

Table 4.8: Contraindications to Lung Transplantation (May Be Centre Specific)

Absolute
- Malignancy in the last two years, with the exception of cutaneous squamous and basal cell tumours
- Untreatable advanced dysfunction of another organ system (although combined lung/other organ transplants can be considered in some centres)
- Active infection – pulmonary mycobacterial infection, chronic active hepatitis B, chronic active hepatitis C (biopsy proven) despite maximal medical therapy
- Congenital or acquired immunodeficiency
- Chronic infection with *Burkholderia cenocepacia* (previous genomovar III)
- Severe chest wall/spinal deformity
- Refractory non-adherence

Relative
- Critical clinical condition, e.g. acute sepsis, invasive ventilation, extracorporeal membrane oxygenation
- Colonised with highly resistant bacteria, fungi or mycobacterium
- Severely abnormal body mass index (high or low)
- Absent or unreliable social support system
- Severe or symptomatic osteoporosis
- Neuromuscular weakness
- Pleurodesis
- Active vasculitis/collagen disorders

increase the risks of infection, post-transplant lymphoproliferative disease (PTLD) and the various side effects of drugs that have a narrow therapeutic window. Patients undergo intense surveillance following transplant to monitor allograft function and to check for complications. Patients are discharged with a hand-held spirometer and asked to measure their lung function on a daily basis, reporting back to the transplant centre if there is a 10% drop in their baseline spirometry. Flexible bronchoscopy with transbronchial biopsy and lavage are required to investigate for acute cellular rejection and infection (see Figures 4.23 and 4.24).

Prognosis

Current international conditional median survival following paediatric lung transplant is 9.1 years (ISHLT registry data). The major impediment to long-term survival is chronic lung allograft dysfunction (CLAD), an umbrella term that encompasses several phenotypes of chronic rejection. The pathophysiology of the development of CLAD is complex and our understanding of the various immune and non-immune factors associated with CLAD is an active research area.

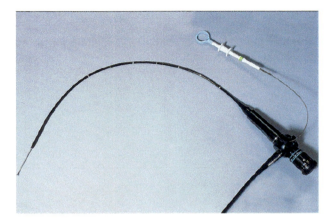

Figure 4.23 A 4.9 mm flexible fibreoptic bronchoscope (Olympus, Japan) with alligator head transbronchial biopsy forceps inserted through the suction channel. Used for monitoring of pulmonary allografts.

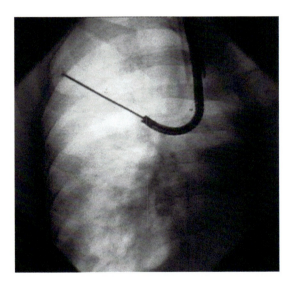

Figure 4.24 Fluoroscopic appearance of position of transbronchial biopsy forceps through the flexible fibreoptic bronchoscope.

Conclusion

Lung transplantation can offer a select group of patients with end-stage lung disease a survival benefit and an excellent quality of life.

FURTHER READING

- Wilmott RW, Bush A, Deterding RR, et al. *Kendig's Disorders of the Respiratory Tract in Children*, 9th Edition. Elsevier; 2019.
- Shteinberg M, Haq IJ, Polineni D, et al. Cystic fibrosis. *Lancet*. 2021 Jun 5;397(10290):2195–2211. doi:10.1016/S0140-6736(20)32542-3. PMID: 34090606.
- Scottish Intercollegiate Guidelines Network, British Thoracic Society. British guideline on the management of asthma. A national clinical guideline. Revised edition published July 2019.
- Bronchiolitis in children: Diagnosis and management. NICE guideline [NG9]. Published: 01 June 2015.

- Harris M, Clark J, Coote N, et al. British Thoracic Society guidelines for the management of community acquired pneumonia in children: Update 2011. *Thorax.* 2011;66(Suppl 2):ii1–23.
- Balfour-Lynn IM, Abrahamson E, Cohen G, et al. BTS guidelines for the management of pleural infection in children. *Thorax.* 2005;60(Suppl 1):i1–21.
- Brugha R, Spencer H. Lung transplantation in children. *Encyclopedia of Respiratory Medicine*, 2nd Edition. Elsevier; 2021.

5 Paediatric Cardiology

Michelle Carr, Florian Moenkemeyer and Michael Quail

CONGENITAL HEART DISEASE

Congenital heart diseae (CHD) is *any* developmental malformation of the heart. The spectrum of disease falling into this classification ranges from simple lesions, for example bicuspid aortic valve through to more complex diseases involving single ventricle lesions such as hypoplastic left-heart syndrome. The underlying causes of CHD remains relatively poorly understood, although the epidemiology suggests a genetic basis contributing to the majority of CHD. Aneuploidies, e.g. Trisomy 21 (Down's syndrome, septal defects) and monosomy X (Turner syndrome, bicuspid aortic valve and coarctation of the aorta) were the earliest identified causes and account for 10–20% of CHD. Copy number variations (small to large deletions or duplications) may also contribute to the development of CHD by altered dosage of genes; an example is 22q11 deletion which causes DiGeorge syndrome (interrupted aortic arch, tetralogy of Fallot, truncus arteriosus). Unfortunately, the cause of CHD in most patients remains unknown.

Clinical Presentation of Congenital Heart Disease

The clinical presentation of CHD in infancy may be dominated by a number of physiological states:

1. Shunts: Anatomical communications between the normally separated pulmonary and systemic circulations may allow for the passage of blood from one side to the other; referred to as a shunt. The location of such communications may be within the heart: atrial septal defects (ASD), ventricular septal defects (VSD), atrioventricular septal defects (AVSD), or between vascular structures: e.g. anomalous pulmonary venous connections, patent ductus arteriosus (PDA) or pulmonary arteriovenous malformations (AVM). The location of the shunt, the direction of flow (left-to-right or right-to-left) and the volume of shunted blood account for the observed signs. The direction and volume of a shunt is influenced by local haemodynamic factors including the relative compliance and resistances on either side of the anatomical communication. For example, an anatomically large PDA may have no significant shunt if the pulmonary vascular resistance (PVR) is equal to the systemic vascular resistance (SVR). With the progressive reduction of PVR after birth below SVR, the ductal shunt will become left to right (aorta to pulmonary artery), the volume of the shunt increasing in proportion to the ratio of PVR and SVR. In patients with persistent pulmonary hypertension of the newborn (PPHN) or Eisenmenger's syndrome, PVR may exceed SVR, and the net shunt will be right to left, resulting in cyanosis.

The direction and volume of a shunt at atrial level is predominately influenced by the compliances of the left and right ventricles. Normally the right ventricle (RV) has higher compliance than the left ventricle (LV), and therefore the net shunt is left to right. In a severely hypertrophied RV (e.g. due to pulmonary stenosis or pulmonary hypertension), the compliance may exceed the LV and the net shunt will be right to left.

2. Increased afterload: Increased ventricular afterload (left or right) can be caused by obstruction to ventricular outflow (outflow tract obstruction, valvar stenosis, or supravalvar stenosis) or increased resistance/obstruction in the vasculature (pulmonary arterial hypertension, or coarctation of the aorta). Increased afterload increases myocardial wall tension and stimulates adaptive concentric hypertrophy. Severely increased afterload beyond the capacity of myocardial adaptation can lead to heart failure. Less severe lesions without accompanying shunts may present with clinical signs such as a murmur due to the obstructive lesion or reduced exercise capacity.

3. Compromised systemic perfusion: This may result from low stroke volume of a systemic ventricle, outflow tract obstruction (critical aortic stenosis) or aortic obstruction (e.g. interrupted aortic arch or coarctation). The clinical picture is one of poor peripheral perfusion, with low pulse volume; patients may be pink or blue (cyanotic). The ductus arteriosus may provide an effective temporary bypass for the obstruction, facilitating systemic perfusion with deoxygenated or mixed blood. However, as the duct closes (some days after birth), life-threatening systemic or lower body hypoperfusion ensues and often also pulmonary venous hypertension. Therapy is directed at maintaining the patency of the arterial duct using intravenous prostaglandins, intensive care for critically ill patients, and planning for surgical relief of the obstruction.

DOI: 10.1201/9781003175186-5

4. Pulmonary venous congestion: Obstruction to pulmonary venous return results in increased pulmonary venous pressure (elevated pulmonary capillary wedge pressure); at progressively higher transvascular gradients, oncotic pressure is exceeded and extravasation of fluid into the interstitial and alveolar space occurs. Obstruction may occur in the pulmonary venous pathway (total anomalous pulmonary venous connection, TAPVD), in the atrium (cor triatriatum) or at the level of the left ventricular inflow (e.g. supravalvular, valvular or subvalvular mitral stenosis). Pulmonary venous congestion may also occur as a consequence of elevated left atrial pressure secondary to LV diastolic dysfunction; increased LV end diastolic pressure (e.g. valve disease, coarctation of the aorta, myocardial disease). The degree of pulmonary venous hypertension determines the clinical presentation. Patients with severe obstruction may present with hypoxia, cyanosis and dyspnoea due to pulmonary oedema, whilst patients with less severe obstruction may remain pink but may present later with failure to thrive.

The following three physiological states predominantly account for patients with cyanosis:

5. Low pulmonary blood flow: Reduction in pulmonary blood flow can be caused by redirection of systemic venous return to the systemic circulation. This commonly occurs in the context of obstruction to right ventricular outflow (tetralogy of Fallot or severe pulmonary stenosis) combined with an intracardiac shunt (e.g. VSD). Obstruction of RV outflow results in a redirection of deoxygenated blood to the left-heart (right-to-left shunt) via a VSD. A similar situation may occur due to impaired filling of the RV due to tricuspid valve stenosis/atresia or RV diastolic disease, with redirection of deoxygenated blood through an ASD. If lung function is normal, pulmonary venous blood returns to the left atrium fully saturated (albeit reduced) and will mix with the shunted deoxygenated systemic venous blood (in the LA or LV). The degree of cyanosis is dependent on the amount of oxygenated and deoxygenated blood in the mix.

6. Parallel circulations: This occurs in transposition of the great arteries, where the aorta arises from the morphological right ventricle and the pulmonary artery from the LV. In this condition, deoxygenated systemic venous return recirculates into the aorta and the oxygenated pulmonary venous return recirculates to the pulmonary artery; a situation clearly incompatible with life. Patients can only survive if there is sufficient mixing of the parallel streams; this can occur best at atrial level through a large interatrial communication, less well at ventricular level (via a VSD) and even less well at great vessel level (via a PDA). Critical cyanosis may be managed medically by maintaining patency of the PDA by prostaglandins, but may require the creation of an artificial interatrial communication, until definitive treatment by surgically switching the great vessels.

7. Intracardiac mixing: Complete intracardiac mixing of blood may occur at atrial level (common atrium), ventricular level (all univentricular hearts), or great artery level (common arterial trunk). Patients are expected to be mildly cyanosed depending on the relative amount of deoxygenated blood in the mix and breathless according to the amount of pulmonary blood flow.

SHUNT LESIONS
Ventricular Septal Defect (VSD)

Prevalence: The prevalence of VSD is 3.1 per 1000 live births and is the commonest form of CHD, representing approximately 35% of all cardiac lesions at birth.

Aetiology and Classification: VSD are one of the most common types of congenital cardiac malformations. They commonly occur in isolation, but are also a common defect in association with genetic syndromes.

Assessment: VSD are increasingly diagnosed antenatally. However, due to the equal pressures of the left and the right ventricle in the foetal circulation, the shunt volume might be low and be missed by foetal echocardiography. With the drop in pulmonary vascular resistance after birth a shunt between the pulmonary and systemic circulation will become more apparent, so frequently a murmur on clinical examination prompts a suspicion for a VSD. Small defects will produce high velocity shunts with a loud holosystolic murmur and potentially a thrill. Larger lesions will not necessarily produce a murmur across the lesion due to an unrestrictive physiology. A mid-diastolic murmur may be audible at the apex originating from the high flow across the mitral valve. Large shunts will increase pulmonary blood flow resulting in heart failure with tachypnoea, recurrent chest infections, feeding difficulties and failure to thrive.

Diagnosis: There may be no electrocardiogram (ECG) or chest x-ray (CXR) abnormalities with small lesions, larger lesions might show ECG changes consistent with left atrial dilatation and left ventricular hypertrophy (LVH). The CXR will show pulmonary plethora and cardiomegaly (Figure 5.1).

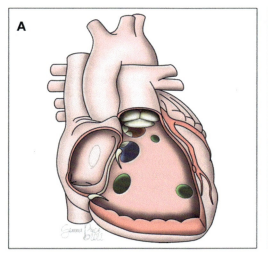
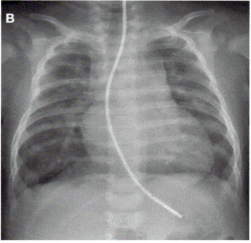

Figure 5.1   A. View into the right ventricle with ventricular septal defects in the different areas of the septum. Not only the size but also the site is important for the assessment of indication for surgery, operability, but also the likelihood of spontaneous closure. B. Chest x-Ray in an infant with large VSD, high pulmonary blood flow and pulmonary plethora.

VSD are suspected clinically and diagnosed with a transthoracic echocardiogram (TTE). The TTE shows the size, location and relationships of the defect. It also can identify additional lesions, assess heart function and estimate shunt volume. TTE is usually sufficient for operative planning to describe the exact location of the VSD and its surrounding structures (Figure 5.1).

Treatment: Larger defects resulting in symptoms of heart failure will need to be treated. Conservative management with diuretics and nasogastric feeding can help growth, but such interventions usually indicate the need for closure. With time adjacent tissue might partially (or completely) obstruct the VSD and reduce the shunt volume. VSDs located in the apical trabeculations tend to close spontaneously. In selected cases an interim solution with a pulmonary artery band might be used to protect the pulmonary circulation in these cases until spontaneous or surgical closure can be obtained.

If indicated most defects are closed surgically on cardiopulmonary bypass, although transcatheter techniques may be used in selected cases with good results.

Prognosis: Many VSD close spontaneously in the first five years of life. Surgical intervention nowadays carries a low risk and acquired heart block for isolated lesions is extremely rare.

Late presentations of unrepaired large VSD are unusual but can present in locations with limited access to healthcare. Untreated high pulmonary blood flow may result in elevation of PVR, pulmonary arterial hypertension, elevation of right-sided pressures and right ventricular hypertrophy (RVH). This physiological situation may preclude any surgical treatment and ultimately lead to Eisenmenger's syndrome (shunt reversal with cyanosis).

Atrial Septal Defect (ASD)

Prevalence: ASDs are amongst the most common congenital heart defects with a prevalence of 1.4 per 1000 births, and represent 15% of all CHD.

Aetiology and Classification: An ASD is the result of a developmental insufficiency of the interatrial septation. The defect should be distinguished from the naturally occurring foramen ovale. The aetiology is unknown, but an ASD is associated with genetic abnormalities, such as Holt–Oram syndrome.

The direction and volume of shunt across the ASD is principally determined by the size of the defect and relative ventricular compliance. Under normal conditions an ASD results in a left-to-right shunt. In certain disease states associated with reduced RV compliance (e.g. pulmonary hypertension, restrictive RV physiology in tetralogy of Fallot) the shunt can be bidirectional or right to left.

The developmental septation of the atria is complex, and failure of particular stages results in a range of specific forms of ASD, in order of decreasing frequency: 1. Ostium secundum ASD; 2. Ostium primum ASD; 3. Sinus venosus defects (superior and inferior); 4. Coronary sinus defects (rare).

Ostium primum defects are part of the atrioventricular septal defect spectrum and are associated with abnormal development of the atrioventricular valves. Sinus venous defects occur in combination with anomalous pulmonary venous connections.

Assessment: Clinical signs and symptoms occur in proportion to the shunt. In a small ASD, no clinical signs may be apparent. Large shunts are associated with fixed splitting of the second heart sound, and a systolic murmur over the right ventricular outflow tract (left upper sternal edge), due in increased flow across the pulmonary valve. Large defects may be associated with decreased exercise capacity in teenagers and adults.

Diagnosis: ASD shunting is associated with right heart dilatation, which may be visible on CXR. The ECG can show signs of right ventricular hypertrophy and (incomplete) right bundle branch block. Diagnosis is reliably made by TTE.

Treatment: Small ASD may not require any treatment, and some may close spontaneously. Borderline defects can be assessed by cardiac MRI to calculate the shunt volume and conform indication for closure. Larger defects can be closed electively, either by transcatheter device closure or if unsuitable by cardiac surgery.

Prognosis: The prognosis is excellent with normal life expectancy if corrective intervention is performed before adulthood.

Patent Ductus Arteriosus (PDA)

Prevalence: The prevalence of PDA is 1 per 1000 births, they represent 10% of all CHD.

Aetiology and Classification: The ductus arteriosus is a normal developmental structure. Pathological patency of the arterial duct is defined as persistence beyond three months of age. A PDA is more common in premature than term babies and also has higher incidence in patients with RDS.

The ductus arteriosus is an essential part of the foetal circulation, facilitating an anatomical bypass of the high resistance pulmonary circulation *in utero*. Indeed, premature closure of the duct in utero can result in severe heart failure and hydrops foetalis. During foetal development the duct is kept open by the low blood oxygen tension and high levels of prostanoids produced by the placenta and its reduced metabolism in the foetal lung.

The ductus arteriosus usually closes in the first hours after birth with increase in blood oxygen tension and decreasing prostaglandin levels resulting in smooth muscle contraction. Subsequently the ductus obliterates, usually in the first two weeks of life, resulting in a fibrous strand of tissue. Failure to close will result in systemic to pulmonary (left-to-right) shunting and depending on the shunt volume, in increased pulmonary blood flow and heart failure.

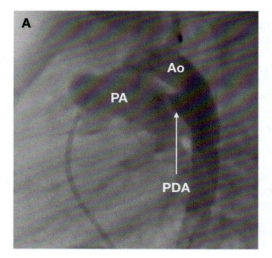 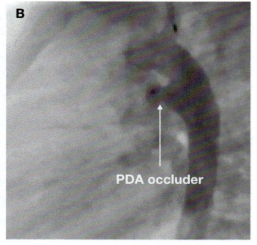

Figure 5.2 Interventional occlusion of a Patent Ductus Arteriosus. A. Injection into the descending aorta fills the pulmonary artery via the PDA due to left-to-right shunting. B. PDA occlusion device has been deployed in the ductus arteriosus, showing no contrast passing into the pulmonary artery from the aorta.

Clinical Presentation: The size of the PDA and the PVR after birth will define the clinical presentation. In the preterm infant increasing oxygen demand can raise suspicion of a patent arterial duct. Most commonly the patients are asymptomatic. A continuous murmur in the high left sternal border is pathognomonic for the presence of a PDA. Larger lesions can result in an active precordium and a wide pulse pressure due to the high stroke volume and the diastolic steal.

Diagnosis: Small PDAs may have no abnormalities on CXR or ECG, larger shunts will result in left atrial and ventricular dilatation, which can be demonstrated on the ECG with increased P-wave amplitude and duration, and electrical signs for LVH. The CXR might show an enlarged LA and cardiomegaly with pulmonary plethora.

TTE is used to confirm the diagnosis and identify associated lesions. Doppler studies are used to calculate the pressure difference between the systemic and pulmonary circulation to evaluate the pulmonary artery pressure.

Treatment: In preterm neonates, the initial treatment to close a PDA with a left-to-right shunt is usually medical with paracetamol or ibuprofen to inhibit prostaglandin synthesis (conversely prostaglandin infusion is used to maintain duct patency if required postnatally).

There is debate if a small PDA without obvious haemodynamic importance requires intervention. Some data suggest a small but elevated life-long risk of endocarditis with a restrictive shunt and recommend closure. A larger PDA with signs of left-heart volume loading requires closure. Nowadays, most PDAs can be addressed with an interventional catheter procedure depending on the morphology of the duct (Figure 5.2). Selected cases might require a surgical ligation from a lateral thoracotomy.

Right-to-left (reversed direction) shunting across a PDA is indicative of abnormal pulmonary vascular resistance, and is a contraindication to closure.

Prognosis: An isolated PDA has an excellent prognosis after either catheter-based or surgical treatment. Both interventions carry a low risk. There will be no limitations in activity or life expectancy. Untreated large PDAs can very rarely result in pulmonary hypertension in early adult life. If the PVR is irreversibly elevated closure of a PDA is contraindicated.

Atrioventricular Septal Defect (AVSD)

Prevalence: The prevalence of AVSD is 0.29 per 1000 births. AVSD is commonly associated with Trisomy 21, with about 30% of patients with this genetic abnormality affected.

Aetiology and Classification: AVSD results from abnormal development of the separation of the atrioventricular junction with fusion of the inlet valves and septation deficits between the atrial primum septum and the ventricular inlet septum (Figure 5.3).

Isolated atrial communications without ventricular component (ostium primum ASD, see above) still include the abnormal fusion of the atrioventricular valves.

More complex lesions can involve ventricular imbalance precluding conventional surgical correction and must be managed as a single ventricle heart.

Clinical Presentation: AVSD can be diagnosed by routine foetal ultrasound. The diagnosis of Trisomy 21 should always prompt postnatal cardiac evaluation. The clinical presentation is mainly dependent on the size of the intracardiac shunts and the severity of regurgitation of the atrioventricular valves. Heart failure (failure to thrive, tachypnoea, increased work of breathing and tachycardia) can occur early in large shunts with the physiological decrease in pulmonary vascular resistance postnatally.

Auscultatory findings are determined by the volume of the shunt. Signs include fixed splitting of the second heart sound and a murmur over the right ventricular outflow Large shunts may have an active precordium and a soft diastolic murmur at the left lower sternal edge reflecting increased flow across the atrioventricular valve.

Diagnosis: The abnormal development of the atrioventricular junction also involves the conduction pathway resulting in a superior axis in the ECG (Figure 5.4). Additional features of ventricular hypertrophy and atrial enlargement can be present dependent on AV valve regurgitation and shunt volume. The CXR abnormalities also range from no changes to pulmonary plethora and cardiomegaly in large shunts with heart failure. The diagnosis is confirmed with TTE which is sufficient to delineate morphological and plan surgical repair.

Treatment: Dependent on signs of heart failure, anti-congestive medical management may be required early to allow sufficient growth. The aim is a surgical repair around 3 to 5 months of age. There is an increased risk of complications for surgery in patients under 5 kg. Small or complex patients with heart failure may require an interim solution with a pulmonary artery band to

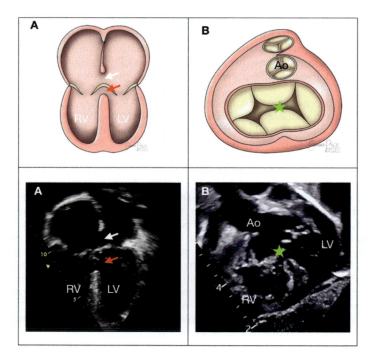

Figure 5.3 A. Four-chamber diagram (above) and corresponding TTE image (below). The whole area of the Atrioventricular junction is abnormally formed resulting in a large primum ASD (white arrow) and inlet VSD (red arrow). B. En face view of the atrioventricular valve structure in AVSD. Instead of two separate orifices the atrioventricular valves are fused. Two bridging leaflets (green star) span the interventricular septum. The aorta (AO) is in a more anterior position.

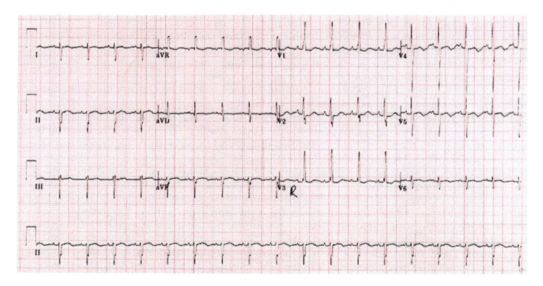

Figure 5.4 A 12-lead ECG in a patient with AVSD. Negative Vector in lead I and aVF indicating a superior QRS axis.

restrict pulmonary blood flow and allow further growth until complete repair. Surgery aims to septate the heart with one or two patches and repair the abnormal valves.

Prognosis: Residual stenosis or regurgitation of the left AV valve is an important prognostic factor. Severe left AV valve dysfunction may require further intervention or valve replacement.

Obstruction of the left ventricular outflow tract is a known complication which may require re-operation.

With improvement of cardio-pulmonary bypass and surgical techniques the current overall survival of AVSD is reported as 85%, 82% and 71% at 10, 20 and 30 years, respectively, after initial complete AVSD repair. Published data show no elevated risk for surgery for patients with Trisomy 21, however, they are at higher risk for pulmonary hypertension.

OBSTRUCTION TO PULMONARY BLOOD FLOW

Obstruction to pulmonary blood flow from the RV may be caused by pulmonary valve stenosis, RV outflow tract obstruction or disease of the pulmonary vasculature (e.g. branch pulmonary artery stenoses or pulmonary vascular disease). This obstruction increases RV afterload, necessitating RV remodelling and hypertrophy. Increased RV afterload beyond the capacity of RV adaptation may cause failure of the right ventricle. In the presence of an intracardiac shunt the obstruction may cause right-to-left shunting and clinical cyanosis.

Pulmonary Stenosis with Intact Interventricular Septum

Prevalence: The prevalence of pulmonary stenosis is 0.55 per 1000 births, representing 6% of CHD. There is an elevated risk of up to 3% for familial recurrence of isolated PS.

Aetiology and Classification: Stenosis can occur below the valve (subvalvar), valvar, supravalvular just above the valve, further in the periphery or a combination of these. Pulmonary stenosis is commonly associated with Noonan's or Williams–Beuren syndrome. Peripheral pulmonary artery stenoses are found in Alagille syndrome. Maternal rubella infection during pregnancy has a high incidence of pulmonary stenosis but is now rare due to immunisation.

Clinical Presentation: Severe stenosis can present in the neonatal period with cyanosis due to right-to-left shunting at atrial level and requires emergency intervention. The pulmonary circulation might be dependent on a patent ductus arteriosus (critical stenosis). Less severe stenosis might not produce any obvious clinical symptoms. Auscultation of valvar stenosis reveals a mid-systolic murmur with an ejection click over the left upper sternal border, that is not radiating into the carotid artery region (in contrast to AS), and splitting of the second heart sound. Left untreated and with hypertrophy of the right ventricle, shunting at atrial level can occur due to restrictive diastolic properties of the RV resulting in cyanosis. With RV hypertrophy the muscle bundles in the right ventricular outflow tract (RVOT) can contribute to dynamic obstruction and be responsible for acute deterioration in severe stenosis.

Diagnosis: Depending on severity, the signs of RVH and RA dilatation might be present on ECG and CXR. TTE is usually sufficient to confirm the diagnosis and identify the exact location of the stenosis. The pressure gradient is estimated using Doppler measurements.

Treatment: Intervention is frequently considered if the transpulmonary pressure gradient is over 64 mmHg (> 4 m/s on Doppler). Symptomatic patients might need individual decisions even at lower gradients. Transcatheter pulmonary valvuloplasty is the treatment of choice in most centres for valvar PS even though some data suggest a better long-term freedom from re-intervention for surgical valvotomy. Severely dysplastic and small pulmonary valves or more complex obstructions frequently require surgical correction.

Prognosis: Prognosis is dependent on the type and location of the obstruction and co-morbidities. Peripheral pulmonary stenosis can resolve spontaneously and tends to improve even in severely affected patients with Williams–Beuren syndrome. Mild to moderate PS frequently remains stable without the need for intervention. Post-interventional re-stenosis can occur and a degree of pulmonary regurgitation after intervention on the valve is common.

Tetralogy of Fallot/Pulmonary Atresia with VSD

Prevalence: The prevalence of tetralogy of Fallot is 0.36 per 1000 births, representing 4.4% of CHD.

Aetiology and Classification: This lesion is an abnormal configuration of the RVOT with malalignment of the outlet septum and subpulmonary stenosis, a VSD with overriding aorta and right ventricular hypertrophy (Figure 5.5A). At the extreme end of the spectrum there is absence of the RVOT and main pulmonary artery resulting in pulmonary atresia with VSD. In pulmonary atresia, pulmonary perfusion is dependent on the PDA or systemic to pulmonary collateral arteries. There is association with a deletion on the short arm of Chromosome 22 (22q11, DiGeorge syndrome). Common additional features include a right aortic arch.

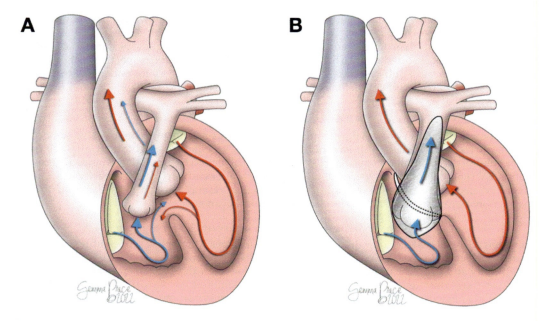

Figure 5.5 A. Unrepaired Tetralogy of Fallot, showing the combination of VSD, RV outflow tract obstruction, RV hypertrophy and the aorta overriding the VSD. B. Repair of Tetralogy of Fallot with VSD closure and transannular patch enlargement of the right ventricular outflow tract and the commonly hypoplastic pulmonary valve.

Clinical Presentation: The clinical presentation depends on the degree of right ventricular outflow tract obstruction. In cases with little obstruction, the presentation may be more akin to a VSD with normal saturations and heart failure ('Pink Fallot'). In severe obstruction there is severe cyanosis including acute life-threatening hypercyanotic spells ('Tet-spells'). Hypercyanotic spelling occur most often in patients with dynamic muscular obstruction of the RVOT. They are aggravated by stress and agitation due to adrenergic activity and can lead to acute life-threatening cyanosis and cardiac arrest.

On examination. patients have an ejection systolic murmur over the left upper sternal border. A parasternal thrill may be present over the pulmonary area. The absence of the murmur in hypercyanotic spells confirms complete dynamic obstruction to pulmonary blood flow.

Diagnosis: Right ventricular hypertrophy is seen on ECG and CXR. Pulmonary oligaemia, small central pulmonary arteries and right ventricular hypertrophy often give the appearance of a boot-shaped heart. TTE is diagnostic and in the vast majority of cases sufficient for comprehensive assessment of the morphology prior to surgery.

Treatment: In symptomatic neonates with significant cyanosis or duct-dependent pulmonary circulation, a palliative intervention to improve pulmonary blood flow may be required: e.g. modified Blalock-Taussig shunt or RVOT stent. Complete repair is usually performed electively in infancy, with closure of the VSD, relief of the right ventricular outflow tract obstruction and pulmonary valve stenosis (Figure 5.5B). The surgical mortality risk is reported as less than 5%.

Prognosis: Surgical repair is associated with excellent short- and medium-term survival rates. The 30-year actuarial survival for patients repaired before their fifth birthday is 90% of the expected survival rate and the annualised risk of death triples in the third postoperative decade. Late morbidity is characterised by atrial and ventricular arrhythmias, and the haemodynamic consequences of pulmonary regurgitation due to surgical relief of RVOT obstruction in infancy.

LEFT HEART OBSTRUCTIVE LESIONS

Left-sided obstructive lesions such as aortic stenosis (AS) and coarctation result in an increase in the pressure proximal to the lesion. Increased ventricular afterload leads to adaptive ventricular hypertrophy. Hypertrophy leads to increased myocardial oxygen consumption and possible myocardial ischaemia and fibrosis.

Aortic Stenosis

Prevalence: The prevalence of AS is 0.19 per 1000 births, accounting for 2.3% of CHD. Aortic valve disease is more common in males than females. A bicuspid aortic valve is seen in 1% of the general population.

Aetiology and Classification: AS can be valvar, subvalvar or supravalvar. Valvar and subvalvar lesions can develop in association with other left-sided obstructive lesions. Subvalvar stenosis may be a discrete membrane or a diffuse tunnel-like obstruction. Most AS is mild and obstruction at any level may be progressive.

Clinical Presentation: Severe AS can present in the neonatal period with signs of cardiac failure, critical aortic stenosis and aortic atresia being significant duct-dependent lesions. Older children with severe lesions may present with syncope or chest pain on exertion. Pulses are weak in severe valvar AS. A thrill may be palpable suprasternally and the apex beat may be hyper-dynamic. An ejection systolic click indicates a stenotic aortic valve. The aortic component of the second heart sound may be reduced and can be delayed until after the pulmonary component (reversed splitting).

Diagnosis: Left ventricular hypertrophy may be identified by high left-sided voltages on ECG. If stenosis is severe, evidence of myocardial ischaemia or strain may be evident (ST depression and T-wave inversion). Echocardiography is used to identify the site and extent of the stenosis.

Treatment and Management: Symptomatic patients or progression of the stenosis warrant intervention to relieve the obstruction. The exact gradient at which these changes become apparent varies between patients. In general, if the pressure gradient between the left ventricle and ascending aorta exceeds 64 mmHg (non-invasively measured by Doppler ultrasonography using the modified Bernoulli equation) treatment is required.

Optimal treatment is the subject of major debate and institutional approaches can vary. Treatment options include transcatheter balloon valvuloplasty or surgical repair. Each case is assessed individually, to decide on the most appropriate course. Currently, at our centre, surgical repair is the favoured initial intervention.

Prognosis: Often the initial intervention is not curative treatment and later in life additional interventions or aortic valve replacement may be required. Valve replacement in younger patients may utilise the Ross procedure rather than using a prosthetic valve. In the Ross procedure the patient's native pulmonary valve is used to replace the damaged aortic valve, and then a homograft connects the right ventricle to the pulmonary artery. This process allows growth of the valves and eliminates the need for anticoagulation.

Coarctation

Prevalence: The prevalence of coarctation of the aorta (COA) is 0.29 per 1000 births. It accounts for 3.6% of congenital heart defects. The condition is more common in boys, with a 2:1 sex ratio. Coarctation may occur in combination with other forms of congenital heart disease, most notably bicuspid aortic valve in approximately 50% of patients (conversely coarctation occurs in approximately 5% of patients with bicuspid valves).

Aetiology and Classification: Morphologically, COA is a localised intraluminal projection of a 'shelf' from the posterior or lateral wall of the isthmus in the region of the ductus arteriosus (Figure 5.6). COA is also often associated with a variable degree of hypoplasia of the transverse arch. Turner syndrome is the most frequent chromosomal abnormality associated with COA. This, together with the male preponderance suggests an X-chromosome dosage effect.

Clinical Presentation: COA may be detected antenatally by foetal echocardiography or present postnatally after ductal closure. As the ductus arteriosus closes after birth, the degree of aortic obstruction becomes progressively more severe, resulting in reduced systemic perfusion, acutely increased afterload and cardiogenic shock. Clinically infants have reduced femoral pulses. In older children and adults, less severe forms of COA may present with secondary hypertension.

Treatment and Management: Initial medical treatment of severe neonatal COA includes resuscitation and initiation of intravenous prostaglandin therapy to maintain or restore ductal patency. Treatment options for correction of COA include surgery, percutaneous balloon angioplasty, and endovascular stent implantation. Whilst surgery is the dominant treatment choice for native COA in neonates, balloon angioplasty and/or stent implantation are commonly used for treatment of recurrent or native COA in older children and adults.

Prognosis: Persistence or recurrence of the COA is a known complication of the repair in a small but significant number of patients. Repeat intervention can be required in 10% of patients.

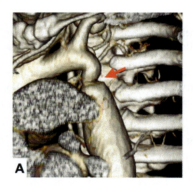
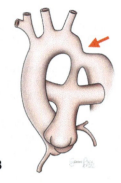
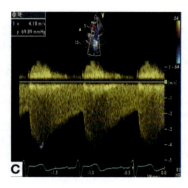

Figure 5.6 A. Volume render of a CT showing coarctation of the aorta (red arrow). B. Diagram of coarctation of the aorta (red arrow), this image also shows a patent ductus arteriosus, which in the neonatal period can provide an anatomical bypass of the obstruction and can be maintained patent with prostaglandin infusions. C. Continuous wave Doppler echo across a severe coarctation, showing the typical pattern of continuous antegrade flow during diastole.

Regardless of the specific intervention the aorta in patients with COArepair remains abnormal. This group of patients remains at risk of complications such as hypertension as well as the need for repeat intervention. Life-long follow-up is necessary to identify and treat these if they occur.

TRANSPOSITION OF THE GREAT ARTERIES (TGA)

Prevalence: TGA is the second most common cyanotic cardiac lesion (after tetralogy of Fallot), with a prevalence of 0.3 per 1000 births, accounting for 3.8% of all congenital heart disease. It is the most common cyanotic lesion to present in the neonate and is more common in males than females.

Aetiology and Classification: TGA exists when the pulmonary artery originates from the LV and the aorta arises from the RV (ventriculo-arterial discordance) (Figure 5.7A). TGA can also be found in a more complex form in in association with other cardiac lesions. The aetiology is unknown and likely multifactorial. In simple TGA, the pulmonary and systemic circulations operate in parallel rather than in series. Deoxygenated blood circulates from the right atrium to the right ventricle into the aorta and around the body returning via the vena cava to the right-sided system; oxygenated blood returns from the lungs into the left atrium, left ventricle and exits via the transposed pulmonary artery back to the lungs.

Clinical Presentation: The presentation is generally cyanosis without respiratory distress soon after birth. It is incompatible with prolonged survival unless mixing of oxygenated and deoxygenated blood can occur. Mixing usually occurs at atrial level via the foramen ovale (or ASD) and through a patent arterial duct. Patency of the arterial duct is achieved through the administration of intravenous prostaglandin after birth. The presence of a large VSD may provide adequate mixing. For some babies with simple TGA, there is only a foramen ovale and they can be very cyanosed at birth. An emergency balloon septostomy may be required in these cases to increase the atrial communication size. This is performed using a balloon catheter from the femoral vein or umbilicus directed across the foramen ovale. The balloon is inflated and pulled back across the septum to create a larger hole in the atrial septum. Many babies have the diagnosis made in foetal life (Figure 5.7B). It remains challenging to predict which babies will have restriction at the atrial level and will require balloon atrial septostomy and they all need careful evaluation after birth.

Differential Diagnosis: Other forms of congenital heart disease with restricted pulmonary blood flow will present with cyanosis. The diagnosis can be aided with the typical clinical findings, a prominent second heart sound as the aorta is more anteriorly placed in the chest with 'egg on a string' appearance on CXR. Definitive diagnosis can be confirmed with an echocardiogram.

Treatment: TGA is incompatible with survival without surgical correction. If there is an antenatal diagnosis, then delivery in a maternity unit where paediatric cardiology is available. Intravenous prostaglandin infusion should be commenced after birth to maintain patency of the ductus arteriosus and a clinical assessment performed to determine if a balloon atrial septostomy is required. Corrective surgery for simple TGA is the arterial switch repair with anatomical correction for the transposed arteries (Figure 5.7C). The transfer of the coronary arteries can

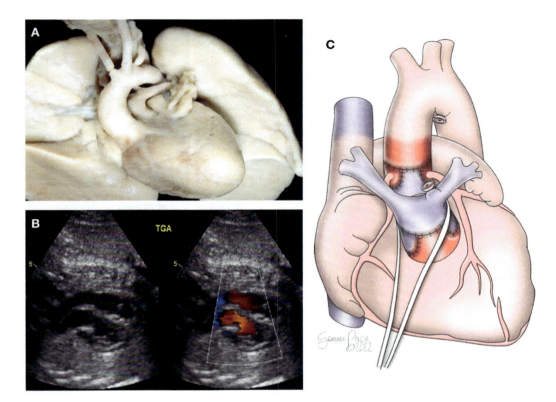

Figure 5.7 A. Post mortem specimen of transposition of the great arteries, the aorta arising from the right atrium and the pulmonary trunk from the left ventricle. B. Foetal echocardiogram of transposition of the great arteries demonstrating the classic parallel great arteries. C. Arterial switch operation for TGA. The aorta and pulmonary arteries are transected and anastomosed to the root of concordant ventricle. The pulmonary artery now lies anterior to the aorta and the branch pulmonary arteries straddle the aorta (the LeCompte manoeuvre). The coronary arteries are dissected and reimplanted to the neo-aortic root.

be technically challenging but over time with increased surgical experience the outcome has improved greatly.

Prognosis: The long-term outlook is very good after surgery in simple TGA with a 96% survival at 20 years. Several long-term consequences are recognised, including neopulmonary stenosis, neoaortic regurgitation and neoaortic root dilatation. Long-term follow up is required in this population and 2–8% of patients may require intervention, including balloon angioplasty, transcatheter stenting or surgical patch arterioplasty of the pulmonary arteries. There has been a high frequency of neurodevelopmental abnormalities reported in these patients. All TGA patients should have neurodevelopmental evaluation ideally in early childhood.

EBSTEIN ANOMALY OF THE TRICUSPID VALVE

Prevalence: The prevalence of Ebstein anomaly is 0.044 per 1000 and represents 0.5% of CHD.

Aetiology and Classification: Ebstein anomaly is a congenital abnormality of the tricuspid valve and RV with the following components: (1) adherence of the tricuspid leaflets to the underlying myocardium (failure of delamination); (2) anterior and apical rotational displacement of the functional annulus; (3) dilation of the 'atrialised' portion of the right ventricle with variable degrees of hypertrophy and thinning of the wall; (4) redundancy, fenestrations and tethering of the anterior leaflet; (5) dilation of the right AV junction (the true tricuspid annulus); and (6) variable ventricular myocardial dysfunction (Figure 5.8A). Maternal use of lithium in the first trimester is associated with a modest increase in the risk of Ebstein anomaly (approximately two additional cases per 100 births).

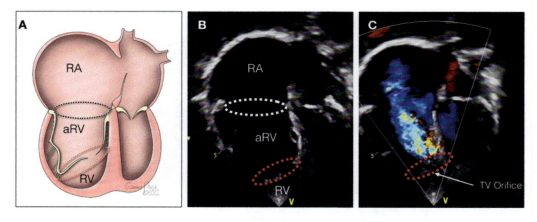

Figure 5.8 A. Echocardiographic image of the Ebstein anomaly. The expected position of the normal tricuspid valve (TV) is illustrated by the white ellipse. In Ebstein anomaly the tricuspid valve is apically displaced and rotated (Red ellipse) producing an 'atrialised' right ventricle (aRV). The overall size of the right atrium (RA) is increased and the functional right ventricle (RV) is reduced. This is associated with severe tricuspid regurgitation. B and C. Echocardiographic appearances are shown as a colour flow map, with regurgitation appearing as a blue jet.

Clinical Presentation: The degree of displacement and the severity of associated tricuspid regurgitation determines the clinical presentation. Mild cases may go undetected or present in adulthood. In severe cases there is gross right atrial enlargement and raised right atrial pressure, which may produce severe cardiomegaly in the neonatal period. The anomaly is usually associated with an ASD and, therefore, right-to-left shunting at the atrial level and subsequent cyanosis may occur. *CXR:* Ebstein anomaly results in gross enlargement of the cardiac contour with a prominent curved right atrial border on the plain chest radiograph. *ECG:* Right atrial enlargement with P-wave enlargement, and right bundle branch block are characteristic. Ebstein anomaly is associated with accessory pathways and may result in a delta wave. *Echocardiography* is sufficient for diagnosis and allows characterisation of the morphological features and assessment of the severity of tricuspid regurgitation (Figures 5.8B and 5.8C).

Treatment and management: Treatment is dependent on the severity of the lesion and the age of the patient. Mild cases may be managed conservatively. Atrial arrhythmia due to atrial dilatation is common in adulthood and may require pharmacological treatment or electrophysiological ablation. Surgical repair of the tricuspid valve may be considered in selected cases.

Prognosis: Prognosis is dependent on the severity of the lesion. Severe neonatal Ebstein anomaly may be life-threatening.

TRUNCUS ARTERIOSUS (COMMON ARTERIAL TRUNK)

Prevalence: The prevalence of truncus arteriosus is 0.078 per 1000 and represents 0.98% of CHD.

Aetiology and Classification: Truncus arteriosus is defined as a single arterial trunk arising the heart, which overrides a large misaligned VSD (Figure 5.9). The pulmonary, systemic and coronary arteries all originate from the trunk. This produces the physiological pattern of cyanosis caused by intracardiac mixing because the simultaneous ejection of both ventricles into the common trunk merges streams of blood. The morphological classification of common arterial trunk depends on the branching pattern of the pulmonary artery. The truncal valve is often abnormal (bicuspid, tricuspid or quadricuspid) with varying degrees of stenosis and regurgitation. Truncus arteriosus is frequently associated with interruption of the aortic arch (~13%)

Clinical Presentation: Cyanosis may be seen immediately after birth. Signs of heart failure may manifest within days to weeks, due to the fall in pulmonary vascular resistance after birth. Antenatal diagnosis or identification of cyanosis at newborn checks are the commonest modes of presentation. Rarely, infants present with dyspnoea or failure to thrive. Occasionally patients may survive to adulthood without treatment, invariably with pulmonary vascular disease. Echocardiography is sufficient to define the morphological features, particularly the characteristics of the truncal valve.

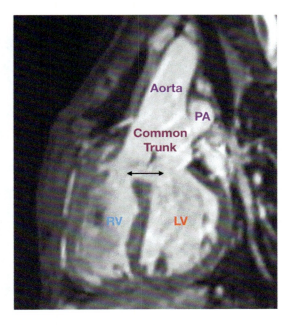

Figure 5.9   Cardiac MRI image of an unrepaired truncus arteriosus in an older child. A single common trunk arises from the heart, overriding a large VSD (double headed arrow). The pulmonary artery (PA) and the aorta arise from the common trunk, receiving mixed blood from the LV and RV.

Treatment and Management: Definitive surgical repair consists of reconstruction of the common trunk to produce a systemic vessel from the left ventricle, patch closure of the VSD and establishment of a right ventricle-to-pulmonary artery conduit.

Prognosis: The prognosis is influenced by morphological features, particularly the function of the truncal valve. Late revision of the right ventricle-to-pulmonary artery conduit is likely.

TOTAL ANOMALOUS PULMONARY VENOUS CONNECTION/DRAINAGE (TAPVD)

Prevalence: The prevalence of TAPVD is 0.08 per 1000 and represents 1.5% of CHD.

Aetiology and Classification: Pulmonary veins may connect abnormally to a site other than the left atrium – usually the right atrium, systemic veins or coronary sinus. If all the veins connect abnormally, then it is described as total anomalous pulmonary venous connection/drainage (TAPVD). In TAPVD, a complete left-to-right shunt causes all of the pulmonary venous return to mix with the systemic venous return, causing cyanosis. Survival is dependent on obligatory right-to-left shunting of the mixed pulmonary venous and systemic venous blood, usually at atrial level.

Morphology: In TAPVD the pulmonary veins coalesce posterior to the left atrium but do not drain into it. Drainage from this venous confluence to the right atrium may be: (a) via either an ascending vein to the innominate vein and then to the SVC (supracardiac, 50% of patients) (Figure 5.10A and 5.10B); (b) the coronary sinus directly into the right atrium (cardiac, 15% of patients); (c) via a descending vein, which passes through the diaphragm into either the IVC or portal venous system (infracardiac, 25% of patients); or (d) a mixture of these routes may co-exist (mixed, 10% of patients) (Figure 5.10C and 5.10D).

Clinical Presentation: The clinical presentation depends on the type of TAPVD, and if there is obstruction to pulmonary venous return (more common in infracardiac TAPVD). In the absence of obstruction, patients may present with mild cyanosis or failure to thrive. TAPVD with venous obstruction has a more severe presentation associated with marked cyanosis, respiratory distress, and pulmonary oedema usually occurring within 24 to 36 hours of birth. Obstructed TAPVD should always be considered in the differential diagnosis of PPHN.

Diagnosis: The CXR is helpful with diagnosis and may show the sites of venous dilation and the presence of pulmonary oedema in obstructed TAPVD. Echocardiography establishes the diagnosis but can be challenging in the case of obstructed infracardiac TAPVD. In complex cases,

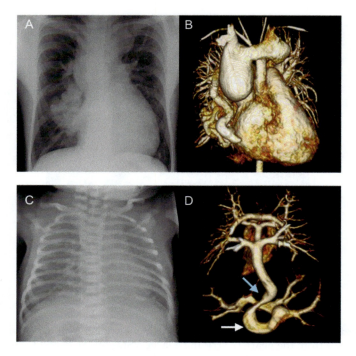

Figure 5.10 Supracardiac total anomalous pulmonary venous drainage (A and B). A. CXR in a teenager with a late presentation of supracardiac total anomalous pulmonary venous connection. (B) MRI from the same patient. Note the dilated SVC and right-sided pulmonary veins, which had some evidence of obstruction. The patient subsequently underwent complete repair. Infracardiac Total Anomalous Pulmonary Venous Drainage (C and D). (C) CXR in a newborn infant presenting with cyanosis and respiratory distress showing pulmonary oedema. (D) MRI showing total anomalous infracardiac drainage of the pulmonary veins in the same patient. Note the narrowing of the veins as they pass through the diaphragm (blue arrow) before draining into the portal vein (white arrow).

cross sectional imaging may be required to identify all the sites of pulmonary venous drainage (Figure 5.10).

Treatment and Management: Medical management is directed towards stabilisation prior to surgical repair, including mechanical ventilation and treatment of pulmonary oedema. Definitive surgical repair depends on the site of the TAPVD but is intended to redirect all pulmonary venous return to the left atrium.

Prognosis: The prognosis following repair of TAPVD is generally good with higher mortality in the early postoperative phase. Patients surviving the first year after operation have an excellent prognosis. Rare complications include residual narrowing at the surgical connection of the pulmonary venous confluence to the LA. Rarely there can be delayed pulmonary vein stenosis requiring re-operation.

SINGLE VENTRICLE CHD

Classification: The term 'single ventricle' covers a wide range of different cardiac morphologies, for example hypoplastic left-heart syndrome (0.18 in 1000 births), tricuspid atresia (0.12 in 1000 births) or pulmonary atresia with intact ventricular septum (0.1 in 1000 births); however, pragmatically, the term can be used to describe a group of patients who, following surgical 'correction', have a circulation supported by one ventricle. Modern palliative management has resulted in long-term survival for many patients who would otherwise have died as infants.

This definition also extends to include some hearts with two ventricles, for example where two ventricles are connected by a large VSD, but which cannot be surgically septated because of AV valve apparatus straddling the ventricular septum (chordae tendinae attached to the septal crest

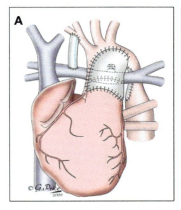
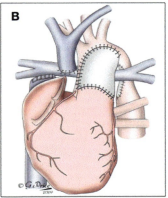
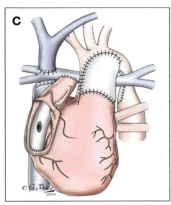

Figure 5.11 Diagrams of the staged palliative correction of single ventricle congenital heart disease, in this example Hypoplastic left-heart syndrome. The first stage occurs after birth, and the final stage is usually completed at 3–5 years of age. A. Norwood operation. B. Bidirectional superior cavo-pulmonary connection (BCPC). C. Total cavopulmonary connection (TCPC).

or opposite ventricle) or when there is significant imbalance of the ventricular chambers, such as in double inlet left ventricle or some forms of atrioventricular septal defect.

Management: The ultimate management goal is the creation of a single ventricle circuit with separation of the systemic and pulmonary circulations a Fontan or total cavopulmonary circulation – such that the single ventricle pumps blood into the systemic circulation and systemic venous return is directed to the pulmonary circulation without a ventricular pump. This is performed in a step-wise surgical fashion involving two or three stages (Figure 5.11).

Prognosis: Short- and medium-term prognosis is strongly influenced by cardiac morphology, and some infants do not survive to the completion of the Fontan circulation. For those who have completed the Fontan, recent data indicates 90% survival at 30 years. However, there is increased morbidity with age, and at 40 years only 40% will be free from a serious adverse event.

MYOCARDIAL DISEASE

Heart muscle (myocardial) disease is less common than congenital heart disease in children.

Myocarditis

Aetiologies for myocarditis include infectious, toxins and autoimmune disease. Viruses are the most common cause particularly enteroviruses (these can be particularly destructive to the myocardium) but parvovirus, coxsackie, adenovirus, influenza, chickenpox and EBV can all cause myocardial inflammation.

Presentation: Clinical presentation ranges from an asymptomatic state to fatigue, palpitations, chest pain, dyspnoea and fulminant congestive cardiac failure. Physical examination includes soft heart sounds, a prominent third sound and often tachycardia. A pericardial friction rub may be heard.

Diagnosis: Endomyocardial biopsy has traditionally been the gold standard diagnostic test for myocarditis (with specimens typically sent for histology, immunohistochemistry and polymerase chain reaction (PCR) for potential infectious agents). It is useful for diagnostic confirmation and in determining the form of myocarditis (e.g. giant-cell myocarditis, lymphocytic or sarcoid). Some patients with suspected myocarditis are considered unsuitable for endomyocardial biopsy. Additionally, myocardial inflammation is often patchy and therefore a biopsy may be non-diagnostic if unaffected tissue is biopsied.

Cardiac magnetic resonance Imaging (CMR) is an important modality for the diagnosis of myocarditis. CMR allows for targeting several features of myocarditis, inflammatory hyperaemia and oedema, necrosis/scar, contractile dysfunction, and accompanying pericardial effusion can all be visualised during a single scan (Figure 5.12).

Treatment: The underlying cause must be identified, treated, eliminated or avoided. Treatment for myocarditis is symptomatic as little evidence for immunosuppression exists. Severe cases may need mechanical circulatory support to allow a period of myocardial rest and hopefully recovery.

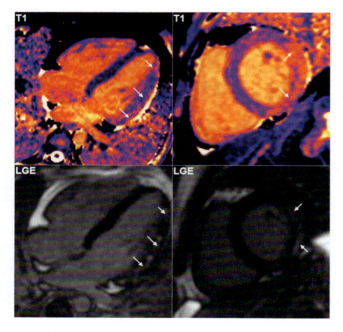

Figure 5.12 A 14-year-old boy presenting with chest pain and elevated troponin (12,000) following COVID-19 vaccination. CMR findings demonstrate elevated myocardial T1 (upper panels, arrows) in the lateral LV consistent with myocardial oedema. The patient also had sub-epicardial late gadolinium enhancement (LGE) suggesting myocardial fibrosis or scarring in the same location (lower panels, arrows).

Myocarditis can cause confusion with Dilated Cardiomyopathy (DCM) as the echocardiography appearances are similar. Typical acute myocarditis however tends to demonstrate less dilatation and lacks the thin walls of DCM.

Pericarditis

The aetiologies are similar to myocarditis, although an isolated pericardial effusion may also be bacterial and purulent.

Clinical Presentation: Typical presentation is with chest pain which is sharp, sudden in onset, retrosternal and pleuritic. Characteristically it worsens when supine and improves upon leaning forward. In 85% of cases a high-pitched scratchy sound or pericardial rub is heard on auscultation. Acute pericarditis has typical diffuse ST elevation seen on ECG, as well as low voltages, PR depression and T-wave inversions. Echocardiography can be used to demonstrate and quantify a pericardial effusion.

Treatment: The mainstay of treatment is symptomatic, bedrest and NSAIDs. Colchicine and corticosteroids are also used as adjuncts. For resistant recurrent pericarditis, specialist advice should be sought, steroids, immune modulating therapies and as a last resort surgical pericardiectomy can be considered.

The main complication is tamponade. Tamponade can occur with an acute accumulation of fluid, clinical findings include tachycardia, hypotension, increased jugular venous pressure (JVP) and pulsus paradoxus. Ultrasound guided pericardiocentesis may need to be performed as a procedure, cardiac output should be maintained using intravenous fluid and avoiding emergency diuretics.

Dilated Cardiomyopathy (DCM)

DCM is the most common myocardial disease, with an incidence of 1 in 2500. In DCM, the heart is dilated and as a result contracts inefficiently. DCM aetiologies include, end stage metabolic disease, exposure to toxins such as anthracyclines, chronic tachycardias or nutritional deficiencies such as vitamin D deficiency and hypocalcaemia.

The majority of cases are probably sporadic or inherited mutations of cardiac structural proteins. Genetic causes are varied with many cases considered isolated lesions, but all modes of inheritance are described. The DCM genetic lesions are associated with over 20 abnormal loci and genes making screening challenging. If clinically suspected, some more common genetic lesions can be screened for; these include Barth syndrome (X-linked with cyclical neutropenia) and lamin A/C mutations (often associated with skeletal myopathy and abnormal rhythms). The cardiomyopathy associated with Duchenne and Becker muscular dystrophy rarely causes symptoms before later teenage years.

In most cases of DCM, symptoms can be controlled with medical therapy for many years, but a few cases do deteriorate more rapidly, resulting in cardiomyopathy being the most common indication for paediatric heart transplantation in Europe. The cornerstone of long-term treatment for cardiac failure is currently with angiotensin converting enzyme inhibitors, beta-blocker and spironolactone. Other treatments are more geared to symptom control such as diuretics and digoxin (if the latter is used in low dose with low levels to reduce the risk of sudden death). End stage heart failure refractory to medical management can be treated with ventricular assist devices, however these patients experience high rates of VAD-related adverse events.

Restrictive Cardiomyopathy (RCM)

This uncommon cardiomyopathy is a myocardial disorder resulting from increased stiffness of the myocardium leading to impaired filling.

The aetiology is heterogeneous with diverse inherited and acquired causes and manifestations. Acquired aetiologies include infiltrative (amyloidosis, sarcoidosis) or storage diseases (Gaucher disease, mucopolysaccharidosis). Inherited mutations are noted in the sarcomere subunits and RCM also associated with some neuromuscular diseases such as BAG-3 abnormalities and myofibrillary problems.

Diagnosis: Enlargement of the atria is typically seen on echocardiogram. Biventricular chamber size and systolic function are usually normal until later stages of the disease. RCM may cause signs or symptoms of left or right heart failure.

Treatment: Treatment is aimed at the underlying aetiology, when known, and heart failure management. Usually the prognosis is poor with complications including arrhythmias, thromboembolic disease, pulmonary hypertension and heart failure.

Hypertrophic Cardiomyopathy

Incidence: Hypertrophic cardiomyopathy (HCM) is a genetic heart disease that causes abnormal thickening of the heart muscle and is associated with an increased risk of sudden cardiac death (SCD). HCM is rare in children, with an estimated prevalence of less than 3:100,000 and annual incidence between 0.24 and 0.47 in 100,000 births.

Aetiology and Pathogenesis: Most cases of HCM are caused by mutations in cardiac sarcomere proteins with autosomal dominant inheritance (albeit with variable and age-related penetrance). However, many other pathophysiological processes may produce an HCM phenotype including neuromuscular disorders, inborn errors of metabolism, or genetic syndromes (e.g. Noonan's syndrome).

Clinical Presentation: Symptomatic presentation may occur at any age, with breathlessness on exertion, chest pain, palpitation, syncope, or SCD. In children and adolescents, the diagnosis is often made during screening of relatives of affected family members. Rare presentations may also occur in the neonatal period with severe LV hypertrophy due to inborn errors of metabolism (e.g. Pompe's disease).

Treatment and Management: Investigations for diagnosis and prognosis include: 12 lead ECG, echocardiography and cardiac MRI (in older children). Arrhythmia monitoring by ambulatory ECG (Holter, implantable loop recorders) may be required to identify malignant arrhythmias. Cardiopulmonary exercise testing is utilised for arrhythmia provocation and assessment of functional capacity. Genetic testing can be used to identify mutations in affected individuals and their first-degree relatives. Management is directed towards 1. Prevention of SCD; 2. Management of symptoms; and 3. Family screening. Prevention and management of malignant ventricular arrhythmias is the cornerstone of SCD prevention. Risk factors for SCD include: previous ventricular arrhythmias (VF/VT), non-sustained VT, unexplained syncope, and extreme LVH. Whilst medical management with beta-blockage is often utilised, implantable cardioverter defibrillators (ICDs) are the primary therapy used to treat malignant ventricular arrhythmias. Unfortunately, children are at increased risk of complications associated with ICD use; therefore, appropriate patient selection is key to preventing of ICD-related morbidity at a group level. Symptom management is dependent on identifying the specific underlying cause, and may include treatment for arrhythmia, left ventricular outflow tract obstruction or heart failure management due to LV diastolic impairment. Family screening of first-degree relatives is a key element of HCM management. This process takes advantage of the autosomal dominant inheritance of sarcomeric protein mutations to identify affected individuals amongst relatives.

Prognosis: The overall five-year survival for children with presumed sarcomeric HCM is estimated at 82%. Survivors of HCM in childhood, have increased cardiovascular complications with age: at age 40 years, 40% of patients experience LV systolic impairment and 20% have atrial fibrillation.

Heart Transplantation

In Europe the main indication for heart transplantation is DCM, although congenital heart disease is an increasingly common indication. Children with severe heart disease might require mechanical support prior to transplantation. In the acute phase a temporary complete cardiopulmonary support with Extracorporeal Membrane Oxygenation (ECMO) is chosen but will need to be exchanged to a long-term solution after a few weeks.

For most children, particularly children under 10 years, an external pneumatic ventricular assist device (VAD) is used to support the LV +/- the RV. There is a high incidence of major thromboembolic complications (up to 30%); particularly in patients requiring prolonged support with extracorporeal devices. More advanced devices using impeller pump technology can be implanted in adults and adolescents. These devices have a much lower risk of thrombosis. Efforts are being made to transfer the technology to smaller children.

The most important limiting factor of a successful heart transplantation is the availability of donor organs. Advances in recent years with the inclusion of donation after circulatory death (DCD) deceased donors have increased the number of available organs substantially. Most children survive heart transplantation and in the current era approximately 60% will survive ten years after transplantation. However, very long-term survival is uncertain as accelerated coronary artery disease limits the allograft survival. Although cellular rejection is now very rare with modern immunosuppression, the drugs themselves may have side effects that include increased risk of infections, chronic kidney disease and malignancy, particularly EBV driven post-transplant lymphoproliferative disorders. Antibody-mediated rejection is more widely recognised as cellular rejection becomes less common and is difficult to treat effectively.

Heart–lung transplantation is rarely performed due to donor organ shortage. Indications are limited. There is instead a tendency to use the lungs and heart separately to benefit two recipients.

Endocarditis

Infective endocarditis (IE) is an infection of the endocardium and/or the heart valves. The infective process involves the production of thrombus (vegetation) and damage to infected tissue or valves.

Incidence: Between 0.05 and 0.12 cases of IE per 1000 paediatric admissions in the United States from 2003 to 2010.

Pathogenesis: The majority of children affected by IE have risk factors, notably pre-existing congenital heart disease, indwelling central venous catheters or rheumatic heart disease. IE arises as a complex interaction between bacteraemia, injured endothelium and components of the clotting system (fibrin and platelets).

A variety of microorganisms can cause IE, however staphylococci and streptococci species are the most common pathogens associated with IE in children, with frequencies influenced by the presence of structural heart disease. *Staphylococcus aureus* IE is associated with a more fulminant course and associated mortality.

Clinical Presentation: Subacute IE is characterised by a prolonged period of low-grade fever, fatigue, malaise, cachexia, sweating, myalgia and other non-specific symptoms. By contrast acute IE has a more rapid and fulminant course. Patients with acute IE are usually systemically unwell with high fever and may have symptoms of heart failure secondary to valve destruction or embolic phenomena.

Diagnosis: Blood cultures are key to diagnosis and are a major diagnostic criteria. *Echocardiography* to identify vegetations should be performed in patients in whom there is a reasonable suspicion of IE (e.g. risk factors of structural heart disease, indwelling central lines or other prosthetic material, persistent bacteraemia or clinical signs of endocarditis).

Treatment: Antibiotic therapy (type, dose and duration) is guided by the results of blood cultures. Surgical treatment may occasionally be required in the presence of severe valve destruction, embolic phenomena or failure of medical management.

Prognosis: Mortality is highest in patients with cyanotic congenital heart disease or infection with *Staphylococcus aureus*.

Kawasaki Disease

Incidence: The age of presentation is less than 5 years old in about 75% of the cases. The incidence is related to race and ethnicity with the highest among Asians and Pacific Islanders (Japan with almost 140 cases per 100,000 children under the age of 5 years).

Aetiology: The cause for Kawasaki disease is unknown, but an infectious cause or trigger is likely. Paediatric patients have developed symptoms with some similarity to Kawasaki disease in paediatric inflammatory multisystem syndrome (PIMS-TS) related to a COVID-19 infection.

Clinical Presentation: Kawasaki disease is an inflammatory disease including high fever, non-exudative conjunctivitis, inflammation of the oral mucosa, rash, cervical adenopathy and findings in the limbs, including swollen hands and feet, red palms and soles, and, later, sub-ungual peeling. Patients can present with carditis and valvulitis, the major cardiac and potential long-term implication result from coronary involvement and the development of coronary aneurysms.

Diagnosis: Clinical diagnosis and investigations for inflammation lead to the diagnosis of (in-)complete Kawasaki disease. TTE is used for cardiac involvement including screening for coronary ectasia or aneurysms. Cross sectional imaging with CT or angiography might be necessary in selected cases with widespread coronary involvement (Figure 5.13).

Treatment: The primary goal of the treatment is the suppression of the inflammatory process with the infusion of immunoglobulins and anti-inflammatory drug treatment. Anti-platelet or anticoagulation is used to reduce the risk of thrombus formation and myocardial infarction in affected coronaries (Figure 5.14).

Prognosis: Prognosis is dependent on severity of coronary involvement and is still not clearly defined long-term. There is concern, that even those without aneurysms may be at risk of accelerated atheromatous disease. Severe coronary involvement carries a significant risk of thrombotic obstruction, myocardial ischaemia and infarction. Rupture of large aneurysms is reported but rare. Interventional treatment with stenting of bypass grafts might be required. Acute myocardial infarction and deaths are reported in severely affected individuals.

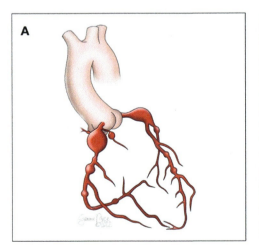 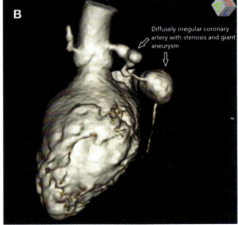

Figure 5.13 A. Diagram of locations of coronary artery aneurysms in a patient with Kawasaki disease. B. CT 3D reconstruction showing the affected coronary artery system with areas of ectasia, stenosis and giant aneurysm.

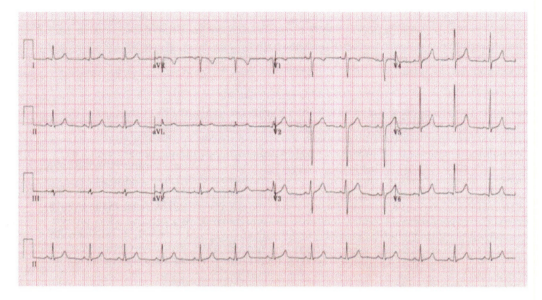

Figure 5.14 12-lead ECG with normal Sinusrhythm, normal conduction and repolarisation. Negative T-waves in the right precordial leads is a normal finding in the paediatric population.

ARRHYTHMIAS

There are various approaches to the classification of arrhythmia including, however a Depending on the resulting ventricular rate rhythm disorders are divided into tachycardic and bradycardic arrhythmias with the latter less frequent in childhood.

Tachyarrhythmias

Aetiology: The majority of tachycardic arrhythmias in otherwise healthy children are supraventricular in origin and are usually associated with a narrow QRS complex.

There are three main mechanisms of supraventricular tachycardias: 1. Re-entrant tachycardias involving the AV node (e.g. Atrioventricular re-entrant tachycardia: AVRT, AV nodal re-entrant tachycardia: AVNRT). 2. Intra-atrial re-entrant tachycardias (atrial flutter or atrial fibrillation [very rare in childhood]). 3. Increased automaticity (ectopic atrial tachycardia).

Ventricular arrhythmias are rare in children and are usually associated with a broad QRS complex tachycardia. Ventricular tachycardias may occur in patients with structural heart disease, cardiomyopathy or inherited arrhythmias (e.g. Long QT syndrome, Brugada syndrome, catecholaminergic polymorphic ventricular tachycardia).

Clinical Presentation: Symptoms vary according to the heart rate and rhythm and can range from mild to life-threatening. Symptoms of palpitations and (pre-)syncope often prompt investigation of arrhythmias. Patients may also present with a family history of arrhythmia or sudden cardiac death.

Diagnosis: ECG is the principal diagnostic tool to diagnose arrythmias. The resting ECG may identify abnormalities such as long QT, pre-excitation (delta wave [Figure 5.15]) or abnormal repolarisation which can be diagnostic for inherited arrhythmia syndromes. During an episode of arrhythmia, the ECG will distinguish between narrow and broad complex tachycardias. Specific monitoring (24-hour Holter, event and implantable loop recorders) can be utilised to diagnose arrhythmias that occur with low frequency. Additional investigations utilised include exercise or pharmacological provocation tests, and invasive electrophysiological studies.

Treatment: Patients presenting in shock need to be treated as per APLS guidelines including cardioversion if indicated. Specific treatments are based upon the underlying arrythmia. The commonest forms of SVT in childhood due to AV re-entrant mechanisms (AVRT and AVNRT) can be successfully interrupted with intravenous adenosine, which transiently slows conduction at the AV node component of the re-entrant circuit. Tachyarrhythmias originating from the

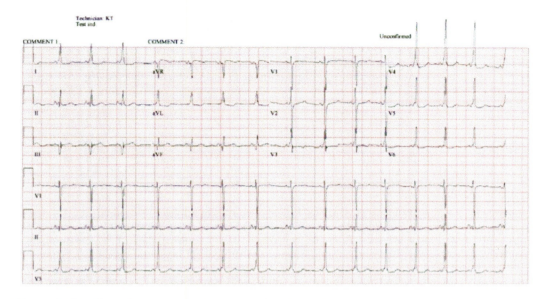

Figure 5.15 Wolff–Parkinson–White syndrome: Pre-excitation, short PR interval and delta wave in the 12-lead ECG in a patient with SVT.

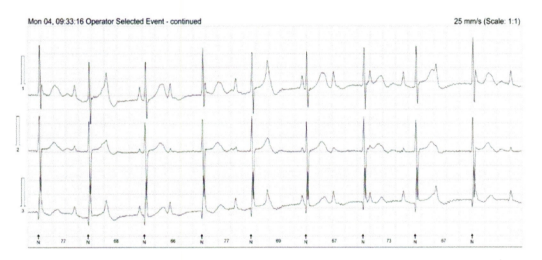

Figure 5.16 A 24-hour Holter ECG monitor with complete heart block. The P-waves have a regular rate, but there is complete atrioventricular dissociation.

atrium (atrial flutter or fibrillation) do not respond to adenosine and require pharmacological or electrical cardioversion. Chronic arrhythmias can often be managed with anti-arrhythmic drugs. Electrophysiological investigations and ablation are reserved for older patients. Patients with high risk of VT or VF might require implantation of a Cardioverter-Defibrillator (ICD) (Figure 5.16).

Prognosis: The prognosis for AVRT and AVNRT is excellent, electrophysiological ablation has a success rate of more than 90%. Other arrhythmias are more difficult to treat and might require life-long drug therapy.

Complex arrhythmias might limit life expectancy especially if associated to abnormalities of the myocardium or related to inherited channelopathies and result in progressive deterioration or sudden cardiac death.

Bradyarrhythmias

Bradyarrhythmias are rare in children. The most frequent form is congenital heart block (CHB) due to maternal autoantibodies against the foetal conduction system (SLE, Sjögren syndrome). AV-block can also occur in patients with congenital heart disease (congenitally corrected transposition of the arteries) or be acquired through damage to the conduction system (e.g. infection or surgery). Sinus node dysfunction is rare. In certain circumstances implantation of a permanent pacemaker might be required.

References

- Baltimore RS, Gewitz M, Baddour LM, et al. Infective endocarditis in childhood: 2015 update: A scientific statement from the American Heart Association. *Circulation*. 2015;132:1487–1515.
- Bondy C, Bakalov VK, Cheng C, Olivieri L, Rosing DR and Arai AE. Bicuspid aortic valve and aortic coarctation are linked to deletion of the X chromosome short arm in Turner syndrome. *Journal of Medical Genetics*. 2013;50:662–665.
- Dennis M, Zannino D, Plessis Kd, et al. Clinical outcomes in adolescents and adults after the fontan procedure. *Journal of the American College of Cardiology*. 2018;71:1009–1017.
- Driscoll D, Michels V, Gersony W, et al. Occurrence risk for congenital heart defects in relatives of patients with aortic stenosis, pulmonary stenosis, or ventricular septal defect. *Circulation*. 1993;87:I114–I120.
- Ginde S, Lam J, Hill GD, et al. Long-term outcomes after surgical repair of complete atrioventricular septal defect. *The Journal of Thoracic and Cardiovascular Surgery*. 2015;150:369–374.
- Jordan LC, Ichord RN, Reinhartz O, et al. Neurological complications and outcomes in the Berlin Heart EXCOR® pediatric investigational device exemption trial. *Journal of the American Heart Association*. 2015;4:e001429.
- Liu Y, Chen S, Zühlke L, et al. Global birth prevalence of congenital heart defects 1970–2017: updated systematic review and meta-analysis of 260 studies. *International Journal of Epidemiology*. 2019;48:455–463.
- Moosmann J, Uebe S, Dittrich S, et al. Novel loci for non-syndromic coarctation of the aorta in sporadic and familial cases. *PloS One*. 2015;10:e0126873–e0126873.
- Nollert G, Fischlein T, Bouterwek S, et al. Long-term survival in patients with repair of tetralogy of fallot: 36-year follow-up of 490 survivors of the first year after surgical repair. *Journal of the American College of Cardiology*. 1997;30:1374–1383.
- Norrish G, Field E and Kaski JP. Childhood hypertrophic cardiomyopathy: a disease of the cardiac sarcomere. *Frontiers in Pediatrics*. 2021;9.
- Patorno E, Huybrechts KF, Bateman BT, et al. Lithium use in pregnancy and the risk of cardiac malformations. *New England Journal of Medicine*. 2017;376:2245–2254.
- Yong MS, Yaftian N, Griffiths S, et al. Long-term outcomes of total anomalous pulmonary venous drainage repair in neonates and infants. *The Annals of Thoracic Surgery*. 2018;105:1232–1238.

6 Dermatology

Maanasa Polubothu

VASCULAR LESIONS – TUMOURS

INFANTILE HAEMANGIOMA

Infantile haemangioma (IH) is a common endothelial cell tumour of infancy. It involutes spontaneously over time but may require treatment depending on the site, size and associated complications (Figures 6.1 to 6.4).

Incidence

IH is the most common benign soft tissue tumour in infancy occurring in approximately 4% of newborns.

Aetiology

The aetiology is unknown, but IH are more common in placental anomalies, advanced maternal age, multiple gestation pregnancy, prematurity, females, low birth and Caucasian infants.

Classification

Superficial, deep or mixed.

- Superficial component is bright red
- Deep component is blue-tinged or may present as a skin-coloured lump

Genetics

Unknown.

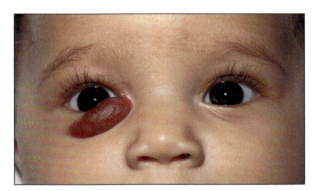

Figure 6.1 Infantile haemangioma: below the right eye threatening vision, requires treatment.

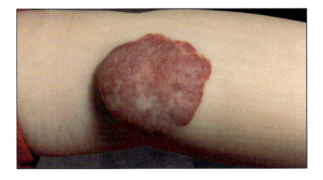

Figure 6.2 Right arm, showing signs of spontaneous resolution.

DOI: 10.1201/9781003175186-6

119

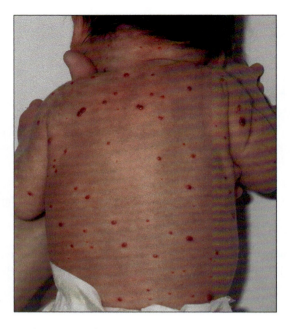

Figure 6.3 Multiple or miliary, consider screening for internal lesions.

Clinical Presentation
Lesions are not present at birth but appear within the first weeks of life. There is an initial rapid growth phase for around six months, after which they stabilise/plateau and involute spontaneously over two to ten years.

Precursor lesions can be present at birth; pallor, telangiectasias and/or ecchymotic macules.
IH is palpable as a soft lump and can be single or multiple.

Differential Diagnosis
The main differential diagnosis is with other congenital vascular tumours.

Patients should be referred if the history is not typical, or examination reveals a hard lump on palpation. Possible diagnoses include rapidly involuting congenital haemangioma (RICH), non-involuting congenital haemangioma (NICH), kaposiform endothelioma, and tufted angioma, but these benign vascular tumours must be differentiated from malignant tumours, such as infantile fibrosarcoma or rhabdomyosarcoma, which can present in the same way. Diagnosis is informed by imaging but usually requires biopsy for definitive diagnosis.

Pathology
Histology shows positive endothelial cell staining for GLUT1 (Glucose transporter-1 protein); this can differentiate IH from other lesions in cases where there is diagnostic uncertainty.

Treatment
Treatment is conservative for the majority, but patients should be referred to a paediatric dermatologist if the lesion is:

- Near important structures, e.g. eye, nose, mouth, subglottic.
- Ulcerated.
  - Ulceration affects approximately 16%; it is more common in lip and perineal IH, most commonly occurring in the first four months during the rapid growth phase.
- Bleeding significantly.
- Multiple – may need further investigation for internal haemangiomas.

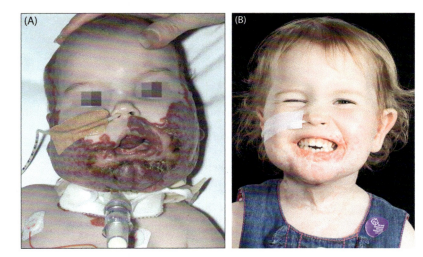

Figure 6.4   Infantile haemangioma: (A) extensive plaque-like haemangioma associated with subglottic lesion requiring tracheostomy, showing resolution with propranolol treatment (B).

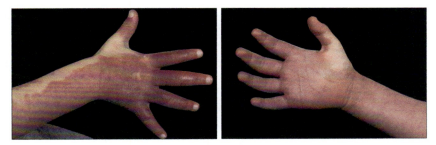

Figure 6.5   Port wine stain of the right hand and forearm.

■ Plaque-like segmental lesions of the head and neck may be associated with intra-cerebral anomalies and/or cardiac or large vessel anomalies (PHACES syndrome), or those of the lumbosacral region may be associated with urogenital or spinal anomalies (LUMBAR syndrome).

  • Small, superficial IHs can have a good response to topical timolol.

  • Systemic treatment of choice is currently oral propranolol.

  • For ulceration +/− bleeding, treatment is wound care.

Prognosis

Prognosis is generally excellent, although up to 15% result in disfigurement, airway or visual obstruction, or ulceration thus highlighting the need to refer to the tertiary care early in these cases.

VASCULAR LESIONS – MALFORMATIONS

STORK MARK (NAEVUS SIMPLEX)

This is a very common flat pink lesion, present at birth in 30–40% of newborns. It is usually located on the forehead, eyelids, occiput, or midline of the back. It may be V-shaped on the forehead/occiput. Facial lesions fade, but occipital tend not to. The lesions are not pathological, so no active management is needed.

CAPILLARY MALFORMATION

This is a relatively common congenital and permanent malformation of capillaries (Figure 6.5). It may be associated with ocular and/or neurological abnormalities (Sturge–Weber syndrome) when affecting the forehead/upper eyelid, or with other genetic conditions (for example, the *PIK3CA*-related overgrowth syndromes, phakomatosis pigmentovascularis).

Prevalence

Prevalence of 0.3%.

Aetiology

Caused by somatic activating genetic mutations thought to be specific to capillary endothelial cells.

Classification

Can be diffuse or localised and segmental.
  Can be clearly demarcated or reticulate (net-like).

Genetics

Somatic activating mutations in *GNAQ, GNA11, PIK3CA* and *PTPN11*.

Clinical Presentation

- Present from birth, it will not grow independently but is permanent.
- Macular (flat), red/purple/pink lesion; changes colour intensity with heat/emotion.
- Well-defined edges or can be reticulate (net-like).
- May be associated with subtle overgrowth of the affected face, including the lip and gingiva, or overgrowth/undergrowth of the affected limb.
- Blanches under pressure.
- Full systems examination to look for any associated abnormalities with a focus on neurological examination, including head circumference due to the association of megalencephaly-capillary malformation syndrome and Sturge–Weber syndrome.
- If present on the forehead, it requires brain MRI with contrast due to the association with Sturge–Weber syndrome.
- Risk of glaucoma with forehead and periocular capillary malformations.

Differential Diagnosis

Differential diagnosis included naevus simplex (stork mark), cutis marmorata (both should fade with time) and infantile haemangioma, arteriovenous malformation, and lympho-venous anomalies in their early stages.

Pathology

Histopathology shows ectatic vessels of variable calibre located in the papillary and upper reticular dermis.

Treatment

- Refer to paediatric dermatology for assessment of response to pulsed-dye laser therapy and camouflage make-up.
- If any lesion affects the forehead or the upper eyelid, refer to the ophthalmologist for urgent assessment to exclude raised intraocular pressure; glaucoma can be present from birth.
- Refer for neurological assessment +/− MRI/MRA of the brain if affecting the forehead or the upper eyelid.
- Skin biopsy (if capillary malformation is not on the face) for genotyping, especially if associated with other abnormalities.
  - Offer psychological support and refer to patient support groups.

Prognosis

Capillary malformations persist throughout life. Hyperplastic skin changes and nodular areas may develop in late adolescence/adulthood and are more common on the face.

VENOUS MALFORMATIONS

Venous malformations (VM) are congenital slow-flow malformations of the veins.

Incidence

Estimated at 1–5 in 10,000.

Aetiology

Somatic activating mutations in key genes involved in angiogenesis or cell growth lead to a focal area of dilated and dysfunctional veins deficient in smooth muscle cells.

Classification

Can be sporadic (> 90%), usually unifocal, or familial, which can be multifocal.

Sporadic VM can be isolated or associated with overgrowth and lymphatic anomalies.

Genetics

Somatic activating mutations in *TEK*, *PIK3CA* in sporadic VM or *TEK, GLOM1* in familial.

Clinical Presentation

- Malformations are present from birth but may not be initially noticed (Figure 6.6).

- Occur as bluish discolouration, lumps, pain or swelling, and change in size with activities and posture, and can be exacerbated by trauma.

- Can occur anywhere in the skin, including mucosal surfaces, soft tissue viscera and even bone.

- Can be localised or extensive.

- Can be associated with overgrowth, such as in segmental overgrowth syndromes (Figure 6.7).

- Complications include pain, restricted movement, thromboses and a bleeding coagulopathy, usually localised intravascular coagulopathy, disfigurement and hemarthroses leading to joint contractures.

- Phleboliths can occur from two years caused by intralesional thrombosis and subsequent calcification.

Differential Diagnosis

Deep infantile haemangiomas, lymphatic anomalies.

Pathology

Ectatic, poorly defined venous channels form a complex network that can permeate normal tissues or enlarged venous channels.

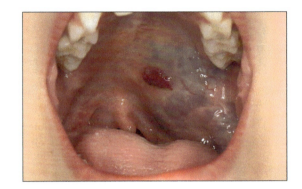

Figure 6.6   Venous malformation involving the palate.

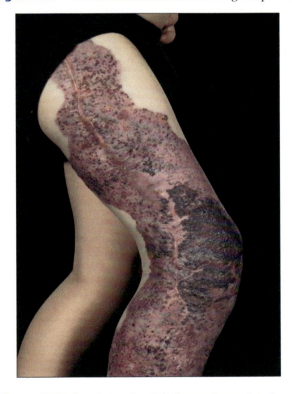

Figure 6.7   Involving the right leg and associated with growth dysregulation and a lymphatic component.

Treatment

- Patients should be referred to a tertiary vascular anomaly centre for investigation.

- Ultrasound Doppler/MRI to assess flow and extent of malformation.

- Assessment of possible associated abnormalities.

- Compression, sclerotherapy or surgery, medical therapy with targeted therapies can be considered in symptomatic progressive cases if required.

- Biopsy for histopathology and genotyping can be helpful; blood for genotyping is recommended if familial presentation.

Prognosis

Venous malformations can slowly dilate with age without intervention.

ARTERIOVENOUS MALFORMATIONS

Extracranial arteriovenous malformations are rare congenital high-flow malformations of arteries and veins. They are often difficult to manage and are associated with significant morbidity.

Incidence

Rare; exact incidence unknown.

Aetiology

Somatic mutations in key genes in angiogenesis, either single somatic activating mutations in sporadic AVM, or second-hit somatic mutations on the background of a germline mutation in familial AVM syndromes.

Classification

Can be sporadic or familial, such as in CM-AVM syndrome or hereditary haemorrhagic telangiectasia syndromes.

Genetics

Somatic activating mutations in *KRAS*, *BRAF* and *MAP2K1* in sporadic AVM, *RASA1* and *EPHB4* in CM-AVM syndrome, and *ENG*, *ACVRL1*, *GDF2* and *SMAD4* in hereditary haemorrhagic telangiectasia syndromes.

Clinical Presentation

- May be evident at birth or present in childhood, with rare cases in in adolescence.

- Present as a vascular stain with increased temperature, a palpable pulsation, audible bruit.

- Progress over time with enlargement, dilated veins, local tissue ischemia and dystrophic skin changes; progression may be exacerbated by puberty.

- Can cause pain and high-pressure bleeding.

- High-output cardiac failure can occur in the final stages; regular cardiac examination is crucial, and should consider baseline ECHO.

Differential Diagnosis

Port wine stain, infantile haemangioma, low-flow vascular anomalies, congenital vascular tumours.

Pathology

Malformed capillaries, venules, arteries and arterioles. Abrupt changes in the thickness of the medial and elastic layers of vessels with abnormal vessel dilatation.

Treatment

- Refer to the tertiary vascular anomaly centre for MDT management, including surgery, interventional radiology, dermatology, genetics and psychology.

- Ultrasound Doppler/MRI/angiography to assess flow, extent of lesion and feeding vessels.
- Embolisation/surgery if possible and genetic testing to determine eligibility for targeted therapies.

Prognosis

AVMs progress and enlarge with acceleration of growth during puberty and pregnancy.

PIGMENTARY LESIONS

POST-INFLAMMATORY PIGMENTARY CHANGES

Normal skin pigmentation can be increased or decreased during and following inflammation.

VITILIGO

Vitiligo is an acquired macular depigmentation associated with autoimmune conditions. Childhood onset may be associated with a better prognosis.

Prevalence

Common; affecting up to 2% of adults and children.

Aetiology

The exact aetiology is unknown, but hypotheses include immune destruction or self-destruction of melanocytes.

Genetics

Exact genetic cause is unknown but likely complex and multifactorial – several HLA types have been associated with vitiligo, and additionally multiple susceptibility loci have been identified through genome-wide association studies (GWAS).

Clinical Presentation

Lesions are not present at birth. Distribution is typically symmetrical, with lesions often coalescing to form large areas of depigmentation. There is a predilection for peri-orofacial and extensor surface skin. Patients may have a family history of autoimmune conditions.

- Complete skin depigmentation – milky white lesions (Figure 6.8)
- Not palpable
- Clear-cut edges
- Usually symmetrical, occasionally segmental

Pathology

Biopsy shows a loss of epidermal melanocytes.

Management

- Refer to a dermatologist for therapy – topical steroids and/or calcineurin inhibitors, light therapy.
- Consider single measurement of thyroid function and autoantibodies.
- Camouflage make-up.
- Psychological support.

HYPOMELANOTIC MACULES

History

Lesions can be present at birth; patients may develop new lesions, but existing lesions are usually static in childhood. They can occur at any site and may be associated with tuberous sclerosis.

Clinical Presentation

- Hypopigmented lesions.
- Classic oval shape (Figures 6.9 and 6.10).

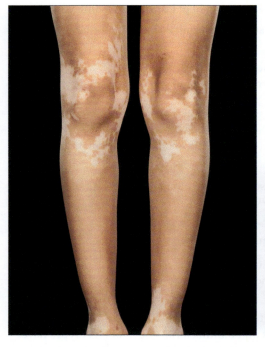

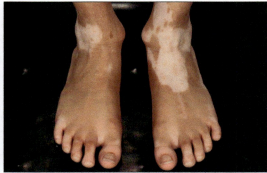

Figure 6.8 Vitiligo affecting knees and feet.

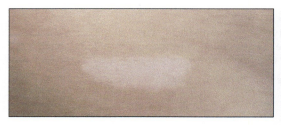

Figure 6.9 Isolated hypomelanotic macule.

- Not palpable.
- Any site but the trunk is uncommon.
- Check for other cutaneous signs of tuberous sclerosis: facial angiofibromas, shagreen patches, periungual fibromas.
- Check neurology, abdomen, heart, blood pressure.

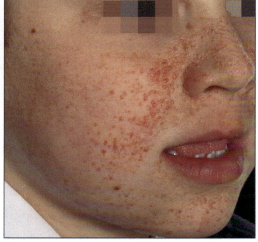

Figure 6.10 Facial angiofibromas (adenoma sebaceum) seen in tuberous sclerosis. These can be treated with topical rapamycin.

Treatment

Refer for a full assessment of tuberous sclerosis:

- MRI of the brain
- Abdominal ultrasound
- Ophthalmological assessment
- Cardiac ECHO and ECG
- Investigation of family members if a diagnosis of TS is confirmed

PIGMENTARY MOSAICISM

Pigmentary mosaicism is an umbrella term used to describe pigmentation, either hypo- or hyper-pigmentation which follows the lines of Blaschko. Described by German dermatologist Alfred Blaschko, lines of Blaschko are a pattern of lines on the skin that represent the developmental growth pattern during epidermal cell migration.

Pigmentary mosaicism can be associated with neurological or ophthalmological problems.

Aetiology

Caused by somatic mosaicism of genes affecting keratinocytes or rarely X-linked conditions, or chromosomal mosaicism.

Genetics

Can be caused by chromosomal mosaicism, somatic variants in *mTOR, KITLG, RhoA* or somatic variants or germline variants (X-linked) in *TFE3, PFH6, USP9X POLA1*; the remainder of the genetic causes are unknown.

Clinical Presentation

Lesions are usually present from birth and may extend later.

- Hypopigmented or hyperpigmented lesions

- Lesions may follow lines of Blaschko – linear on limbs, whorled on the trunk

- Not palpable

- Check neurology, teeth, eyes, head circumference

Treatment

- Refer to a paediatric dermatologist.

- Ophthalmology and neurology assessments.

- Consider a brain MRI if there are any neurodevelopmental or neurological concerns.

- Consider skin biopsy and blood tests for genetic analysis.

CAFÉ-AU-LAIT MACULES

Café-au-lait macules (CALMs) can be present at birth; patients may develop new lesions, but existing lesions are static. Lesions can appear at any site and size (Figure 6.11). Patients may have a family history of neurofibromatosis or other genetic conditions. Neurofibromatosis is a common cause of multiple CALMs, but CALMs have been described in over 200 genetic conditions, so a complete systems examination is important.

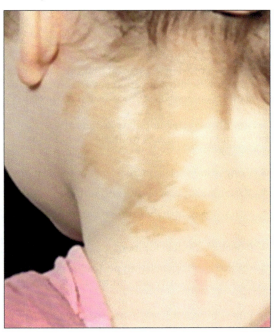

Clinical Examination

- Hyperpigmented lesions.

- Variable shape, size and site.

- Flat, not palpable.

- Check for other signs of neurofibromatosis Types 1 (NF1) and 2: axillary/inguinal freckling, cutaneous neurofibromas, plexiform neuromas, peripheral schwannomas, raised BP, scoliosis, pseudoarthroses and a full neurological examination.

Figure 6.11 *Café-au-lait* macule on the neck.

- Check for signs of early puberty and bony abnormalities seen in McCune–Albright syndrome.
- Plot growth parameters including head circumference, and look for any dysmorphic features.

Treatment

- Refer to a paediatric dermatologist for monitoring of CALMs.
- Annual ophthalmological assessment for signs of neurofibromatosis 1, plus annual BP measurement.
- MRI brain scans are not done routinely but could be considered if there are any neurological signs or developmental delay.
- If it is NF1, it usually would have six CALMs of the appropriate size (> 0.5 mm prepubertal) by the age of 6 years.

CONGENITAL MELANOCYTIC NAEVI

Congenital melanocytic naevi are moles present at birth.

Incidence

Single CMN are common and seen in 1 in 100 newborns. In severe cases CMN are multiple and extensive, seen in 1 in 20,000 people.

Aetiology

Somatic mosaicism for MAPK pathway mutations in neural crest-derived melanocytes.

Classification

CMN can be single or multiple. When multiple at birth, they can be associated with extracutaneous manifestations, including neurological and endocrine abnormalities, characteristic facies and melanoma

CMN with an extracutaneous manifestation is termed CMN syndrome.

Genetics

Somatic activating mutations in *NRAS*, *BRAF* and mosaic gene fusions.

Clinical Presentation

Lesions are present at birth, at any site, size and number, in the most severe cases affecting up to 80% of the cutaneous surface area (Figures 6.12 to 6.14).

Patients may develop new lesions after birth, and in the case of multiple CMN this is expected.

- Congenital moles, increased skin markings.
- Variable shape, size, site and number.
- Usually palpable, but sometimes not if < 0.5 cm.
- Check neurodevelopment.
- Colour heterogeneity, hypertrichosis, rugosity and nodularity are common.
- CMN tend to lighten with age, more so in the fair-skinned; this is particularly notable in scalp CMNs, which tend to blend seamlessly with the surrounding hair.

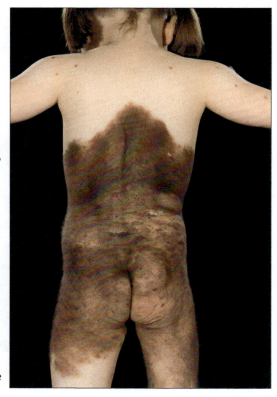

Figure 6.12 Multiple lesions in congenital melanocytic naevi.

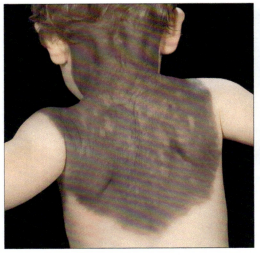

Figure 6.13 Spontaneous lightening in congenital melanocytic naevi.

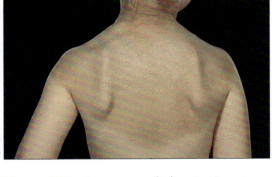

Figure 6.14 Spontaneous lightening in congenital melanocytic naevi.

Treatment

- Conservative if one lesion; refer to a paediatric dermatologist for assessment and follow-up for melanoma if:
  - More than one lesion at birth.
  - Cosmetic implications.
  - Neurodevelopmental abnormalities.
- MRI brain and whole spine with contrast if more than one lesion, to look for associated neurological melanosis/structural abnormalities/tumours.

Prognosis

- Single CMN do not tend to cause any problems.
- For multiple CMN, MRI CNS is the best indicator of prognosis with regards to neurological problems and risk of melanoma; a normal MRI CNS confers low risk.
- Absolute risk of melanoma in childhood is 1–2%.

BLISTERING CONDITIONS

EPIDERMOLYSIS BULLOSA

Epidermolysis bullosa is a group of rare genetic conditions of mucocutaneous skin fragility. Presentation and clinical course are highly variable depending on the type (simplex, junctional dystrophic, mixed) and the underlying genetic mutation.

Prevalence

Estimated at 5–20 per million for localised and 2 per million for generalised.

Aetiology

Caused by genetic changes in genes affecting key proteins which affect the attachment of layers of the skin.

Genetics

Autosomal dominant or recessive mutations in *KRT5, KRT14, PLEC, COL17A1, COL7A1, DST, EXPH5* and *KLHL24*.

Clinical Presentation

The condition is present from birth, with skin and/or mucosal fragility and blistering in response to minor skin trauma. There may be a family history of epidermolysis bullosa and this may be associated problems such as pain, hoarse cry, failure to thrive, difficulty feeding or secondary infection.

- Blistering/skin denudement in sites of handling/trauma (Figures 6.15 and 6.16), with scarring in some subtypes.

- Small white papules (milia) are present in areas of healing.

- Signs of bacterial superinfection.

- Full systems examination with minimal handling.

Management

- Immediate referral to a specialist centre for optimisation of skin care, exact diagnosis and MDT management.

- Minimise handling/procedures/ observations.

- Pain control, optimisation of nutrition.

- Skin biopsy and genetic testing for diagnosis, genetic counselling.

IMMUNOBULLOUS DISORDERS

These are rare, acquired blistering conditions, secondary to immunological attack on skin integrity and often difficult to manage. Conditions include linear IgA disease, pemphigus, pemphigoid and epidermolysis bullosa acquisita. Skin biopsy with immunostaining is diagnostic and informs further management.

INFLAMMATORY CONDITIONS

ECZEMA

Eczema is common in childhood and mainly affects atopic individuals.

Incidence

Prevalence is 10–30% of children in developed countries.

Aetiology

Complex polygenic traits and environmental influences.

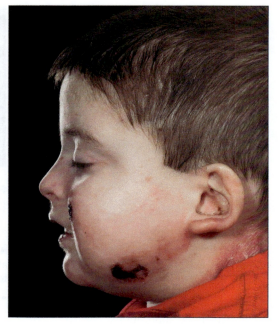

Figure 6.15 Blistering and erosions on the face in epidermolysis bullosa.

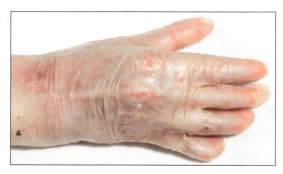

Figure 6.16 Scarring leading to 'mitten-hand' deformity in dystrophic epidermolysis bullosa.

Classification

Infantile eczema presents at three months or earlier, tends to affect the scalp and face first, spreading to the limbs and trunk, with the napkin area spared.

Childhood eczema tends to be flexural.

In puberty onwards, eczema predominantly affects the face, hands, wrists, back and dorsal feet.

Genetics

Polygenic aetiology, but genetic causes of impaired skin barrier, e.g., loss-of-function mutations in filaggrin (FLG), predispose. Multiple susceptibility loci have been identified through GWAS.

Differential Diagnosis

Seborrheic dermatitis, psoriasis, contact dermatitis, fungal infections or scabies.

Pathology

Spongiotic tissue reaction with intercellular oedema within the dermis, intraepidermal vesicles, infiltration of the epidermis with lymphocytes and parakeratosis. It can have acanthosis and hyperkeratosis. Varying degrees of oedema are seen in the dermis and a superficial lymphohistiocytic perivascular infiltrate.

Clinical Presentation

Eczema is not present at birth, but there may be a family history of atopy, +/- ichthyosis vulgaris. The severity should be assessed – sleep disrupted, faltering growth, school absence, the impact of chronic itch, steroid requirement.

Several validated eczema scores exist to assess the impact on quality of life and assess clinical severity; they should be used to monitor and assess the efficacy of treatment.

- Red, dry rash (Figures 6.17 and 6.18).

- Often flexural in childhood, but may be widespread (Figure 6.19).

- Lichenification, excoriation, oedema, weeping papules, papulovesicles and erosions, ill-defined erythema, xerosis.

- Post-inflammatory hypo/hyper-pigmentation can occur.

- Superficial bacterial infections – bright red, shiny, may have yellow crusting, warm to touch (Figure 6.20).

- Look for vesicles, roofless or crusted ulcers as signs of eczema herpeticum.

- Look out for vesicubullous eruptions which scab and can be present on affected and also unaffected skin in eczema coxsackium (enteroviral infection caused most commonly by Coxsackie A6 and A16).

- Measure growth parameters.

Treatment

- Daily baths with lukewarm water, using oily bath additives and soap substitutes.

- Regular emollients.

- Appropriate potency of topical steroid.

- Treat secondary infections where necessary.

- Refer to a paediatric dermatologist for further management if unresponsive, for:

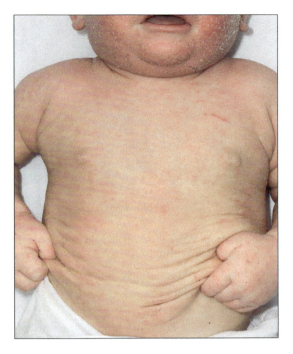

Figure 6.17   Eczema is intensely pruritic.

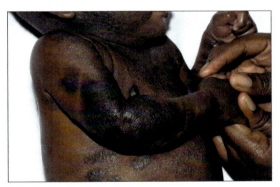

Figure 6.18   It may not appear erythematous on darker skin

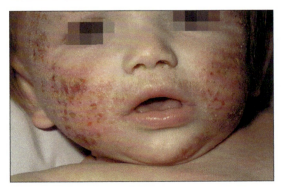

Figure 6.19   Facial eczema.

131

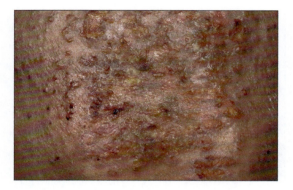

Figure 6.20 Close-up of infected eczema.

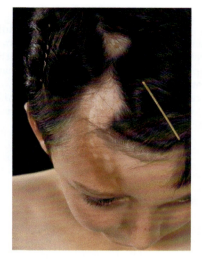

Figure 6.21 Morphea *en coup de sabre.*

- For more potent topical steroids +/– topical calcineurin inhibitors.

- Inpatient wet wrap dressings.

- Systemic treatment – azathioprine, methotrexate, rarely oral prednisolone or ciclosporin.

- Biologics – A novel recombinant human monoclonal antibody that inhibits interleukin-4 and interleukin-13 signalling (Dupilumab) is now licensed in the United Kingdom for children > 6 years who have failed systemic therapy.

■ Psychological support for children and families.

■ Use of patient support groups.

Prognosis
The majority of cases gradually improve with age, with over half of children clear by adolescence.

MORPHOEA (LOCALISED SCLERODERMA)
This is a rare, chronic scarring inflammatory disease of the skin that can affect underlying tissues. The aetiology is unknown.

Clinical Presentation
Morphoea is not normally present at birth. Lesions are initially red/pink/purple, particularly at the edges, and subsequently pale with scarring. The linear form is most common in childhood. The condition is slowly progressive. Lesions are usually asymptomatic, but long-standing lesions can lead to disability with contractures and wasting. The most severe type is *'en coup de sabre'* affecting the scalp, and can be associated with neurological problems (Figure 6.21).

■ Red/pink/purple/pale areas.

■ Poorly defined borders.

■ Older lesions are atrophic and scarred.

■ May be plaque-like or linear.

■ Growth of underlying tissues is restricted, particularly in the linear form, leading to deformity or asymmetry.

Treatment

■ Refer to a paediatric dermatologist.

■ May require systemic anti-inflammatory treatment: steroids (short-term) and methotrexate.

■ Ultrasound/MRI to assess any effects on underlying tissues.

PSORIASIS

Psoriasis is a chronic inflammatory disease of the skin. It is less common in childhood but may be under-diagnosed as eczema.

Incidence

Incidence is 40 per 100,000 in children.

Genetics

Strong family history in many cases suggests a significant genetic component. Various susceptibility loci have been identified on GWAS. HLA-Cw6 and HLA-B17 may be associated with increased susceptibility.

Aetiology

The exact cause is unknown but is characterised by epidermal hyperproliferation with a loss of differentiation, dilatation and proliferation of dermal blood vessels and inflammation.

Clinical Presentation

The child may have a family history of psoriasis. The guttate type may be triggered by a bacterial infection, classically streptococcal.

- Well-defined red patches with silvery overlying scale (Figure 6.22).

- May be in plaques, classically extensor joint surfaces/scalp, also nappy area (Figure 6.23).

- May be guttate (rain-drop-like).

- Check nails for pitting and onycholysis.

- Joints may be affected (psoriatic arthropathy).

Differential Diagnosis

Eczema, pityriasis rubra pilaris, fungal infections, seborrheic dermatitis.

Treatment

- Screen for streptococcal infection if guttate.

- Topical treatment of skin lesions with moisturisers, vitamin D analogues, steroids, coal-tar derivatives, dithranol.

- Obesity is the most common co-morbidity – refer for weight management.

- Screening for psoriatic arthritis.

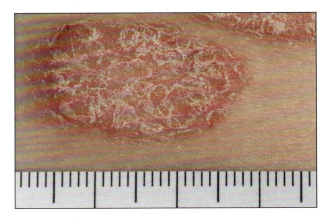

Figure 6.22   Close-up of abdominal plaque psoriasis.

133

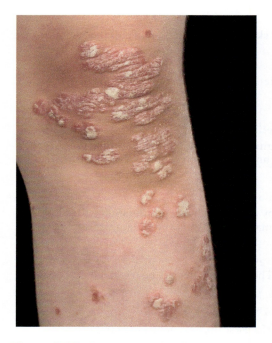

Figure 6.23 Extensor surface lesions in psoriasis.

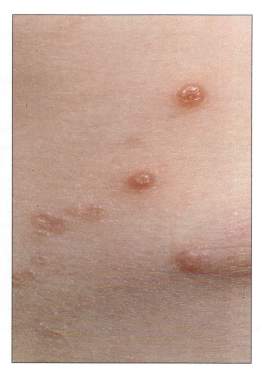

Figure 6.24 Molluscum contagiosum – papular lesions showing umbilication.

- Topical treatment of scalp lesions with oil-based moisturisers, tar-based shampoo, topical steroids or vitamin D analogues.

- Refer to a paediatric dermatologist if the patient fails to respond to conventional topical treatment or if there is a sudden deterioration and the child is systemically unwell (erythroderma or generalised pustular psoriasis).

- Options for systemic treatment include methotrexate, acitretin, ciclosporin and the newer biological anti-tumour necrosis factor (TNF) agents, as well as Interleukin 12/23 and Interleukin-17A inhibitors.

- Psychological support should be offered.

LUMPS AND BUMPS

MOLLUSCUM CONTAGIOSUM

Chronic localised infection with Molluscum contagiosum virus, a poxvirus.

History

Lesions are not normally present at birth and are progressive, with the appearance of papular, dome-shaped, flesh-coloured lesions. They are itchy and occasionally secondarily infected. There is often a contact history. Lesions can be severe in the immunocompromised child.

Examination

- Groups of flesh-coloured umbilicated papules (Figure 6.24).

Management

- Conservative for the majority, but may take two years to resolve.

- Ablative treatment with cryotherapy is of limited value.

- Imiquimod application may be appropriate for the immunocompromised child.

SEBACEOUS NAEVUS

History

Naevus is present from birth, often on the scalp but can be elsewhere. It usually flattens after six months and then remains static in childhood until puberty.

Examination

- Yellowish/skin-coloured raised naevus (Figure 6.25)
- Well-defined edges
- Slightly shiny/oily
- No overlying hair

Management

It is usual to refer for removal before the age of puberty, as rarely can it become malignant thereafter; whether this is absolutely necessary is questionable.

APLASIA CUTIS

History

This is present from birth, usually on the scalp. There is absent skin, usually healed with scarring at birth, but occasionally open at birth.

Examination

- Defect of scalp skin, atrophic/sunken once healed (Figure 6.26).
- No overlying hair.
- Well-defined edges.
- Can be single or multiple, any size.

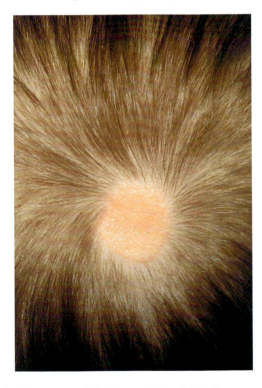

Figure 6.25 Sebaceous naevus in scalp.

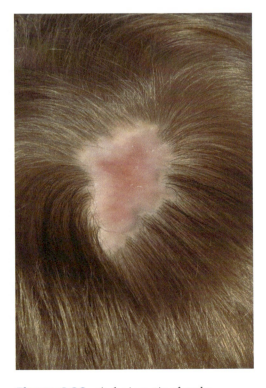

Figure 6.26 Aplasia cutis of scalp.

- Check neurology and perform a general examination for other defects if linear sebaceous naevus is present.

Management

- Consider skull x-rays, +/− MRI to look for underlying bony defects and intracerebral abnormalities if the lesions are large or multiple, or there is a clinical impression of a bony defect.

- If only a skin defect, management is conservative, but if large it may require plastic surgery.

- Skin biopsy for genotyping is necessary if associated with extracutaneous abnormalities.

OTHER IMPORTANT CONDITIONS

ACRODERMATITIS ENTEROPATHICA

This is a rare skin condition of infancy caused by the failure of zinc absorption (genetic – true acrodermatitis enteropathica), or as a result of acquired dietary zinc insufficiency, and is reversed by zinc supplementation.

Genetics

Autosomal recessive mutations in the *SLC39A4* gene, which encodes a protein that appears to be involved in the zinc transporter protein ZIP4.

Clinical Presentation

Progressive skin lesions affecting the nappy area, face and hands/feet are not present at birth but often begin after the child is weaned onto solid food. Lesions are unresponsive to any topical therapies.

- Well-defined erythematous encrusted skin lesions (Figures 6.27 and 6.28)

- Child may be failing to thrive with diarrhoea

- Alopecia is common

Differential Diagnosis

Primary immunodeficiencies, atopic eczema, epidermolysis bullosa, biotinidase deficiency, malnutrition, and severe seborrheic dermatitis.

Treatment

- Confirm the diagnosis by measuring the serum zinc level.

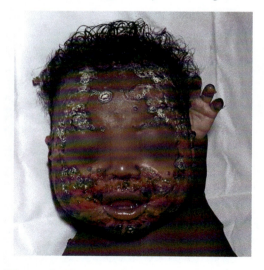

Figure 6.27 Facial lesions in acrodermatitis enteropathica.

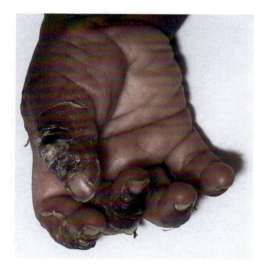

Figure 6.28 Acral lesions in acrodermatitis enteropathica.

- Oral zinc supplementation reverses skin findings within days to weeks.

- Monitor zinc levels – may require supplementation for life.

- Blood DNA for genotyping if a genetic cause suspected.

Prognosis

Prognosis is excellent with timely diagnosis and zinc supplementation.

INCONTINENTIA PIGMENTI

This is an X-linked dominant genetic condition lethal to males. It is mosaic in females and is caused by mutations in the *IKBKG* gene.

Clinical Presentation

There are four stages of skin lesions, which can overlap:

- Blistering and erythematous lesions appear in the first few weeks of life.

- Verrucous in the first few months.

- Hyperpigmented flat lesions appear in the first few years.

- Hypopigmented atrophic lesions in later childhood/adulthood.

Patients may have problems with teeth, eyes, hair growth and neurology and there may be a family history on the mother's side.

- First two stages of skin lesions follow lines of Blaschko – linear on the limbs, whorled on the trunk (Figures 6.29 and 6.30).

- Possible alopecia.

- Check teeth, eyes, neurology.

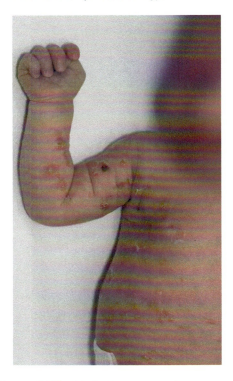

Figure 6.29 Vesiculoverrucous lesions following Blashko lines in incontinentia pigmenti.

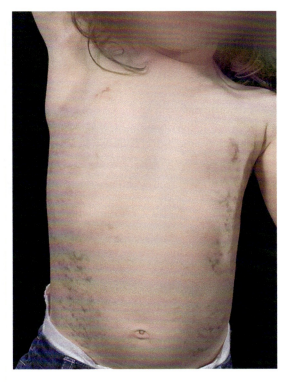

Figure 6.30 Chinese-figurate pigmentation phase in incontinentia pigmenti.

137

Treatment

- Conservative for skin lesions.

- Refer for genetic testing and counselling.

- Refer to ophthalmology, dentistry, neurology for appropriate imaging and follow-up.

CUTANEOUS MAST CELL DISEASE

This is a rare skin condition characterised by the accumulation of mast cells in tissues, either locally (solitary mastocytoma) or widespread (urticaria pigmentosa, diffuse cutaneous mastocytosis), which very rarely affects other organ systems. It is generally less severe than the adult disease and usually improves with age.

Prevalence

Prevalence is 1 in 10,000.

Genetics

Caused by mutations in *KIT*.

Clinical Presentation

The disease may be present at birth, with single (solitary mastocytoma [SM]) or multiple (urticarial pigmentosa [UP]) itchy lesions anywhere on the skin, and diffuse erythema, blistering, thickening of skin and itch (diffuse cutaneous mastocytosis [DCM]). Lesions are persistent over the years. If severe, the patient may have flushing, diarrhoea, abdominal pain and wheezing, which do not necessarily indicate systemic mastocytosis, but rather systemic effects of cutaneous mast cell release.

- SM or UP lesions are red/brown and thickened, urticate upon stroking (Darier's sign).

- Hyperpigmented macules in urticaria pigmentosa.

- DCM is Darier positive over the whole skin and the child may be generally unwell.

- Multiple triggers, including emotional, physical, infective and pharmacological.

- Check for lymphadenopathy and hepatosplenomegaly.

- Serum tryptase levels have been suggested to indicate risk of anaphylaxis.

Treatment

- Oral antihistamines and mast cell stabilisers.

- Avoid known precipitants of mast cell degranulation, including codeine, certain anaesthetic drugs and radiological contrast. Refer to a textbook for a full list of drugs and other agents.

- May cause anaphylaxis; consider EpiPen prescription if appropriate.

- Patient support groups can provide support and comprehensive documentation for parents on trigger avoidance.

Prognosis

Those with onset at less than 2 years of age have an excellent prognosis with lesions resolving by adolescence. Childhood mastocytosis is largely (> 90%) limited to the skin, unlike adult which tends to present with systemic features.

Ichthyosis

Ichthyosis is a group of genetic skin conditions in which there is dry, scaly skin from birth. Ichthyosis vulgaris is common and associated with atopic eczema. The other ichthyoses are rare and include recessive X-linked ichthyosis and autosomal recessive congenital ichthyoses.

Incidence

Ichthyosis vulgaris is the most common, affecting 1 in 250 births. X-linked ichthyosis is the next most common, affecting 1 in 6000 male births. Autosomal congenital recessive ichthyoses are rare with an overall incidence of 1 in 200,000 births.

Aetiology

Abnormalities in proteins influence epidermal structure, leading to epidermal hyperplasia accompanied by abnormal desquamation, resulting in dry and scaly skin.

Classification

Classified as either non-syndromic, affecting the skin, or syndromic, in which there is extracutaneous involvement. Non-syndromic types are rare and outside the scope of this chapter.

Genetics

Ichthyosis vulgaris is associated with genetic variants in the filaggrin gene. Recessive X-linked ichthyosis is caused by mutations in the steroid sulfatase (STS) gene. Genetic causes of ARCI include *ABCA12, ALOX12B, LOXE3A, CERS3, CYP4F22, NIPAL4, PNPLA1, SDR9C7, SULT2B1, TGM1*.

Clinical Presentation

The more severe forms can be associated with collodion baby (collodion membrane at birth, shed after a few weeks) – see the section 'Collodian Baby and Harlequin Ichthyosis'. Dry scaly skin, often from birth, is present in rarer forms. Patients have difficulty regulating body temperature, and there may be a build-up of skin scales in the ears. There may be a family history of ichthyosis.

- Dry, scaly skin may be worse in certain areas dependent on type (Figures 6.31 to 6.33).
- Skin may be normal colour or red or blistered, depending on type.
- Scalp may be involved with hair growth reduction.
- Palms may be hyperlinear.
- Check neurology as rare types are associated with neurological abnormality.

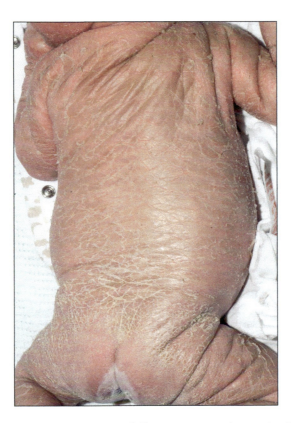

Figure 6.31 Hyperkeratosis and scaling in different autosomal recessive ichthyosis.

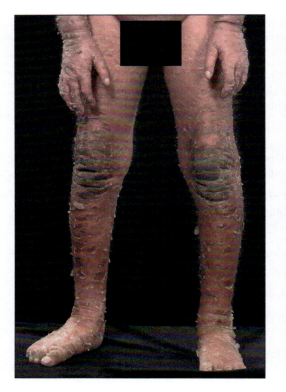

Figure 6.32 Hyperkeratosis and scaling in different autosomal recessive ichthyosis.

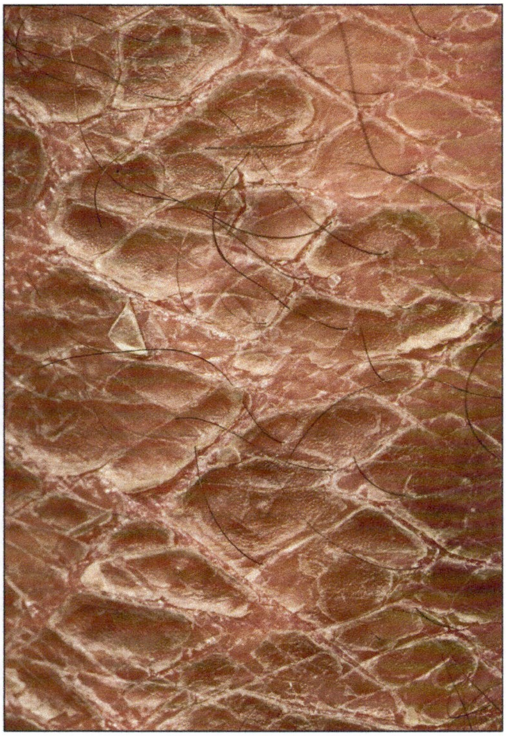

Figure 6.33 Hyperkeratosis and scaling in different autosomal recessive ichthyosis.

Pathology
Increase in the stratum corneum and loss of the normal basket weave pattern.

Management
- For ichthyosis vulgaris, moisturisers only.
- For the more severe forms, refer to a paediatric dermatologist.
- Intensive moisturising regime, oral retinoid therapy for severe ichthyosis if indicated.
- Genetic testing and counselling.

Prognosis
Ichthyoses are not curable and persist throughout life. There is a risk of transmission to offspring; thus, genetic counselling should be offered.

LINEAR EPIDERMAL NAEVI
This is a heterogeneous group of congenital lesions assumed to be caused by genetic mosaicism, which can be associated with other abnormalities. Different types are related to the cell of origin, e.g. keratinocytic or adnexal.

Genetics
Somatic activating mutations in *HRAS, KRAS, PIK3CA, FGFR, AKT1, KRT1, KRT10.*

Incidence
Occurs in 1–3 out of every 1000 births.

Aetiology

Benign hamartomatous growth of epidermal cells and structures caused by somatic activating mutations occurring during normal development.

Classification

Can be isolated to the skin or have extracutaneous associations as in epidermal naevus syndromes or in segmental overgrowth syndromes. Can involve only the keratinocytes or may also involve epidermal structures such as hair follicles, sebaceous glands and apocrine and eccrine glands.

Pathology

Hyperkeratosis, acanthosis (thickening of the epidermis and elongation of the rete ridges) and papillomatosis (projection of dermal papilla above the surface of the skin). Epidermolytic hyperkeratosis describes lysis of epidermal cells above the basal layer associated with marked hyperkeratosis – this variant is suggestive of somatic mutations in keratin 1 (*KRT1*) and keratin 10 (*KRT10*), clinically of importance as it can be passed to germline in cases of gonadal mosaicism, leading to a rare autosomal dominant germline genodermatosis.

Clinical Presentation

Epidermal naevi are usually present from birth and can extend after birth. They can be associated with other congenital abnormalities.

- Follow Blaschko's lines (Figure 6.34).
- Palpable epidermal lesions.
- Variable colour and texture dependent on type (Figure 6.35).
- Check for other abnormalities, bone abnormalities and growth parameters.

Management

- Laser therapy can be useful in certain types.

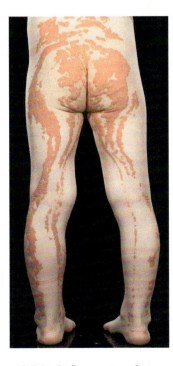

Figure 6.34 Inflammatory linear epidermal naevi.

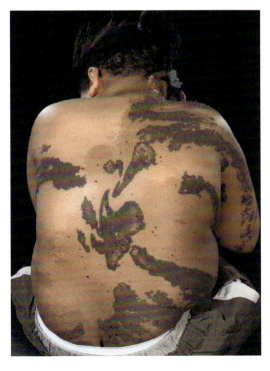

Figure 6.35 Pigmented sebaceous naevi.

141

■ Surgical excision is possible for small lesions.

■ Skin biopsy to look for epidermolytic hyperkeratosis and genetic testing – refer for genetic counselling.

Prognosis

Epidermal naevi persist throughout life and can spread. There is a possibility of gonadal mosaicism with certain types, thus inheritance in a germline fashion to offspring.

ECTODERMAL DYSPLASIA

Ectodermal dysplasia is a heterogeneous group of over 100 genetic conditions defined clinically as abnormalities of two of the following ectodermal structures: skin, hair, nails and teeth. It is very variable in severity and can be part of a broader syndrome.

Incidence

Incidence is estimated at 1–2 per 10,000 for hypohidrotic ectodermal dysplasia. Other types are very rare, and the exact incidence is unknown.

Aetiology

Abnormalities in key proteins required for developmental ectodermal appendage formation.

Classification

The most recent classification system groups disorders based on the major developmental pathway involved (*EDA*, *WNT* or *TP63*), phenotypic features and mode of inheritance.

Genetics

Classic ectodermal dysplasias are caused by genetic variants affecting the ectodysplasin signal transduction pathway (*EDA*, *EDAR*, *EDARADD*, and *IKBKG*, *GJB6*, and *WNT10A*). *TP63* related ectodermal dysplasia is caused by genetic variants in *TP63* and is associated with cleft palate/lip and limb defects.

Clinical Presentation

There may be a family history with variable inheritance patterns. Abnormalities may be obvious from birth or not until early childhood. Hair may have no or reduced rate of growth or increased breakage. Sweating may be reduced, leading to over-heating or febrile convulsions. The child may have reduced vision or hearing and may have reduced tear production and recurrent conjunctivitis.

■ Child and other family members, if appropriate.

■ Dystrophic nails.

■ Sparse or brittle hair, absent eyebrows/lashes/body hair.

■ Skin may be dry or eczematous.

■ Can be associated with immune deficiency.

■ Teeth may be reduced in number and/or abnormal in shape (Figure 6.36).

■ Characteristic facial features in X-linked hypohydrotic type (Figure 6.37).

■ Check for other congenital abnormalities, e.g. clefting, limb defects.

■ Faltering growth.

Management

■ Ophthalmology and hearing check.

■ Moisturisers for skin.

■ Education for parents in avoiding hyperthermia for hypohidrotic type children.

■ Dental assessment and long-term management.

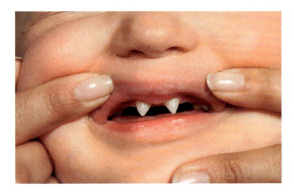

Figure 6.36 Reduced and abnormal teeth in ectodermal dysplasia.

■ Referral to relevant surgical teams for cleft and limb defects.

■ Prompt referral to immunology if a suspected immune deficiency.

■ Refer the family to genetics for counselling.

PAEDIATRIC DERMATOLOGICAL EMERGENCIES

STEVENS–JOHNSON SYNDROME AND TOXIC EPIDERMAL NECROLYSIS

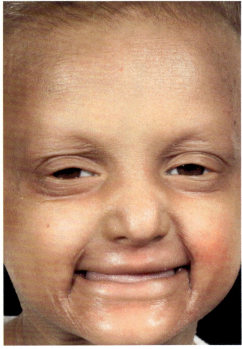

Figure 6.37 Reduced hair, dry skin and characteristic facial features in X-linked hypohydrotic ectodermal dysplasia.

These conditions comprise a rare but severe mucocutaneous reaction to infectious agents or drugs (most commonly NSAIDs, antibiotics and anticonvulsants) characterised by extensive necrosis and detachment of the epidermis. Toxic epidermal necrolysis (TEN) is usually more rapid in onset than Stevens–Johnson syndrome (SJS), more severe, affects more of the skin surface and has a poorer outcome.

Incidence

Approximately one to two per million children per year, SJS is more common than TEN 3:1 ratio.

Risk is increased in children with underlying malignancy (particularly hematological malignancies), HIV, certain HLA types, and children with genetic polymorphisms related to drug metabolism.

Classification

■ < 10% skin involved in SJS, > 30% in TEN, between 10–30% is termed SJS/TEN overlap

Clinical Presentation

There is a preceding infection or history of medication. SJS is often caused by *Mycoplasma pneumoniae* in children; TEN is usually caused by a drug (as listed above). The child becomes systemically unwell before the onset of mucocutaneous signs, with a prodrome of fever, malaise and myalgia, and arthralgia which may be accompanied by early photophobia, conjunctival irritation and difficulty swallowing. There is a sudden onset of rash and mucous membrane involvement with worsening of the clinical picture (Figures 6.38 to 6.40)

Child is unwell – can be severely toxic.

■ Skin lesions are initially red, may be target-like, subsequently large areas of blistering and skin necrosis.

■ At least two mucous surfaces are involved in SJS, always including the mouth with characteristic crusting of the lips.

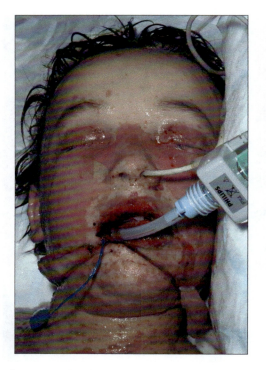

Figure 6.38 Stevens–Johnson syndrome and toxic epidermal necrolysis: acute phase followed by gradual resolution.

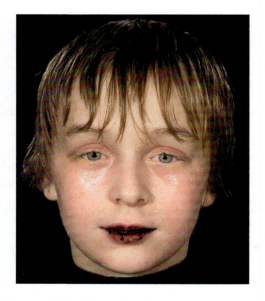

Figure 6.39 Typical oral lesions.

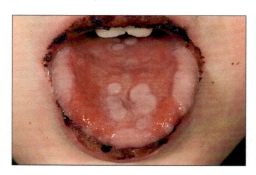

Figure 6.40 Typical oral lesions.

Genetics

As above, increased incidence in those with certain HLA types and those with genetic polymorphisms related to drug metabolism.

Differential Diagnosis

Erythema multiforme, erythroderma and erythematous drug eruptions, linear IgA bullous dermatosis, staphylococcal scalded skin syndrome.

Pathology

Histopathology shows keratinocyte necrosis, which can be partial or full thickness. Subepidermal bullae and a patchy perivascular, lymphohistiocytic, inflammatory infiltrate may be seen.

Treatment

- Urgent admission; TEN requires intensive care or a burns unit.
- Stop potentially causative medications.
- Treat with appropriate antibiotic(s) if infection is considered a likely cause.
- Fluid and temperature management.
- Pain control.
- Wound care.
- Refer to an ophthalmologist.
- Scrupulous eye and oral care.
- Skin and blood cultures for sepsis.

- For TEN, treatment options include intravenous immunoglobulin, methylprednisolone and anti-TNF biological agents.

Prognosis

Up to 10% mortality in children (greater in adults) and risk of recurrence upon re-exposure to the trigger.

STAPHYLOCOCCAL SCALDED SKIN SYNDROME

Haematogenous dissemination of exotoxin following Staphylococcus Aureus infection primarily affects children, most commonly under 6 years.

Incidence

Eight cases per million in all children, rising to 45 cases per million in children less than two years.

Aetiology

Caused by infection with exotoxin-producing strains of *Staphylococcus aureus* leading to haematogenous dissemination of exfoliative/epidermolytic exotoxins.

Clinical Presentation

There may be a history of preceding skin lesion/infection. The patient has a sudden onset fever and systemic illness with diffuse redness of the skin and the development of blistering/desquamation. Early skin signs include pain and erythema, which may initially be more prominent in the skin folds, progressing to widespread erythema within 48 hours. Later, shallow erosions or large flaccid bullae develop.

- Toxic, unwell child.

- Diffuse erythema, +/− superficial skin peeling.

- Nikolsky's sign is positive (minimal shearing pressure causes skin separation).

- May be the focus for staphylococcal entry.

- Hypovolemia and temperature instability.

Pathology

Biopsy of blisters shows subcorneal cleavage.

Treatment

- Urgent admission

- Specialist dermatology nursing

- Skin swabs and blood cultures

- IV antibiotics to cover *Staphylococcus* spp.

- Fluid management

- Pain management

Prognosis

With prompt and appropriate treatment, the prognosis is excellent, with full recovery within weeks and no scarring, although post-inflammatory pigmentary changes can occur.

COLLODION BABY AND HARLEQUIN ICHTHYOSIS

These are two distinct clinical entities; however, they have in common a similar approach to basic management soon after birth. A collodion baby is encased in a so-called collodion membrane at birth. The condition is usually associated with underlying genetic ichthyosis (of variable severity). The most severe is harlequin ichthyosis (HI). HI is potentially fatal, but good early management optimises the chance of survival.

Incidence

The incidence of autosomal recessive ichthyosis is one in 200,000, but the incidence is higher in areas of high consanguinity.

Clinical Presentation

A thickened membrane is present around the skin at birth, which eventually sheds. There may be a family history of ichthyosis.

- Child's temperature may be unstable.
- Membrane may be red, cracking, forming plates (HI).
- Edges of facial orifices may be retracted (ectropion, eclabion).
- Chest/limb digits may be constricted (HI).

Management

- Refer to a paediatric dermatologist.
- Specialist dermatology nursing in regulated temperature and humidity settings.
- Scrupulous eye care – ophthalmology opinion.
- Occasionally, the skin is near normal after the collodion membrane is shed, but if not, refer family to a geneticist for gene testing and counselling.

Early referral to plastic surgery if limb/digit constriction occurs.

- For HI, consider early oral retinoid therapy.
- Optimise fluid balance; provide nutritional support if feeding is difficult.

Psychological support for the family.
   Pain management and early referral to palliative care are appropriate.

Prognosis

For Harlequin ichthyosis, mortality was previously estimated at approximately 50%, but improvements in neonatal care may improve this.

ECZEMA HERPETICUM

There is a herpes simplex viral infection on a background of eczema. It carries significant mortality.

Clinical Presentations

There is a history of preceding eczema and of familial herpes simplex infection.

- Vesicles or roofless blisters, characteristic 'punched out' lesions
- Child may be systemically unwell.

Management

- Admission for IV acyclovir and treatment of underlying eczema.

GENERALISED PUSTULAR PSORIASIS

This is rare in childhood but potentially very serious. It may be the presenting episode of psoriasis.

History

There may be a history of preceding psoriasis, with acute exacerbation/onset of the skin condition. The child is systemically unwell.

Examination

- Erythroderma (redness all over) and scaling, with multiple overlying multiple sterile superficial pustules.

- Child is toxic and unwell.

Management

- Urgent admission
- Systemic ciclosporin/methotrexate/biologicals
- Specialist dermatology nursing
- Genetic testing for interferonopathies

MALIGNANT SKIN CONDITIONS

Langerhans' Cell Histiocytosis

- Proliferation of Langerhans cells in the skin and/or other organs.
- Skin lesions tend to be truncal +/− in the scalp, similar in appearance to seborrheic dermatitis.
- Skin biopsy is diagnostic.
- Clinical presentation and course are highly variable.
- Management varies between topical treatments and systemic chemotherapy.

Malignant Melanoma

Malignant melanoma is very rare in childhood. Known predisposing factors are very large or multiple congenital melanocytic naevi, familial melanoma syndromes, and DNA repair defects.

Others

Other malignant conditions include cutaneous leukaemic deposits, rare vascular tumours (see above), squamous cell carcinomas, basal cell carcinomas and cutaneous T-cell lymphoma.

ACKNOWLEDGEMENTS

The author would like to thank Professor Veronica Kinsler for her contribution to the previous edition upon which this chapter was based and for her kind permission to re-use images.

FURTHER READING

- (2021). Executive summary: Consensus recommendations for the use of retinoids in ichthyosis and other disorders of cornification in children and adolescents. *Journal of the American Academy of Dermatology.*
- Solman, L., et al. (2018). Oral propranolol in the treatment of proliferating infantile haemangiomas: British Society for Paediatric Dermatology consensus guidelines. *The British Journal of Dermatology* 179, 582–589.
- Kinsler, V.A., et al. (2019). Mosaic abnormalities of the skin – Review and guidelines from the European Reference Network for rare skin diseases (ERN-Skin). *The British Journal of Dermatology.*
- McPherson, T., et al. (2019). British Association of Dermatologists' guidelines for the management of Stevens-Johnson syndrome/toxic epidermal necrolysis in children and young people, 2018. *The British Journal of Dermatology* 181, 37–54.
- Has, C., et al. (2021). Practical management of epidermolysis bullosa: consensus clinical position statement from the European Reference Network for Rare Skin Diseases. *Journal of the European Academy of Dermatology and Venereology* 35, 2349–2360.
- Has, C., et al. (2020). Consensus reclassification of inherited epidermolysis bullosa and other disorders with skin fragility. *The British Journal of Dermatology* 183, 614–627.
- Smith, C.H., et al. (2020). British Association of Dermatologists guidelines for biologic therapy for psoriasis 2020: A rapid update. *British Journal of Dermatology* 183, 628–637.
- Solman, L., and Glover, M. (2019). Management of atopic dermatitis. In *Harper's Textbook of Pediatric Dermatology,* pp 253–264.
- Seyger, M.M.B. (2019). Psoriasis. In *Harper's Textbook of Pediatric Dermatology,* pp 368–375.
- Langan, S.M., and Williams, H.C. (2019). Clinical features and diagnostic criteria of atopic dermatitis. In *Harper's Textbook of Pediatric Dermatology,* pp 193–211.

- Kinsler, V. (2019). Congenital melanocytic naevi. In *Harper's Textbook of Pediatric Dermatology*, V.K. Peter H. Hoeger, Albert C. Yan, John Harper, Arnold P. Oranje, Christine Bodemer, Margarita Larralde, David Luk, Vibhu Mendiratta, and Diana Purvis ed. Wiley-Blackwell.
- Schaffer, J.V. (2021). Pediatric mastocytosis: Recognition and management. *American Journal of Clinical Dermatology* 22, 205–220.
- Waelchli, R., Aylett, S.E., Atherton, D., Thompson, D.J., Chong, W.K., and Kinsler, V.A. (2015). Classification of neurological abnormalities in children with congenital melanocytic naevus syndrome identifies magnetic resonance imaging as the best predictor of clinical outcome. *The British Journal of Dermatology* 173, 739–750.
- Waelchli, R., et al. (2014). New vascular classification of port-wine stains: Improving prediction of Sturge-Weber risk. *The British Journal of Dermatology* 171, 861–867.
- Douzgou, S., et al. (2021). A standard of care for individuals with PIK3CA-related disorders: An international expert consensus statement. *Clinical Genetics*.
- Kinsler, V.A., et al. (2017). Melanoma in congenital melanocytic naevi. *The British Journal of Dermatology* 176, 1131–1143.
- Sabroe, R.A., et al. (2021). British Association of Dermatologists guidelines for the management of people with chronic urticaria 2021. *The British Journal of Dermatology*.
- ISSVA Classification of Vascular Anomalies ©2018. International society for the Study of Vascular Anomalies. Available at "issva.org/classification". Accessed January 2021.
- Paller, S., and Mancini, A.J. (2020). *Hurwitz Clinical Pediatric Dermatology*, 6th Edition. Elsevier.

7 Ophthalmology

Richard Bowman, Sohaib R Rufai, Sri Gore, Robert H Henderson and Ken Nischal

Ophthalmology in a children's hospital often plays a key role in diagnosis, disease surveillance and timing of therapeutic intervention. This chapter should allow the paediatrician to understand these many roles.

ANATOMY OF THE EYE

See Figures 7.1 to 7.3 for terminology of eye anatomy.
See Figure 7.4 for description of eye movements.

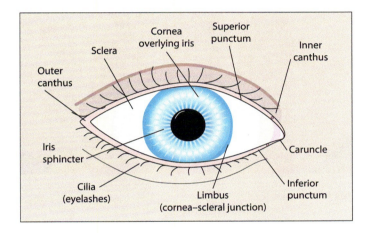

Figure 7.1   External landmarks of the eye and periocular region.

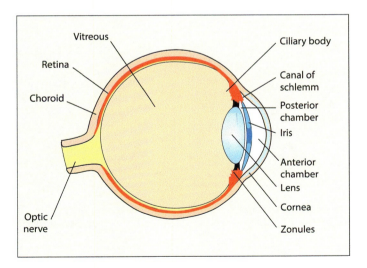

Figure 7.2   Cross-section of the globe.

DOI: 10.1201/9781003175186-7

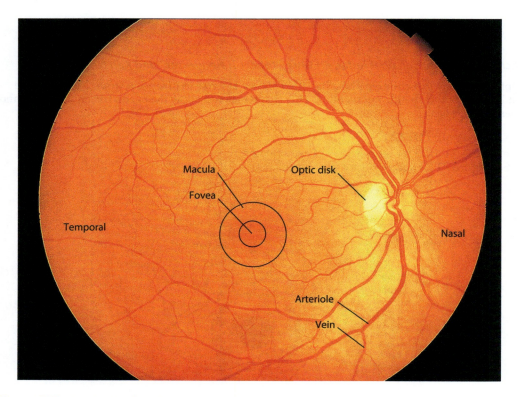

Figure 7.3 Fundus landmarks.

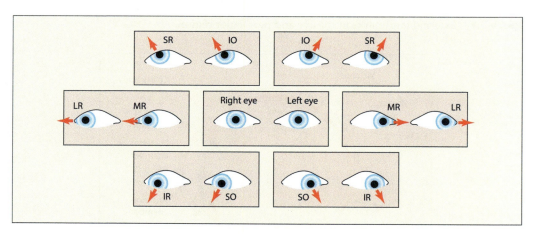

Figure 7.4 Schematic showing the field of action of the extraocular muscles. IO – inferior oblique; IR – inferior rectus; LR – lateral rectus; MR – medial rectus; SO– superior oblique; SR – superior rectus.

VISUAL DEVELOPMENT

Visual Milestones

Figure 7.5 provides an easy guide to important milestones. Delayed visual maturation (DVM) may be seen in otherwise healthy children, which resolves by 6 months of age. Complex DVM occurs where there is pathology explaining a degree of visual impairment, but the child is exhibiting additional delay.

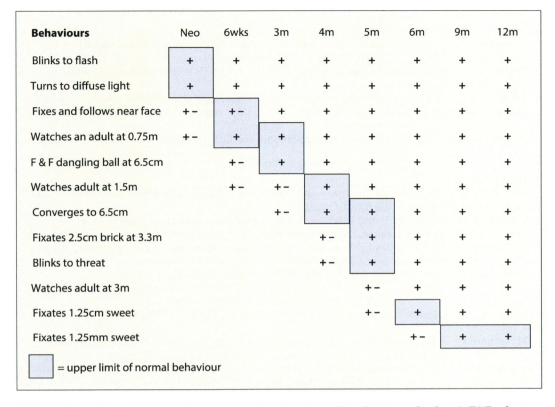

Behaviours	Neo	6wks	3m	4m	5m	6m	9m	12m
Blinks to flash	+	+	+	+	+	+	+	+
Turns to diffuse light	+	+	+	+	+	+	+	+
Fixes and follows near face	+ –	+ –	+	+	+	+	+	+
Watches an adult at 0.75m	+ –	+	+	+	+	+	+	+
F & F dangling ball at 6.5cm		+ –	+	+	+	+	+	+
Watches adult at 1.5m		+ –	+ –	+	+	+	+	+
Converges to 6.5cm			+ –	+	+	+	+	+
Fixates 2.5cm brick at 3.3m				+ –	+	+	+	+
Blinks to threat				+ –	+	+	+	+
Watches adult at 3m					+ –	+	+	+
Fixates 1.25cm sweet					+ –	+	+	+
Fixates 1.25mm sweet						+ –	+	+

☐ = upper limit of normal behaviour

Figure 7.5 Observable visual behaviour (after Blanche Stiff and Patricia Sonksen). F&F – fixates and follows.

Amblyopia

This is the most common cause of decreased vision in childhood, affecting 1.44% of children worldwide. It occurs when the neural pathways between the affected eye and the brain fail to develop, usually due to lack of stimulation. The earlier the onset of amblyopia, the greater the depth of the deficit. The critical period for visual development is probably between the first and eighth weeks of life; visual disruption during this period can cause dense amblyopia.

Amblyopia has numerous causes; the commonest are strabismus, visual deprivation (e.g. due to congenital cataract) and significant refractive error. Amblyopia is reversible by treating the cause (e.g. prescribing spectacles) and occlusion therapy or atropine penalisation of the better eye, with early detection and treatment offering the best outcome.

LIDS

Blepharitis

Incidence: Very common.

Aetiology: Inflammation of the eyelid margin

Clinical Presentation: erythematous eyelid margins with or without eyelid crusting, itching, light sensitivity, eye rubbing, ocular foreign body sensation and recurrent chalazia (see below).

Differentials: Conjunctivitis (see the section 'Conjunctiva').

Association: Usually isolated but may be associated with acne rosacea.

Treatment: Lid hygiene. Topical antibiotics, mild steroids and occasionally systemic tetracyline antibiotics may be needed. Treatment is necessary for severe disease to prevent corneal complications such as infection and scarring.

Prognosis: Usually good if recognised, assessed and treated appropriately.

Chalazion/Stye

Incidence: Very common.

Aetiology: Chalazia are blocked and inflamed meibomian glands. Styes are blocked and infected eyelash follicles. Both are associated with blepharitis.

Differentials: Molluscum, herpes simplex, milia (for styes). Pilimatrixoma and juvenile xantho-granolomas for chalazia.

Treatment: Chalazia require warm compresses, massage, topical antibiotics +/− incision and curettage if persisting for many months. Styes may require removal of a buried eyelash and topical/oral antibiotics.

Prognosis: Both have a high rate of resolution with medical treatment and rarely need surgery.

Congenital Ptosis

Incidence: Rare.

Aetiology: 'Ptosis' describes the drooping of the upper lid and, in children, is commonly due to a congenital dysfunction of the levator muscle.

Clinical: Usually unilateral and from birth. The severity can vary from mild to severe.

Treatment: Ptosis, of any cause, may cause disruption of visual development in child and thus requires referral even if mild. Children may require glasses, patching and some require surgery. Surgical treatments may include a levator muscle resection or brow suspension.

Prognosis: Good if under specialist ophthalmology/multidisciplinary teams.

Rarer Causes of Ptosis and Associations

Neurogenic ptosis: Ptosis can be associated with third nerve palsy and Horner syndrome (Figure 7.6).

Myasthenia gravis: The ptosis (usually bilateral) can be the only ocular symptom but can include brow abnormalities and can present asynchronously with systemic signs or symptoms. The gold standard test is muscle electrophysiology.

Myopathies: For example, mitochondrial and muscular dystrophies. These are usually bilateral, can be progressive and associated with eye movement abnormalities.

Associations: Lots of conditions can be associated with ptosis such as blepharophimosis. This condition usually involves bilateral ptosis, epicanthus inversus and ectropion.

Epiblepharon

Aetiology: Rotation of the eyelashes towards the eye. This is not an entropion.

Incidence: Commoner in babies and children of Asian ethnicity.

Presentation: Children may be asymptomatic or present with ocular pain, redness, eye rubbing and light sensitivity.

Treatment: Monitoring, ocular lubricants and/or eyelid surgery.

Prognosis: Good. This can resolve spontaneously as children grow.

Entropion and Ectropion

Incidence: Rare in children.

Aetiology: Entropion (lid margin turned inwards) and ectropion (lid margin turned out) are usually associated with other syndromes or conditions.

Examples: Cicatrising viral conjunctivitis causing entropion, ectropion associated with ichthyosis.

Epicanthal Fold

This is a fold of skin at the medial canthus. This can be common among young children of Asian origin but can also be present in some syndromes. These can give the impression of an esotropia (in-turning squint).

Treatment: Usually not necessary. These usually become less prominent when the child's nasal bridge develops.

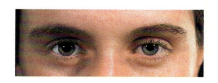

Figure 7.6 Left Horner syndrome with the left pupil slightly smaller and the left lid slightly ptotic (droopy).

Epiphora (Watery Eye)

Incidence: Very common (one in three births).

Aetiology: Most commonly due to congenital lacrimal duct obstruction, and can also occur due to over-production of tears.

Clinical Presentation: Watery and/or sticky eye from birth. Symptoms can be variable and fluctuate depending on the environment or situation (worse in windy, cold weather and when the child has nasal congestion).

Treatment: More than 90% resolve before the age of 1 year. Keeping the eyelids clean with boiled cooled water may be all that is necessary. Lacrimal sac massage is advised for those with copious mucous to reduce the risk of dacryocystitis; massage is not proven to cause resolution. Syringe and probe procedures may be advised for children between 1 and 4 years if their symptoms are significant. Rarely, children may require a dacryocystorhinostomy.

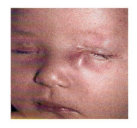

Figure 7.7 Dacryocoele in a baby. If this becomes infected it is termed dacryocystitis.

Note: A dacryocystocoele (Figure 7.7) is usually seen in a newborn as a blue swelling at the medial canthus and has an additional anatomical abnormality to simple nasolacrimal duct obstruction. These children require urgent assessment by a paediatric ophthalmologist due the risk of respiratory distress. They can often resolve with sac massage but may need oral or IV antibiotics if they become infected.

Note: a watery eye can be a sign of glaucoma.

Preseptal Cellulitis – Infective

Incidence: not uncommon.

Aetiology: This is inflammation and infection caused by a condition on the surface of the lids, such as trauma/insect bite or a lesion, e.g. chalazion.

Clinical Presentation: redness and swelling of the eyelids but no involvement of the eye or orbit. Vision is usually unaffected unless the upper eyelid is swollen and impinging on the visual access. Eye movements and optic nerve function is unaffected.

Treatment: Oral antibiotics are usually enough, but IV antibiotics may be required in severe cases.

Lid Coloboma

Incidence: Rare.

Aetiology: Developmental anomaly.

Clinical Presentation: Gap in the eyelid (upper or lower) (Figure 7.8).

There is an association with oculo-auricular-vertebral syndrome (formerly known as Goldenhar) and upper lid colobomas. Amniotic band syndrome and other clefting syndromes usually affect the lower lid.

Treatment: Lubrication in the first instance to prevent exposure keratopathy. Early referral to oculoplastic surgeon to perform lid reconstruction.

Prognosis: Good once repair is achieved.

Lid Lesions
Molluscum Contagiosum

- **Aetiology:** Common eyelid tumour (see also the chapter 'Dermatology') caused by a poxvirus.

- **Clinical Presentation:** Often situated on the lid margin. Should be looked for in cases of follicular or chronic conjunctivitis. The lesions are small umbilicated nodules (Figure 7.9).

- **Treatment:** Usually self-limiting, but if conjunctivitis is troublesome then curettage of lid lesions may be needed.

- **Prognosis:** Good.

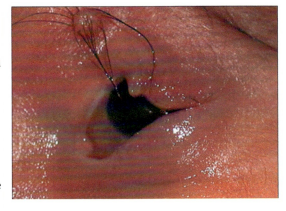

Figure 7.8 Upper lid coloboma.

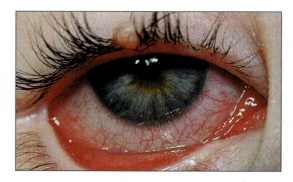

Figure 7.9 Molluscum contagiosum – raised papillomatous lesion with a central core containing virus particles.

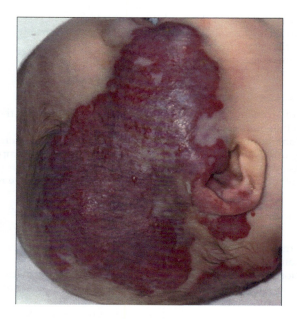

Figure 7.10 Flat haemangioma in PHACES.

Herpes Simplex

See the section 'Conjunctivitis' and the chapter 'Dermatology'.

Capillary Haemangioma

These are vascular tumours which can involve any part of the body. If they involve the periocular area they may interfere with visual development and hence should be referred to a multidisciplinary team. They may also be present within the orbit causing proptosis, eye movement limitation and rarely optic nerve compromise. Suspect PHACES association (Posterior fossa abnormalities, Haemangioma, Arterial lesions, Cardiac abnormalities, Eye problems, Sternal notch) if they are bilateral, flat with wide distributions (Figure 7.10). See the chapter 'Dermatology' for more details on treatment.

Port Wine Stain

Clinical Presentation: The lesion is a dermal capillary vascular anomaly that may occur in the periocular region; see also the chapter 'Dermatology'.

Systemic associations include Sturge–Weber syndrome and cutis marmorata telangiectasia congenita.

Treatment/Prognosis: The highest risk factors for glaucoma in these patients include: a diagnosis of Sturge–Weber syndrome, diffuse periocular involvement, and ocular involvement. These patients require glaucoma screening.

CORNEA

Keratoconus

Incidence: 0.13%.

Aetiology: Unclear but may be hereditary and induced by chronic rubbing.

Classification: Based on anterior and posterior radius of curvature, thinnest corneal thickness and corrected distance visual acuity (ABCD Grading System).

Presentation: Central or paracentral thinning of the cornea, leading to poor visual acuity due to irregular and/or high astigmatism as the cornea bulges outward in a cone shape.

Associations: Atopy, aniridia, blue sclera, congenital cataracts, ectopia lentis, microcornea, Leber's congenital amaurosis, retinitis pigmentosa, retinopathy of prematurity and vernal conjunctivitis.

Treatment: In mild to moderate cases, contact lenses can correct the visual loss. In cases of acute hydrops, topical dehydrating, lubricating and steroid agents are needed. In severe cases, penetrating or deep lamellar corneal transplant is required. Collagen cross-linking using ultraviolet A (UVA) light can slow the progression of keratoconus.

Prognosis: Generally good with early recognition and prompt intervention.

Rare Corneal Developmental Disorders

Microcornea is defined as any cornea less than 10 mm in horizontal diameter. No active treatment is needed other than surveillance for complications.

Cornea plana is characterised by a flat cornea with a curvature of less than 43 diopters. Patients must be reviewed to exclude glaucoma and correct any refractive error.

Megalocornea is characterised by a cornea with a horizontal diameter greater than 13 mm. Children often need lubrication, especially at night. If the cornea is enlarged in the presence of congenital glaucoma (Figure 7.11), it is not defined as megalocornea.

Corneal Dystrophies

See Table 7.1. Only dystrophies commonly affecting children are described.

Corneal Deposits

Corneal deposition in the paediatric age group can vary from the simple deposition of iron in the epithelium, with no visual complications, to a full-thickness corneal opacification that can lead to profound amblyopia or even blindness.

Corneal deposition can be metabolic or non-metabolic. The metabolic causes include the mucopolysaccharidoses (not MPS III – Sanfillippo), the mucolipidoses, glycogen storage disorders (namely Von Gierke disease), sphingolipidoses (namely Fabry disease), Gaucher disease, gangliosidoses, cystinosis, Wilson disease, tyrosinaemia Type II, alkaptonuria, Niemann–Pick disease, LCAT deficiency and metachromatic leukodystrophy. Non-metabolic causes include corneal blood staining (seen after blunt trauma with blood in the anterior chamber), band-shaped keratopathy (Figure 7.12) (from calcium deposition in the cornea), amyloid deposition and neoplastic causes (i.e. monoclonal gammopathy).

Keratitis

Keratitis is an inflammation of the cornea. It may affect the epithelium, subepithelium or stroma. Most causes of keratitis are due to infections such as herpes simplex keratitis or bacterial keratitis, but there are also non-infection-related causes such as neurotrophic ulcer or dry eye.

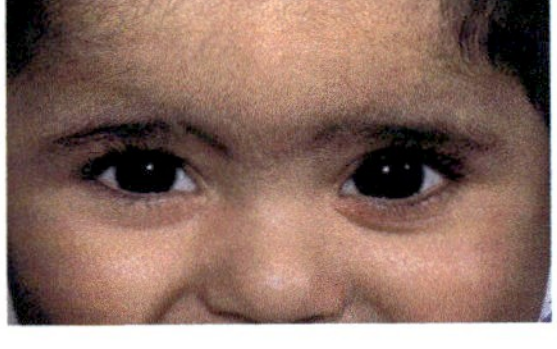

Figure 7.11 Bilateral congenital glaucoma with the left eye bigger than the right eye. Large corneas associated with congenital glaucoma are not termed megalocornea.

Insufficient Tear Production (Dry Eye)

This is insufficient production of aqueous tears leading to epithelial erosions, filamentary keratitis and secondary corneal vascularisation. It is rare in children.

Table 7.1: Differential Diagnosis of Neonatal Corneal Opacity

Aetiology	Age of onset	Corneal signs	Other
INFECTIOUS DISEASE			
Herpes simplex (Type II)	4–10 days	Unilateral corneal ulcer, positive fluorescein staining, often in a geographic configuration	Viral culture for herpes
Rubella	Birth	Diffuse corneal oedema, often associated with cataracts	Serology including IgM
Neisseria gonorrhoeae	2–3 days	Diffuse punctate staining with possible corneal ulceration	Gram stain and culture
TRAUMA			
Tears in Descemet's membrane	Birth	Vertical corneal striae with oedema in the area of breaks in Descemet's membrane	History of forceps delivery often associated with soft tissue injury of the face
Corneal perforations with amniocentesis	Birth	Local corneal opacity with possible iris adhesions	Amniocentesis; traumatic cataract
DYSGENESIS SYNDROMES			
Peters' anomaly	Birth	Central corneal opacity may extend to the limbus; iridocorneal strands	60% with glaucoma
Sclerocornea	Birth	Peripheral corneal opacity associated with flattening of the cornea	May be associated with other anterior segment anomalies
Limbal dermoid	Birth	Limbal mass; yellow-white in appearance; may also have hair follicles	May be isolated or associated with Goldenhar syndrome
DYSTROPHIES			
Congenital hereditary endothelial dystrophy (CHED)	Birth to several months	Bilateral diffuse corneal oedema; corneal thickening; corneal diameter normal	Attenuated or absent endothelium; autosomal dominant or recessive
Posterior polymorphous dystrophy (PPD)	Infrequently at birth to first few years of birth	Deep linear opacities and thickening of Descemet's membrane (snail tracks); deep posterior vesicles; corneal oedema	Usually autosomal dominant
Congenital hereditary stromal	Birth	Diffuse, flaky stromal central anterior stromal haze with deeper involvement	
METABOLIC			
Mucopolysaccharidoses (Hurlers-MPS-IH most severe form)	Unusual at birth	Diffuse ground-glass appearance through all layers; bilateral and symmetrical	Urinary glycosaminoglycans; autosomal recessive
Mucolipidoses (Type IV)		Anterior and epithelial clouding	Autosomal recessive
Cystinosis (rare)	Rarely at birth, usually first year	White needle-like crystals within corneal stroma; ground-glass appearance	Renal impairment; crystals also in conjunctiva; glaucoma; autosomal recessive
Tyrosinaemia	Neonate	Corneal epithelial deposits	Tyrosine in blood and urine; hyperkeratosis of skin
CONGENITAL			
Congenital glaucoma	Birth to first 6 months of life	Buphthalmos corneal oedema; Haab's striae (horizontal curvilinear breaks in Descemet's membrane due to stretch injury)	Increased ocular pressure; myopic shift; increased cupping

It may be associated with Riley–Day syndrome (familial dysautonomia), ectodermal dysplasia, keratoconjunctivitis sicca (KCS) usually due to primary or secondary Sjögren syndrome and radiation therapy.

Treatment is with adequate lubricating drops and in some cases temporary lacrimal punctal occlusion with silicone punctal plugs to decrease tear drainage. Tarsorraphy should also be considered. Prognosis is reasonable if treated early.

Non-Infection-Related Keratitis

The hereditary type is very rare. Aetiology includes autosomal dominant keratitis (*PAX 6*, homeobox gene mutation), ectrodactyly, ectodermal dysplasia and cleft lip and palate syndrome (EEC), ectodermal dysplasia, keratitis–ichthyosis–deafness syndrome (KID), Riley–Day syndrome (familial dysautonomia), epidermolysis bullosa, keratopathy (corneal erosions, epithelial defects) and corneal vascularisation. The child is usually photophobic and has reduced visual acuity (Figure 7.13).

Treatment depends on the cause, but lubrication is the mainstay together with punctual plugs and/or tarsorraphy.

Inadequate Spreading of Tears

Inadequate spreading of tears is rare and leads to epithelial erosions or dellen (an area of corneal dessication). This is most commonly seen in lid colobomas, corneal limbal dermoids (Figure 7.14) most commonly seen in Goldenhar syndrome, facial palsy and Moebius syndrome. Treatment involves adequate ocular surface lubrication and removal of the cause if possible (e.g. limbal dermoid removal or lid coloboma repair).

Increased Evaporation of Tears

This is usually present when there is proptosis or when the lids do not close adequately when the child is asleep. Seen in shallow orbits (craniosynostoses), lid colobomas, lagophthalmos, comatosed patients and lid ectropion (e.g. in cases of lamellar ichthyosis). Treatment involves eye ointment to exposed eyes when the child is asleep and regular daily lubrication. Tarsorraphy and a moist chamber may be needed.

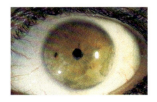

Figure 7.12 Band-shaped keratopathy, secondary to uveitis, in a patient with juvenile chronic arthritis. Note also a small, irregular pupil due to posterior synechiae (adhesions of the iris to the anterior capsule of the lens).

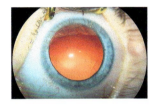

Figure 7.13 Keratitis affecting the superior half of the cornea. This was present from birth and progressive.

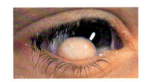

Figure 7.14 Very large limbal dermoid, causing difficulty in closure of the eyelids.

Trauma (Including Corneal Anaesthesia)

The aetiology may be congenital, e.g. familial dysautonomia, Goldenhar syndrome, oculofacial syndromes and leprosy, or acquired, e.g. damage to the trigeminal nerve due to herpes zoster, herpes simplex, intra-cranial tumours both pre- and/or post-operatively, especially cerebellopontine angle tumours. Repetitive trauma is the main cause of chronic keratitis and the presence of corneal anaesthesia allows repetitive trauma. The accompanying reduced blink reflex reduces corneal wetting and exacerbates such a keratitis. Treatment is with lubricating agents. Tarsorraphy or botulinum toxin-induced ptosis may be needed.

Avitaminosis A

This is common in some under-developed countries and is due to a deficiency of dietary vitamin A intake. It is characterised by a thickening of the corneal epithelium, keratinisation of the epithelium and a diffuse corneal opacity. Secondary pannus and corneal vascularisation can occur. In addition to corneal pathology, white triangular keratinised lesions (Bitot's spots) of the temporal conjunctiva occur. The treatment is protein, calorie and vitamin A replacement. Prognosis depends on how soon replacement is initiated, as corneal changes can be permanent.

Vernal Keratoconjunctivitis

Vernal keratoconjunctivitis presents with mucoid discharge and lumps on the superior tarsal conjunctiva (papillae) (Figure 7.15). Rarely, these can cause trauma to the superior half of the cornea leading to corneal epithelial erosions, shield ulcers (3–11% of patients) and corneal vascularisation (micropannus).

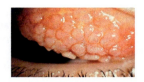

Figure 7.15 Giant papillae in vernal keratoconjunctivitis.

Treatment is with topical anti-allergic medication, usually with topical steroid therapy and lubricating agents. Supratarsal steroid injection or topical cyclosporin drops may also be needed in severe cases. Prognosis is good if treated aggressively.

Infection-Related Keratitis

Herpes Simplex

Herpes keratitis can occur at almost any age in children, as even neonates can become infected as they pass through the birth canal. Neonatal herpes simplex keratitis may be the only sign of systemic herpes simplex. Any child who will not open an eye should be considered to have either herpes simplex or a foreign body until proven otherwise. Viral cultures from scrapings taken from the edge of any ulcer are necessary. However, PCR for HSV may be performed even on tears or conjunctival swabs from the affected eye. Herpes simplex keratitis (epithelial) is treated with topical aciclovir while stromal and/or endothelial disease with intact epithelium is treated with topical aciclovir and topical steroids. Systemic aciclovir should be considered if systemic herpes simplex is a possibility.

Varicella-Zoster

Corneal involvement is extremely rare, but ocular findings include swollen lids, vesicular lesions of the lids, and varying degrees of keratoconjunctivitis. Infrequently superficial punctate keratitis of the cornea occurs. Treatment is with oral aciclovir, and topical cycloplegic drops for eye comfort. Prognosis is usually good.

Chlamydia Trachomatis

Trachoma is a cause of blindness worldwide. The causative organism is *Chlamydia trachomatis*, an intracellular parasite. A chronic follicular conjunctivitis results from infection with secondary corneal scarring. Treatment is with a single oral dose of azithromycin and topical erythromycin eye ointment.

Bacterial

Bacterial keratitis is rare and usually seen in children with some type of predisposing factor such as: neurotrophic cornea, contact lenses, trauma, dry eyes, HSV, immunosuppression, immunodeficiency or vitamin deficiency. Keratitis is usually stromal with or without accompanying hypopyon (pus in the anterior chamber). Culture and gram stain are required, followed by appropriate intensive topical and oral antibiotics. Prognosis is variable as residual scarring can severely affect vision.

Fungal

Fungal keratitis is very rare. The infection may be due to filamentous fungi such as *Aspergillus* or *Fusarium* spp. or to yeast-like fungi such as *Candida* spp. Most traumatic fungal ulcers are the result of filamentous organisms, while infection by yeasts are most common in patients with immunosuppression or dry eyes. Culture and gram stain are required. Treat with systemic and topical antifungal agents. Visual prognosis is often guarded and corneal graft may be needed.

CONJUNCTIVA

Infection-Related Conjunctivitis
Neonatal Conjunctivitis

- **Incidence:** Varies from 1 to 21% depending on the region of the world.
- **Aetiology:** Chemical, gonococcal, HSV type II, chlamydia and bacterial.

■ **Clinical Presentation:** Conjunctival inflammation occurs during the first month of life (ophthalmia neonatorum – Figure 7.16). This is a notifiable condition.

■ **Treatment:** Swabs and appropriate topical and, if gonococcal or chlamydial, systemic antibiotics.

■ **Prognosis:** Good if treated promptly.

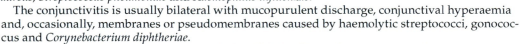

Figure 7.16 Ophthalmia neonatorum caused by *Chlamydia* spp.

Bacterial Conjunctivitis

This is very common, with the commonest causes being *Staphylococcus aureus*, *Streptococcus pneumoniae* and *Haemophilus influenzae*.

The conjunctivitis is usually bilateral with mucopurulent discharge, conjunctival hyperaemia and, occasionally, membranes or pseudomembranes caused by haemolytic streptococci, gonococcus and *Corynebacterium diphtheriae*.

Treatment is with broad-spectrum topical antibiotics. If membranes or pseudomembranes are present these should be physically removed and an anti-inflammatory topical drop added to the antibiotic.

Swabs should be taken if the discharge is copious or persistent despite topical antibiotics.

Viral Conjunctivitis

Viral conjunctivitis is a common, contagious, usually bilateral condition with the most common causes being adenovirus, HSV, enterovirus and EBV. Adenoviral conjunctivitis presents with watery discharge, conjunctival hyperaemia, follicular conjunctivitis, preauricular lymphadenopathy and pseudomembranes in severe cases.

Treatment is with topical antibiotics to prevent secondary bacterial infections.

Chronic Conjunctivitis

This is uncommon. It is usually unilateral but may be bilateral chronic red eye. It may be caused by *Molluscum contagiosum*, toxic conjunctivitis (aminoglycoside antibiotics, antivirals, glaucoma medication, eye makeup and preservatives), Parinaud's oculoglandular syndrome and blepahrokerato conjunctivitis.

Chlamydia Conjunctivitis

This usually unilateral condition causes follicular conjunctivitis with preauricular lymphadenopathy. Treatment includes taking appropriate swabs and treating with topical and systemic erythromycin, exclusion of pneumonitis and referral to genitourinary medicine to exclude other sexually transmitted diseases. Single-dose azithromycin may also be used with topical erythromycin ointment.

Non-Infection-Related Conjunctivitis
Allergic Conjunctivitis

Allergic conjunctivitis is a very common, bilateral seasonal or perennial condition.

There is often chemosis, watery discharge and conjunctival hyperaemia with a history of hayfever.

Topical anti-allergic medication includes mast cell stabilisers or antihistamines or dual action eyedrops. Systemic antihistamines may also be needed.

Atopic Keratoconjunctivitis

A not uncommon condition associated with lid eczema, inflammation of the lid margins (blepharitis) and mucoid discharge. Cataracts, keratoconus and retinal detachments may occur. Secondary glaucoma may occur if periocular steroids are used to treat the skin.

Lubricating agents and, if necessary, anti-allergy topical and systemic medication may be needed.
Prognosis depends on complications that may occur.

Conjunctival Pigmentation
Benign Melanosis

Brown-black patches are seen near the limbus and sometimes in the interpalpebral bulbar conjunctiva. The patches move very easily over the globe and are most commonly seen in pigmented races.

No treatment needed as there is no risk of malignant change.

Flat Deep Pigmentation

A not uncommon condition in pigmented races. It is due to unilateral subepithelial melanocytosis and as such the pigmentation cannot be moved over the globe. There is a slate-grey appearance, which may be isolated to the eye (melanosis oculi), isolated to the periocular skin (dermal melano-cytosis) or involve both eye and skin (oculodermal melanocytosis or naevus of Ota). Naevus of Ota is associated with an increased risk of glaucoma and increased risk of uveal melanoma. Oculo-(dermal) melanocytosis is nine times more common in young patients with uveal melanoma than in the general population with uveal melanoma.

Regular observation is needed.

Elevated Conjunctival Lesions
Pigmented Nodules
Naevus

Naevus is a common solitary, well-defined, slightly elevated lesion, which moves freely over globe. Most (75%) are pigmented. Naevi usually are present at the limbus, plica, caruncle and lid margin.

There is a rare malignant transformation to melanoma. Rapid growth may be seen around puberty; an excisional biopsy may be needed to confirm the diagnosis.

Non-Pigmented Small Nodules
Phlycten

Phlycten is an uncommon, straw-yellow, slightly elevated lesion usually at or near the limbus, sur-rounded by hyperaemia.

The commonest cause is *Staphylococcus aureus* hypersensitivity seen in blepharitis. If associated with blepharitis then topical antibiotic and topical steroid therapy is used.

Non-Pigmented Large Nodules
Epibulbar Dermoid

An uncommon solid, elevated, congenital lesion, usually located at the limbus. It may have hairs on the surface (Figure 7.14).

Ocular associations include lid coloboma, ocular coloboma, microphthalmos and aniridia, Goldenhar, Treacher–Collins and Franchescetti syndromes.

If the lesion is very large or causing ocular surface wetting problems, it must be removed.

Plaque-Like Conjunctival Lesions
Pterygium

A wing-shaped, very common fleshy lesion usually at the nasal limbus seen in equatorial regions. It occurs mainly in adults but may be seen in teenagers.

Treatment is rarely needed in teenagers. In adults, if it encroaches on the corneal central axis it should be removed.

Bitot Spot

These are rare foamy plaques temporal to the limbus, seen in avitaminosis A. Vitamin A replace-ment is needed.

Diffusely Elevated Conjunctival Lesions
Lymphoma

A very rare diffuse subconjunctival fleshy lesion, which may be bilateral. Smaller patches have been termed 'salmon patches'. It is most commonly associated with non-Hodgkin's or Burkitt's lymphoma.

Excision biopsy followed by systemic therapy from the oncology team is needed.

Plexiform Neurofibroma

An uncommon diffuse, very smooth, elevated lesion extending from the lid to the superior bulbar conjunctiva. It is almost always associated with NF1.

Usually no treatment is needed but occasionally debulking has been considered.

SCLERA

Pigmentation of the Sclera

This is uncommon and can be due to metabolic and non-metabolic causes. Metabolic causes include alkaptonuria, haemochromatosis and jaundice, while non-metabolic causes include osteogenesis imperfecta I, Marshall–Smith, Russell–Silver, Roberts, and Ehlers–Danlos VI syndromes, all of which may be associated with blue sclera. It may also be seen in Marfan, Hallermann–Streiff, Bloch–Sulzberger, Turner and Kabuki syndromes and in high myopia.

Scleral Inflammation

Episcleritis

An uncommon inflammation of the episclera. Unlike scleritis, the eye is not tender to touch.

Simple episcleritis often follows a viral illness and is self-limiting. Nodular and diffuse disease may be associated with systemic lupus erythematosus (SLE), juvenile idiopathic arthritis, spondyloarthropathy, inflammatory bowel disease, rheumatic fever, relapsing polychondritis, polyarteritis nodosa and inflammatory bowel disease.

Topical mild steroids can be used to treat episcleritis and while this can be recurrent, prognosis is usually good.

Scleritis

Scleritis is an uncommon inflammation of the sclera that is tender to touch. It may be diffuse, nodular or necrotising.

Causes include idiopathic, infections, surgically induced (necrotising or diffuse), rheumatic diseases, connective tissue disorders, enteropathies, vasculitides, granulomatous diseases and certain skin disorders.

Treatment includes treating underlying conditions and using anti-inflammatory drugs systemically (non-steroidal or steroidal) to treat the eye initially. Prognosis is guarded if necrotising, but this is extremely rare in children.

DEVELOPMENTAL ANOMALIES OF THE GLOBE

Microphthalmia and Anophthalmia

Very rare developmental anomalies. In anophthalmia, the eye fails to form very early in development (week 3) and microphthalmia is a spectrum of conditions where ocular tissues form but to varying degrees. Both these ocular anomalies can be unilateral or bilateral, be associated with orbital cyst as well as varying degrees of orbital and eyelid malformation. Microphthalmia can be associated with anterior segment anomalies, congenital cataract, glaucoma, strabismus and refractive error. Visual potential is variable and dependent on multiple factors such as the level of malformation and the vision in the other eye.

Microphthalmia and anophthalmia have been associated with numerous systemic conditions some with known genetic mutations.

Patients with bilateral ocular malformations have a higher rate of brain and systemic malformations compared to those with the unilateral condition but all patients must be assessed comprehensively in a specialist multidisciplinary team setting. Visual potential must be assessed, and treatment offered if appropriate.

Orbital and eyelid tissues may require expansion by specialist teams such as oculoplastic surgeons and prosthetists for optimal aesthetic results. The eyes are an important focal point for social interaction and acceptance into society and thus socket rehabilitation is more than 'cosmetic surgery'.

Nanophthalmos

In this rare developmental anomaly, the eye is small in its overall dimensions but is not affected by other gross developmental defects nor accompanied by other systemic congenital anomalies. There is high hypermetropia, with short axial length (16–18.5 mm) and a crowded anterior chamber predisposing to glaucoma. Glaucoma occurs later in life, as do choroidal effusions because of the thickened inelastic sclera. Systemic associations include Kenny–Caffey syndrome. Treatment includes correction of refractive error and review for glaucoma and choroidal effusions.

IRIS

Congenital Iris Defects
Iris Coloboma

An uncommon developmental anomaly due to nonclosure of the embryonic fissure in the fifth week of gestation. Typical iris colobomas occur in the inferonasal quadrant and may involve the ciliary body, choroid, retina and optic nerve.

Iris colobomas may be isolated or associated with ocular features such as retinochoroidal/optic nerve coloboma, microcornea, microphthalmosor both, or microphthalmos with cyst. Nystagmus and/or cataracts may be seen. Although iris colobomas can be associated with almost any chromosomal abnormality, they are frequently seen in branchio-oculo-facial, cat-eye, CHARGE, 13q deletion, Goltz, triploidy, Patau (trisomy 13), Wolf–Hirschhorn (4p-) and Walker–Warburg syndromes.

Patients should be reviewed for correction of refractive error and cataract progression if lens opacity is present.

Aniridia

The prevalence of aniridia is 1:72000 (as determined in Sweden and Norway), with most causes due to mutations in *PAX6*.

Aniridia (autosomal dominant) is a panocular, bilateral disorder. The most obvious presenting sign is the absence of much or most of the iris tissue. In addition to iris involvement, foveal and optic nerve hypoplasia may be present, resulting in congenital sensory nystagmus and leading to reduced visual acuity to 6/30 or worse. Anterior polar cataracts, glaucoma, and corneal opacification often develop later in childhood and may lead to progressive deterioration of visual acuity. Glaucoma occurs in up to half of all cases.

Associations include Wilm's tumour, genitourinary abnormalities and retarded growth or development (AGR triad) or both (WAGR), or associated with ataxia and neurodevelopmental delay (Gillespie syndrome).

All children with sporadic aniridia should have repeated abdominal ultrasonographic and clinical examinations; molecular genetic evaluation reveals intragenic mutation only. Aniridia is commonly associated with glaucoma (46–70%) and nearly keratopathy in adulthood (78–96%) due to limbal stem cell deficiency.

Changes in Iris Colour
Brushfield Spots

These occur in approximately 67% of patients with Down's syndrome. Very similar iris findings may occur in normal individuals (Wolfflin nodules).

Juvenile Xanthogranuloma

Juvenile xanthogranuloma (JXG) is a rare condition and iris involvement occurs almost exclusively in infants. Usually unilateral yellow nodules or diffuse infiltration may be seen. It may present with spontaneous hyphaema (blood in the anterior chamber) and/or unilateral glaucoma may occur.

All children with JXG should have ocular screening because even asymptomatic ocular lesions may be associated with glaucoma. Most ocular lesions will regress with topical steroids, but some require systemic steroids and others a small dose of radiotherapy treatment. Prognosis is usually good.

Langerhans Cell Histiocytosis

See also the chapters 'Dermatology' and 'Oncology'.

Although similar to JXG, which is systemically benign, Langerhans cell histiocytoses are systemic malignancies and need appropriate chemotherapy. They are rare and usually limited to orbital involvement but iris nodules or choroidal involvement may rarely occur in Letterer–Siwe disease.

Patients should have routine ophthalmic examination and treatment of underlying disease.

Heterochromia Irides

The differential diagnosis of paediatric heterochromia irides (Figure 7.17) is extensive but may be classified as congenital or acquired and whether the affected eye is hypopigmented or hyperpigmented.

Hypochromic Heterochromia

- Congenital causes: Horner syndrome; Waardenburg syndrome; piebaldism trait.

- Acquired causes: Fuch's heterochromic cyclitis – a rare type of unilateral iritis; non-pigmented iris tumours.

Hyperchromic Heterochromia

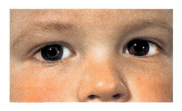

Figure 7.17 Heterochromia irides. This child had Waardenburg syndrome.

- **Congenital Causes:** Iris mammillations – unilateral villiform protuberances that may cover the iris usually in association with oculodermal melanosis or neurofibromatosis (NF); congenital iris ectropion; unilateral iris coloboma (affected iris is darker); port wine stain.

- **Acquired Causes:** Cataract surgery in children – operated on eye can be darker in eyes operated on early in life; topical medication (e.g. latanoprost, which is a prostaglandin analogue and causes darkening of the iris of the eye being treated); pigmented iris tumours; rubeosis iridis, iris neovascularisation – causes include retinopathy of prematurity, retinoblastoma, Coats' disease, and iris tumours; siderosis – due to intraocular metallic foreign body.

Leukaemia/Lymphoma

See also the chapter 'Haematology'.

Leukaemia iris infiltrates, although rare, have been reported with most types of childhood leukaemia and lymphoma. Acute lymphoblastic leukaemia (ALL) is both the most common form of childhood leukaemia and the most likely to be associated with iris infiltration.

Anterior chamber aspiration or iris biopsy may be needed to exclude an infectious aetiology. Chemotherapy may not be effective and low-dose external radiation has been used successfully despite potential for cataract development.

PUPIL ANOMALIES

Leukocoria

A white pupil reflex. It may be caused by:

- Congenital cataract (may be unilateral or bilateral) (Figure 7.18).

- Persistent foetal vasculature (a rare congenital, usually unilateral, condition).

- Inflammatory cyclitic membrane.

- Retinal dysplasia (very rare)

- Tumours and granulomas – retinoblastoma, retinal astrocytoma and Toxocara granuloma.

- Retinal detachment – Retinopathy of prematurity, retinoblastoma, Coats' disease, Toxocara granuloma, and Stickler syndrome.

- Miscellaneous – extensive retinal nerve fibre myelination and large chorioretinal coloboma.

Dyscoria

A rare abnormality of the pupil shape. Congenital causes include persistent pupillary membranes, iris coloboma, iris hypoplasia and ectopia lentis et pupillae (see below). Acquired causes include posterior synechiae seen in iritis or trauma.

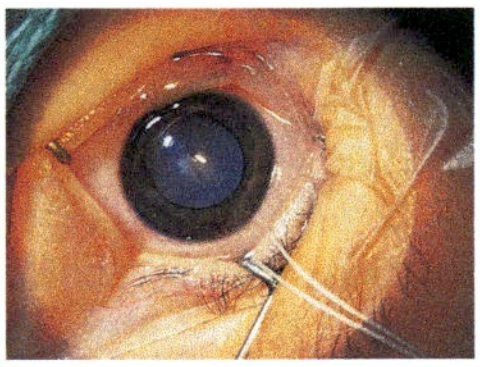

Miosis

Uncommonly a pupil or pupils may be less than 2 mm, and may react poorly to dilating drops. This may be due to congenital miosis (microcoria) when there is an absence of the dilator pupillae muscle or fibrous contraction secondary to persistent pupillary membrane. It can be seen in congenital rubella syndrome, Marfan syndrome, in 20% of Lowe (oculocerebrorenal) syndrome and in *ectopia lentis et pupillae*.

Figure 7.18 Leukocoria due to a congenital cataract, at operation.

If visual development is thought to be hindered, surgical enlargement of the pupil can be performed. Appropriate management of visual development usually results in good vision.

Mydriasis

Rarely a large pupil, usually greater than 4 mm, may be present. This may be congenital but blunt trauma causing iris sphincter rupture, ciliary ganglionitis (unilateral most commonly after chicken pox – also known as Adie's pupil) or acquired neurological disease must be excluded, especially third nerve palsy.

If there is ciliary ganglionitis, accommodation can be affected and the child will need a reading prescription.

Correctopia

An uncommon displacement of the pupil. Normally, the pupil is displaced inferonasally about 0.5 mm from the centre of the iris.

Causes include sector iris hypoplasia, colobomas, ectopia lentis et pupillae and Axenfeld–Rieger anomaly. Intermittent corectopia, with pupils shifting from central to eccentric positions, have been reported during coma and may represent a sign of rostral midbrain dysfunction.

Very rarely if the pupil is very eccentrically displaced then pupilloplasty may be needed to improve the visual axis.

Anisocoria

In this relatively common condition, there is a difference in size between the two pupils. The three main causes in childhood that need to be considered are physiological, Horner syndrome and Adie's pupil (ciliary ganglionitis).

The child should be examined in bright light and then in the dark. If the anisocoria is physiological then the difference will remain constant and will be no more than 2 mm. If the anisocoria is accentuated in bright surroundings this suggests that the larger pupil is at fault and cannot constrict. The commonest cause for this is ciliary ganglionitis (Adie's pupil). If the anisocoria is accentuated in the dark, this suggests that the smaller pupil is at fault. The commonest cause for this is Horner syndrome.

Horner Syndrome

Horner syndrome comprises miosis, with ipsilateral ptosis and sometimes anhidrosis (Figure 7.19). Congenital Horner syndrome is associated with hypopigmentation of the affected side. Acquired Horner syndrome may be due to: central (first-order neurone) lesions; preganglionic (second-order) lesions; postganglionic (third-order) lesions; metastatic neuroblastoma perhaps causing a congenital Horner syndrome.

Even if there is heterochromia irides, metastatic neuroblastoma should be excluded.

Adie Syndrome

This presents with mydriasis with vermiform iris movements on slit-lamp examination.

The commonest association is chicken pox infection but other viral infections may also cause ciliary ganglionitis.

Accommodation is usually affected and the child may need reading spectacles.

LENS ANOMALIES

Aphakia

Aphakia is the absence of the lens, most commonly iatrogenic after congenital cataract extraction. Rare causes are spontaneous resorption of a cataract (may be seen in Lowe syndrome and Hallerman–Streiff syndrome), spontaneous complete dislocation of the lens and, rarely, congenital primary aphakia.

Refractive correction of aphakia is needed and surveillance to exclude glaucoma, which can develop any time in the patient's life.

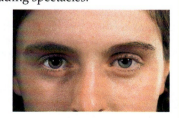

Figure 7.19 Left Horner syndrome with the left pupil slightly smaller and the left lid slightly ptotic (droopy).

Abnormal Shape

Coloboma

Coloboma is rare, but may be associated with other colobomatous ocular defects.

Aetiology is often unclear but refractive treatment is necessary as astigmatism is common.

Lentiglobus

A rare unilateral condition, which usually causes myopia. This may be associated with posterior polar cataract.

Dislocated Lens

This is uncommon but may be seen with ocular associations such as: megalocornea, severe buphthalmos, very high myopia and aniridia, familial ectopia lentis, *ectopia lentis et pupillae*, isolated familial microspherophakia. *Ectopia lentis et pupillae* is an autosomal recessive condition in which there is displacement of the pupil and lens in opposite directions.

Dislocated lens may be seen in systemic associations such as Marfan, Weil–Marchesani, Ehlers–Danlos, Stickler, Kniest syndromes, mandibulofacial dysostosis and osteogenesis imperfecta. Metabolic disorders include homocystinuria, hyperlysinemia and molybdenum cofactor deficiency.

Treatment includes the exclusion of systemic association. Careful observation with refractive correction to ensure adequate visual development is needed. The child may need lensectomy to improve visual function.

Lens Opacity

Lens opacities may be classified in terms of the age at which it occurs or in terms of characteristic lens opacities for certain systemic associations.

Congenital or Infantile Cataract

(See Figures 7.18 and 7.20)

The British Congenital Cataract Interest Group found that two-thirds of congenital cataracts are bilateral and one-third are unilateral; 31% are associated with systemic disease (6% unilateral and 25% bilateral); 61% are associated with ocular disease (47% unilateral and 14% bilateral). No underlying cause or risk factor can be found in 92% of unilateral and 38% of bilateral cases. Hereditary disease is associated with 56% of bilateral and 6% of unilateral cases.

In all bilateral cases, unless there is a hereditary risk or associated ocular disease, the following investigations should be considered depending on the child's systemic condition:

- Cataract gene panel testing.

- Urine: Reducing substances (galatosaemia), dipstick for proteinuria (Alport), amino acids (Lowe).

- Serology: TORCH, RBC galactokinase activity, RBC galactose-1-phosphate uridyltransferase activity, serum ferritin, karyotype, calcium, glucose, VDRL phosphorus, alkaline phosphatase.

Possible associations include:

- Hereditary.

- Ocular: Persistent hyperplastic primary vitreous, aniridia, iris coloboma, microphthalmos.

- Systemic:

  - Infection: intrauterine infection.

  - Metabolic disease: galactosaemia, neonatal hypoglycaemia, hypocalcaemia.

  - Renal disease: Lowe syndrome, congenital haemolytic syndrome.

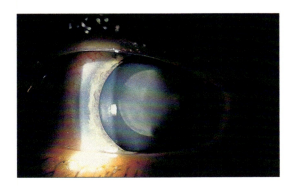

Figure 7.20 Congenital lamellar cataract.

- Chromosomal disorders: Trisomy 13 (Patau syndrome) and 18 (Edward syndrome).

- Neurological disease: Marinesco–Sjögren syndrome (ataxia), Smith–Lemli–Opitz, Zellweger and Sjögren–Larsson syndromes.

- Skeletal disorders: Conradi syndrome.

- Skin disorders: Ectodermal dysplasia, Rothmund–Thomson, incontinentia pigmenti and Cockayne syndromes.

- Miscellaneous: Norrie, Rubinstein–Taybi, Turner and Hallermann–Streiff syndromes.

The IOLunder2 Study evaluated outcomes following primary intraocular lens implantation in children aged under 2 years with congenital or infantile cataract. The study found that intraocular lens implantation did not deliver better visual outcomes or protect against postoperative glaucoma, rather it was associated with increased risk of requiring earlier reoperation. Conventional treatment involves aphakic correction with glasses or contact lenses. Lensectomy with sparing of the capsule for possible secondary implantation performed between 6–10 weeks of age is now considered the preferred treatment option, but lens removal with intraocular implantation is still common. Amblyopia therapy with correction of the refractive state is essential.

Juvenile Cataract

These may be:

- Hereditary.

- Ocular: Coloboma, ectopia lentis, aniridia, retinitis pigmentosa and posterior lenticonus.

- Systemic:

  - Renal disease: Alport syndrome.

  - Skeletal disease: Marfan syndrome.

  - Skin disease: Atopic dermatitis, Marshall syndrome, lamellar ichthyosis.

  - Chromosomal disorders: Trisomy 21.

  - Metabolic disease: Galactokinase deficiency, Fabry disease, Refsum disease, mannosidosis, diabetes mellitus, hypocalcaemia.

  - Neurological disorders: Myotonic dystrophy, Wilson disease.

  - Miscellaneous: Chronic uveitis, drug-induced (steroids), NF2, Stickler syndrome.

Lens aspiration with implantation is the usual method of treatment. Prognosis is good as long as the visual pathway is otherwise unaffected.

RETINAL ANOMALIES

BOX 7.1   RETINOPATHY OF PREMATURITY

Retinopathy of prematurity is a disease that can affect premature babies. It is caused by abnormal vessel growth, which can lead to scarring and retinal detachment. Current UK guidelines for the screening and treatment of retinopathy of prematurity recommend that babies less than 32 weeks gestational age or less than 1501g birthweight should be screened for ROP.

The International Classification of Retinopathy of Prematurity, third edition (ICROP3) is used to describe location, extent and stage of the disease and indication for and commencement of screening. This has been standardised by dividing the retina into three zones. Zone I is an area centred on the optic disc and extending from the disc to twice the distance between the disc and the macula. Zone II is a ring concentric to Zone I that extends to the nasal ora serrata (the edge of the retina on the side of the eye toward the nose). Zone III is the remaining crescent of retina on the temporal (toward the temple) side. ROP is a progressive disease. It begins with some mild changes in the vessels, and may progress to more severe changes. The stage of ROP describes how far in this progression the vessels have reached. Low birthweight, prolonged supplemental oxygen and respiratory distress syndrome are risk factors for ROP.

- Stage 1 is characterised by a demarcation line between the normal retina nearer the optic nerve and the non-vascularised retina more peripherally.
- Stage 2 ROP has a ridge of scar tissue and new vessels in place of the demarcation line.
- Stage 3 ROP features extraretinal neovascular proliferation extending from the ridge into the vitreous.
- Stage 4 refers to a partial retinal detachment. The scar tissue associated with the fibrovascular ridge contracts, pulling the retina away from the wall of the eye. This can be subdivided into Stage 4a (fovea spared) and 4b (fovea involved) – the visual potential may be good in the former but is markedly decreased in the latter.
- Stage 5 ROP implies a complete retinal detachment, usually with the retina pulled into a funnel-shaped configuration by the fibrovascular scar tissue. Eyes with Stage 5 ROP usually have no useful vision, even if surgery is performed to repair the detachment.

Plus disease is characterised by dilation and tortuosity of retinal vessels, and preplus disease is characterised by abnormal vascular dilation, tortuosity insufficient for plus disease, or both. This is used as a means of determining the need for treatment.

Aggressive ROP (AROP) is characterised by significant vascular tortuosity and dilatation but without the characteristic ridge typical of Type 1 disease. This will rapidly progress to Stage 4 ROP without urgent treatment.

TREATMENT

If ROP does develop, it usually occurs between 34 and 40 weeks after conception, regardless of gestational age at birth. Treatment modalities include either injection of anti-VEGF agents or laser photocoagulation. The laser treatment is applied to the retina anterior to the vascular shunt that does not yet have a blood supply. The purpose of the treatment is to eliminate VEGF drive and reduce abnormal vessels before they fibrose and produce a tractional retinal detachment.

Haemorrhages

Haemorrhages may be intragel, preretinal (subhyaloid), retinal and subretinal.

Preretinal haemorrhages are between the posterior vitreous face and the retina. They may be seen in sickle cell retinopathy, trauma, subarachnoid haemorrhage (Terson syndrome) and non-accidental injury (widespread retinal and subretinal haemorrhages also seen with or without retinal schisis).

Retinal haemorrhages may be flame-shaped, dot and blot or Roth spots (superficial retinal haemorrhage with white centre).

Flame-shaped haemorrhages are seen in retinal vein occlusions, acute papilloedema, optic disc drusen, acute hypertensive retinopathy and retinal perivasculitis (especially early CMV retinitis). Dot and blot haemorrhages may be seen in diabetes mellitus-related retinopathy. They may be seen in shaken baby syndrome in association with superficial and subretinal haemorrhages (Figure 7.21) (see the chapter 'Child Protection'). Roth spots are seen in severe anaemias, leukaemia, bacterial endocarditis and may also be seen in trauma.

Subretinal haemorrhages are red, raised areas over which the retinal vessels are clearly visible. They are seen in sickle cell anaemia, Coats' disease (retinal telangiectasia), trauma, shaken baby syndrome and, rarely, choroidal neovascularisation.

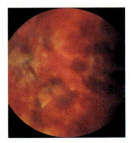

Figure 7.21 Widespread retinal haemorrhages in a proven case of shaken baby syndrome.

Treatment is targeted to the cause. Prognosis depends on severity and depth of haemorrhage.

Exudates

Rarely, yellow waxy deposits may occur, which may be retinal (focal, diffuse or macular star) or subretinal. Focal or diffuse exudates may be seen in diabetic retinopathy (unusual to see in children), old branch retinal vein occlusion (very rare in children), radiation retinopathy or retinal telangiectasia.

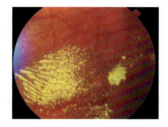

Figure 7.22 Exudates due to Coats' disease.

A macular star (stellate pattern of exudates centred on the macula) may be seen in malignant hypertension, papilloedema, neuroretinitis and very rarely retinal angioma (Von Hippel–Lindau syndrome or idiopathic).

Subretinal and intraretinal exudates may be seen in Coats' disease, Familial Exudative vitreo-retinopathy (Figure 7.22), or rarely with *Toxocara canis* retinochoroiditis.

Treatment for Coats' disease comprises laser direct to leaking vessels, and areas of retinal non-perfusion. Drainage of subretinal fluid is indicated in Stage 3b or worse detachment.

Foveal Hypoplasia

A rare underdevelopment of the fovea, commonly associated with nystagmus. This can be diagnosed using optical coherence tomography (Figure 7.23). The Leicester Grading System for foveal hypoplasia can be used to grade the severity of foveal hypoplasia and predict future visual acuity.

Electrodiagnostics may help elucidate albinism as a cause. If foveal hypoplasia is mild but visual acuity poor, then suspicion for other visually limiting pathology should be raised and investigations carried out as appropriate.

Maculopathy

Very rarely, there may be an abnormality of the macula and fovea. Causes include epiretinal membrane, macula oedema, a bull's eye appearance secondary to macula or retinal dystrophy or crystalline/exudative deposits.

Epiretinal Membrane

Striated appearance radiating out from the fovea, which causes a drop in vision. Idiopathic is the commonest cause but may also be seen in juvenile retinoschisis, Bardet–Biedl syndrome and chronic intraocular inflammation.

Vision is often poor and treatment options are limited.

Bull's Eye Maculopathy

This rare condition is characterised by hyperpigmentation in the centre of the macula, surrounded by a hypopigmented zone, concentric to which is a final hyperpigmented zone.

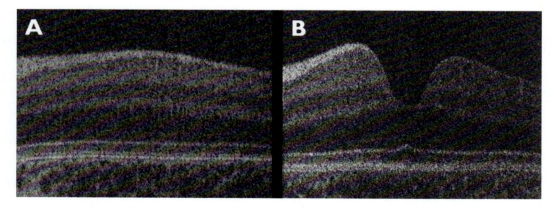

Figure 7.23 Optical Coherence Tomography demonstrating A. foveal hypoplasia and B. normal fovea. Adapted from Rufai et al., *Ophthalmology*, 2020 April; 127(4): 492–500.

Causes include long-term chloroquine use, some types of cone dystrophy (Figure 7.24), cone–rod dystrophy, rod–cone dystrophy, juvenile neuronal ceroid lipofuscinosis, benign concentric annular macular dystrophy (usually late onset) and Stargardt disease (macular dystrophy starting in childhood).

Prognosis is often guarded. If due to chloroquine the drug should be stopped.

Coloured Macular Lesions

These are all very rare.

Yellow lesions may be seen in Best's vitelliform macular dystrophy, a dominantly inherited condition that starts in childhood. In the early stages there may be no lesion at the macula but usually there is an egg yolk-like lesion at the macula (Figures 7.25 and 7.26).

There is no treatment and prognosis is guarded with time.

Cherry-red spots are due to a change in the nerve fibre layer surrounding the fovea, such as ischaemia or deposition of abnormal metabolic by-products, resulting in an accentuation of the normal deep red colour of the fovea.

Causes in children are metabolic disorders such as Tay–Sachs disease, Sandhoff disease, Niemann–Pick disease, generalised gangliosidosis and sialidosis I and II and central retinal artery occlusion. Prognosis is poor.

Atrophic macula lesions include infectious causes such as congenital toxoplasomosis, or genetic causes such as North Carolina Macula Dystrophy.

Pale Retinal Lesions
Inflammatory Lesions

These are all rare in children but it is important to consider them in a differential diagnosis of a yellow/white lesion in the retina.

- Single focal lesions: toxoplasmosis (Figure 7.27), toxocariasis (Figure 7.28), candidiasis and cryptococcus. Occasionally pars planitis ('snowbanks' in the inferior peripheral retina) may also be seen. All are accompanied by vitritis, which makes the view of the fundus hazy.

- Multiple focal lesions: candidiasis, sarcoidosis, Lyme disease, choroidal pneumocystosis, presumed ocular histoplasmosis syndrome, Behçet disease, Vogt–Koyanagi–Harada (VKH) syndrome, sympathetic ophthalmitis and tuberculous choroiditis.

- Diffuse lesions: CMV retinitis (Figure 7.29), acute retinal necrosis, herpes simplex retinitis and measles retinitis.

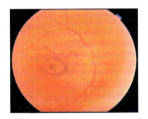

Figure 7.24 Bull's eye maculopathy seen in a case of cone retinal dystrophy.

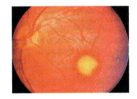

Figure 7.25 Yolk-like appearance of Best disease.

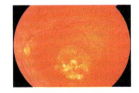

Figure 7.26 Scrambled egg appearance of Best disease.

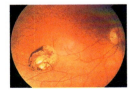

Figure 7.27 Extrafoveal toxoplasmosis scar.

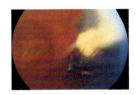

Figure 7.28 Peripheral *Toxocara* granuloma.

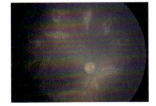

Figure 7.29 Cytomegalovirus retinitis.

169

In all the above cases, appropriate serological investigations and radiological examinations need to be undertaken. Joint ophthalmic and rheumatological evaluation improves the management of these cases. Prognosis depends on the diagnosis, with the worst prognosis being for retinal necrosis or inflammation affecting the macula.

Non-Inflammatory Lesions
Most are uncommon with some very rare.

Focal Pale Lesions
These may be due to coloboma of the retina and choroid, 'polar bear tracks', retinal astrocytoma and retinoblastoma.

Coloboma of retina and choroid: usually a circular or oval-shaped lesion that may be associated with a coloboma of the optic disc or iris. It is due to incomplete closure of the foetal ocular fissure. Retinochoroidal colobomas may be associated with a serous or rhegmatogenous retinal detachment.

Retinal astrocytoma: a hamartoma seen in 50% of patients with tuberous sclerosis. In children, a pale, almond-shaped lesion lies in the nerve fibre layer. In adults it becomes calcified, showing a mulberry-like lesion. It is usually unilateral.

Early retinoblastoma: small pale lesion, flat, elevated or nodular depending on how early it is detected (see below).

Diffuse Pale Lesions
Non-hereditary: Myelinated nerve fibres, high myopia, large coloboma of the optic disc and retina, retinal ischaemia and commotio retinae ('bruising' of the retina after blunt trauma).

Hereditary: Albinism and choroidal dystrophies such as choroideraemia and diffuse choroidal atrophy.

Multiple Focal/Discrete Lesions
Hereditary: Typical/atypical retinitis pigmentosa, retinitis pigmentosa-like retinal dystrophy with systemic associations, female carriers of X-linked ocular albinism and female carriers of choroideraemia and angioid streaks. (See Table 7.2, for systemic associations of retinitis pigmentosa.)

Retinal Detachment
Retinal detachment is very uncommon in children. It may be **rhegmatogenous** (due to a retinal hole or tear); serous or **exudative** (from leaking vessels, or rarely a defect in the optic nerve); **tractional** (due to traction on the surface of the retina from fibrosis in the attached vitreous) or **solid** (due to a tumour). A choroidal detachment is most commonly seen in hypotony following intraocular pressure-lowering operations such as trabeculectomy or trauma.

In a child with high myopia and retinal detachment, the possibility of Stickler syndrome must be excluded; the presence of congenital myopia and/or specific vitreous anomalies seen on slit-lamp examination can support the diagnosis.

Folds in the Fundus
These are uncommon and may be fine and multiple or falciform (large and single). Chorioretinal folds may be seen in ocular hypotony, swollen optic discs, choroidal tumours, hypermetropia, orbital pseudotumour or tumour, Falciform folds are seen in familial exudative vitreoretinopathy, Norrie disease, retinopathy of prematurity and Persistent Foetal Vasculature (PFV). Vitreoretinal evaluation is necessary and prognosis depends on diagnosis.

THE OPTIC DISC

Optic Disc Swelling
Unilateral optic disc swelling is not common but may be due to longstanding ocular hypotony (from any cause), uveitis, posterior scleritis, papillitis/neuritis, neuroretinitis, acute phase of Leber's hereditary optic neuropathy, papilloedema (very rarely unilateral), optic nerve glioma and other compressive lesions.

Table 7.2: Systemic Disorders Associated with Retinitis Pigmentosa or Retinal Pigmentary Retinopathy

1 Hearing difficulties:
- Usher syndrome. USH 1: Retinitis pigmentosa onset by age 10 years; cataract; profound congenital sensory deafness; labyrinthine defect. USH 2: Retinitis pigmentosa onset in late teens; childhood sensory deafness. USH 3: Postlingual, progressive hearing loss; variable vestibular dysfunction; onset of retinitis pigmentosa symptoms, usually by the second decade.
- Alstrom syndrome: Retinal lesion causes nystagmus and early loss of central vision – in contrast to loss of peripheral vision first, as in other pigmentary retinopathies; dilated cardiomyopathy (infancy)/ congestive heart failure; atherosclerosis; hypertension; renal failure; deafness; obesity; diabetes mellitus.
- Infantile refsum disease (early onset): Mental retardation; minor facial dysmorphism; retinitis pigmentosa; sensorineural hearing deficit; hepatomegaly; osteoporosis; failure to thrive; hypocholesterolemia.
- Classical refsum disease (late onset): Cardinal clinical features of Refsum disease are retinitis pigmentosa, chronic polyneuropathy and cerebellar signs.
- Cockayne dwarfism: Precociously senile appearance; pigmentary retinal degeneration; optic atrophy; deafness; marble epiphyses in some digits; photosensitivity; and mental retardation; subclinical myopathy.
- Mucopolysaccharidosis (MPS).
- Kearns–Sayre ophthalmoplegia: Pigmentary degeneration of the retina; deafness and cardiomyopathy are leading features.

2 Skin disorders:
- Refsum disease.
- Cockayne syndrome.

3 Renal disorders:
- Senior–Loken syndrome: Renal dysplasia; retinitis pigmentosa; retinal aplasia; cerebellar ataxia; sensorineural hearing loss.
- Rhyns syndrome: Retinitis pigmentosa; hypopituitarism; nephronophthisis; mild skeletal dysplasia.
- Bardet–Biedl syndrome: Obesity; rod–cone dystrophy; onset by end of second decade hypogonadism; renal anomalies; polydactyly; learning disabilities
- Cystinosis.
- Alstrom syndrome.

4 Skeletal disorders:
- Bardet–Biedl syndrome.
- Cockayne syndrome.
- Jeune syndrome: Chondrodysplasia that often leads to death in infancy because of a severely constricted thoracic cage and respiratory insufficiency; retinal degeneration.
- MPS 1H, 1S, 11,111.
- Infantile refsum disease.

5 Hepatic disorders:
- Zellweger syndrome: Hypotonia; seizures; psychomotor retardation; pigmentary retinopathy and cataracts.

6 Neurological/neuromuscular:
- Kearns–Sayre syndrome.
- Chronic progressive external ophthalmoplegia: Retinitis pigmentosa and restricted eye movements.
- Neuronal ceroid lipofuscinosis: Characterised by intralysosomal accumulations of lipopigments in either granular, curvilinear, or fingerprint patterns; progressive dementia, seizures and progressive visual failure.
- Hallervorden–Spatz syndrome: Retinitis pigmentosa and pallidal degeneration.
- Joubert syndrome: Hypoplasia of the cerebellar vermis; saccadic initiation failure; hyperpnea intermixed with central apnoea in the neonatal period; retinal dystrophy.
- Infantile refsum disease.
- Abetalipoproteinemia (Bassen–Kornzweig syndrome): Coeliac disease; pigmentary degeneration of the retina; progressive ataxic neuropathy; acanthocytosis.

Bilateral optic disc swelling may be seen more commonly than unilateral and may be due to buried optic disc drusen (Figures 7.30 and 7.31), papilloedema (Figure 7.32), malignant hypertension, cavernous sinus thrombosis and bilateral papillitis. In papillitis, vision is always affected but not in papilloedema unless it is chronic or severe. Papilloedema may be due to a CNS tumour, idiopathic intracranial hypertension or in children with craniosynostosis.

Prognosis is dependent on the cause.

Optic Atrophy

Optic atrophy occurs due to loss of neuronal axons. It may be **compressive, secondary, consecutive, ischaemic, primary hereditary, secondary hereditary** or **metabolic**

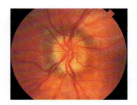

Figure 7.30 Swollen optic disc due to optic disc drusen; note the increased retinal vessels crossing the optic disc margins.

Compressive Optic Atrophy

Neuro-imaging is important in any case of optic atrophy. Surveillance with colour vision, visual field analysis and electrodiagnostic testing may be necessary in cases of optic gliomas. Differential diagnoses include optic pathway glioma, treated with chemotherapy or increasingly biological, craniopharyngioma or pituitary tumours. Prognosis may be guarded for vision.

Consecutive Optic Atrophy

Consecutive optic atrophy is caused by diseases of the inner retina or its blood supply, such as retinitis pigmentosa cone dystrophy, diffuse retinal necrosis (e.g. CMV retinitis, acute retinal necrosis and Behçet disease), cherry-red spot at macula syndromes and mucopolysaccharidoses.

Prognosis for vision is usually poor.

Ischaemic

Anterior ischaemic optic neuropathy is very rare in children and usually associated with labile blood pressure and renal failure. Far more common is optic atrophy associated with neonatal encephalopathy and cerebral visual impairment. This may be due to similar hypoxic factors, which cause brain damage or retrograde degeneration.

Secondary Optic Atrophy

Secondary optic atrophy is preceded by swelling of the optic nerve head (Figure 7.33) as a result of swelling, ischaemia, or inflammation, i.e. chronic papilloedema, papillitis. Prognosis depends on the severity of the primary disease.

Primary Hereditary Optic Atrophy

This is usually mitochondrial though the genetic mutation may be in the mitochondrial genome, e.g. Leber's optic neuropathy,

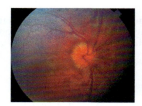

Figure 7.32 Papilloedema.

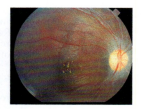

Figure 7.33 Optic atrophy following papilloedema.

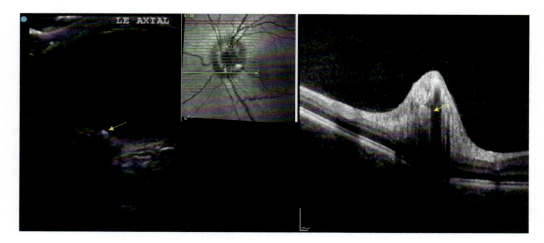

Figure 7.31 Optic disc drusen evident on ultrasound examination (left) and optical coherence tomography (right), denoted by yellow arrows. On ultrasound examination, optic disc drusen are visible as an increased echogenicity at the optic nerve head due to calcification. On optical coherence tomography, optic disc drusen are identified as hyporeflective stuctures +/– a hyperreflective border, located above the lamina cribrosa. Image courtesy of OR Marmoy, Great Ormond Street Hospital for Children, London.

or the nuclear genome, e.g. *OPA1* dominant optic atrophy. Prognosis is variable and new pharmacological and gene therapy treatments are being developed.

Secondary Hereditary Optic Atrophy

A variety of non-mitochondrial neuro-degenerative conditions can cause optic atrophy especially diseases affecting predominantly white matter such as the adrenoleukodystrophies.

Prognosis for vision is guarded.

Metabolic Optic Atrophy

A variety of conditions include propionic acidaemia and some of the mucopolysaccharidoses. Optic atrophy has also been described with vitamin B12 and folate deficiency.

Small Optic Disc

The optic nerve may appear small (hypermetropia) or actually be smaller than it should be (tilted disc and optic nerve hypoplasia – Figure 7.34). The latter is uncommon but if seen the possibility of endocrine dysfunction must be excluded in cases of optic disc hypoplasia – classically seen in septo-optic dyplasia. Nystagmus is invariably seen with bilateral optic disc hypoplasia.

Endocrine replacement is important. Visual prognosis depends on the degree of hypoplasia.

Large Optic Disc

This is seen commonly in myopia, congenital optic disc pit, optic disc coloboma (Figure 7.35) and morning glory anomaly.

Bilateral cases of optic coloboma should be investigated with neuroimaging for midline defects. Morning glory anomaly is almost always associated with intracranial abnormalities – even if unilateral.

Large Optic Disc Cup and Glaucoma

Most normal discs have a cup-to-disc ratio of 0.3 or less. Physiological cupping (a cup-to-disc ratio greater than 0.7) is present in about 2% of the normal population, and glaucomatous cupping (Figure 7.36), where there is raised intraocular pressure, with or without increased corneal diameter, increased myopia, Haab's striae and increased axial length. Glaucoma is characterised by damage to the optic nerve and can cause vision loss.

Treatment depends on severity of the glaucoma but varies from medical topical treatment to laser treatment or surgery. Prognosis for glaucoma depends on how early the glaucoma presents: Neonatal and infantile presentation is a worse prognosis than later presenting (juvenile glaucoma).

Optic Disc Vascular Abnormalities

These may be **congenital** (prepapillary loop, Bergmeister papilla, persistent hyaloid artery, increased disc vessel numbers) or **acquired** (optic disc collaterals, neovascularisation, opticociliary shunts, dragged optic disc vessels). No treatment is needed but in acquired cases the cause must be sought. All causes are rare.

Optic Disc Haemorrhages

These are not uncommon and may be due to acute papilloedema, papillitis, infiltrative optic neuropathy, and optic disc drusen. Investigation, including optic disc imaging and visual field analysis, to exclude early papilloedema is important.

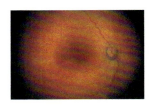

Figure 7.34 Optic nerve hypoplasia.

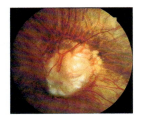

Figure 7.35 Marked optic disc coloboma.

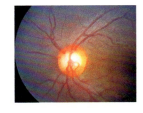

Figure 7.36 Optic disc cupping in juvenile glaucoma.

Lesions Obscuring the Optic Disc

These are all rare and include primary optic disc tumours, such as capillary angioma (rare, Figure 7.37) and melanocytoma; retinal tumours such as astrocytoma or combined hamartoma of the retina and RPE; infiltrative lesions due to leukaemia (Figure 7.38), tuberculosis granuloma or sarcoid. Treatment is dependent on the diagnosis, as is prognosis.

THE ORBIT

Abnormalities of Globe Position

Enophthalmos

Enophthalmos describes the globe positioned more posteriorly in the orbit giving an appearance of a sunken eye with a deep upper lid sulcus and ptosis. This appearance is rare in children; significant orbital wall fracture, orbital radiotherapy/proton therapy or incessant eye rubbing are possible aetiologies. Pseudo-enophthalmos is caused by a relatively small eye volume such as in microphthalmia or pthtisical eye.

Treatment depends on the cause but reconstruction of the orbit to restore volume, fat grafting and prosthetic shells are options.

Proptosis

Proptosis describes the globe positioned more anteriorly in an orbit. It may be axial (forward without any displacement in any other direction) or non-axial. Axial proptosis can be caused by lesions within the cone of extraocular muscles, while non-axial proptosis is caused by lesions outside this cone. The commonest cause of proptosis in children is infective orbital cellulitis. Rarer causes include orbital haemorrhage secondary to lymphatic malformation and other vascular anomalies, orbital inflammation and tumours.

Pseudoproptosis is caused by a large globe (e.g. high myopia, buphthalmos [congenital glaucoma]), lid retraction, or a shallow orbit, such as in children with Crouzon, Apert and Pfeiffer syndromes.

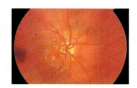

Figure 7.37 Retinal capillary angioma on the optic disc in a child with Von Hippel–Lindau syndrome.

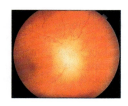

Figure 7.38 Leukaemic infiltration of the optic disc.

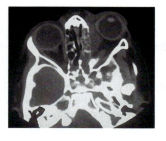

Figure 7.39 CT scan showing ethmoid sinusitis and contiguous orbital cellulitis with proptosis.

Infective Orbital Cellulitis

Incidence: Common.

Aetiology: The most common cause is from adjacent sinus disease.

Clinical Presentation: Eyelid swelling and redness may be the first signs. Progression to intraorbital disease may be heralded by eye movement restrictions, proptosis or vertical/horizontal displacement of the globe, redness and swelling of the conjunctiva and disruption in optic nerve function (Figure 7.39). Patients are also at risk of progression to intracranial abscesses and cavernous sinus thrombosis and thus may present with neurological signs and symptoms.

Differentials: Orbital inflammation, orbital tumours and vascular anomalies.

Treatment: Prompt assessment by a multidisciplinary team involving paediatrics, ENT and ophthalmology is recommended. Usually patients require admission, IV antibiotics and sinus decongestants. Imaging with MRI or CT is preformed if the clinical picture is not improving with IV antibiotics. Surgical drainage of subperiosteal or orbital abscesses may be required. The use of corticosteroids for these patients remains uncertain.

Prognosis: Usually good if assessment and management is prompt.

Orbital Inflammation

Paediatric orbital inflammatory disease (POID) encompasses the specific and non-specific non-infectious inflammatory conditions which involve the orbit. Subgroups of PIOD include specific disease entities such as thyroid eye disease, whereas non-specific refers to conditions such as myositis, idiopathic orbital inflammation and dacryoadentitis where there are no histological or immunological markers. Non-specific conditions can be considered interim diagnoses until biomarkers underlying pathological processes can be unravelled.

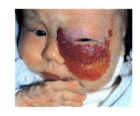

Figure 7.40 Left proptosis due to orbital and periorbital capillary haemangioma.

Benign Orbital Tumours
Orbital Dermoid

Incidence: Rare.

Aetiology: Congenital choristomas containing hair follicles and sebaceous material. Usually located at the level of the lateral brow. They may be superficial or have deeper extension into the orbit.

They are benign and rarely rupture spontaneously.

Differential: Pilomatrixoma, encephalocoele (particularly if located in the medial orbit).

Treatment: Small cysts may be monitored but surgeons recommend excision if diagnosis is uncertain or there is a risk of rupture through trauma. Cysts should ideally be removed unruptured to prevent post-operative inflammation.

Capillary Haemangiomas

Incidence: Common.

Clinical Presentation: These lesions in the orbit have a natural history like those elsewhere in the body, but may not be noticed unless they grow in infancy or are picked up as incidental findings. They may present with progressive proptosis (Figure 7.40).

Treatment: See the chapter 'Dermatology'. Medical treatment is advised.

Teratoma

These are very rare germ cell tumours which can contain heterogenous tissues such as muscle, hair, bone. These have malignant potential and are locally destructive. Assessment by the MDT team is advised..

Optic Nerve Glioma

Optic nerve glioma may be isolated or associated with NF1. Monitoring with colour vision, electrodiagnostics and visual fields is important to evaluate visual function, while neuroimaging is needed to monitor growth of the tumour.

Plexiform Neurofibroma

See also section on NF2.

These can present in children from early infancy into late childhood. Lesions can infiltrate tissues of the orbit and eyelid causing visual loss, proptosis (usually non-axial) and disfigurement. Surgical resection should be planned in an MDT setting.

Langerhans Cell Histiocytosis

This is a progressive disease process which can occur at any age but usually under 10 years. It can be unifocal or multifocal. A CT scan would demonstrate a soft tissue mass with adjacent bony lysis. Treatment involves excision biopsy and/or corticosteroids and chemotherapy.

Malignant Tumours of the Orbit

See also the chapter 'Oncology'.

Incidence: these are all extremely rare.

Presentation: Mass effect within the orbit causing proptosis, chemosis, eye movement disturbances and optic nerve dysfunction. Some can present as infective orbital cellulitis, e.g. rhabdomyosarcoma and neuroblastoma.

Treatments: Tailored treatments including surgery, chemotherapy, immunotherapy and radiotherapy is planned on a case-by-case basis in a MDT setting. Imaging and tissue biopsy is key to management planning.

Rhabdomyosarcoma

Peak presentation is approximately 7 years of age with proptosis. Progresses rapidly and is highly malignant.

Metastatic neuroblastoma

Presents in a similar manner to rhabdomyosarcoma but usually at a younger age (under 5 years) with the primary tumour in the abdomen. Forty percent of metastases affect both orbits.

Acute leukaemia

Usually presents around 7 years of age with rapid onset proptosis and ecchymosis (bruising in the lids).

Retinoblastoma

See intraocular tumours.

Orbital Vascular Malformations

Spectrum versus separate entities, these lesions may comprise lymphatic, venous and arterial or a combination of the latter. Different rates of flow though the channels.

Lymphatic Malformation

Incidence: Rare.

Aetiology: Lymphatic malformation (formerly known as lymphangioma) are vascular anomalies, not tumours. Microcystic, macrocystic and combined forms exist.

Clinical Presentation: They exhibit commensurate growth but can fluctuate in size during viral illness or cause acute bleeds. Within the orbit they may cause symptoms of proptosis, eye movement abnormalities, periocular swelling and ptosis and optic nerve compromise. There is no increase of the lesion on Valsalva, unlike venous malformations.

Assessment: Ultrasound to check flow and MRI scan to exclude intracranial developmental vascular anomalies.

Treatment: Mainstay is sclerotherapy and possibly surgical debulking if required.

Prognosis: Variable.

EYE MOVEMENT DISORDERS

See also the chapter 'Neurology'.

These may be classified as disorders in primary position of gaze, anomalous eye movements and nystagmus. All cases should be referred for ophthalmic opinion.

Ocular Deviation in Primary Gaze

If a deviation remains stable regardless of the position of the gaze of the eyes, it is called comitant. If it does change it is termed non- or in-comitant.

Esodeviation

This is a turning in of one or both eyes.

Pseudodeviation

Epicanthic folds: Symmetric corneal reflexes confirm the absence of true esotropia.

Narrow interpupillary distance seen in hypotelorism.

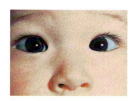

True Esodeviation

Commitant Esotropia

Infantile esotropia (Figure 7.41) develops before the age of 6 months with a large and stable angle, crossfixation (child uses right eye to look to left and *vice versa* as the eyes are so convergent) and normal refraction for age.

■ Non-accommodative esotropia: esotropia after 6 months of age with normal refraction.

Figure 7.41 This child has epicanthic folds but the corneal light reflex on the right cornea is central, while the reflex in the left eye is off the pupil, indicating the presence of a left esodeviation.

- Refractive accommodative esotropia: Onset is usually between two and three years, associated with hypermetropia (long-sightedness).

- Non-refractive accommodative esotropia: Onset after six months but before three years. No significant refractive error but excessive convergence for near (called high accommodative convergence: accommodation ratio – AC/A ratio).

- Sensory esotropia: Due to reduction in vision, with one eye much worse than the other, which disrupts fusion, e.g. in unilateral cataract.

- Convergent spasm: Intermittent esotropia with pseudomyopia and miosis due to accommodative spasm, which may be seen after trauma or due to a posterior fossa tumour but usually has a functional element.

Incomitant Esotropia

- VI nerve palsy: May be congenital or acquired (associated with raised intracranial pressure). Esotropia gets worse when looking in the distance.

- Möbius syndrome: Bilateral gaze palsies, with esotropia in 50% of cases (due to superimposed VI nerve palsies). There is usually bilateral VII nerve palsies and may be associated V, IX and X nerve palsies and brainstem abnormalities.

- Duane syndrome: Usually due to hypoplasia of the sixth nerve(s) and miswiring of the horizontal rectus muscles which leads to cocontraction of the medial and lateral recti.

Exodeviation (the Eyes Diverge in Primary Position)
Pseudo-Exodeviation

Hypertelorism: Look for symmetry of corneal light reflexes.

True Exodeviation
Comitant Exotropia

Intermittent exotropia: A common condition with exotropia more commonly present for distance than for near (Figure 7.42). In bright sunlight the child will characteristically close the diverging eye.

- Sensory exotropia: Much less common in children than sensory esodeviation.

- Convergence insufficiency: Usually seen in older children. Convergence exercises may help but there should be a low threshold to neuroimage if there are any neurological signs or worsening despite convergence exercises.

Incomitant Exotropia

- Congenital III nerve palsy: Exodeviation and hypodeviation of the affected eye, with ptosis and sometimes pupil enlargement. There is a limitation of upgaze and adduction.

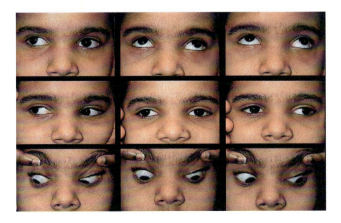

Figure 7.42 Exotropia.

- Acquired III nerve palsy (Figure 7.43): Rare. The same signs as in the congenital condition but the pupil is dilated.

- Duane syndrome Type II: See above.

Anomalous Eye Movements
Upshoots in Adduction (On Version Testing)

- Inferior oblique overaction: may be primary (usually bilateral and seen with esotropia but also with exotropia occurring in childhood) or secondary (to a superior oblique palsy) (Figure 7.44).

- Duane syndrome: See above. Upshoots occur due to a leash effect of a tight lateral rectus muscle secondary to co-contraction of the medial rectus muscle.

- Dissociated vertical deviation: A bilateral condition most commonly seen in association with infantile esotropia. At moments of inattention the eye will move up and then move down to its original position while the fixating eye remains still. It differs from inferior oblique overaction in that the eye may elevate in any position of gaze.

- Craniosynostoses (Figure 7.45): In the syndromic craniosynostoses, e.g. Apert, Pfeiffer, Crouzon, the extraocular muscles are excyclorotated such that the medial rectus now acts as an elevator as well as an adductor.

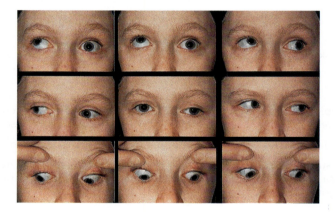

Figure 7.43   III nerve palsy (left side).

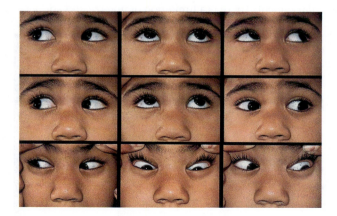

Figure 7.44   Right superior oblique palsy. The right eye does not depress in adduction as well as it should do. There is also a mild right inferior oblique overaction (there is a slight upshoot of the right eye in adduction).

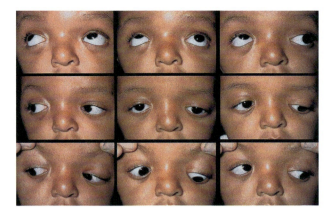

Figure 7.45 Child with Apert syndrome who shows anomalous eye movements with upshoots in adduction and coincident downshoots in abduction. This child also demonstrates a V pattern: when the child looks up, the eyes diverge, compared to when the child looks down. There is also a right depression deficit.

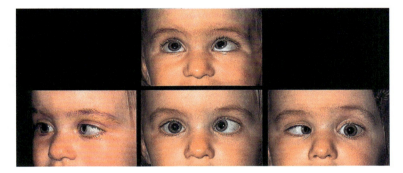

Figure 7.46 Left esotropia due to left VI nerve palsy (left abduction deficit).

Downshoots in Adduction (On Version Testing)

- Duane syndrome: See above.

- Brown syndrome: This is not an uncommon condition where the tendon of the superior oblique muscle is unable to pass freely through its pulley (the trochlea, at the superomedial orbital rim). This results in restriction of elevation in upgaze usually just in the adducted position. As a result there may be a coincident downshoot in adduction on version testing. It is usually idiopathic but may be acquired due to inflammation at the trochlea or trauma.

- Superior oblique overaction: May be primary and usually seen with intermittent exotropia in older children (late teens).

Limitation of Abduction

- VI nerve palsy (Figure 7.46): There is always an esotropia in the primary position of gaze. In Duane I and II there may not be an esotropia in primary position of gaze.

- Any restrictive myopathy of the medial rectus: Myositis, pseudotumour, and, very rarely, thyroid eye disease.

Limitation of Adduction

- III nerve palsy (Figure 7.43): May be congenital or acquired (see above).

- Internuclear ophthalmoplegia (INO): A lesion in the medial longitudinal fasiculus leading to ipsilateral adduction limitation and contralateral eye abducting nystagmus.

- Myasthenia gravis: Very rare but may mimic adduction deficit.

- Acute myositis: restriction of movement in the direction of the field of action of the affected muscle.

- Duane syndrome II and III.

Limitation of Horizontal Versions or Gaze Palsies

- Any lesion of the paramedian pontine reticular formation (PPRF) causes ipsilateral gaze palsy.

- One-and-a-half syndrome: A lesion of the PPRF/abducens nucleus and adjacent medial longitudinal fasiculus causing an ipsilateral gaze palsy and ipsilateral INO. A right-sided neurological lesion would lead to inability for either eye to look to the right, the right eye could not adduct (part of the INO) but the left eye could abduct but only with a nystagmus.

- Bilateral pontine lesions result in total horizontal gaze palsies.

- Fisher syndrome: A rare variant of Guillain–Barré syndrome, which may present in children with ophthalmoplegia, ataxia and areflexia, though the initial presentation may be one of horizontal gaze palsy or an INO.

Limitation of Vertical Eye Movement (One or Both Eyes)

- Palsy of a muscle: Superior rectus, inferior oblique (upgaze affected) and inferior rectus, superior oblique palsy (downgaze affected).

- Orbital floor fracture: Causing entrapped inferior rectus muscle and restriction of elevation.

- Orbital space occupying lesion, e.g. capillary haemangioma, plexiform neurofibroma.

- Symblepharon: Attachment of lid to globe will cause restriction of elevation or depression.

- Brown syndrome: See above. Deficit in elevation.

- Monocular elevation deficit: Formerly called double elevator palsy. This may be due to idiopathic tightening of the inferior rectus muscle or idiopathic with no evidence of inferior rectus tightening.

Vertical Gaze Palsy

- Parinaud syndrome: Decreased upgaze, large pupils, convergence insufficiency and convergence-retraction nystagmus. In children, one of the commonest causes is a pinealoma.

- Hydrocephalus: Stretching of the posterior commissure results in loss of upgaze with or without tonic downward deviation of the eyes ('sunset' sign).

- Metabolic causes: May affect vertical eye movements. Tay–Sachs disease may cause impairment of vertical and later horizontal gaze. Niemann–Pick variants may also cause vertical gaze anomalies.

Generalised Limitation of Ocular Movements

This may be due to multiple ocular motor palsies or to other causes.

Due to Multiple Ocular Motor Palsies

- Cavernous sinus lesions
- Superior orbital fissure lesion
- Brainstem lesions

Due to Other Causes

- Chronic progressive external ophthalmoplegia (mitochondrial disease)
- Myotonic dystrophy
- Acquired saccadic initiation failure (ocular motor apraxia)

- Metabolic causes: Tay–Sachs disease, and occasionally other lipid-storage diseases
- Congenital fibrosis syndrome (often a congenital dysinnervation syndrome affecting the third cranial nerve).

Nystagmus

Nystagmus is characterised by involuntary, rapid and repetitive eye movements.

Character of Nystagmus

- Horizontal jerk: A combination of slow drift with fast corrective phase. The 'nystagmus' direction is the same as the fast corrective phase.
- Pendular: Nystagmus velocity is the same in both directions but on lateral gaze this usually develops a horizontal jerk component.
- Oblique: Due to a combination of horizontal and vertical directions of pendular nystagmus.

Early onset nystagmus – this is usually classified as infantile nystagmus which can be purely motor or associated with foveal hypoplasia and other ocular conditions (see below) and latent or fusional maldevelopment nystagmus associated with early loss of binocularity. Does not usually require neuro-imaging.

- Manifest nystagmus is usually benign but may be acquired. It is uniplanar, dampens on convergence and worsens on eccentric fixation.
- Latent nystagmus: No nystagmus with both eyes open but horizontal jerk nystagmus is seen when one eye is covered. Most commonly seen with infantile esotropia but may be seen with other early onset deviations. The fast phase is towards the uncovered fixating eye.
- Manifest-latent nystagmus: Usually seen with infantile esotropia and dissociated vertical deviation. The nystagmus becomes worse when one eye is occluded.
- Spasmus nutans: An early onset (3–18 months) unilateral or bilateral small amplitude high frequency horizontal nystagmus often associated with head nodding. It is most often idiopathic with resolution by 3 years of age but it may be due to an optic pathway glioma.
- Roving nystagmus: Severe disruption of visual function may lead to this and the commonest causes are Leber's congenital amaurosis (severe retinal dystrophy) or optic nerve hypoplasia (bilateral).

Later Onset Nystagmus (Does Usually Require Neuro-Imaging)

- Coarse horizontal jerk nystagmus: Usually seen in cerebellar disease, with fast phase ipsilateral to the lesion.
- Torsional nystagmus: If pure then this is usually only seen in central vestibular disease such as syringomyelia or syringobulbia associated with Arnold–Chiari malformation, demyelination and, very rarely, lateral medullary syndrome in children.
- Downbeat nystagmus: Usually seen in lesions at the craniocervical junction (e.g. Arnold–Chiari malformation), drug toxicity (phenytoin, carbamazepine), trauma, hydrocephalus and demyelination.
- Upbeat nystagmus: Usually seen in cerebellar degenerations (e.g. ataxia telangiectasia) and encephalitis; in babies a retinal dystrophy should be excluded (especially cone dystrophy).
- Gaze-evoked nystagmus: May be seen with lesions of the vestibulocerebellum axis, brainstem or cerebral hemispheres or after a gaze palsy or with drug toxicity (phenytoin and carbemazipine).
- Periodic alternating nystagmus: The direction of the nystagmus reverses. It may be congenital idiopathic but is usually seen with Arnold–Chiari malformation or cerebellar disease, trauma or demyelination.
- Rebound nystagmus: Attempt to maintain eccentric gaze results in gaze-evoked nystagmus, which dampens and sometimes reverses direction. On returning to primary gaze a transient nystagmus develops. It is usually seen in cerebellar disease.

- See-saw nystagmus: Pendular nystagmus in which one eye elevates and intorts while the other eye depresses and extorts and then the eyes reverse. The commonest cause is chiasmal or parasellar tumours but it may also be seen in albinism as a transient finding, head trauma and syringobulbia.

- Internuclear ophthalmoplegia: The abducting eye has nystagmus (see above) and is due to a lesion in the medial longitudinal fasiculus.

- Monocular nystagmus: May be seen in spasmus nutans, unilateral deep amblyopia, superior oblique myokymia and optic nerve glioma.

- Convergence-retraction nystagmus: Seen in Parinaud syndrome (see above).

Ocular Causes of Nystagmus

Disruption of vision will lead to nystagmus. There may be obvious (usually bilateral) ocular disease such as corneal opacities, congenital cataract, microphthalmos, aniridia and oculocutaneous nystagmus or less obvious ocular disease such as retinal dystrophy (usually cone dystrophy or Leber's congenital amaurosis), ocular albinism, X-linked congenital stationary night blindness, optic nerve hypoplasia and early onset optic atrophy.

Depending on the cause, nystagmus may be improved with drugs or surgery. The null position is a position of the eyes where the nystagmus is most dampened; in this position the child sees better. The child may adopt an abnormal head position so that the eyes are in the null position. Abnormal head posture may be improved by surgical repositioning of the extraocular muscles.

REFERENCES

- Belin MW, Duncan JK. Keratoconus: the ABCD grading system. *Klin Monbl Augenheilkd*. 2016 Jun;233(6):701–707.
- Bonini S, Bonini S, Lambiase A, et al. Vernal keratoconjunctivitis revisited: a case series of 195 patients with long-term followup. *Ophthalmology*. 2000 Jun;107(6):1157–1163.
- Chiang MF, Quinn GE, Fielder AR, et al. International classification of retinopathy of prematurity, third edition. *Ophthalmology*. 2021 Jul 8:S0161–6420(21)00416-4.
- Edén U, Iggman D, Riise R, et al. Epidemiology of aniridia in Sweden and Norway. *Acta Ophthalmol*. 2008 Nov;86(7):727–729.
- Fu Z, et al. Global prevalence of amblyopia and disease burden projections through 2040: a systematic review and meta-analysis. *Br J Ophthalmol*. 2020 Aug;104(8):1164–1170.
- Gupta N, Dhawan A, Beri S, D'souza P. Clinical spectrum of pediatric blepharokeratoconjunctivitis. *J AAPOS*. 2010 Dec;14(6):527–529.
- Harding P, Moosajee M. The molecular basis of human anophthalmia and microphthalmia. *J Dev Biol*. 2019 Aug 14;7(3):16.
- Harding P, Moosajee M. The molecular basis of human anophthalmia and microphthalmia. *J Dev Biol*. 2019 Aug 14;7(3):16.
- Hashemi H, Heydarian S, Hooshmand E, et al. The prevalence and risk factors for keratoconus: a systematic review and meta-analysis. *Cornea*. 2020 Feb;39(2):263–270.
- Hingorani M, Nischal KK, Davies A. Ocular abnormalities in Alagille syndrome. *Ophthalmology*. 1999 Feb;106(2):330–337.
- Landsend ECS, Lagali N, Utheim TP. Congenital aniridia – A comprehensive review of clinical features and therapeutic approaches. *Surv Ophthalmol*. 2021 Mar 4:S0039–6257(21)00065-5.
- Machen L, MacIntosh P. Considerations in pediatric proptosis. *JAMA Ophthalmol*. 2018 Oct 1;136(10):1197–1198.
- Postolache L, Parsa CF. Brushfield spots and Wölfflin nodules unveiled in dark irides using near-infrared light. *Sci Rep*. 2018 Dec 21;8(1):18040.
- Rahi JS, Dezateux C. Congenital and infantile cataract in the United Kingdom: underlying or associated factors. British Congenital Cataract Interest Group. *Invest Ophthalmol Vis Sci*. 2000 Jul;41(8):2108–2114.
- RCPCH. Screening and treatment of retinopathy of prematurity – clinical guideline. 2020; Available from: https://www.rcpch.ac.uk/resources/screening-treatment-retinopathy-prematurity-clinical-guideline. Accessed August 2021.
- Rennie CA, Chowdhury S, Khan J, et al. The prevalence and associated features of posterior embryotoxon in the general ophthalmic clinic. *Eye*. 2005 Apr;19(4):396–399.

- Rufai SR, Thomas MG, Purohit R, et al. Can Structural grading of foveal hypoplasia predict future vision in infantile nystagmus?: A longitudinal study. *Ophthalmology*. 2020 Apr;127(4):492–500.
- Solebo AL, Cumberland P, Rahi JS; British Isles Congenital Cataract Interest Group. 5-year outcomes after primary intraocular lens implantation in children aged 2 years or younger with congenital or infantile cataract: findings from the IoLunder2 prospective inception cohort study. *Lancet Child Adolesc Health*. 2018 Dec;2(12):863–871.
- Wadhwani M, D'souza P, Jain R, et al. Conjunctivitis in the newborn- a comparative study. *Indian J Pathol Microbiol*. 2011 Apr–Jun;54(2):254–257.
- Weaver DT. Current management of childhood ptosis. *Curr Opin Ophthalmol*. 2018 Sep;29(5):395–400.
- Woo KI, Kim Y-D. Management of epiblepharon: state of the art. *Curr Opin Ophthalmol*. 2016 Sep;27(5):433–438.

8 Neurology

Noelle Enright and Anoushka Alwis

CRANIAL NERVE EXAMINATION

Although it can be difficult to undertake a cranial nerve examination in the correct order in small children, it is essential to perform the core component. Much of the examination can be done through careful observation of the child at play but some areas such as visual acuity and fundoscopy much be formally tested. Below is a description of the cranial nerve examination in detail. Further detail on the eye examination can be found in ophthalmology (see the chapter 'Opthalmology').

CONDITIONS TYPICALLY PRESENTING WITH CRANIAL NERVE ABNORMALITIES

Ptosis: This is defined as an abnormal drooping of the upper eyelid in front of the eye, it may be partial or complete, covering the whole eye. Ptosis can be unilateral or bilateral, congenital or acquired.

Causes of Unilateral Ptosis

1. Simple congenital ptosis. This is the most common cause, and is most prevalent in males.

2. Horner's syndrome partial ptosis, miosis and anhidrosis due to disruption of the sympathetic nerve supply. If congenital it will be accompanied by heterochromia iridis in a brown eyed child (Figure 8.13).

3. Third nerve palsy (Figure 8.1). The ptosis is usually severe. In a complete third nerve palsy, there is associated dilatation of the pupil and the eye will be positioned 'down and out', due to involvement of the superior, inferior and medial rectus and the inferior oblique muscles. Causes include a space occupying lesion of the orbit or midbrain, uncal herniation, inflammation of the base of the skull, or an aneurysm of the base of the skull.

4. Marcus–Gunn jaw winking phenomenon causing intermittent ptosis (Figure 8.3).

Causes of Bilateral Ptosis

1. Congenital, look for evidence of dysmorphic features as it can be associated with genetic conditions such as Noonan's.

2. Neuromuscular disease such as congenital myopathy.

3. Myasthenia – see further details below (Figure 8.4).

MYASTHENIA

There are three broad categories of myasthenic syndromes (Figure 8.5).

Neonatal myasthenia occurs in the infants of mothers with acetylcholine receptor (AChR) or MuSK antibodies and is usually transient (Figure 8.6).

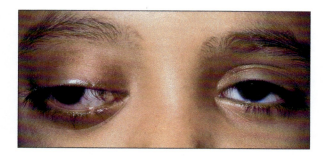

Figure 8.1 Third nerve palsy and exophthalmos secondary to an orbital tumour. There is severe ptosis and the eye is 'down and out'; the pupillary dilatation cannot be seen.

DOI: 10.1201/9781003175186-8

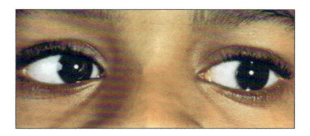

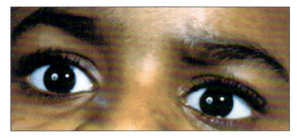

Figure 8.2, 8.3 Left sixth nerve palsy as a false localising sign of intracranial hypertension in a boy who also has an upgaze palsy.

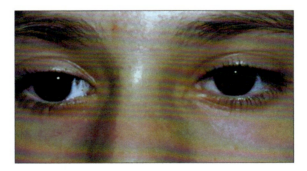

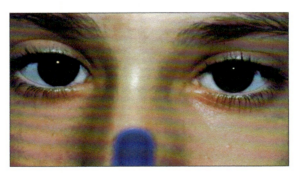

Figure 8.4, 8.5 Lateral gaze palsy in a girl with an operable brainstem tumour; although she cannot look to the left with either eye on command, the eyes do move to converge.

Congenital myasthenic syndromes (CMS) are inherited genetic conditions, typically autosomal recessive inheritance patterns are seen, although not exclusively. To date 35 genes have been reported as associated with CMS. Variants in these genes, which are expressed at the neuromuscular junction, cause impaired neuromuscular signal transmission. These patients often present before 2 years of age, although neonatal onset, and later onset of symptoms can occur. Clinically they present with muscle fatigue, weakness, and hypoplasia, eye signs such as ophthalmoplegia

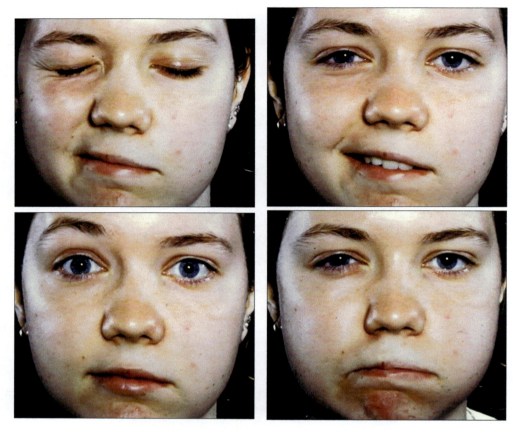

Figures 8.6–8.9   Left lower motor neuron facial palsy in a child. 8.6: Her mouth does not move on the left when asked to show her teeth; 8.7: She cannot fully close the left eye; 8.8: Her left eyebrow does not move when asked to look surprised; 8.9: the left cheek does not move when asked to blow out her cheeks. Note the very obvious abnormality involving both upper and lower face.

and ptosis. They may also have arthrogryposis from birth, and respiratory complications such as repeated apnoeas or respiratory infections due to bulbar involvement. Some patients may have some distinctive facial features such as a high arched palate or low set ears. Diurnal fluctuation in muscle strength is not always a feature, some patients may have no eye signs at all and are termed 'limb girdle' CMS. Diagnosis is typically done through single fibre EMG and genetic testing once there is a clinical suspicion. Treatment options include pyridostigmine, ephedrine, salbutamol, amifampridine (3,4-diaminopyridine), quinidine, fluoxetine, and acetazolamide but need to be targeted to the specific underlying genetic cause. It is important to be aware of the risk of respiratory complications and recurrent infections and the potential need for increased respiratory support during intercurrent infections, as well as the possibility of developing bulbar involvement and feeding difficulties (Figure 8.7 to 8.15).

Juvenile myasthenia gravis (MG) is an autoimmune disorder that leads to dysfunction of the AChR. it similar to the adult form, but younger children are more likely to have purely ocular symptoms and be AChR antibody negative. Ocular symptoms are the most common presenting symptom in particular ptosis. Other possible presenting symptoms are limb weakness, bulbar weakness, respiratory muscle weakness, and generalised fatigue. Diagnosis is made through a combination of clinical suspicion, antibody testing for AChR and muscle-specific kinase (MUSK) antibodies, a single fibre EMG, and if needed performing an Edrophonium (tensilon) test. Consider performing genetic testing for CMS in those who are antibody negative. Treatment options include – anticholinesterase drugs (e.g. pyridostigmine, or neostigmine in neonates). Early thymectomy in cases of AChR antibody positive disease with generalised weakness, especially with bulbar involvement. Immunosuppression with alternate day steroids (+/- azathioprine) for

Table 8.1: **Cranial Nerve Examination**

Cranial Nerve	Function	Testing
CN II (Optic)	Visual acuity	Formal assessment requires a Snellen chart but difficulty counting fingers, seeing hand movements, or with perception of light suggests increasing severity of impairment.
	Visual fields	These should be assessed by confrontation using wriggling fingers, or if available a white pin for peripheral visual fields and a red pin for central visual fields.
	Pupillary light reflexes	First observe the size, shape and symmetry of both pupils. Direct light reflex. Consensual light reflex. Swinging light test, for Relative Afferent Pupillary Defect (RAPD). Accommodation reflex
	Fundoscopy	Check the red reflex first. Then observe the optic disc colour and edges. Finally scan the retina
CN III, IV, VI (Oculomotor, Trochlear, Abducens)	Eye movements and eyelid elevation	First, observe the eye in primary position by asking them to fixate on a pen help 50 cm from the nose. Look for ptosis, nystagmus and strabismus. Ask about diplopia. CN III palsy – eye down and out (Figure 8.1), due to involvement of the superior, inferior and medial rectus and the inferior oblique muscles. The eyelid may be completely closed. CN IV palsy – This is extremely rare. It causes paralysis of the superior oblique muscle (SO4). Head tilt is often prominent and the patient has difficulty looking down (e.g. when walking downstairs). It is usually idiopathic but may be due to a pseudotumour. CN VI palsy – The eye is unable to look laterally because of paralysis of the lateral rectus muscle (LR6) (Figure 8.2) Ophthalmoplegia – Paralysis of third, fourth and sixth nerves. Upward gaze palsy – The child is unable to look upwards (Figure 8.3). This implies pressure on the midbrain. Lateral gaze palsy – The child is able to look to one side but not the other (Figure 8.4). Convergence is preserved (Figure 8.5).
CN V (Trigeminal)	Sensation to the face	Test ophthalmic (V1), maxillary (V2) and mandibular (V3) sensory branches with cotton wool.
	Motor supply to masseter, pterygoid, and temporalis muscles	Inspect for wasting then ask the patient to clench their jaw and to open their jaw against resistance.
	Reflexes	Corneal reflex – afferent V1, efferent VII. Jaw-jerk – afferent V3, efferent motor V
CN VII (Facial)	Facial movement	The child is asked to show their teeth (Figure 8.6), screw up their eyes voluntarily (Figure 8.7) and against resistance, look surprised (Figure 8.8) and blow their cheeks out (Figure 8.9). The facial expression (e.g. on smiling spontaneously) should also be noted. Lower motor neuron facial palsy – presents as an obvious weakness of the face with involvement of the eye (Figures 8.6 to 8.9). Upper motor neuron facial palsy – An upper motor neuron facial palsy is often mild (Figure 8.10). The eye is usually not involved because of the bilateral innervation of the upper part of the face (Figure 8.11). The child usually smiles normally (Figure 8.12). Upper motor neuron facial palsies may also be bilateral.
CN IX X, XI, XII (Vestibulocochlear, Glossopharyngeal, Vagus, Spinal Accessory, Hypoglossal)	Hearing	Lesions are often bilateral and involving several cranial nerves. Hearing assessment
	Gag reflex	Assess speech quality and volume for hoarseness and quietness (dysarthria, dysphonia).
	Palatal movement	Ask the patient to open their mouth and say 'Ahhhh' checking for palatal asymmetry.
	Motor function to trapezius and sternocleidomastoid	Check the left and right gag reflex.
	Motor supply to tongue muscle	Shrug their shoulder, and push their head to the right and left against resistance. Finally, inspect the tongue for wasting, fasciculations, and deviation.

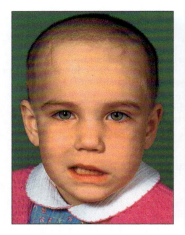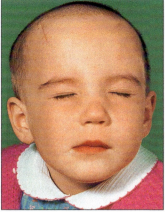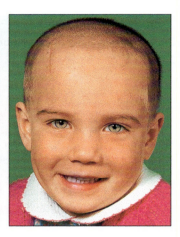

Figure 8.10–8.12   Upper motor neuron facial palsy. Unilateral in a child recovering from a cerebral abscess. The asymmetry of the lower face is obvious when the child is asked to show her teeth (8.10), but the upper face is not involved, and she is able to close both eyes normally (8.11), and the palsy is not obvious with spontaneous emotion (e.g. when she smiles, 8.12).

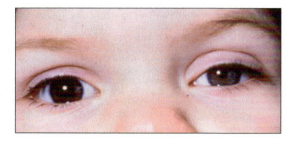

Figure 8.13   Congenital ptosis with heterochromia iridis (left eye is blue; right eye is brown).

severe symptoms not controlled with pyridostigmine. Immunoglobulin or plasma exchange for acute exacerbations, especially with respiratory compromise.

MOTOR SYSTEM

As with the cranial nerves, adaptations may often be required when examining the motor system in young children or those with a neurological disability. However, a broad understanding of what should be done and what abnormalities you may find will be useful to adapt as necessary.

PYRAMIDAL DISORDERS

The pyramidal tracts are a system of efferent nerve fibres that carry signals from the cerebral cortex, mainly the primary motor cortex, through the corona radiata, internal capsule, cerebral peduncles, pons and upper medulla to either the brainstem or spinal cord. It is divided into the corticospinal tract and the corticobulbar tract. Lesions to the pyramidal tract lead to signs and symptoms similar to an upper motor neuron (UMN), hyperreflexia, spasticity, and upgoing plantars. Although acutely they may present with hypotonia and hyporeflexia. Any injury to the pyramidal tracts will cause these symptoms but the most classic description of this is cerebral palsy.

Cerebral Palsy

Cerebral palsy (CP) is a non-progressive disorder of permanent motor dysfunction caused by an injury to the developing foetal or infant brain. It should be noted that although the underlying cause may be non-progressive the effect on motor function may change with time as the central

Table 8.2: **Motor System**

Area of Examination	Findings to watch for
General Observation – observe the patient, the room, and the family. If possible, remove clothing down to underwear to allow close observation of breathing, muscle bulk, joint position, and skin.	Look for any equipment – evidence of ankle foot orthosis suggesting tight ankles, wheelchair suggesting reduced mobility. Wasting – look for muscle wasting and the pattern it appears in, e.g. Figure 8.14 showing wasting of the right hand in a child with hemiplegia. Movements – observe for any evidence of a movement disorder such as chorea or tremor, also observe for a paucity of movement due to a possible hemiplegia or weakness. See table 8.1 for a more complete description of abnormal movements. Finally, observe the pattern of breathing - Diaphragmatic breathing may be seen in spinal muscular atrophy, due to weak intercostal muscles and a stronger diaphragm causing the abdomen and not the chest to expand during inhalation. Paradoxical breathing (indrawing of the intercostal muscles on inhalation) may be seen in diaphragmatic weakness.
Gait	This should include observing the child walking without shoes and socks, if possible, as well as tiptoe, heal, and heal toe walking. Observe hopping and jumping if the child is able. Abnormal gait patterns may include: • Hemiplegia causing circumduction of the affected foot and dystonic posturing of the hand. • Cerebellar ataxia may cause a broad-based unsteady gait, whereas those with proprioceptive difficulties may study their feet closely to compensate. • Diplegia may present as both legs circumducting and the feet being inverted. • A high stepping gait is commonly seen with foot drop. • A waddling gait is commonly associated with proximal lower limb weakness (such as Duchenne muscular dystrophy). Finally, ask the patient to rise quickly from sitting on the floor to standing to observe for evidence of proximal muscle weakness (Gower's sign).
Posture	Ask the child to stand with their feet together, to stretch their arms and fingers out, and keep their eyes closed. Even young children can maintain this for a few minutes. The following may be observed: • Inability to maintain the posture. • Drift downwards and dystonic posturing of one arm in a unilateral pyramidal lesion (hemiparesis). • Dyskinetic posturing, e.g. in Wilson disease. • Chorea or ballismus. • Tremor, e.g. pill-rolling in Wilson disease. • Falling over in a child with loss of position sense.
Co-ordination	Finger-to-nose testing and heel-to-shin testing: ask the child to touch his nose and then your finger with the index finger of the same hand to bring out ataxia (with past pointing) or dystonia.
Formal examination of all four limbs	Again, closely observe each limb for evidence of asymmetry, wasting, fasciculations, or abnormal movements. Then perform formal testing of tone, power, and reflexes. Remember to compare left and right for each part of the examination.

nervous system matures. The overall prevalence ranges from 2–4 per 1,000 live births, depending on where in the world the child is.

The diagnosis can be made clinically but it is important to remember to look for the underlying cause to ensure that a diagnosis such as hereditary spastic paraplegia is not being missed. A normal brain MRI should immediately be a cause for concern about a potential missed diagnosis.

Causes to consider:

■ Perinatal

• Prematurity – intraventricular haemorrhage and periventricular leukomalacia

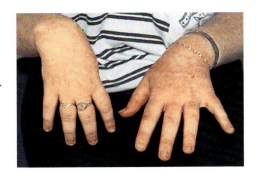

Figure 8.14 Wasting of the right hand in a child with hemiplegia.

Table 8.3: Classification of CP by Pattern of Motor Involvement

	Subtype	Common Clinical Features	
		Less than 5 years old	Older than 5 years
Spastic	Spastic Subtype	• Signs of UMN lesions – brisk reflexes, upgoing plantars, clonus • Increased tone • Contractures	
	Hemiplegic – one side of the body is affected due to a unilateral brain injury such as a neonatal stroke.	Early hand dominance and motor asymmetry. Difficulty using both hands in the midline. When prone, the affected upper limb provides less support, and the affected leg moves less. Over 1–2 years the movement of the affected side reduces until increased tone and UMN signs appear.	The arm is typically more affected than the leg. The arm is adducted at the shoulder and flexed at the elbow, the forearm is pronated, and the wrist and fingers are flexed with the hand closed. The hip is partially flexed and adducted, and the knee and ankle are flexed; the foot may remain in the equinovarus or calcaneovalgus position. In more mildly affected patients postural abnormalities can be brought out by walking or running.
	Diplegic – lower limbs are most affected, typically associated with pre-term infants who have periventricular leukomalacia.	Initially, hypotonia of the lower limbs. By 6 months, spasticity of the lower limbs develops. They typically commando crawl.	Lower limbs are most affected. Flexion, adduction and internal rotation of the hips with contractures of the hip flexors and hamstring muscles. Reduced muscle bulk in the lower limbs.
	Quadriplegic – typically associated with congenital infection or peri/postnatal events such as HIE.	Delayed gross motor milestones. Poor head control. Spasticity often develops by 2–3 months and by 9 months they may have scissoring of the lower limbs.	All limbs are affected. Upper limbs may be more affected than lower limbs but not always. These children often have a severe functional impairment with co-morbidities. These may include seizure disorders and respiratory/swallowing difficulties.
Dyskinetic	Term infants with severe perinatal asphyxia with basal ganglia and thalamic injury. Kernicterus can also cause choreoathetoid CP.	Reduced spontaneous movements. Swallowing difficulties. Persistent primitive reflexes. Delayed motor milestones. Abnormal involuntary movements typically become more prominent by 2–3 years.	Can be dystonic or choreoathetoid. Primitive reflexes may be retained. Clonus and extensor plantar responses may be absent. Abnormal movements often worsened by illness, stress or excitement.
Ataxic	Typically due to an event in the early prenatal period. Can have an underlying genetic cause such as cerebellar hypoplasia, Joubert's syndrome, Granule cell deficiency.	Hypotonia. Delayed development.	Ataxia which improves with time. Speech can also be affected and is jerky and slow.

- Perinatal factors – placental pathology, intrauterine growth restriction, multiple births, antepartum haemorrhage

- Jaundice causing kernicterus

- Perinatal asphyxia – it is important to take a clear birth history

- Postnatal
  - Encephalitis, meningitis, severe gastroenteritis with dehydration or hypoglycaemia
  - Head injury – both accidental and non-accidental
  - Hypoxic ischaemic injury for any cause
  - Neurovascular insult – arterial ischaemic stroke, haemorrhagic stroke or venous sinus thrombosis
- More specific causes
  - Genetic causes – for example, arginase deficiency or cerebellar hypoplasia
  - Structural brain malformations
  - Teratogens – foetal alcohol syndrome
  - Congenital infections – toxoplasmosis, cytomegalovirus, Zika virus

CP is typically classified according to the pattern of motor involvement (Table 8.3), although this has limitations and classification based on function, especially using the Gross Motor Functional Classification System (GMFCS), is also now quite commonly used.

CP is managed by a therapy team of physiotherapists, occupational therapists, speech and language therapists, community paediatricians, neurodevelopmental paediatricians and social workers. They manage the many co-morbidities these children often develop, such as:

1. Feeding difficulties and management of reflux, aspiration and drooling.

2. Epilepsy occurs in 25–50% of children with CP and in many cases can be complex.

3. Management of movement disorder including management of contractures and of hyperkinetic movement disorders.

4. Learning difficulties including speech and communication difficulties.

EXTRAPYRAMIDAL DISORDERS

Extrapyramidal disorders are those that are associated with the motor tracts that do not travel through the pyramids of the medulla but are involved with the regulation and modulation of anterior horn cells. They are in turn modulated by other areas of the CNS including the nigrostriatal pathway, the basal ganglia, the cerebellum, the vestibular nuclei and areas of the cerebral cortex, thus injuries to any of these areas can present with extrapyramidal symptoms.

Extrapyramidal symptoms are movement disorders which typically improve with sleep, Table 8.4 may help in distinguishing the different movement disorders.

Wilson Disease

This is an autosomal recessive disorder of copper metabolism due to a variant of the intracellular copper transporter gene ATP7B. The prevalence is 1 in 30,000. The age of onset is 4–50 years (neurological presentation is rare under 8 years, but possible in patients over 4 years of age).

Table 8.4: Distinguishing Between Movement Disorders

		Tremor	Chorea	Dystonia	Tics	Myoclonus	Ataxia
Action	Rest	+	+	+	+	+	
	Action		+	+		+	+
Speed	Fast	+	+		+	+	
	Slow			+			+
Complexity	Simple	+			+	+	+
	Complex		+	+			
Site	Proximal	+	+	+	+	+	
	Distal		+		+	+	+
Type	Stereotyped	+			+	+	+
	Variable		+	+			

Clinical Presentation:

- Facial immobility

- Rigidity

- Dyskinesia

- Dysarthria

- Dysphagia

- Tremor – especially of the wrist and shoulder (typically pill-rolling)

- Behavioural difficulties with aggression, euphoria and immaturity

- Kayser–Fleischer ring at the limbus of the cornea (always in patients with neurological presentation) (Figure 8.15)

- Liver disease

- Haemolytic anaemia

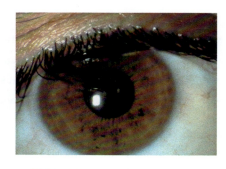

Figure 8.15 Wilson disease. Kayser–Fleischer ring in a child.

Sydenham's Chorea

A movement disorder associated with Group A streptococcal infection and rheumatic fever. It is less common in countries with easy access to antibiotic treatment but is more common in resource-limited countries. It occurs in approximately 18–36% of cases of rheumatic fever but can occur without cardiac involvement.

Clinical features include:

- Chorea – typically bilateral, but may be more prominent on one side.

- Dystonia.

- Behaviour abnormalities and emotional lability.

- Rheumatic heart disease should be considered.

Investigations

- Throat swab, Antistreptococcal titre (ASO) and anti-DNase B.

- ECHO and ECG.

- Neuroimaging is not essential unless another diagnosis is being considered.

Treatment

- Long-term penicillin to eradicate group A strep and prevent recurrence.

- Psychiatric and psychological support.

- Carbamazepine or sodium valproate for treatment of chorea.

- In more severe cases of chorea consider haloperidol.

- Immunosuppression with prednisolone can be considered in more severe cases also.

GENETIC DYSTONIA

Dystonia is a rare movement disorder occurring in 16 per 100,000 population. Over 200 genes have been identified as causes for genetic dystonia and these can present from infancy to adulthood, affecting one or multiple body parts. Most commonly they are generalised and present in childhood.

Table 8.5: Genetic Dystonia

Dystonia	Older Classification	Genetic Classification	Inheritance
Isolated Dystonia	DYT1	DYT-TOR1A	AD
	DYT5A		
	DYT6	DYT-THAP1	AD
	DYT24	DYT-ANO3	AD
	DYT25	DYT-GNAL	AD
	DYT28	DYT-KMT2B	AD
Combined (+myoclonus)	DYT11	DYT-SGCE	AD
Combined (+parkinsonism)	DYT5a	DYT-GCH1	AD/AR
	DYT4b	DYT-TH	AR
	-	DYT-SPR	AR
	DYT3	DYT-TAF1	XL
	DYT16	DYT-PRKRA	AR
	DYT12	DYT-ATP1A3	AD
Paroxysmal + other dyskinesia	DYT8	PxMD-PNKD	AD
	DYT10	PxMD-PRRT2	AD
	DYT18	PxMD-SCL2A1	AD
	-	PxMD-ECHS1	AR

Segawa Syndrome (DYT5a or DYT-GCH1)

This syndrome is autosomal-dominant with reduced penetrance. The mutation is in the gene coding for guanosine triphosphate cyclohydrolase I, the rate-limiting step for tetrahydrobiopterin (cofactor for phenylalanine, tyrosine and tryptophan, monooxygenases).

Clinical Features

- Dystonia often worse in the evening
- Equinovarus posturing of the foot
- Gait disturbance
- Ankle clonus
- Extensor posturing of the big toe (Figure 8.16)

Table 8.6: Treatable Causes of Extrapyramidal Abnormalities

Condition	Diagnostic Test	Treatment
Wilson disease	Plasma copper, caeruloplasmin	Penicillamine
Sydenham chorea	Antistreptococcal titre, anti-DNase B	Penicillin
Segawa syndrome	Trial of L-DOPA, guanosine triphosphate cyclohydrolase I gene	L-DOPA
Anti-NMDA receptor encephalitis	Anti-NMDA antibodies	Steroids, immunoglobulin, plasma exchange
Systemic lupus erythematosus	Antinuclear antibodies, anti-double-stranded DNA autoantibodies	Immunosuppression
Moyamoya (see 'Stroke')	MR angiography	Revascularisation
Arteriovenous malformation	Contrast CT, MRI, conventional arteriography	Surgery, embolisation, radiotherapy
Tumour	Neuroimaging	Radiotherapy
Glutaric aciduria type I	Urinary organic acids	Protein restriction, carnitine
Homocystinuria	Plasma total homocysteine, methionine	Pyridoxine, methionine restriction, betaine
Infections	Mycoplasma, CMV, HIV	Antimicrobials
Drugs and toxins	Urine and blood screening	Withdrawal
Conversion disorder (hysteria)	Exclusion of alternatives, observation	Rehabilitation
Sandifer syndrome (reflux)	pH studies, barium swallow	Omeprazole, Nissen fundoplication

Investigations

- Exclude alternative causes, especially Wilson disease
- DNA for genetic testing
- Trial of Levodopa

Treatment

- Levodopa/carbidopa in doses of up to 100/25mg TDS

CAUSES OF DYSTONIA AND/OR CHOREA

- Hypoxic-ischaemic damage (may be delayed or worsen after initial stability)
- Bronchopulmonary dysplasia
- Post cardiopulmonary bypass
- Intracranial trauma (may be delayed)
- Wilson disease (Figure 8.15)
- Anti-NMDAR antibody encephalitis
- Extensor toe in a teenager suggests Segawa syndrome (Figure 8.16)
- Poststreptococcal
- Cerebrovascular disease, e.g. moyamoya
- Ataxia telangiectasia (see 'Ataxia', Figure 8.17)
- GM1 and GM2 gangliosidoses
- Mitochondrial disease (e.g. Leigh syndrome)
- Pantothenate kinase-associated neurodegeneration (PKAN): an autosomal recessive disorder of coenzyme A homeostasis caused by defects in mitochondrial pantothenate kinase 2 gene (previously known as Hallervorden–Spatz disease)
- Huntington chorea

MANAGEMENT

- Clinical: prepare an accurate description of movement disorder and any associated behavioural manifestation (video and further opinions may be helpful); slit-lamp examination by an ophthalmologist for Kayser–Fleischer rings.
- Initial investigations: neuroimaging (including magnetic resonance angiography, MRA), plasma copper and caeruloplasmin, antistreptolysin O titre, plasma amino acids, urine organic acids, plasma lactate, alpha fetoprotein. May need CSF lactate, white cell enzymes, pH studies and barium swallow and DNA testing for Huntington chorea or ataxia telangiectasia if clinically indicated.
- Long-term: appropriate treatment of underlying cause (Table 8.2), trial of levodopa for dystonia, anticholinergics (e.g. trihexyphenidyl). In severe extrapyramidal disorders, appropriate seating and treatment of Sandifer syndrome, i.e., gastro-oesophageal reflux, may produce improvement and diazepam may reduce dystonic spasms while oral baclofen may reduce associated spasticity. For severe dystonia, intrathecal baclofen or deep brain stimulation may be offered in specialist centres.

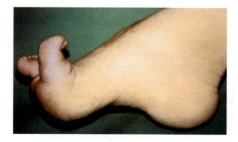

Figure 8.16 Extensor toe in a teenager suggests Segawa syndrome.

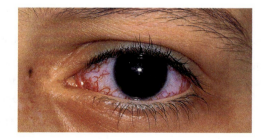

Figure 8.17 Ataxia telangiectasia; conjunctival telangiectasia.

Table 8.7: Causes of Ataxia

Acute Ataxia	Non-Progressive Chronic Ataxia	Progressive Chronic Ataxia
Posterior fossa space-occupying lesion (may be accompanied by head tilt) • Tumour • Extradural or subdural haematoma • Cerebral infarction	Cerebellar malformations	Ataxia telangiectasia (AT) (Figure 8.17)
Acute cerebellitis (e.g. mycoplasma)	Ataxic CP (often accompanied by epilepsy and parietal lesions on neuroimaging)	Ataxia–oculomotor apraxia (also abnormality of AT gene)
Postinfectious cerebellitis (e.g. chickenpox)	Intermittent ataxia due to mutation in a channelopathy gene such as CACNA1A	Metachromatic leukodystrophy, other leukodystrophies
Guillain–Barré syndrome (see 'Acute weakness')		Friedreich ataxia (FA) – abnormality of frataxin gene (Figure 8.18)
Drugs and toxins (e.g. phenytoin, carbamazepine, lead)		Early onset ataxia with preserved deep tendon reflexes (also abnormality of frataxin gene)
Acute Disseminated Encephalomyelitis (ADEM)		Hereditary sensory and motor neuropathies (Figure 8.19) (see also 'Chronic progressive weakness')
		GM1 and GM2 gangliosidoses

Table 8.8: Treatable Causes of Intermittent or Progressive Ataxia

Condition	Diagnosis	Treatment
Posterior fossa tumour	Neuroimaging	Surgery, VP shunt, chemo/ radiotherapy
Drugs and toxins	Urine drug screen	Stop use of drugs
Glucose transporter deficiency	Low CSF to plasma glucose ratio or variant in SLC2A1 gene	Ketogenic diet
Biotinidase deficiency (see 'Epilepsy')	Urine organic acids Plasma biotinidase	Biotin
Primary vitamin E deficiency	Plasma vitamin E	Vitamin E
Secondary vitamin E deficiency	Plasma vitamin E Acanthocytosis	Vitamin E (+A+K)
Abetalipoproteinaemia	Plasma triglycerides	
Hypobetalipoproteinaemia	Plasma lipoproteins	
Alpha-tocopherol transfer protein	Genetics	
Friedreich ataxia	Frataxin gene	Nicotinamide Erythropoietin
Hartnup disease	Urine amino acids	Nicotinamide
Maple syrup urine disease	Urine amino acids	Thiamine
Hereditary paroxysmal cerebellar ataxia	Genetic testing	Acetazolamide
Refsum disease	Plasma phytanic acid	Dietary
Pyruvate dehydrogenase complex deficiency	Plasma/CSF lactate Enzyme assay Gene on Xp22	Thiamine may help

Ataxia

Although ataxia implies a cerebellar lesion, it may be difficult to distinguish cerebellar ataxia from peripheral neuropathy, action myoclonus or dystonia in a young child. Horizontal nystagmus and past-pointing suggest the involvement of the cerebellum, whereas areflexia indicates peripheral neuropathy (see also 'Extrapyramidal disorders').

Investigations

- Neuroimaging. This should be urgent if there is reduced visual acuity (secondary to raised intracranial pressure), vomiting or headache. It should be avoided if the patient is areflexic and clinically has peripheral neuropathy or telangiectasia in view of the chromosomal fragility in AT.

- CSF glucose to exclude glut-1 deficiency.

- Biotinidase.

- Nerve conduction studies to diagnose peripheral neuropathy and to distinguish from FA.

- Alpha-fetoprotein and immunoglobulins to screen for AT.

- White blood cell chromosome fragility (AT), DNA for genetic testing if a high index of suspicion of AT or FA; urine amino and organic acids, plasma amino acids; plasma and CSF lactate, biotinidase; phytanic acid; triglycerides and lipoproteins; white cell enzymes.

- Ataxia gene panel to look for underlying genetic cause such as a channelopathy.

FRIEDREICH ATAXIA (FA)

FA occurs in 1 in 8,000. It is autosomal recessive, with reduplication of the GAA sequence in intron 1 of the frataxin gene on 9q. Reduplication reduces frataxin, the protein associated with mitochondrial membranes and crests. It may reduce oxidative stress by preventing iron accumulation. The size of expansion (120–1,700 repeats) is related to the patient's age at onset.

Clinical Signs

- Ataxia – mixed sensory and cerebellar
- Speech – scanning dysarthria, then slurred
- Intention tremor, clumsiness of hands
- Nystagmus (relatively rare)
- Fatigue
- Cardiac symptoms secondary to cardiomyopathy
- Pes cavus (Figure 8.18)
- Loss of position and vibration sensation, particularly in the legs
- Loss of tendon jerks (classically absent at ankle, brisk at knee)
- Extensor plantar responses (pyramidal involvement, as for brisk knee jerks)
- Scoliosis
- Diabetes
- Optic atrophy
- Deafness

Diagnosis

- ECG, ECHO
- Nerve conduction – reduced amplitude sensory nerve action potential; reduced velocity motor and sensory conduction
- Frataxin gene on 9q

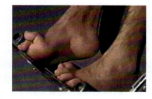

Figure 8.18 Pes cavus in Friedrich ataxia.

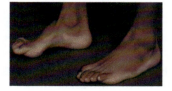

Figure 8.19 Pes cavus in hereditary sensory motor neuropathy (CMT).

Management

- Multidisciplinary, treating cardiomyopathy, scoliosis, motor disorder and diabetes.

- Omaveloxolone was approved by the FDA as the first therapy for FA in over 16 year olds in 2023.

Death from cardiac complications occurs in early or middle adult life.

ACUTE GENERALISED WEAKNESS IN A PREVIOUSLY WELL CHILD

The child may be generally unwell with signs of infection or may have other symptoms such as rash or pain to aid in the differential diagnosis. It is important to perform a thorough examination, especially of power and reflexes to localise the lesion, and to examine the cranial nerves to understand if they are involved.

Causes:

- Guillain–Barré syndrome

- Cervical cord lesion (e.g. transverse myelitis, stroke, trauma, tumour – Figure 8.20).

- Poliomyelitis (including vaccine-associated; usually asymmetrical weakness) and other viruses, e.g. non-polio enterovirus such as Coxsackie and Echo, adenoviruses, Japanese B encephalitis virus

- Dermatomyositis (Figure 8.21)

- Viral myositis

- Myasthenia Gravis (see 'Ptosis')

- Botulism – associated with fixed, dilated pupils

- Other toxins (e.g. lead, vincristine)

- Acute presentation of chronic weakness (e.g. hereditary sensory motor neuropathy, Charcot–Marie–Tooth disease [CMT] – Figure 8.19)

Clinical Features

- Ascending weakness, starting in feet and legs and progressing to hands and arms and then to respiratory muscles and cranial nerves, strongly suggests Guillain–Barré syndrome.

- Descending weakness starting in cranial nerves strongly suggests the rarer Miller–Fisher variant of Guillain–Barré syndrome.

- Spinal cord disease should be excluded as quickly as possible if there is acute flaccid weakness with rapid onset, especially if there is bladder involvement.

- Asymmetrical flaccid weakness suggests viral infection secondary to polio and non-polio enteroviruses.

- Pain suggests myositis in acute viral myositis, polymyositis or dermatomyositis (Figure 8.21), although there may be pain in Guillain– Barré syndrome.

Investigations

- MRI spine with contrast. This should be done urgently if there is any bladder involvement to suggest a spinal cord lesion.

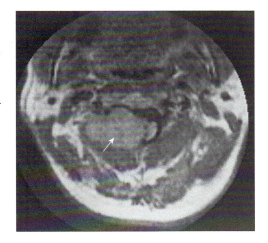

Figure 8.20 A neurofibroma at C1 pushing the cord over. This type of lesion can occasionally cause a flaccid quadriparesis and if there is any doubt about the diagnosis of Guillain–Barré, MRI of the neck should be considered, especially if there is bladder involvement.

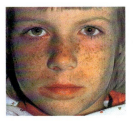

Figure 8.21 Dermatomyositis; heliotrope rash in a child. Note the characteristic serious expression.

- Creatine phosphokinase (CPK) and EMG to help diagnose dermatomyositis or viral myositis.

- Nerve conduction studies to diagnose Guillain– Barré syndrome; may be normal in the initial phase of illness and in the Miller–Fisher variant; other conditions (e.g. botulism) may have characteristic neurophysiological features.

- Exclusion of myasthenia (see 'Bilateral ptosis').

- CSF is not usually necessary if the clinical diagnosis is clearly ascending weakness consistent with Guillain–Barré syndrome as the protein is not raised until a few days after onset, but should be considered with PCR for a variety of viruses if there are unusual features, e.g. asymmetry suggestive of polio or other viral causes of acute flaccid paralysis.

- Throat and rectal swabs for enterovirus.

- Spirometry should be performed regularly in ascending Guillain–Barré syndrome if the child remains unventilated and can co-operate.

Treatment

- Initial management should focus on ensuring supportive management is in place, including evaluation for the need for respiratory support. Proceeding to ventilation if there is a deterioration.

- Treatment of the specific underlying cause (e.g. urgent surgery for spinal cord tumour, immunosuppression for dermatomyositis (Figure 8.21), immunoglobulin (and/or plasmapheresis) for Guillain–Barré syndrome.

- Physiotherapy and occupational therapy, and an assessment of swallow with possible nasogastric feeding if there is bulbar involvement.

GUILLAIN–BARRÉ SYNDROME

Incidence is 0.6–1.1 per 100,000 children. Guillain–Barré syndrome is an inflammatory demyelinating polyradiculoneuropathy in most patients. Preceding infections include Campylobacter, CMV and EBV.

Presenting Features

- Pain
- Ascending weakness
- Ataxia
- Respiratory weakness
- Bulbar weakness
- Bilateral facial weakness
- Ophthalmoplegia

Investigations

- MRI spine with contrast shows thickening and enhancement of the anterior spinal nerve roots.
- Nerve conduction studies may be consistent with demyelination.

Management

- Admission and close observation, particularly of respiratory and cardiac function.
- Intravenous immunoglobulin is the first line of treatment.
- Plasmapheresis if immunoglobulin does not arrest deterioration or lead to improvement.
- Ventilation for respiratory failure.
- Pacing for cardiac dysrhythmias.
- Physiotherapy to prevent contractures and aid mobilisation during recovery.

Spinal Cord Disorders

- Acute spinal cord injury usually occurs in the context of trauma. As there may be no bony injury, all children involved in significant trauma should be nursed flat and in a stiff collar until they are conscious enough to confirm that there is no pain in the neck or back indicative of ligamentous injury and instability.

- Chronic spinal cord injury may occur in children with skeletal deformities and may present with the insidious onset of pyramidal and/or lower motor neuron and sensory signs (Figure 8.22).

- Tumours (Figure 8.23), e.g. extradural in the context of neurofibromatosis or intradural (extra- or intramedullary), may present with pain, stiffness, focal neurological deficit or bladder symptoms. Diagnosis is usually made with an MRI of the spine, which is indicated urgently in a unit where the child can be surgically decompressed if there is recent deterioration.

- Syringomyelia (Figure 8.24) may occur spontaneously or secondary to tumours.

- Transverse myelitis may be clinically similar, but can be distinguished on MRI. Methylprednisolone should be given as soon as possible and further immunosuppression should be considered if there is no improvement.

- Discitis is usually painful.

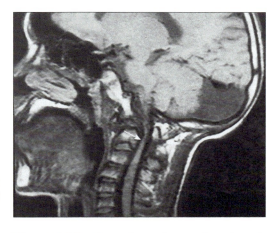

Figure 8.22   Conradi syndrome; thinning of the cord in the high cervical region.

Predisposing Conditions

- Down syndrome
- Neurofibromatosis
- Mucopolysaccharidoses
- Achondroplasia

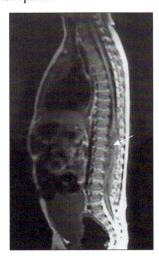

Figure 8.23   Cord tumour, probably ependymoma.

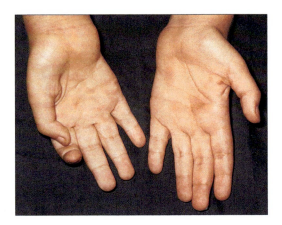

Figure 8.24   Syringomyelia. Wasting of the small muscles of the hands, worse on the right.

- Goldenhar syndrome
- Klippel–Feil syndrome
- Conradi syndrome
- Coffin–Lowry syndrome

HYPOTONIA IN INFANCY

CAUSES OF WEAKNESS IN INFANCY

- Congenital myotonic dystrophy (Figure 8.25)
- SMA types 1 and 2 (Figure 8.26)
- SMARD1 (SMA with respiratory distress due to diaphragmatic weakness)
- Congenital muscular dystrophies: Ullrich (UCMD), merosin deficient (MDC1A)
- Dystroglycanopathies (muscle–eye–brain disease, Walker Warburg syndrome)
- Congenital myopathies:
  - Pompe disease (glycogen storage disease type II)
  - Nemaline myopathy
  - Myotubular myopathy
- Congenital and neonatal myasthenia
- Botulism
- Congenital hypomyelinating neuropathies
- Spinal cord disease:
  - Birth trauma
  - Congenital malformation
- Central:
- Chromosomal
- Down syndrome: trisomy 21
- Prader–Willi: genomic imprinting with interstitial deletion in paternal
- 15q1.1-1.3 and uniparental disomy
- Metabolic
- Peroxisomal: Zellweger syndrome (Figure 8.27), neonatal adrenoleukodystrophy
- Amino acidurias
- Organic acidurias
- Mitochondrial disorders
- Structural brain malformation
- Cerebral haemorrhage
- Sepsis

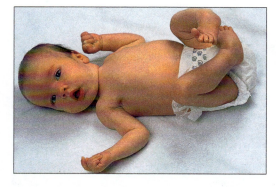

Figure 8.25   Infant with myotonic dystrophy with characteristic decreased tone, bilateral talipes and fish-shaped mouth.

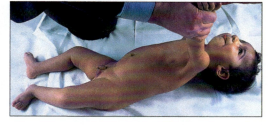

Figure 8.26   Infant with spinal muscular atrophy showing truncal and limb hypotonia, bell-shaped chest, frog-legged posture and preserved facial movement with alert expression; tongue fasciculation is also characteristic.

Clues towards diagnosis in history and exam:

- History of maternal illness (e.g. MG, myotonic dystrophy), pregnancy and birth history, foetal movements and presence of polyhydramnios

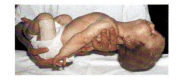

- Examination of infant, noting alertness, ability to fix and follow, any distinctive features (e.g. trisomy 21, Prader–Willi syndrome), ptosis, facial and bulbar weakness (difficulty feeding/ swallowing secretions), tongue fasciculation (in SMA), posture, presence of contractures/scoliosis, degree of truncal and limb weakness, reflexes

Figure 8.27 Zellweger disease: infant with profound hypotonia.

- Examination of the mother for signs of myotonic dystrophy (ability to bury eyelashes, grip myotonia although the ward setting may be too warm to demonstrate difficulty in releasing grip) or myasthenia (ptosis and fatigable weakness)

Investigations:

- Genetic studies for characteristic conditions (e.g. myotonic dystrophy, SMA, Prader–Willi) and congenital myopathy gene panel by whole genome sequencing.

- As there are now treatment options for SMA (gene therapy and Nusinersen), if this diagnosis is considered then an urgent Multiplex ligation-dependent probe amplification (MLPA) should be sent.

- Plasma CK.

- ECHO (e.g. for Pompe).

- X-ray of the knee to look for patellar calcification/stippling in peroxisomal disorders, e.g. Zellweger syndrome (Figure 8.27).

- Appropriate biochemistry for metabolic conditions (e.g. very long chain fatty acids for peroxisomal disorders [Figure 8.27] or plasma/CSF lactate for mitochondrial disease).

- EMG and nerve conduction studies. Stimulation single fibre EMG +/−repetitive nerve stimulation for myasthenia.

- Neuroimaging of the brain to exclude structural brain abnormality, either isolated or in association with muscle disease (e.g. Walker Warburg congenital muscular dystrophy, muscle–eye– brain disease) and of the spine to exclude birth trauma.

- Muscle biopsy may be needed if diagnosis cannot be secured by an alternative method.

- Stool for clostridium botulinum.

MYOTONIC DYSTROPHY (DM1)

Myotonic dystrophy is a clinically heterogeneous disorder occurring between 1 in 7,400 to 1 in 10,700 in Europe; the most severe form is congenital DM1. It is autosomal dominant and due to the expansion of a triplet repeat (CTG) in the 3′-untranslated region of the DMPK (myotonin protein kinase gene) on chromosome 19q13, disrupting mRNA metabolism. Congenital DM1 is maternally inherited.

Clinical Presentation

DM1 may present in the neonatal period (congenital myotonic dystrophy) with severe weakness, respiratory insufficiency, facial weakness (Figure 8.25) with characteristic 'tent-shaped' mouth and arthrogryposis (talipes equinovarus is particularly common, Figure 8.25). As it is maternally inherited, examine the mother's hand grip for myotonia and to see if she can bury her eyelashes. Limb weakness improves during infancy, but facial weakness persists, and these children have learning difficulties, which may be severe. The milder, 'adult' form of myotonic dystrophy (paternal > maternal inheritance) usually presents in later childhood with mild distal limb and characteristic facial weakness, grip myotonia with difficulty releasing the clenched fist (worse in cold weather), early cataracts, cardiac arrhythmias and often mild learning difficulties. In males, frontal balding and testicular atrophy develop in adulthood.

Diagnosis

- DMPK gene analysis should be obtained in characteristic cases.

- EMG shows myopathic features with myotonic discharges ('dive bomber') in older children and adults.

Management

- Management of congenital DM1 is supportive and respiratory involvement is the leading cause of death. Ventilation requirement past 4 weeks of life has a mortality of over 25%.

- Management of later onset disease is targeted at the specific symptoms the child develops, including respiratory support, physiotherapy and occupational therapy.

- In older teenagers and adults mexiletine can be considered for treatment of myotonia. It is contraindicated in those with 2nd–3rd degree heart block.

SPINAL MUSCULAR ATROPHY (SMA)

SMA is a neuromuscular condition caused by degeneration of the anterior horn cells in the spinal cord and motor nuclei in the lower brainstem, resulting in progressive muscle weakness and atrophy. It is an autosomal recessive condition due to a biallelic deletion of exon 7 of the survival motor neuron (SMN1) gene on chromosome 5q13. There are 5 subtypes of classical 5q related SMA 0–4. The difference is in part due to modifying effect of another gene SMN2 which is close to SMN1, the more copies of SMN2 a person has the milder the phenotype of SMA they appear to have. The incidence ranges from 5–13 per 100,000 live births.

SMA type 0

This is prenatal onset of SMA and affected neonates have severe weakness, areflexia, facial weakness and cardiac anomalies. They do not achieve any motor milestones and typically die by one month of age due to respiratory failure. These infants have only one copy of SMN2.

SMA type 1

Patients with SMA 1 typically have two or three copies of SMN2. There is progressive proximal weakness of the limbs from birth or soon afterwards (Figure 8.26). Paralysis of the intercostal muscles leads to narrowing of the chest ('bell-shaped' chest) and abdominal breathing. Clinical features include: alert baby with normal eye and facial movement, severe axial and limb weakness (legs > arms, 'frog posture') with small chest, diaphragmatic breathing, tongue fasciculation and areflexia.

The diagnosis should be considered in any infant with unexplained weakness or hypotonia. Urgent Multiplex ligation-dependent probe amplification (MLPA) target mutation analysis for homozygous deletions of exon 7 of SMN1. If this is negative, then SMN1 sequencing can be done to look for rarer point mutation. An EMG would show a neurogenic pattern but should not be needed in most cases given the ease of access to genetic testing in the UK at present.

Disease modifying treatment is now available for SMA1 and for all these treatments the earlier the treatment is started the better the outcome. Thus, the importance of urgent genetic confirmation of the diagnosis and referral to a neuromuscular centre. For infants with SMA1 gene therapy with onasemnogene abeparvovec. For those over 20kg or who cannot have an adenoviral vector, the options include Nusinersen, an antisense oligonucleotide that modifies the splicing of SMN2 to increase the production of normal SMN protein. This is an intrathecally delivered medication. An oral medication known as Risdiplam is also available. This is an SMN2 splicing modifier that corrects the splicing deficit of SMN2, leading to increased levels of full-length SMN protein. All treatments have been shown to increase ventilation-free survival and have improved motor outcomes. Management of associated conditions such as feeding difficulties, scoliosis and respiratory complications continues to be very important for these children.

SMA types 2, 3 and 4

SMA 2 accounts for approximately 20% of SMA cases, SMA 3 for 30% and SMA 4 for less than 5%. SMA 2 infants typically sit unaided but without treatment are unlikely to stand. Onset is typically within the first year of life but after 6 months of age. They usually have three copies of SMN2. SMA 3 children have onset of symptoms between 18 months and adulthood and have three or four copies of SMN2. In SMA 4 onset is in adulthood and although not clearly defined is typically thought to be over 30 years of age. They have four to eight copies of SMN2. There may be some regression of motor skills at onset, then a relatively stable course with survival to adulthood with optimal surveillance and management of scoliosis and respiratory and nutritional complications. Clinical features include severe axial and limb weakness (legs > arms) with areflexia, tongue fasciculation and hand tremor (very evident as baseline tremor in 12 lead ECG limb leads). SMA2 children are usually of normal intelligence and verbal but have variable bulbar weakness causing feeding difficulty, intercostal weakness with a weak cough, prominent diaphragmatic breathing and susceptibility to chest infections and nocturnal respiratory insufficiency requiring the use of non-invasive ventilation.

Treatment with onasemnogene abeparvovec is not yet available via the NHS for SMA 2–4. Although studies are underway to investigate its use in SMA 2. Both Nusinersen and Risdiplam are available. Supported management for any respiratory, feeding or orthopaedic complications of the disease continues to be important.

DUCHENNE AND BECKER MUSCULAR DYSTROPHY (DMD AND BMD)

Muscular dystrophies are a group of inherited progressive myopathic disorders where the primary symptom is muscle weakness. DMD and BMD are dystrophinopathies caused by a variant of the dystrophin gene which results in progressive muscle weakness due to muscle fibre degeneration. The dystrophin gene is a large gene on the X chromosome. DMD occurs in 1 in 3,500; BMD in 1 in 30,000 male births. DMD (severe) involves 'out of frame' deletions, duplications or point mutations, which lead to the absence of dystrophin. BMD (milder, allelic form) has 'in frame' mutations, which result in reduced quantities of abnormal, but partially functional dystrophin. Rarely girls may be affected, either as manifesting carriers due to skewed X inactivation or Turner syndrome (XO) or have a chromosomal translocation involving Xp21.

Clinical Presentation

Children have an abnormal gait aged 3–4 years, are unable to run, have frequent falls and often demonstrate language delay and other cognitive or behavioural problems. Some present earlier with global developmental delay.

Table 8.9: Chronic and Progressive Weakness in the Older Child

	Causes	Clues to diagnosis	Investigations
Spinal Cord Disorders	See under 'Acute generalised weakness'	Bladder or bowel involvement	MRI spine with contrast
Muscle Disease	Duchenne and Becker Muscular Dystrophy	Positive Gower's sign (Figure 8.28), calf pseudohypertrophy	Elevated CK Genetic testing for dystrophin deletion, duplication and point mutation studies
	Limb Girdle Dystrophies	Scapular winging or pelvic weakness with preservation of distal muscles and facial muscles.	May have moderately elevated CK EMG – myopathic changes Diagnosis is confirmed with genetic testing
	Myotonic Dystrophies	Facial involvement, myotonia and family history	EMG – myotonic discharges Confirmed with genetic testing
	Congenital Myopathies	A high arched palate and facial hypotonia may give a clue.	Diagnosis is confirmed with genetic testing
	Metabolic Myopathies	Dynamic symptoms especially if triggered by exercise (although can be static or progressive)	Elevated CK and recurrent episodes of myoglobinuria
Congenital and Autoimmune Myasthenia	See under 'Ptosis'		
Anterior Horn Cell Disease	SMA 3 – see 'SMA'		
Neuropathies	Demyelinating and axonal neuropathies	Examine the feet and hands of both parents	See CMT below

- Duchenne: show progressive weakness with loss of ambulation by 8–12 years. The children develop cardiomyopathy (usually asymptomatic) and nocturnal hypoventilation requiring nocturnal non-invasive ventilation (NIV) in their mid-teens. Late swallowing difficulty may occur, which may necessitate gastrostomy feeding. With optimum cardiorespiratory management, the mean age of survival is now in the late 20s. Survival beyond the fourth decade is very unlikely.

- Becker: usually presents later with cramps and/or weakness, with slower progression. Children walk beyond 16 years and often have a normal lifespan. They may develop severe cardiomyopathy which if untreated is the main cause of early death.

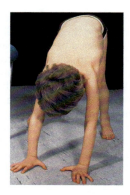

Figure 8.28 A boy with DMD executes Gowers manoeuvre, which demonstrates muscular dystrophy and proximal weakness.

There is an anaesthetic risk in both DMD and BMD with inhalation anaesthetics and suxamethonium.

Management

- Physiotherapy to maintain full-range movements.

- Night ankle/foot orthoses to prevent tendoachilles shortening.

- DMD: oral steroids (prednisolone or deflazacort) either daily, or intermittent 10 day on 10 day off dose.

- Ischial weight-bearing knee–ankle–foot orthoses (KAFOs) to prolong ambulation.

- Once non-ambulant, good postural management is needed in a powered wheelchair with a spinal brace or spinal surgery for scoliosis.

- Regular respiratory monitoring with FVC, yearly sleep study and ECHO; nocturnal NIV when there is evidence of sleep hypoventilation and an ACE inhibitor +/− beta-blocker when ECHO shows signs of cardiomyopathy.

- Maintain optimal nutritional status including vitamin D and calcium status for bone health, especially if the child is taking steroids.

- Endocrine referral for osteopenia, delayed puberty or growth restriction.

- Learning and behavioural support as necessary.

HEREDITARY MOTOR AND SENSORY NEUROPATHY (CHARCOT-MARIE-TOOTH – CMT)

CMT is a group of disorders caused by variants in genes that are expressed in myelin or axons and so are thought of as either demyelinating or axonal. The majority are due to variants in one of these four genes: PMP22, MPZ, GJB1 and MFN2, but over 40 genes have been identified with autosomal dominant, recessive and even X-linked inheritance patterns. There are seven subtypes (CMT 1–7). CMT1A is the most common form of CMT presenting in childhood, in 1 in 26,000. It is an autosomal dominant mutation; CMT2 and recessive and X-linked forms of CMT1 may be clinically similar. Commonly it involves a 1.5 megabase duplication within band 17p11.2 on chromosome 17. Duplication leads to three copies of the gene encoding peripheral myelin protein 22 (PMP-22). Occasionally there is point mutation in the PMP-22 gene. Deletion in PMP22 is associated with the condition hereditary neuropathy with liability to pressure palsies (HNPP).

Clinical Presentation

CMT usually presents at under 10 years, with gait disturbance – instability, high-stepping, difficulty in running, frequent falls; foot deformity with pes cavus (Figure 8.19; the child may also have hammer toes) or pes planus and valgus deformity, symmetrical wasting of the peroneal muscles, calves or lower thighs, reduced or absent reflexes and subtle sensory abnormalities. Later, weakness and sensory loss may develop in the hands.

Diagnosis

■ Nerve conduction: motor and sensory conduction velocities are reduced to <50% of normal in CMT1A with increased distal latencies.

■ Genetic studies: typically gene panels include PMP22 if CMT1 is suspected or without if not.

Management

Often none is needed, but includes careful foot care, physiotherapy and orthotic review, occupational therapy assessment for fine motor problems, e.g. handwriting difficulty, with access to a keyboard and extra time in exams if necessary. Orthopaedic surveillance and intervention may be needed for progressive foot deformity.

Prognosis

Typically CMT is compatible with a normal lifespan and the child is usually ambulant throughout; however, they may need to use orthoses or walking aids in later life.

SPINA BIFIDA

Spina bifida is a type of open neural tube defect and the incidence varies greatly around the world. In Europe, the incidence of neural tube defects is approximately 9 per 10,000 births and the incidence has decreased due to the practice of women of childbearing age taking pre-conception and antenatal folic acid, as well as antenatal diagnosis with ultrasound. Genetic factors are important. The risk of having a further affected child if one is already affected is 1 in 30. The risk of having a third affected child if two are affected is 1 in 6.

Definitions

■ Meningocoele (Figure 8.29): cord is usually normal, lesions are covered with skin, neurology is often normal.

■ Myelocoele or myelomeningocoele (Figure 8.30): cord is exposed and abnormal, with only a thin covering if any; the risk of neurological impairment is very high.

■ Spina bifida occulta: spinal cord is covered with bone and skin, but usually marked with a sacral pit, hairy patch or lipoma. Children usually present later with bladder problems or minor gait disorders.

Site

The defect most commonly occurs in the lumbosacral area, less commonly in the dorsal region and uncommonly in the cervical region. Only 10% of lesions affect the skull (encephalocoeles).

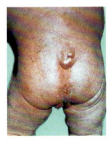

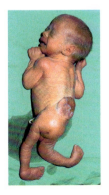

Figure 8.29 Meningocoele with relatively normal legs.

Figure 8.30 Myelocoele with flaccid, wasted legs.

Complication and Co-morbidities

- Loss of sensation: sensory loss in the skin can lead to ulceration as the child may not know that they have burnt or cut themselves. The ability to recognise a full rectum or bladder may also be lost.

- Bladder problems: most children with lumbosacral myelomeningocoeles are incontinent to a degree. The bladder sphincters are often innervated abnormally and this may lead to a neuropathic bladder, which does not empty properly. The pressure inside the urinary tract may be high because of this and the child is also subject to frequent urinary tract infections. There is a risk of chronic renal failure in the long term if the bladder is not appropriately managed.

- Hydrocephalus: usually secondary to Arnold–Chiari malformation of the brainstem. It occurs in patients with high lesions – e.g. thoracolumbar myelomeningocoele.

- Paralysis: with a lumbosacral lesion, the legs will be partially paralysed (Figure 8.30) to an extent dependent on the site of the lesion and the degree of damage to the spinal cord. Secondary syringomyelia may lead to deterioration.

- Limb deformities: if the limbs are partially paralysed, there will be muscular imbalance and limb deformities may be present from birth (Figure 8.30) or develop at a later stage.

- Kyphoscoliosis: the vertebral column may be abnormal and children are at high risk of kyphoscoliosis.

Management

- Early closure of the spinal defect. Today this is done in the majority of instances, although surgical treatment may not be appropriate in some children with extensive neurological damage or severe hydrocephalus.

- Management of hydrocephalus: a shunt will usually be inserted.

- Management of the bladder: it is essential that the child has a urodynamic study to examine the nature of the neuropathic bladder. Intermittent catheterisation is usually used to improve continence and prevent infection. Children will need regular urine tests performed and adequate treatment of the urinary tract infections. With careful management, it is now unusual for children to develop chronic renal failure.

- Physical management: many children with flaccid limbs can be given appropriate orthoses and can walk. Other children may be wheelchair dependent. It is important to prevent kyphoscoliosis with an appropriate spinal brace if indicated.

HEADACHE IN CHILDREN AND YOUNG PEOPLE

Headache is a common paediatric complaint, indeed in a class of 30 at least one child will have a headache problem. Encouragingly, on account of absence of nociceptors from parenchyma, the 'brain does not feel pain', hence childhood headache rarely indicates dangerous intracranial pathology. However, the presence of any red flag signs or symptoms (Table 8.10) should alert the clinician to precisely this possibility. Brain tumours are amongst the most common cancers of childhood (Table 8.10).

Table 8.10: Some Headache Red Flags

- Young child (< 4 years) or learning difficulties
- Sudden onset
- Increasing frequency/severity
- Increased by coughing or straining
- Early morning or waking from sleep
- Nausea +/– vomiting
- Increasing head circumference (infant)
- New neurological signs, including squint
- Head tilt
- Occipital location
- Neck stiffness
- Behaviour change

RECOMMEND NEURO-IMAGING

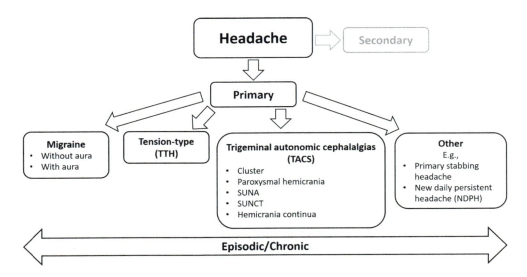

Figure 8.31 Headache classification

DEFINITIONS AND CLASSIFICATION (FIGURE 8.31)

- **Primary headaches** refer to a distinct group of disorders with condition specific pathophysi-ologies. Common examples in childhood include migraine and tension-type headache (TTH); trigeminal autonomic cephalalgias (TACS) are rare

- Primary headaches are **episodic** or **chronic**, e.g. episodic migraine is classified as < 15 headache days/month whilst chronic migraine is ≥ 15 headache days/month for > three consecutive months

- **Secondary headache** is a symptom caused by (i.e. secondary to) another disorder. Examples include head and/or neck trauma, intracranial infection or inflammation and raised intracra-nial pressure. Often additional signs and symptoms are present

HEADACHE HISTORY AND EXAMINATION

Pain is a difficult sensation to describe and localise, especially for a very young child. Here are a few tips:

- *Be child and young person focussed* – consider the clinic room environment; aim to gather as much detail from the patient as possible, using parental observations to supplement.

- *Parental history* – in particular seek information regarding family headache history and early life markers of migraine.

- *Be structured* – consider using a proforma. This encourages a systematic, relevant and detailed approach. Table 8.11 has a helpful mnemonic ('LQIDFOE') for reference.

- *Use inference*, e.g. in a young child unable to score pain (i.e. 'X out of 10') it may be possible to infer severity from their behaviour. For example, continued routine activities during an attack could be assumed mild pain. Whereas, extreme withdrawal or taking themselves off to bed is likely to indicate moderate to severe pain.

- *Tools*:
  - Drawing – asking a child or young person to draw their headache and/or aura can be really helpful in informing phenotype (Figure 8.32).
  - Diaries and smartphone apps (e.g. 'Migraine Buddy') to record symptoms, frequency, associations/triggers, administration of medication, response to medication, medication changes, etc.
  - Paediatric Migraine Disability Assessment (PedMIDAS).

Table 8.11: **Headache History Mnemonic**
'LQIDFOE'
- Location
- Quality
- Intensity
- Duration
- Frequency
- Others
- Effect on activity

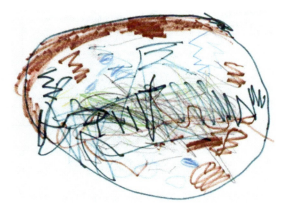

Figure 8.32 A 5-year-old girl had a one year history of headache. There was family history of brain tumour and migraine. Her drawing illustrates the 'zigzags', 'squiggly lines' and 'spots' she sees during an attack. She received a subsequent diagnosis of migraine. An MRI brain scan was normal.

- Revised Children's Anxiety and Depression Scale (RCADS).
- Paediatric Quality of Life Inventory (PedsQL).

■ Conduct a thorough examination (detailed elsewhere in this chapter/handbook) with particular focus on red flag signs e.g. impaired GCS, systemic disturbance, meningism, new focal neurological deficit, signs of raised intracranial pressure; don't forget to measure BP and undertake fundoscopy for papilloedema.

SECONDARY HEADACHE
Table 8.12 gives an overview of some important secondary headache diagnoses, examination features and investigation findings.

Medication – Overuse Headache (MOH)
This is often unrecognised, poorly evaluated and yet a common cause of chronic headache. Consider this in children with a prior primary headache diagnosis, who develop a *new-type* of headache or *worsening* of pre-existing headache. Associations include:

■ Use of ergots, triptans, opioids, but also paracetamol and NSAIDs

■ Alone or in combination for ≥ ten days/month

■ ≥ three months use

Most children respond to an abrupt discontinuation of all overused medication, but may experience an initial deterioration in symptoms. Improvement is generally seen after two months.

PRIMARY HEADACHE
Common Management Advice
■ Promote lifestyle measures – good sleep hygiene, regular exercise, routine meals, adequate fluid intake

Table 8.12: Some Causes of Secondary Headache in Children and Young People

Condition	History	Examination	Investigations
Post-traumatic	Close temporal relationship to head +/– neck injury (may be minor) May resemble TTH or migraine	May be unremarkable. Scalp soft tissue swelling/haematoma Skull deformity Impaired GCS or mental state	May be negative. Soft tissue swelling/skull fracture (plain x-ray) Intracranial haematoma or parenchymal contusion (CT or MRI)
Infection	Recent URTI, cold sore (HSV) or TB exposure May be incompletely or unvaccinated Systemic features e.g. fever, vomiting, rash	Fever; haemodynamic disturbance. Meningism, photophobia, vesicular or petechial rash (meningoencephalitis). Mastoid swelling (mastoiditis) +/– focal neurological deficit (e.g. cranial nerve palsy, lateralised weakness with UMN signs)	Abnormal inflammatory markers. Abnormal CSF (e.g. ↑ WBC, ↓ glucose, ↑ protein). Cerebritis, leptomeningeal +/– intracranial contrast MRI enhancement (meningitis, abscess, epidural collection)
Demyelination	Subacute onset; visual, sensorimotor, cognitive +/– sphincter disturbance; seizures Recent febrile illness	Dysautonomia, impaired GCS or mental state, focal neurological deficit +/– optic neuritis, sensory level, urinary retention (NMSOD spectrum)	Positive antibodies (MOG/AQP4; blood/CSF) CSF pleocytosis in some. Patchy white +/– grey matter hyperintensity/swelling (CT/MRI)
Raised intracranial pressure (ICP), including SOL and IIH	Persistent; early morning waking; exacerbated by coughing, straining, leaning forward May resemble TTH or migraine	Cushing's triad. Impaired GCS. Papilloedema. Focal neurological deficit	SOL, including tumour (CT/MRI). Elevated CSF manometry opening pressures (IIH). Radiological papilloedema, empty sella, cerebellar tonsillar descent
Vascular	Sudden onset, severe (ICH) Features of raised ICP (ICH and CVST) May resemble migraine or TTH (ischaemic stroke)	Neurocutaneous markers (e.g. NF1, CM AVM, HHT) Cushing's triad, impaired GCS, papilloedema, focal neurological deficit ('FAST positive'). Heart murmur	ICH, vascular malformation, CVST or AIS (CT/CTA or MR/MRA head and neck). Congenital heart disease/right-to-left shunt (echocardiogram). Bleeding diathesis/prothrombosis (FBC/clotting screening)
Medication overuse	High usage of acute analgesia (paracetamol, NSAIDs, triptans) on > two days/week, usually for previous headache	Within normal limits	Not usually indicated

AQP4, aquaporin-4 antibody; CM AVM, capillary malformation arterio-venous malformation syndrome; CTA, CT angiogram; CVST, cerebral venous sinus thrombosis; HHT, hereditary haemorrhagic telangiectasia; ICH, intracranial haemorrhage; IIH, idiopathic intracranial hypertension; MOG, myelin oligodendrocyte glycoprotein antibody; MRA, MR angiogram; NF1, neurofibromatosis type 1; NMSOD, neuromyelitis optica spectrum disorder; SOL, space occupying lesion; TTH, tension-type headache

- *Early* use of simple analgesia (i.e. paracetamol +/– ibuprofen); avoid opioids

- Counsel regarding medication overuse headache

Migraine

From 3 to 10% of UK children are estimated to live with migraine with prevalence increasing in adolescence. There is often a positive family history and vulnerability to motion sickness. Early life markers include infantile colic and benign paroxysmal torticollis, benign paroxysmal vertigo and cyclical vomiting. It is best thought of as recurrent attacks of complex neural dysfunction, including a premonitory fatigue and mood change, headache and postdromal 'grogginess' lasting 2 to 72 hours. Headache is more likely bilateral in children, moderate to severe with a pulsating/throbbing quality aggravated by routine activity. There is associated nausea and/or vomiting plus photo- and phonophobia.

A minority of children experience migraine with aura. These are typically visual (e.g. 'zig-zags' and scotoma), but are also sensory, involve speech, brainstem and/or motor (hemiplegic migraine). *Familial* hemiplegic migraine is associated with mutations in brain ion channel genes (e.g. *CACNA1A, ATP1A2, SCN1A* and *PRRT2*).

Migraine is a life-long condition with inherent fluctuations in course. Most children and adolescents improve overtime. A proportion develop chronic migraine and complications such as status migrainosus.

Management

- Acute.

  - To abort attack or minimise symptoms.

  - First line (early use); paracetamol or ibuprofen; second line triptan.

  - Consider an anti-emetic.

- Prophylaxis.

  - To prevent attacks; usually considered for ≥ three attacks/month.

  - Common first line agents include pizotifen, propranolol or topiramate; choice of agent determined by formulation options and co-morbidities.

  - Supplements (e.g. riboflavin, melatonin, magnesium) show efficacy in some and have an excellent safety profile.

  - Occipital nerve block (steroid and local anaesthetic) is considered in refractory cases.

- Non-pharmalogical management includes behavioural therapies, acupuncture and neuromodulation devices.

- Clinical trials are underway for novel treatments based on increased understanding of migraine biology and the adult experience. These include anti-calcitonin gene-related peptide (CGRP) monoclonal antibodies, gepants and lasmitidan.

Tension-Type Headache (TTH)

Features typically bilateral, mild to moderate pressing or tightening pain that lasts for at least 30 minutes. Unlike migraine, it is not aggravated by physical activity but there may be associated photophobia or phonophobia (but not both). A high incidence of mood disturbance, academic stress and functional symptoms have been reported in association.

Trigeminal Autonomic Cephalalgias

- Uncommon in childhood, but important diagnoses as some respond absolutely to indomethacin

- Classification according to duration

- Headache associated with ipsilateral cranial autonomic symptoms; conjunctival injection/lacrimation, nasal congestion/rhinorrhoea, eyelid oedema, facial sweating, miosis/ptosis

- Short-Lasting Unilateral Neuralgiform Headache Attacks With Conjunctival Injection And Tearing (SUNCT) and Short-Lasting Unilateral Neuralgiform Headache Attacks With Cranial Autonomic Symptoms (SUNA)

- Unilateral, trigeminal territory; neuralgiform headache, 1–600 seconds duration, attacks are isolated or in series

- Associated ipsilateral conjunctival injection and lacrimation (SUNCT); other cranial autonomic symptoms (SUNA)

Paroxysmal Hemicrania

- Typically strictly unilateral, severe supra orbital, orbital and/or temporal headache; 2–30 minutes duration, numerous attacks/day, associated ipsilateral cranial autonomic symptoms

- In children pain may be bilateral and > 30 minutes duration

- Excellent response to indomethacin

Cluster Headache

- Strictly unilateral, 'excruciating' supra orbital, orbital and/or temporal headache; 15–180 minutes duration (untreated), up to eight times/day; associated restlessness/agitation and ipsilateral autonomic symptoms

- Acute treatment – consider early triptans and high-flow oxygen

- Prophylaxis – consider melatonin, topiramate, short course of steroids, greater occipital nerve injection or verapamil (requires close cardiac monitoring); recommend specialist paediatric headache opinion

Hemicrania Continua

- Strictly unilateral headache; > three months duration, associated restlessness/agitation and ipsilateral autonomic symptoms

- Should show good response to indomethacin

MACROCEPHALY AND NEUROSURGICAL CONDITIONS

MACROCEPHALY

Definitions and Terminology

Macrocephaly is defined as a large head with an occipitofrontal circumference (OFC):

- > two standard deviations (SD) above the mean for a given age and sex *or*

- > 99.6th centile for age

Differential diagnosis is broad (Table 8.13), ranging from benign entities (e.g. isolated macrocephaly or familial macrocephaly) to more serious, acquired causes requiring urgent neurosurgical intervention (e.g. progressive hydrocephalus). The cranium contains skull bones, brain parenchyma, cerebrospinal fluid (CSF) and blood – expansion of any of these compartments can cause macrocephaly.

Macrocephaly may be *mild* (OFC + 2 – 3 SD) or severe (OFC > 3 SD); *severe* macrocephaly has frequent association with co-morbidities and neurogenetic conditions of intellectual disability and autism spectrum disorders.

Relative macrocephaly (apparently large head) is defined as OFC < 2 SD, but disproportionately above that for body stature. Consider conditions of intrauterine growth restriction (placental insufficiency, postnatal growth failure e.g. Silver–Russell syndrome), frontal bossing (e.g. vitamin D deficiency rickets), skeletal dysplasias (e.g. achondroplasia) and calvarial thickening (e.g. beta thalassaemia).

Table 8.13: **Some Causes of Macrocephaly**

GENETIC
- **Familial**
- **Autism spectrum disorder**
- **Syndromic**
  + *Cutaneous features* – NF1, PTEN hamartoma syndromes, tuberous sclerosis
  + *Overgrowth* – Sotos, Beckwith-Wiedemann syndromes
  + *RASopathy* – Noonan, Costello, LEOPARD syndromes
  + *Intellectual disability* – Fragile X
- **Metabolic**
  + *Leukodystrophy* – Alexander, Canavan, megalencephalic leukoencephalopathy with cysts
  + *Other white matter* – Glutaric aciduria Type 1, infantile lysosomal storage disorders (Figure 8.44)
- **Bone hyperostosis**
- **Hydrocephalus**

NON-GENETIC
- **Post-infective or haemorrhagic hydrocephalus**
- **Subdural effusions** (Figure 8.45)

OTHER
- **Intracranial vascular malformation** (Figure 8.46)

Table 8.14: **Macrocephaly Clinical Tips**

- OFC measurement – most prominent part of the glabella to most prominent area of occiput *or* largest measurable; largest of three measurements
- Use a narrow, non-stretch measuring tape (dedicated OFC tape preferable)
- Thick hair, distinctive head shape and skull hyperostosis may impact measurement
- Is it isolated? For instance, there are no associated developmental or health concerns.
- Plot height and weight – is macrocephaly part of a generalised growth disorder?
- Measure parental OFC (familial macrocephaly assessment).
- Plot serial OFC measurements (progressive macrocephaly assessment).

Table 8.15: **Some Indications for Genetic Investigation of Macrocephaly**

- Distinctive and/or coarse facial features
- Neurodevelopmental difference
- Epilepsy/seizures
- Neurocutaneous or other skin lesions (café-au-lait, hypopigmented macules, capillary haemangiomata or papillomata around the nose/mouth)
- Congenital malformations
- Intellectual disability
- Skeletal dysplasia, asymmetry or syndactyly
- Signs of inborn errors of metabolism
- Signs of an overgrowth syndrome
- MRI brain findings suggestive of megalencephaly, hydrocephalus or a wider neurogenetic disorder

A systematic clinical approach (Table 8.14), combined with neuroradiological, metabolic and/ or genetic evaluation (Table 8.15) in some, is advised to delineate most likely cause and inform subsequent management.

SOME IMPORTANT CLINICAL ENTITIES

Megalencephaly

This refers to brain overgrowth. Aetiologies includes metabolic (e.g. Alexander; Figure 8.33 and Canavan diseases) and developmental (e.g. *PI3K/AKT/mTOR* signalling pathway dysfunction).

Benign Enlargement of Subarachnoid Spaces (BESS)

Consider this if macrocephaly is isolated, non-syndromic and not associated with features of raised intracranial pressure (ICP), neurodevelopmental delay, regression or seizures. BESS

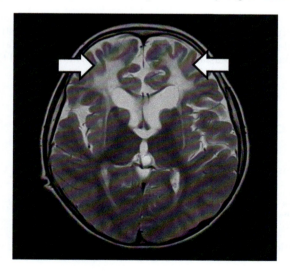

Figure 8.33 Alexander disease. A 13-year-old male with infancy onset developmental delay presents with neurological regression, epilepsy and progressive four-limb spastic-dystonic movement disorder. There was relative macrocephaly; OFC 50th centile; length and weight 0.4th–2nd centile. Axial intracranial MRI T2 sequence shows bilateral anterior predominant white matter changes (white arrows), frontal volume loss and ventricular prominence

represents enlargement of subarachnoid spaces, typically along frontal convexities +/− mild ventriculomegaly. Clinically there is rapid increase in OFC at approximately 6 months of age, stabilisation at 18 months and resolution by 2–3 years. It is usually self-limiting although there is increased risk of subdural haemorrhage thought to be related to stretching of bridging veins. Arachnoid villi immaturity and impaired CSF resorption has been postulated as a likely mechanism.

Familial Macrocephaly (FM)

Consider this where there is a family history of macrocephaly, particularly if traceable through several generations. Birth OFC may be in high normal percentiles and > 2 SD by 1 year. Dolichocephalic head shape is described in infancy, which resolved by adulthood with OFC remaining > 2 SD. Multifactorial and autosomal dominant modes of inheritance have been proposed.

Autism Spectrum Disorder (ASD) and Macrocephaly

ASD is a neurodevelopmental disorder with heterogenous aetiology and a feature of underlying genetic or metabolic disease in a proportion. Multifactorial inheritance is likely causative in some. Macrocephaly is a well described association and occurs in 15–35% of children with ASD. This is typically not present at birth with accelerated brain growth manifesting in first 1–3 years of life. The cause for this remains unclear.

HYDROCEPHALUS

Anatomy

CSF is produced at a relatively constant rate by choroid plexuses, flows caudally through the ventricular system and is reabsorbed by arachnoid granulations and central nervous system (CNS) lymphactics.

Definition

Hydrocephalus is a heterogenous disorder of CSF homeostasis with hallmarks of abnormal CSF accumulation in and pathological expansion of cerebral ventricles. Secondary raised intracranial pressure threatens permanent brain injury with sequelae including visual loss, significant motor and cognitive impairments. Acute hydrocephalus is a medical emergency, left untreated brain herniation and death may ensue.

Causes and Classification

Hydrocephalus is most common in infancy. This is predominantly congenital or post-haemorrhagic secondary to prematurity associated intraventricular haemorrhage. Congenital forms are associated with CNS malformations (e.g. Arnold–Chiari, Dandy–Walker syndrome) and more likely have a genetic/syndromic basis (e.g. X-linked Bickers–Adams–Edwards syndrome – aqueductal stenosis, intellectual disability and adducted thumbs).

In *obstructive* hydrocephalus ventricular CSF pathways are blocked or *'non-communicating'*, e.g. by a congenital stenosis, brain tumour or intraventricular bleed (Figure 8.34).

In *non-obstructive hydrocephalus* ventricular CSF pathways are patent or *'communicating'*, but there is impaired CSF resorption (e.g. subarachnoid haemorrhage, meningitis; Figure 8.35, leptomeningeal disease) or CSF hypersecretion (choroid plexus hyperplasia or non-obstructive tumours e.g. choroid plexus papilloma).

Normal pressure hydrocephalus is more prominent in adults.

Clinical Presentation

Clinical presentation is largely determined by the age of the child and degree of cerebral compliance. Infants present with tense/bulging fontanelle, increasing OFC, sutural diastasis and 'sun setting' (Figure 8.36). Older children present with features of raised ICP (e.g. morning headache, vomiting, visual disturbance, motor impairments, altered GCS, seizures).

Diagnosis, Treatment and Prognosis

Clinical suspicion is supported by a number of diagnostic and ancillary investigations. Intracranial CT/MRI is key in demonstrating cause (e.g. intracranial haemorrhage, tumour, infection) and/or features of raised ICP (e.g. transependymal oedema, bowing of the third ventricle, cerebellar tonsillar descent). Other useful investigations include CSF manometry for opening

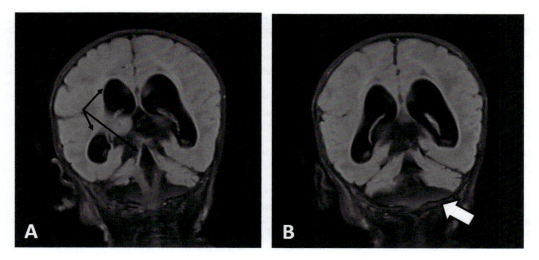

Figure 8.34 Tetraventricular obstructive hydrocephalus. A 10-week-old male infant with Krabbe disease develops new irritability, tonic limb posturing and increasing OFC. Intracranial coronal MRI T2 qTSE sequence shows enlargement of the anterior and temporal horns of the lateral, third and fourth ventricles (A; black arrows). The fourth ventricle appears to be draining into a retro-vermian cyst with ventricular outlet obstruction.

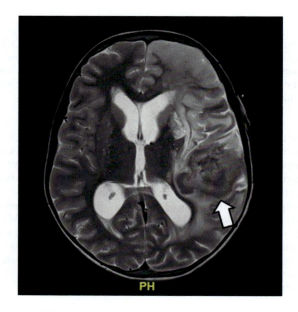

Figure 8.35 Tuberculous (TB) meningoencephalitis. A 14-year-old male presents with a three-week history of headache, weight loss and increasing confusion following recent travel to North Africa and TB exposure. He was hypertensive, tachycardic and had a GCS of 10. Axial intracranial MRI T2 sequence shows ventriculomegaly, left hemisphere oedema and a left fronto-insulo-temporal tuberculoma (white arrow). CSF was positive for acid fast bacilli and Mycobacteria growth indicator tube.

pressure and analysis for infection and protein concentration. In shunted patients, a skull x-ray ('shunt series') is used to assess ventriculoperitoneal shunt (VPS) integrity. Genetic investigation (chromosomal microarray, whole genome sequencing) has a diagnostic role in congenital hydrocephalus. Treatment is symptomatic and includes ventricular tapping (infants), CSF diversion (e.g.

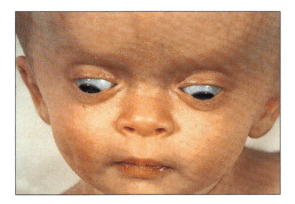

Figure 8.36 'Sun setting' sign in an infant with hydrocephalus.

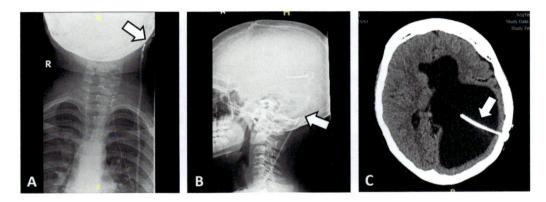

Figure 8.37 Ventriculoperitoneal shunt (VPS) disconnection. 15-year-old male with pre-exisiting VPS for congenital hydrocephalus develops lethargy, new onset squint and is found to have papilloedema. Shunt series shows proximal VPS disconnection (A and B; white arrows). Intracranial axial CT shows the trans-parietal shunt catheter in a markedly dilated left lateral ventricle (C; white arrow).

external ventricular drain, VPS insertion, endoscopic third ventriculostomy) +/− choroid plexus cautery. Related morbidity and prognosis is determined by cause and complications of intervention, including shunt related infection (typically *S. epidermidis*), blockage, disconnection (Figure 8.37) and peritonitis.

BRAIN TUMOURS

(See also the chapter 'Oncology'.)

Over 400 children a year are diagnosed with CNS tumours in the United Kingdom. They represent the second most prevalent group of cancers in childhood (approximately 25%).

CLINICAL PRESENTATION

Raised Intracranial Pressure

- Decreased conscious level
- Headache – early morning or waking from sleep; increased by coughing or straining
- Nausea +/− vomiting – in particular early morning
- Increasing head circumference (infant)
- Diplopia and squint related to VI nerve palsy (false localising sign; Figure 8.38)

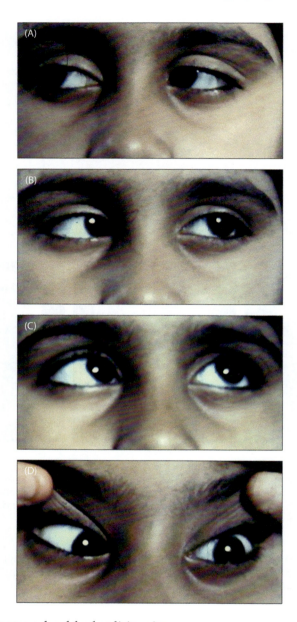

Figure 8.38 Sixth nerve palsy, false localising sign.

- Reduced visual acuity – infer from visual behaviour in a young child who may not report this
- Papilloedema

Top Three Signs and Symptoms by Tumour Location

- *Supratentorial* (e.g. some gliomas) – raised ICP, seizures, papilloedema
- *Central* (e.g. craniopharyngioma) – headache, abnormal eye movements/squint, nausea and vomiting
- *Posterior fossa* (e.g. medulloblastoma, astrocytoma, ependymoma) – nausea and vomiting, headache, abnormal gait and co-ordination difficulties
- *Spinal cord* – back pain, abnormal gait or co-ordination difficulties, spinal deformity

- Brain *stem* (e.g. diffuse mid-line glioma) – abnormal gait and co-ordination difficulties (including hemiplegia), cranial nerve palsies (VI and VII), pyramidal signs

Other

- *Parinaud syndrome* – upgaze palsy, retraction nystagmus, dissociation pupillary response to light and accommodation in pineal tumours

- *Diencephalic syndrome* – emaciation, accelerated skeletal growth, hypotension, hypoglycaemia and hyperactivity in hypothalamic gliomas (Figure 8.39)

COMMON TYPES

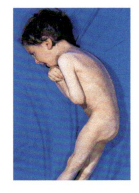

Figure 8.39 Diencephalic syndrome.

Gliomas (CNS Glial Cell Tumours) – Includes Astrocytomas and Ependymomas

Astrocytoma

- Most common type of brain and spinal cord tumour in children; develop at multiple sites

- Present at any age with symptoms determined by location, e.g. epilepsy if supratentorial

- Male and females equally affected

- Most are low grade; 15–20% are linked to neurofibromatosis type 1 (NF1) and pilocytic astrocytomas (typically cerebellar) are prominent (Figure 8.40)

- Diffuse mid-line glioma are a high-grade astrocytoma considered incurable. Most children die within months of diagnosis, < 10% live longer than two years.

Ependymoma

- Third most common type of brain tumour in childhood

- Fourth ventricle location (25% supratentorial; rarely in spinal cord)

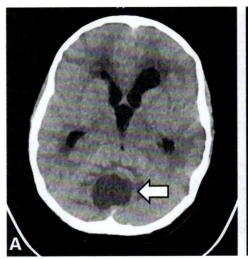
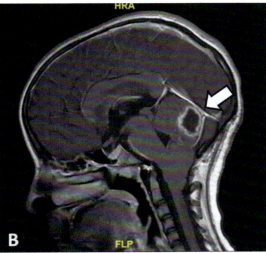

Figure 8.40 Astrocytoma. A 14-year-old female with NF1 presents with a two month history of headache, vomiting and blurred vision. She is found to have papilloedema. Intracranial axial CT (A) and sagittal contrast MRI T1 sequence (B) shows triventricular hydrocephalus, cerebellar tonsillar descent and 'crowding' of the neuronal structures at the foramen magnum. There is a right cerebellar cystic, peripherally enhancing mass close to the cerebellar vermis (white arrows). Tissue histology confirmed a pilocytic astrocytoma.

- Predominant in those < 5 years with presentation including vomiting, headache, head tilt/torticollis (Figure 8.41), ataxia

- Higher occurrence in males

- 60% of children with ependymoma survive ≥ 5 years

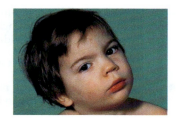

Figure 8.41 Head tilt in posterior fossa tumour.

Medulloblastoma (CNS Embryonal Tumour) (Figure 8.42)

- Most common high-grade childhood brain tumour – metastasis via CSF along the neuroaxis, including spine

- Cerebellar location

- Typical presentation between 3 and 8 years of age with headache, vomiting and ataxia

- Higher occurrence in males

- Survival rates are approximately 60–70% for metastatic and non-metastatic disease, respectively

Craniopharyngioma (Figure 8.43)

- 8% of childhood brain tumours

- Sellar/parasellar location

- Low grade

- Presentation aged 5–15 years due to mass effect – headache, endocrine dysfunction and visual disturbance (reduced visual acuity, visual field defect)

- Most cured by surgery and radiotherapy; complications such as hormone deficiencies can be serious and long term (Figure 8.44)

General Principles of Management

- *Neurosurgery* – biopsy (diagnostic), debulking or resection to remove as much tumour as is safely possible, CSF diversion to treat hydrocephalus

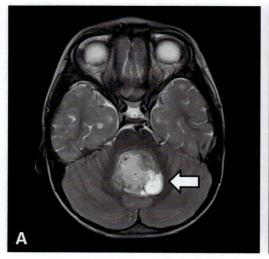
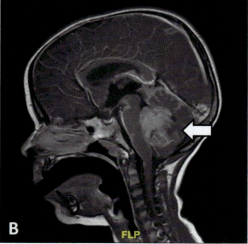

Figure 8.42 Medulloblastoma. A 2-year-old female presents with a one week history of early morning vomiting and ataxia. Intracranial MRI T2 axial (A) and T1 contrast sagittal sequences (B) show an intraventricular posterior fossa tumour causing obstructive hydrocephalus (white arrows). There was associated intracranial and intraspinal leptomeningeal spread. She died three weeks later following rapid progression of metastatic disease. Histology confirmed a large cell/ anaplastic medulloblastoma.

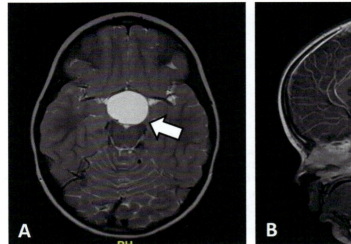

Figure 8.43 Craniopharyngioma. 3-year-old female presents with a history of worsening daily headache, visual impairment and weight gain. Intracranial MRI T2 axial (A) and T1 contrast sagittal sequences (B) show a sellar and suprasellar predominantly cystic mass which is displacing the optic chiasm anteriorly. Tissue histology was consistent with an adamantinomatous craniopharyngioma.

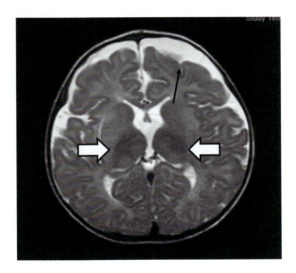

Figure 8.44 Lysosomal storage disorder. An 11-month-old male with a history of parental consanguinity presents with global developmental delay, poor feeding and hepatosplenomegaly. There was relative macrocephaly; OFC 50th centile and weight < 0.4th centile. Axial intracranial MRI T2 sequence shows bilateral dark thalami (white arrows) and a left convexity chronic subdural collection (black arrow). White cell beta-galactosidase activity in blood was very low and a pathogenic homozygous mutation in the GLB1 gene detected, confirming a diagnosis of GM1 gangliosidosis.

- *Radiotherapy* – inoperable tumours, to treat residual tumour post-surgical resection. Not given to children < 3 years of age due to long-term effects on growth, hormonal sufficiency and cognition

- *Proton beam therapy* – select cases (nationally approved list of indicated tumours; generally smaller, well demarcated tumours or those close to critical structures e.g. spinal cord or optic nerve)

219

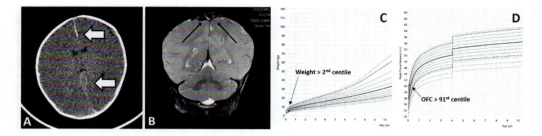

Figure 8.45 Abusive head trauma. A 2-month-old male presents with an out of hospital arrest. Axial intracranial CT shows diffuse cerebral oedema and interhemispheric blood (white arrows; A). Coronal intracranial MRI STIR sequence shows bilateral subdural haemorrhages (black arrows; B). Growth parameters show relative macrocephaly (weight > 2nd centile; C and OFC > 91st centile; D). There were also bilateral, multi-layered, numerous retinal haemorrhages and multiple rib fractures.

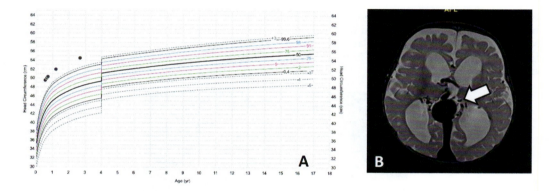

Figure 8.46 Vein of Galen malformation. A 7-month-old female presents with progressive, severe macrocephaly since birth (> 3 SD above 99.6th centile; A). Axial intracranial MRI STIR sequence shows a Vein of Galen malformation (white arrow) and associated ventriculomegaly.

- *Chemotherapy* – pre-operative (to reduce tumour bulk), post-operative (to minimise recurrence), treatment of recurrences, inoperable tumours, in combination with radiotherapy

Prognosis

Depends on tumour type, grading and location. Average five-year survival rate is 74% in England, with wide variance between tumour subgroups. It remains the greatest cancer-related cause of death in children.

SPINA BIFIDA

See also the chapters 'Orthopaedics and Fractures' and 'Neonatal and General Paediatric Surgery'.

Incidence/Aetiology

Spina bifida occurs in approximately 1 in 500, but is very variable geographically. There is reduced incidence since the introduction of folic acid supplementation in pregnancy and antenatal diagnosis with α-fetoprotein and ultrasound.

Genetic factors are important. The risk of having a further affected child if one is already affected is 1 in 30. The risk of having a third child if two are affected is one in six. Environmental factors are also important, particularly poor intake of folic acid in the first trimester.

Definitions

- Meningocoele (Figure 8.47): Cord is usually normal, lesion is covered with skin, neurology is often normal.

- Myelocoele or myelomeningocoele (Figure 8.48): Cord is exposed and abnormal, with only a thin covering if any; the risk of neurological impairment is very high.

- Spina bifida occulta: Spinal cord is covered with bone and skin, but usually marked with a sacral pit, hairy patch or lipoma. Children usually present later with bladder problems or minor gait disorders.

Site

The defect most commonly occurs in the lumbosacral area, less commonly in the dorsal region and uncommonly in the cervical region. Ten percent of lesions affect the skull (encephalocoeles).

Complications of Spina Bifida

- **Loss of sensation:** Sensory loss in the skin can lead to ulceration (Figure 8.49) as the child may not know that he has burnt or cut himself. The ability to recognise a full rectum or bladder may also be lost.

- **Bladder problems:** Most children with lumbosacral myelomeningocoeles are incontinent to a degree. The bladder sphincters are often innervated abnormally and this may lead to a neuropathic bladder, which does not empty properly. The pressure inside the urinary tract may be high because of this and the child is also subject to frequent urinary tract infections. There is a risk of chronic renal failure in the long term if the bladder is not appropriately managed.

- **Hydrocephalus:** Usually secondary to Arnold–Chiari malformation of the brainstem. It occurs in patients with high lesions – e.g. thoracolumbar myelomeningocoele.

- **Paralysis:** With a lumbosacral lesion, the legs will be partially paralysed (Figure 8.48) to an extent dependent on the site of the lesion and the degree of damage to the spinal cord. Secondary syringomyelia may lead to deterioration.

- **Limb deformities**: If the limbs are partially paralysed, there will be muscular imbalance and limb deformities may be present from birth (Figure 8.48) or develop at a later stage.

- **Kyphoscoliosis:** The vertebral column may be abnormal and children are at high risk of kyphoscoliosis.

Management

- Early closure of the spinal defect. Today this is done in the majority of instances although surgical treatment may not be appropriate in some children with extensive neurological damage or severe hydrocephalus.

- Management of hydrocephalus: A shunt will usually be inserted.

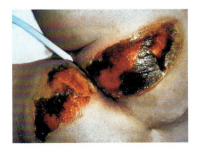

Figure 8.49 Pressure sores secondary to poor sensation in spina bifida. Although bladder problems are common, patients now intermittently catheterise rather than having indwelling catheters.

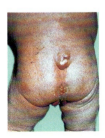

Figure 8.47 Meningocoele with relatively normal legs.

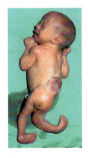

Figure 8.48 Myelocoele with flaccid, wasted legs.

Table 8.16: ILAE Seizure and Epilepsy Classification

Seizures	Focal	Aetiology
	Generalised	• Structural
	Unknown	• Genetic
Epilepsy	Focal	• Infectious
	Generalised	• Metabolic
	Focal and generalised	• Immune
	Unknown	• Unknown
Epilepsy Syndrome		

■ Management of the bladder: It is essential that the child has a urodynamic study to examine the nature of the neuropathic bladder. Intermittent catheterisation is usually used to improve continence and prevent infection. Children will need regular urines performed and adequate treatment of the urinary tract infections. With careful management, it is now unusual for children to develop chronic renal failure.

■ Physical management: many children with flaccid limbs can be given appropriate orthoses and can walk. Other children may be wheelchair dependent. It is important to prevent kyphoscoliosis with an appropriate spinal brace if indicated.

EPILEPSY

Epilepsy affects up to 1 in 200 children and up to one-third is pharmacoresistant. In recent years the International League Against Epilepsy have redesigned the classifications for seizures, epilepsy, and epilepsy syndromes. The newer guidelines have a focus on these elements as well as considering the underlying aetiology for these children's epilepsy – see Table 8.16.

Causes
Neonate

■ Hypoglycaemia; hypocalcaemia; hyponatraemia; hypernatraemia

■ Infection – meningitis, systemic

■ Birth asphyxia, birth trauma, intraventricular haemorrhage

■ Drug withdrawal

■ Stroke – venous sinus thrombosis, arterial

■ Structural brain malformations (e.g. lissencephaly), cortical dysplasia

■ Metabolic conditions (e.g. hyperglycinaemia; pyridoxine deficiency/dependency); biotinidase deficiency); peroxisomal disorders; mitochondrial disorders; Menke kinky hair disease

Child

■ Genetic syndromes (e.g. Angelman – Figure 8.50)

■ Neurocutaneous syndromes, e.g. tuberous sclerosis, hypomelanosis of Ito, linear sebaceous naevus, or incontinentia pigmenti; Sturge–Weber syndrome (Figures 8.51)

■ Metabolic (e.g. mitochondrial, glucose transporter deficiency)

■ Primary/secondary tumour – glioma dysembryoblastic neuroepithelial tumour

■ Structural brain abnormality – neuronal migration defects, such as lissencephaly, double cortex, polymicrogyria, or hemi-megalencephaly, hippocampal sclerosis (Figure 8.52)

Clinical Evaluation

■ A clear and careful history of the events is the most important part of the evaluation. Epilepsy is a clinical diagnosis and investigations should be used to determine the underlying cause and the specific epilepsy syndrome.

■ This can help to both diagnose the events as seizures and determine the epilepsy syndrome.

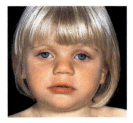

Figure 8.50 Angelman's Syndrome.

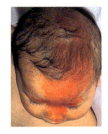

Figure 8.51 Capillary haemangioma in the ophthalmic division of the fifth cranial nerve; Sturge–Weber syndrome is diagnosed when there is underlying pial angioma over the surface of the brain seen on MRI brain with contrast. This may lead to epilepsy, contralateral hemiparesis and learning difficulties. Epilepsy surgery (e.g. hemispherectomy) may improve seizures if epilepsy is severe.

- Ask about the seizures themselves (do they know a seizure is coming, what is the first thing the parents see, and then what happens), as well as the post-ictal phase (tiredness, speech, limb weakness).

- Seizure pattern – triggers, frequency, time of day, age of onset.

- Questions to determine the underlying cause – birth history, development, family history, other medical issues.

- Examination – look for any neurocutaneous markers (Figure 8.51), measure head circumference, determine focal neurology suggesting a CNS lesion, e.g. hemiplegia.

Investigations

- ECG – should be done at diagnosis in all children to exclude arrhythmias.

- EEG – Used to confirm whether epilepsy is generalised or focal, or give clues to the epilepsy syndrome. Initially awake and if not helpful a sleep EEG may be needed. If there is a diagnostic need to capture events then video telemetry may be useful.

- Magnetic resonance imaging (MRI) brain – Not needed in children with easily controlled generalised epilepsy or in those with a clear diagnosis of self-limited epilepsy of childhood. Should be done in all other types of epilepsy.

- Genetic testing – If there are any clues to a specific genetic epilepsy syndrome (SCN1A testing in those with recurrent prolonged febrile convulsions). Microarray in any children with a learning difficulty, ring chromosome 20 in any child with non-convulsive status. Whole genome testing with an epilepsy gene panel should be considered in any child with pharmacoresistant epilepsy.

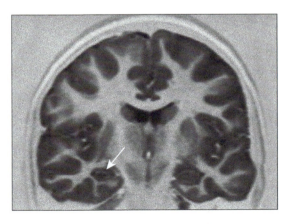

Figure 8.52 MRI scan showing R hippocampus with signal change and atrophy compatible with hippocampal sclerosis (arrow). Around 70% are seizure-free after surgery.

- In infants biotinidase and urine α-aminoadipic semialdehyde (AASA) should be sent and all infants commenced on biotin and pyridoxine until the results are found to be normal.

- Consider lumbar puncture with testing of CSF glucose (Glucose transporter GLUT1 deficiency) amino acids (hyperglycinemia), lactate (mitochondrial syndrome).

Management

- See Table 8.17 below for anti-seizure medications.

- Iron supplementation in reflex anoxic seizures.

- Family education around sudden unexpected death in epilepsy (SUDEP), seizure triggers, medication, and emergency management of seizures.

- If children have failed two anti-seizure medications they should be considered pharma-coresistant and referred to a tertiary epilepsy clinic for consideration of:

  - Epilepsy surgery – considered in anyone with focal epilepsy

  - Ketogenic diet – first line in GLUT 1 deficiency

  - Vagus nerve stimulator

CONDITIONS WITH NEUROLOGICAL DETERIORATION

The majority of children who deteriorate neurologically and cognitively do not have a recognisable degenerative disease. Here we discuss specific neurological diseases with progressive symptoms.

Suggested list of investigations for children presenting with neurological regression (not exhaustive):

- EEG (awake and asleep)

- Blood film to look for evidence of storage in Lymphocytes

- MRI head and possibly spine, MRA, magnetic resonance venography (MRV)

- Biotinidase and trial of biotin

- Plasma lactate

- Plasma amino acids

- Urine organic acids

- Plasma ammonia

- Acyl carnitine

- CSF lactate, glucose, measles antibodies, neurotransmitters

- Electroretinogram (ERG), visual evoked potentials (VEPs)

- Nerve conduction studies

- Very long chain fatty acids

- White cell enzymes

- Skin biopsy, e.g. to exclude Nieman–Pick

- Genetics: chromosomes, array-CGH, Whole genome sequencing

MULTIPLE SCLEROSIS

Multiple sclerosis (MS) is rare in childhood, and uncommon in adolescence (5% of all cases present < 18 years, < 1% before 10 years). It typically presents with a clinically isolated syndrome of optic neuritis (but most cases of optic neuritis do not have MS), transverse myelitis, or brainstem syndrome. Less often they may present with encephalopathy and mimic acute disseminated encephalomyelitis (ADEM). MS has an unpredictable course.

Table 8.17: Common Epilepsy Syndromes in Childhood

Syndrome	Age of Onset	Seizure Types	EEG	Treatment
Childhood Absence Epilepsy	2–12 years	Absence Seizures – Generalised 10 seconds May develop GTC seizures later in life	3 Hz generalised spike and wave	Ethosuximide Sodium Valproate Lamotrigine
Juvenile Absence Epilepsy	8–12 years	Generalised – Absence seizure GTC Myoclonic seizures	Generalised spike-and-wave, fragments of generalised spike-and-wave or polyspike-and-wave	Ethosuximide (for absence seizures only) Lamotrigine Levetiracetam Sodium Valproate
Juvenile Myoclonic Epilepsy	8–25 years	Myoclonic seizures GTC seizure Photoparoxysmal seizures in < 10% May have infrequent, short absence seizures	Generalised spike and wave with polyspike. One-third have photoparoxysmal response. HV may induce absence seizures	Sodium Valproate Levetiracetam Brivaracetam Clobazam Clonazepam Lamotrigine Phenobarbitone
Generalised Tonic Clonic Seizures	5–40 years (peak 11–23 years)	GTC seizures alone	Generalised spike-and-wave or polyspike-and-wave, may only be in sleep	Sodium Valproate Lamotrigine Levetiracetam Clobazam Perampanel Topiramate
Self-limited Epilepsy with Centrotemporal Spikes	3–14 years	Focal motor seizures with hemifacial involvement	Bilateral centro-temporal spike wave discharges	May not require treatment Lamotrigine Levetiracetam
Panayiotopoulos Syndrome	1–14 years	Focal occipital seizures with autonomic features which are prolonged	High amplitude focal discharges activated by sleep	Typically none needed
Infantile Spasms (West Syndrome)	3–12 months	Epileptic spasms typically in clusters on waking	Hypsarrhythmia background – high amplitude and disorganised.	Prednisolone + Vigabatrin Ketogenic diet Levetiracetam Nitrazepam Sodium Valproate Topiramate
SCN1A related Epilepsy (Dravet Syndrome)	< 1 year	Prolonged febrile seizures – GTC Hemiclonic Focal Status epilepticus Myoclonic Absences Atonic	Initially may be normal, generalised slowing and generalised spike wave may develop with time	Sodium Valproate Clobazam Stiripentol Cannabidiol Fenfluramine Ketogenic diet Topiramate Levetiracetam NB – Avoid sodium channel blockers
Myoclonic Seizures in Infancy (Several syndromes)	Under 1 year – Under 4 years all children with myoclonic seizures should be thoroughly investigated	Myoclonic seizures – May go on to have focal seizures and epileptic spasms	May be severely abnormal in myoclonic encephalopathy or normal in myoclonic seizures of infancy	Levetiracetam Clobazam Lamotrigine Pyridoxine in some cases
Lennox-Gastaut Syndrome	1–7 years	Generalised – GTC Tonic Atonic Atypical absences Myoclonic-atonic Focal seizure Epileptic spasms	Slow (< 2.5 Hz) spike-and-wave and paroxysmal fast activity (10 Hz or greater) in slow sleep	Sodium Valproate Lamotrigine Clobazam Typically refractory and very difficult to treat
Landau Kleffner Syndrome	2–8 years	Subacute onset of acquired aphasia 20–30% have no seizures Focal Seizures Atypical Absences Atonic	High amplitude epileptiform activity in temporo-parietal regions = ns activated in sleep	Steroids Ethosuximide Clobazam Sodium Valproate

GTC – generalised tonic clonic seizures; HV – hyperventilation, EEG – electroencephalogram

Table 8.18: Other Important Event Types

Syndrome	Age of onset	Event types	Investigations	Treatment
Febrile seizures	6 months to 5 years	Simple febrile seizures – GTC lasting < 15 minutes, single seizure in 24 hours, no neurological deficit before or after Complex febrile seizures – GTC > 15 minutes, focal seizure of any length, neurological deficit before or after	Determine the underlying infective cause In complex febrile seizures consider EEG, MRI and if over 30 minutes consider genetic testing for SCN1A variants.	None is typically required Consider giving family rescue buccal midazolam for children with frequent seizures or who have had more than one prolonged seizure.
Reflex anoxic seizures	Early infancy and remit by pre-school age	Typically after a sudden stimulus (e.g. bang to the head) profound vagal discharge with a dramatic drop in the heart rate and transient asystole. Child may briefly cry, then become pale, and lose consciousness. May have posturing mimicking a tonic seizure.	Video of events if possible ECG	None is typically needed **Rarely** in very frequent episodes atropine or cardiac pacing has been used
Breath-holding attacks	Pre-school children	After an episode of upset/distress the child will stop breathing in expiration, this looks like a silent cry or expiratory grunt. The child's face then becomes blue with deep cyanosis. They may then recover or go on to syncope and may have an episode of posturing similar to that in a reflex anoxic seizure	Videos of events ECG Testing for iron deficiency anaemia	Iron supplementation if needed
Day-dreaming/inattention	Any age	Can be misdiagnosed as absences. Typically longer and have no associated loss of body tone. They are situational (when child is tired or relaxed), child can be distracted out of them. More common in children with ASD or LD	None needed, should be diagnosed with a clear history	None needed
Infantile Gratification	From infancy onwards	Rhythmic hip flexion and adduction may be accompanied by a distant expression, a flushed face and sometimes followed by sleepiness. More common in a car seat, high chair, or when bored.	Typically can be diagnosed with a good home video	None needed
Non-epileptic Seizures	Typically older children	Can resemble focal non-motor, or motor seizures, or GTC seizures. Clues may include eye closure with resistance to passive opening, there may be a prominence of proximal or truncal movements.	Video of events is the most useful	Psychology involvement is the most useful

GTC – generalised tonic clonic seizures; ECG – electrocardiogram; ASD – autism spectrum disorder; LD – learning disability

Diagnostic Criteria

The diagnosis of MS can be made by fulfilling any one of the following:

■ Two or more non-encephalopathic (ie, unlike ADEM) clinical CNS events with presumed inflammatory cause, separated by more than 30 days and involving more than one area of the CNS.

- One non-encephalopathic episode typical of MS that is associated with MRI findings consistent with 2017 McDonald criteria (Table 8.19) for dissemination in space and in which a follow-up MRI shows at least one new enhancing or nonenhancing lesion consistent with criteria for dissemination in time.

- One ADEM attack followed by a non-encephalopathic clinical event, three or more months after symptom onset, that is associated with new MRI lesions that fulfil the 2017 McDonald dissemination in space criteria.

- A first, single, acute event that does not meet ADEM criteria and for which MRI findings are consistent with the 2017 McDonald criteria for dissemination in space and dissemination in time; this applies only to children ≥ 11 years of age.

Treatment

Any child with a suspected demyelinating disease should be referred to a tertiary paediatric neurology centre. Treatment of initial presentation is with intravenous methylprednisolone. Those who do not respond to methylprednisolone during the acute recurrence can be considered for intravenous immunoglobulin as a second line treatment.

For relapsing-remitting MS disease modifying treatment is recommended with agents such as rituximab, or fingolimod.

ADRENOLEUKODYSTROPHY

X-linked gene (*ABCD1*) at *Xq28*, coding for peroxisomal membrane protein is at fault. Pathogenic variants in the gene result in accumulation of very long chain fatty acids (VLCFAs) in all tissues. In males onset is commonly between the ages of 4 and 8 years. The child shows deterioration in gait with cognitive decline and pyramidal, extrapyramidal and cerebellar signs. Adrenocortical insufficiency is present in about 10% of cases (pigmentation is very rare) and so the diagnosis should be considered in those presenting with this even without the neurological symptoms. Female carries often go on to develop myelopathy and polyneuropathy symptoms during adulthood. About 90% will develop this by 60 years of age.

Diagnosis

- Neuro-imaging – white matter abnormality.

- Elevated very long chain fatty acids.

- DNA testing.

Management

- Allogeneic bone marrow transplantation (BMT) for pre or early symptomatic cerebral disease (few lesions on MRI and performance IQ > 80) or autologous BMT transfected with *ABCD1* for advanced cerebral disease.

Table 8.19: 2017 McDonald Criteria

Dissemination in space	Objective clinical evidence of at least two lesions or objective clinical evidence of one lesion with reasonable historical evidence of a prior attack involving a different CNS site.	
	At least one T2 lesion in at least two of four MS-typical regions of the CNS:	• Periventricular • (Juxta)cortical • Infratentorial • Spinal cord
Dissemination in Time	At least two attacks separated by a period of at least one month	
	Simultaneous presence of gadolinium-enhancing and nonenhancing lesions at any time	
	A new T2 and/or gadolinium-enhancing lesion on follow-up MRI, irrespective of its timing with reference to a baseline scan	
	Demonstration of CSF-specific OCBs (as substitute for demonstration of DIT)	

CNS – central nervous system; CSF – cerebrospinal fluid; MRI – magnetic resonance imaging; OCB – oligoclonal bands

- Steroid replacement therapy for adrenal insufficiency.

- Dietary manipulation for asymptomatic patients has not been shown to be clinically effective and is not recommended.

- Symptomatic management for those with advanced neurological manifestations.

KRABBE DISEASE

This is an autosomal recessive lysosomal storage disorder due to a pathogenic variant in a gene on *14q* coding for α-galactocerebrosidase. The infantile form (onset < 12 months) is most common but it may present at later ages.

Clinical Signs

- Restlessness, irritability, progressive pyramidal and extrapyramidal hypertonia and reduced reflexes

- Seizures often develop as the disease progresses

Diagnosis

- Measurement of galactocerebrosidase (GALC) activity in leukocytes (send white cell enzymes)

- The diagnosis can be confirmed by genetic testing

- Neuro-imaging is often non-specific (usually not a white matter abnormality)

Treatment

- Supportive treatment with early involvement of symptom care teams.

- Trials for early symptomatic infants to determine the efficacy of gene therapy are underway.

METACHROMATIC LEUKODYSTROPHY

Due to an autosomal recessive gene on *22q* coding for cerebroside sulfatase. Prevalence ranges from

- 1:40,000 to 1:100,000 in northern Europe and North America. There are infantile, juvenile and adult forms.

- Infantile (0–25 months): irritability; gait disturbance; spasticity in legs; reduced tendon reflexes.

- Juvenile (4–16 years): mental regression; movement disorder (mixed pyramidal and peripheral neuropathy); seizures.

- Adult (> 17 years): dementia and behavioural issues.

Diagnosis

- White cell enzymes will show deficiency of arylsulfatase A (ARSA) enzyme activity in leukocytes.

- Genetic testing will confirm the diagnosis.

Treatment

- Gene therapy with Libmeldy is now available through the NHS for those who are diagnosed early enough. Early testing and pre-symptomatic screening of siblings is vital.

- Supportive care for those whose disease is too advanced for gene therapy.

NEURONAL CEROID LIPOFUSCINOSIS (NCL)

A group of progressive lysosomal storage disorders. There are four subtypes; infantile, late infantile, juvenile, and adult (although classification by genetic cause is now recommended). Together they are the most prevalent neurodegenerative disorders of childhood. The incidence ranges from 0.6 to 13.6 per 100,000 depending on geographic location. At present at least 13 different genes have been identified as causative of NCL.

INFANTILE (NCL) – HALTIA-SANTAVUORI DISEASE

This affects infants aged from 6 to 12 months, causing developmental regression and ataxia. The patient has stereotyped hand movements, with progressive microcephaly and optic atrophy.

Diagnosis

- Extinguished ERG
- Progressive slowing and flattening on EEG
- Cerebral atrophy on neuro-imaging
- Genetic testing

LATE INFANTILE NCL – JANSKÝ–BIELSCHOWSKY DISEASE

This affects children between 18 months and 4 years, causing developmental regression, ataxia and eventually epilepsy and macular and retinal degeneration.

Diagnosis

- EEG shows spike in response to photic stimulation synchronous with flash.
- ERG extinguished (not necessarily at presentation).
- Skin shows curvilinear bodies in cytosomes.
- Genetic testing.

JUVENILE NCL – BATTEN DISEASE

This affects children between 4 and 7 years of age, causing progressive visual loss and behavioural disturbance, with slow cognitive deterioration. Dysarthria, and extrapyramidal, pyramidal and cerebellar signs gradually supervene.

Diagnosis

- Vacuolated lymphocytes in peripheral blood
- EEG shows pseudoperiodic bursts of slow waves
- ERG and VEP are decreased
- Atrophy and calcification on neuro-imaging
- Skin shows fingerprint profiles
- Genetic testing

Management of All Ceroid Lipofuscinoses

- Seizure control (lamotrigine, sodium valproate).
- Management of progressive movement disorder (see Figure 8.61), visual loss and behavioural problems.
- Patients with CLN2 disease who are age 3 years and older, may benefit from treatment treatment with recombinant human cerliponase alfa (Grade 1B).

TAY–SACHS DISEASE

Due to an autosomal recessive gene on chromosome 15 causing hexosaminidase A deficiency. It is common in Ashkenazi Jews. The child is startled by loud noises, with developmental regression, hypotonia, then hypertonia and seizures. A cherry-red spot at the macula is a characteristic early sign (Figure 8.53). Diagnosis is from white cells (hexosaminidase A).

NIEMANN–PICK DISEASE TYPE C

An autosomal recessive disease (95% are homozygous for *NCP1* gene on chromosome 18); lysosomal cholesterol storage. Children show poor school progress, ataxia, hepatomegaly and vertical

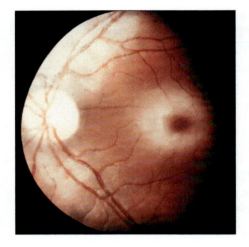

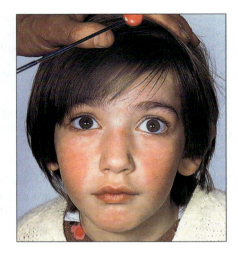

Figure 8.53 Cherry-red spot in the fundus of a child with Tay–Sachs disease.

Figure 8.54 Difficulty in looking up in a patient with Niemann–Pick Type C.

gaze palsy (Figure 8.54). Miglustat appears to slow the progression of neurological symptoms in those who have already developed symptoms.

LEIGH DISEASE (SUBACUTE NECROTISING ENCEPHALOMYELOPATHY)

This is due to mitochondrial disorders (pyruvate carboxylase deficiency, pyruvate dehydrogenase deficiency, respiratory chain enzyme deficiencies). Children show progressive movement disorders, usually extrapyramidal, ptosis and ophthalmoplegia and seizures. Prognosis in those with symptom onset before 2 years of age is poor, although in those with later onset disease life expectancy is longer.

Diagnosis

- Neuro-imaging shows low density in the putamen and caudate. Raised blood and CSF lactate.

- DNA for mitochondrial mutations.

- Muscle biopsy for respiratory chain enzyme analysis if genetic testing is non-diagnostic.

- Skin biopsy for pyruvate dehydrogenase deficiency and respiratory chain enzymes, again only if genetic testing is not diagnostic.

Treatment

Some studies report a positive effect of coenzyme Q in particular mutations. In general treatment is supportive only.

ACUTE DECREASED CONSCIOUS LEVEL (COMA), ENCEPHALOPATHY AND ENCEPHALITIS DEFINITIONS

Coma, encephalopathy and encephalitis are sometimes used interchangeably for conditions impacting conscious level (Table 8.20). Presentation is frequently undifferentiated and the clinician is tasked with delineating cause and providing treatment, often urgently. Recognising important distinctions and overlap can help guide appropriate investigation, diagnosis and management.

- **Decreased conscious level ('DeCon') or coma** can be defined as responding only to voice, pain or being unresponsive on the Alert, Voice, Pain, Unresponsive (AVPU) scale *or* a score of ≤ 14 on the Glasgow Coma Scale (> 5 years) or modified Glasgow Coma Scale (< 5 years). It is an acute neurological emergency with potential for an underlying brain insult to result in significant morbidity or even death.

- **Encephalopathy** can be defined as a syndrome of global brain dysfunction where altered mental state is prominent. This may include behaviour change, cognitive impairment and/or mood

Table 8.20: Causes and Examples of Encephalopathy and DeCon

Cause	Examples
Systemic	Sepsis, shock, hypoxia, liver failure, hypertensive encephalopathy
Intracranial infection	Infectious (meningo)encephalitis, empyema, abscess
Trauma	Accidental, abusive
Intoxication	Alcohol, recreational drugs; accidental inhalation (e.g. CO), ingestion or overdose; self-harm, unusual reaction (sedation, analgesia, anaesthesia), drug toxicity (e.g. AEDs), deliberate poisoning
Metabolic	Acidosis, hypoglycaemia, hyponatraemia, hyperammonaemia, uraemia
Cerebrovascular	Stroke (haemorrhagic, AIS), CVST +/− venous infarction
Neuroimmune encephalitis	CNS inflammation (AE; NMDAR, limbic, Hashimoto's), demyelination (MOG, AQP4 antibodies), post/parainfectious syndromes, CNS vasculitis
Raised ICP	Cerebral oedema (various causes), hydrocephalous, space occupying lesion, IIH
Seizure or epilepsy – related	Prolonged convulsion, post-ictal state, SE (CSE, NCSE)
Decompensation of previously diagnosed condition	Epileptic encephalopathy, VP-shunt blockage, metabolic (e.g. mitochondrial disease), DKA (DM)
Aetiology unknown	Consider seronegative AE if phenotype appropriate

AE, autoimmune encephalitis; AEDs, anti-epileptic medications; AIS, arterial ischaemic stroke; AQP4, aquaporin-4; CO, carbon monoxide; CSE, convulsive status epilepticus: CVST, cerebral venous sinus thrombosis; DKA, diabetic ketoacidosis; DM, diabetes mellitus; IIH, idiopathic intracranial hypertension; MOG, myelin oligodendrocyte glycoprotein; NMDAR, n-methyl-d-aspartate receptor; NCSE, non-convulsive status epilepticus; SE, status epilepticus; VP, ventriculoperitoneal

disturbance with or without DeCon. Additional neurologic symptoms and signs may provide clues to an underlying cause, frequently an encephalitis.

- **Encephalitis** can be defined as brain inflammation. Common causes are infectious and autoimmune. Encephalitis may result in encephalopathy and/or DeCon.

SOME IMPORTANT SECONDARY CAUSES OF ENCEPHALOPATHY AND DECON
Hyperammonaemia

High levels of ammonia (hyperammonaemia) are neurotoxic and can quickly cause irreversible neurological damage. Presentation is with progressive encephalopathy, typically vomiting, seizures and apnoea. Causes are primary (e.g. organic aciduria, urea cycle and fatty acid oxidation defects) or secondary (e.g. duct dependent cardiac lesions, acute liver failure and drug toxicity). Treatment is supportive, including treating infection, stopping sources of protein and neuroprotection plus targeted ammonia scavenging. Haemofiltration may also be necessary. Test ammonia in any unwell child with unexplained encephalopathy and seek urgent attention if > 150 (neonate) or > 50–100 in an older child.

Non-Convulsive Status Epilepticus (NCSE)

NCSE has been defined as a persistent change in mental state with continuous EEG epileptiform discharges. It is observed in specific childhood epilepsy syndromes (e.g. Dravet, Lennox-Gastaut, ring chromosome 20), acute illnesses (e.g. brain injury, encephalitis, metabolic derangement) and learning difficulties. Diagnosis is difficult but important, e.g. as a treatable cause of DeCon, including following CSE. Treatment includes of the underlying cause e.g. antimicrobials and/or immunotherapy for encephalitis, correction of metabolic disturbances. Anti-epileptic drug (AED) strategy may be influenced by NCSE subtype, e.g. more aggressive use in comatose patients. Prognosis varies from relatively benign to sometimes fatal, influenced by aetiology.

Posterior Reversible Encephalopathy Syndrome (PRES)

Paediatric PRES is a relatively rare clinic-radiological syndrome presenting with seizures, headache, altered mental state and/or visual impairment. Predisposing conditions include malignancy, renal disease and major haemoglobinopathies. Hypertension and/or significant BP fluctuations plus transplant, chemotherapeutic and immunosuppressant agents appear significant. Proposed

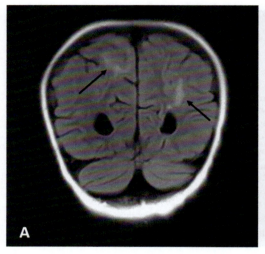 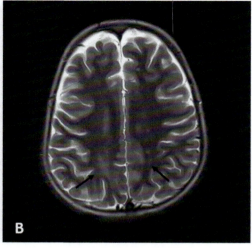

Figure 8.55 Posterior Reversible Encephalopathy Syndrome (PRES). A 4-year-old boy with genetic enteropathy and chronic kidney disease has fluctuating BP, DeCon and seizures on intensive care. EEG showed moderate encephalopathy and a subclinical seizure. Contrast MRI brain scan T2 weighted images (A; coronal and B; axial) show patches of predominantly subcortical white matter change posteriorly in the parietal lobes (black arrows). Infection screen was negative.

pathogenesis includes blood brain barrier disruption, dysregulated cerebral circulation and endothelial dysfunction. Diagnosis is supported by MRI posterior brain vasogenic oedema (Figure 8.55) and EEG slowing (diffuse or focal). Treatment is supportive, including of seizures, hypertension and as far as possible modifiable disease/treatment factors. Prognosis is generally favourable, although long-term sequelae (e.g. epilepsy, residual brain lesions) are described in some.

INFECTIOUS ENCEPHALITIS

Most infectious encephalitides are viral with active replication in brain parenchyma. Common pathogens include herpes simplex virus (HSV), varicella zoster virus (VZV) and enteroviruses, in particular *EV71*. Presenting features include encephalopathy, headache, seizures and focal deficits with fever prominent. Diagnosis is supported by CSF pleocytosis, viral isolation, encephalopathic EEG and typical MRI features, e.g. HSV frontal and temporal lobe predilection. Encephalitis can also be caused by bacteria, fungi and parasites. Treatment includes antimicrobials and management of complications, e.g. neurosurgical management of raised ICP, empyema or abscess. Prognosis is related to organism, time to treatment and related complications.

NEUROIMMUNE DISORDERS WITH ENCEPHALOPATHY IN CHILDREN
Highlights

1. Heterogenous group of conditions characterised by inflammatory, acquired demyelinating syndromes (ADS), post-and parainfectious entities. Traditionally those targeting white matter are deemed ADS, whilst disorders of grey matter are termed autoimmune encephalitis (AE).

2. Triggered by an infective or paraneoplastic process e.g. ovarian teratoma associated N-methyl-d-aspartate receptor (NMDAR) antibody encephalitis. Mechanisms include antibody mediated (e.g. against extracellular ion channels, receptors or other synaptic proteins) and immune cell dysregulation.

3. The most frequently detected antibodies in paediatric AE are anti-NMDAR and MOG. These should be tested in the serum and CSF of all children where AE is suspected.

4. A neuroimmune disorder is *not* excluded by a normal brain MRI or absence of detectable antibodies (i.e. seronegative autoimmune encephalitis).

5. Onset is acute or subacute following a prodrome of viral-type symptoms and/or subtle altered mental state.

6. Children are often polysymptomatic and severe, e.g. encephalopathy, seizures, psychiatric disturbance, movement disorder, speech impairments, dysautonomia.

7. Acute features are difficult to distinguish from infective encephalitis. Antimicrobial treatment, sometimes in parallel with first line immune therapy, e.g. steroids, intravenous immunoglobulin (IV Ig), plasma exchange (PLEX) is recommended until excluded by investigation.

8. Appropriate and timely immunotherapy is reported to improve clinical outcomes.

NMDAR AE

Encephalitis typically presents with encephalopathy and prominent neuropsychiatric symptoms. Seizures, movement disorder and irritable insomnia are also observed. Paraneoplastic (Figure 8.56) and non-paraneoplastic forms are described. Symptoms can be severe, necessitating intensive neurocritical care in some. Diagnosis is by detection of NMDAR antibodies in CSF and serum. Brain MRI is unremarkable and EEG frequently encephalopathic, sometimes with extreme delta brush. Treatment is supportive, including anti-epileptic – dystonic and – psychotic agents. First line immunotherapy includes steroids, IV Ig and PLEX with second line rituximab in refractory cases. Recovery can take months, with some risk of relapse which is often less severe than original presentation.

MOGAD

MOGAD includes an acute disseminated encephalomyelitis (ADEM) phenotype. Triggering events may be recent infection or vaccination, followed by prodromal fever, headache and lethargy. Encephalopathy and/or DeCon ensues in association with various neurological deficits. MRI may be normal initially or show white matter and/or cortical T2 weighted hyperintensities (Figure 8.57). CSF may show pleocytosis and oligoclonal band positivity. Serum and CSF MOG is positive. Acute management is symptomatic, including intensive care for some. Disease targeting immunotherapy includes steroids, IV Ig and PLEX. MOGAD is usually monophasic. A proportion relapse and require chronic immunotherapy. Prognosis varies with prompt immunomodulation recognised to improve clinical outcomes.

Limbic Encephalitis

Presentation is polysymptomatic with prominence of seizures and memory difficulties. Brain MRI may demonstrate mesial temporal or claustral changes and EEG is encephalopathic. Paraneoplastic (e.g. Type I anti-neuronal nuclear antibody) and non-paraneoplastic antibodies (leucine rich glioma inactivated 1 and contactin-associated protein-like 2) are infrequent in contrast

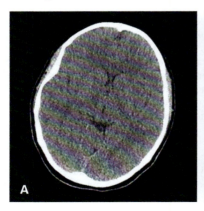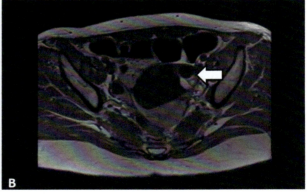

Figure 8.56 Paraneoplastic N-methyl-d-aspartate receptor (NMDAR) antibody encephalitis. A 14-year-old girl with prodromal headache followed by behaviour change, insomnia, confusion, hallucinations, facial grimacing and GCS 11. Axial CT brain (A) shows cerebral oedema. EEG was moderately encephalopathic. CSF oligoclonal bands were positive. Serum and CSF was NMDAR antibody positive. Axial pelvic MRI T2 image (B) shows an ovarian teratom.

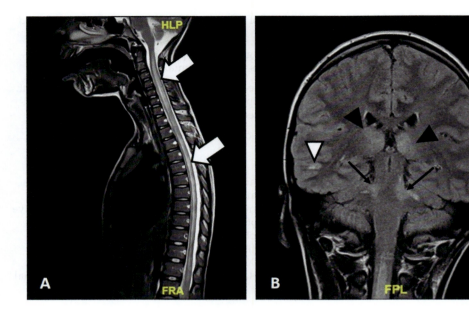

Figure 8.57 Myelin oligodendrocyte glycoprotein acquired demyelination (MOGAD). A 11-year-old boy with acute encephalopathy, fever, headache, visual impairment and urinary incontinence following recent infection. CSF was pleocytic (*WBC85*) with positive oligoclonal bands. Contrasted whole spine MRI sagittal T2 weighted image (A) shows extensive transverse myelitis (white arrows). Contrasted brain MRI coronal T2 weighted image (B) shows bilateral signal abnormalities in the thalami (black arrow heads), brainstem, and cerebellum (black arrows) plus cortex (white arrow head). He also had bilateral optic neuritis. Serum was MOG antibody positive.

to adults. First line immunotherapy includes steroids, IV Ig, PLEX and rituximab in some centres. Long-term morbidity is common with high rates of seizures and cognitive impairment.

The relationship between neuroimmune disorders, environmental and genetics factors is complex. Examples include non-paraneoplastic NMDAR AE following HSV infection and influenza-mediated Acute Necrotising Encephalopathy of Childhood (ANEC; Figure 8.58) associated with RAN Binding Protein 2 (*RANBP2*) gene mutations.

'BRAIN ATTACKS' AND VASCULAR STROKE SYNDROMES IN CHILDHOOD

'Brain attack', sudden onset focal neurological symptoms, are a common presentation to acute paediatrics. Up to 50% are caused by non-stroke disorders ('stroke mimics'). These include migraine, seizures, intracranial infection, inflammation, and tumours. Over 400 UK children a year, however, have a vascular stroke. These conditions are time-critical regards potential brain and life-saving interventions and are therefore primary diagnoses to consider. The main syndromes include arterial ischaemic stroke (AIS), haemorrhagic stroke (HS) and cerebral venous sinus thrombosis (CVST) with venous infarction. Collectively they present significant risk of life-long neurodisability and mortality. Lack of awareness, low clinical suspicion and numerous logistic obstacles continue to challenge recognition and timely diagnosis.

HAEMORRHAGIC STROKE

HS refers to non-traumatic intracranial haemorrhage. Underlying vascular abnormalities (arterial aneurysm, arterio-venous or cavernous malformations) are prominent (Figure 8.59). Severe congenital haemophilia and other rare coagulation disorders also present as HS. Rare autosomal recessive conditions (factor XIII deficiency, Glanzmann's thrombasthenia and alpha 2 anti-plasmin deficiency) are not detected by full blood count or standard clotting screen and should be considered in parental consanguinity. HS is a significant cause of morbidity and mortality in immune thrombocytopenia. All HS requires urgent neurosurgical discussion plus haematologist guided blood product or factor administration in bleeding diathesis. Endovascular, surgical, or conservative vascular malformation management should be evaluated by a specialist neurovascular multidisciplinary team.

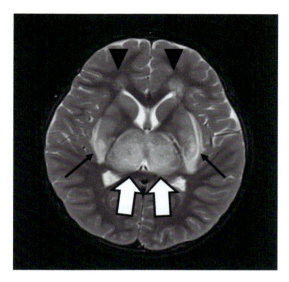

Figure 8.58 Acute Necrotising Encephalopathy of Childhood (ANEC). A 2-year-old boy with progressive encephalopathy and GCS 6 following recent respiratory tract infection. Nasopharyngeal aspirate was influenza A positive. Contrasted brain MRI axial T2 weighted image shows symmetrical swelling and hyperintensity of the thalami (white arrows), posterolateral lentiform nuclei (black arrows) and frontal periventricular white matter (arrow heads).

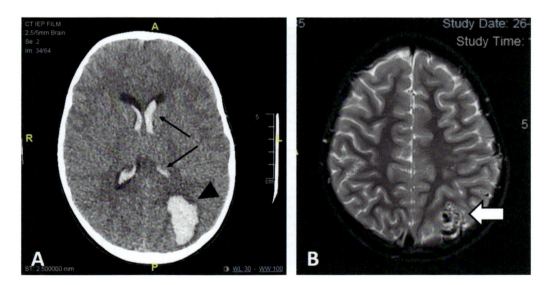

Figure 8.59 Haemorrhagic stroke. A 9-year-old boy develops severe headache, neck stiffness, vomiting and papilloedema 48 hours after a minor head injury. He has a right temporal visual field defect. Axial plain CT (A) shows a left parieto-occipital haemorrhage (black arrow head) with intraventricular extension (black arrows). Axial intracranial MRI T2 sequence shows underlying left parieto-occipital arterio-venous malformation (B; white arrow).

ARTERIAL ISCHAEMIC STROKE

AIS is an acute focal neurological disorder with imaging evidence of cerebral infarction in a corresponding arterial distribution. Most children are 'FAST' positive (Face, Arms, Speech, Time). Caveats to this include younger children and those with sickle cell anaemia, who may present with more diffuse symptoms (e.g. encephalopathy) or 'soft signs', respectively. Transient focal neurological deficits *with* brain infarction are well described in children, hence the term 'TIA' is less relevant in the absence of known vascular disease. Arteriopathy (inflammatory and genetic) plus congenital heart disease (in particular with right-to-left shunt) are aetiologically prominent. Rate of recurrence, prevention and surveillance strategies are determined by cause.

AIS Acute Diagnosis and Management

Figure 8.60 highlights key recommendations from the RCPCH Stroke in childhood clinical guidelines for diagnosis, management, and rehabilitation (2017). Note use of the Pediatric National Institutes of Health Stroke Scale (PedNIHSS), a score of AIS severity in 2- to 18-year-olds, to inform decisions around acute management (Table 8.21). This is in addition to GCS/AVPU measurement, which scores conscious level. Any drop in GCS or increase in PedNIHSS requires urgent discussion with a neurosurgical team to consider life-saving haematoma evacuation (HS) or decompressive craniectomy (DC) for malignant middle cerebral artery (MCA) territory AIS (Figure 8.61). Hyperacute thrombolysis or thrombectomy *may* be considered in children aged 2 to 8 years or *could* be considered in those > 8 years, providing they fulfil criteria and there are no contraindications.

Childhood AIS Aetiologies

Sickle cell (SCD) is the most common AIS risk factor worldwide. Proposed pathophysiology includes anaemia, abnormal red cell morphology, endothelial injury and arteriopathy. Ischaemia is clinical and silent with risk of progressive focal neurological and cognitive deficits over time. The Stroke Prevention Trial in Sickle Cell Anaemia (1998) evidenced blood transfusion as preventative in those delineated high risk by abnormal transcranial Doppler ultrasound (TCD). Annual TCD was made standard of care for 2- to 16-year-olds and regular transfusion offered to those with TCD ≥ 200 cm/s.

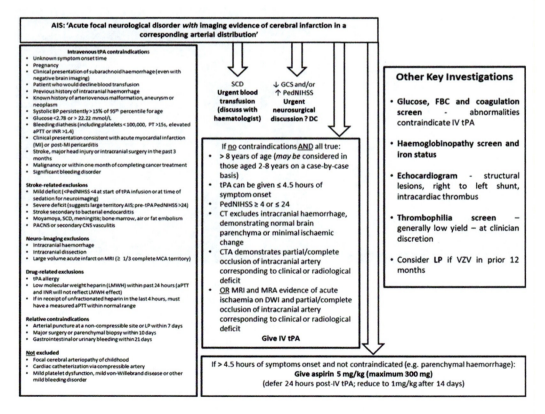

Figure 8.60 AIS hyperacute management. Data from 2017 RCPCH Stroke in childhood guidelines (refer for full recommendations).

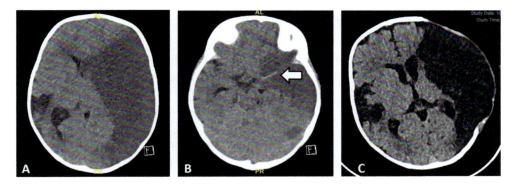

Figure 8.61 Cardio-embolic malignant AIS. A 11-month-old male develops irritability, bulging anterior fontanelle and right hemiparesis post-prosthetic mitral valve (MV) revision. Axial plain CT showing; acute infarction of the entire left MCA territory with mass effect and midline shift to the right (A); hyperdense left MCA due to intraluminal thrombus (B); and left hemisphere decompression following hemicraniectomy and expansion duraplasty. Echocardiography was suspicious for a MV-associated thrombus. Malignant MCA AIS is a life-threatening condition in which space occupying cerebral oedema develops 24 to 96 hours post-large MCA territory infarction; treatment is with urgent decompressive hemicraniectomy.

Focal cerebral arteriopathy (FCA) is a unilateral terminal internal carotid artery (ICA) and/or proximal MCA stenosis. It is the most common arteriopathy seen in previously well children. Post-varicella zoster virus (VZV) FCA is a prominent subtype (Figure 8.62). This rare complication of chickenpox typically presents with basal ganglia infarction in a young child who has had VZV in the previous year. Following primary infection, the virus is hypothesised to spread via the trigeminal ganglion to cause internal carotid circulation vessel wall inflammation. CSF examination, including for VZV PCR and intrathecal antibody synthesis ratio, is recommended. If positive a prolonged course of acyclovir is advised given until cleared (reassess at three months with repeat LP and imaging). It is typically monophasic, although there is risk of recurrence without adequate antiviral treatment. Aspirin is continued at least until vessels have normalised, which occurs in some but not all cases.

Moyamoya (MM) is a progressive occlusive, usually bilateral, intracranial arteriopathy of the terminal ICAs and/or proximal MCAs (Figure 8.63). Sequelae include recurrent AIS, transient ischaemic attacks, cognitive decline and headache. There are numerous genetic, syndromic, and other disease associations, including neurofibromatosis Type 1, Down syndrome and SCD. Cerebral perfusion becomes exquisitely reliant on systemic BP to drive a pressure-passive collateral circulation. Hypertension, unless secondary to renovascular disease, is likely centrally driven to increase cerebral perfusion pressure. Artificial BP lowering (e.g. with anti-hypertensives) may provoke transient or permanent ischaemia and in general should be avoided. Affected children should not be hyperventilated, e.g. for EEG, and should receive intravenous hydration for fasting or fluid losses. Revascularisation surgery may be a more definitive treatment to reduce stroke risk in selected cases.

Craniocervical Arterial Dissection refers to traumatic or spontaneous vessel wall injury resulting in thrombus formation, propagation and downstream embolisation ('showering'). New neurological deficit accompanied by head or neck pain after even seemingly innocuous activities or new Horner's syndrome should raise suspicion. A predilection may be posed by underlying connective tissue disease (e.g. Ehlers–Danlos or Marfan syndromes). Radiological demonstration of an intimal flap or 'flame' sign is challenging on MR and may require CT or catheter angiogram to confirm (Figure 8.64). Treatment trials have indicated non-superiority of anticoagulation over antithrombotic treatment; anticoagulation is generally avoided in intracranial dissection due to potential subarachnoid haemorrhage. Vertebral artery dissection, often bilateral ('mirror'), account for a significant proportion of posterior circulation AIS, particularly in school-age males. Lateral flexion/extension cervical spine x-ray is recommended to screen for vertebral body or articulation abnormalities. Early clinical course tends to be recurrent and often necessitates escalation to anticoagulation.

Table 8.21: Pediatric National Institutes of Health Stroke Scale (PedNIHSS)

PedNIHSS Score

PedNIHSS Definitions	Scale Definition
1a. Level of Consciousness:	0 = Alert; keenly responsive 1 = Not alert, but arousable by minor stimulation 2 = Not alert, requires repeated stimulation to attend, or is obtunded and requires strong or painful stimulation to make non-stereotyped movements 3 = Responds only with reflex motor or autonomic effects or totally unresponsive
1b. LOC Questions: *Tested by asking age and 'where is XX?', XX referring to the name of the parent or other familiar family member present (> 2 years)*	0 = Answers both questions correctly 1 = Answers one question correctly 2 = Answers neither question correctly
1c. LOC Commands: *Tested by asking to open/close the eyes and to 'show me your nose' or 'touch your nose' (> 2 years)*	0 = Performs both tasks correctly 1 = Performs one task correctly 2 = Performs neither task correctly
2. Best Gaze: *Horizontal eye movements tested*	0 = Normal 1 = Partial gaze palsy 2 = Forced deviation/complete gaze palsy
3. Visual: *Test by visual threat (2–6 years) confrontation, finger counting (> 6 years)*	0 = No visual loss 1 = Partial hemianopia 2 = Complete hemianopia 3 = Bilateral hemianopia (including cortical blindness)
4. Facial Palsy: *Tested by patient showing teeth or raising eyebrows/ close eyes*	0 = Normal symmetrical movement 1 = Minor paralysis (flattened nasolabial fold, asymmetry on smiling) 2 = Partial paralysis (total or near total paralysis of lower face) 3 = Complete paralysis of one or both sides
5 and 6. Motor Arm and Leg: *Tested by patient extending arms 90° (if sitting) or 45° (if supine), and the leg 30°*	5a. Left Arm, 5b. Right Arm 0 = No drift for full 10 seconds 1 = Drift ≤ 10 seconds 2 = Some effort against gravity 3 = No effort against gravity 4 = No movement 5 = Amputation 6a Left Leg, 6b Right Leg 0 = No drift for full 10 seconds 1 = Drift ≤ 10 seconds 2 = Some effort against gravity 3 = No effort against gravity 4 = No movement 5 = Amputation
7. Limb Ataxia: *Tested for by reaching for toys/kicking a toy (< 5 years); finger – nose – finger/heel – shin test (> 5 years)*	0 = Absent 1 = Present in one limb 2 = Present in two limbs
8. Sensory: *Observe behavioural response to pinprick*	0 = Normal; no sensory loss 1 = Mild to moderate sensory loss 2 = Severe to total sensory loss
9. Best Language: *Tested by observing speech and comprehension (2–6 years); describe picture (> 6 years)*	0 = Normal; no sensory loss 1 = Mild to moderate aphasia 2 = Severe aphasia 3 = Mute, global aphasia
	Total Score: /42

Childhood primary angiitis of the central nervous system (cPACNS) is a rare, primary inflammatory condition of cerebral arteries without systemic inflammation. Presentation includes diffuse and focal neurologic deficits. Blood inflammatory markers are usually unremarkable; CSF may show elevated protein and/or pleocytosis. Brain MRI shows white and/or grey matter lesions; MRA may detect large vessel stenoses. Cerebral CA may suggest vasculopathic features in larger vessels but may not detect small vessel disease. Brain biopsy is often necessary to confirm vessel wall

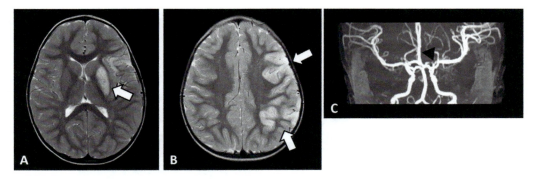

Figure 8.62 Post-VZV FCA. A 4-year-old girl develops right-sided weakness, aphasia and ataxia six weeks after chickenpox. Axial brain MRI T2 sequences show left MCA territory infarction with local gyral swelling and mass effect (A and B; white arrows). Intracranial MR angiogram shows left terminal ICA, MCA and anterior cerebral artery stenosis (C; black arrow head), in keeping with FCA. CSF VZV PCR was positive.

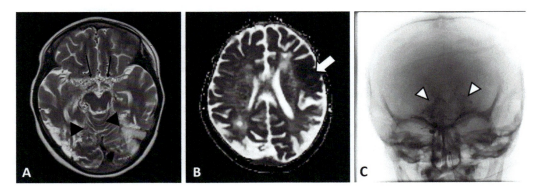

Figure 8.63 Moyamoya. A 9-year-old girl with trisomy 21 presents with right-body focal motor seizures and post-ictal weakness in the context of a febrile influenza A illness, vomiting and diarrhoea. Axial MRI brain T2 sequence (A) shows multiple, bilateral chronic infarcts, mainly in watershed zones, including parieto-occipital areas (black arrow heads) and base of skull collateral vessels (black arrows). Apparent diffusion coefficient MRI sequence (B) shows acute left anterior MCA territory infarction (white arrow). Selective angiography of the right internal carotid artery (C) shows severe, bilateral occlusive vasculopathy of both ICAs with numerous 'puff of smoke' moyamoya collaterals (white arrow heads).

inflammatory infiltration. Management includes aspirin in conjunction with immunomodulatory agents.

CEREBRAL VENOUS SINUS THROMBOSIS AND VENOUS INFARCTION

CVST results in outflow obstruction, increased venous pressure, regional cytotoxic oedema, and ischaemic infarction susceptible to haemorrhage. Peak incidence is in neonates with risk factors of perinatal complications, dehydration, and sepsis. Presentation is with lethargy, seizures, and apnoea. Risk factors in older children include head trauma, ENT infection, hypercoagulable conditions (leukaemia, inflammatory bowel, and nephrotic syndromes) and procoagulant drugs (e.g. asparaginase). Presentation is with raised intracranial pressure (headache, sixth nerve palsy and papilloedema). Diagnosis is by intracranial CT or MRI plus venography (Figure 8.65). CT may be falsely positive in neonates (higher haematocrit levels may mimic thrombus in a normal sagittal sinus). Consider thrombophilia screening, particularly if unprovoked or in familial prothrombosis. Measure CSF opening pressures where lumbar puncture is performed. Management includes treating provoking factors and anticoagulation to prevent thrombus propagation. There is risk of

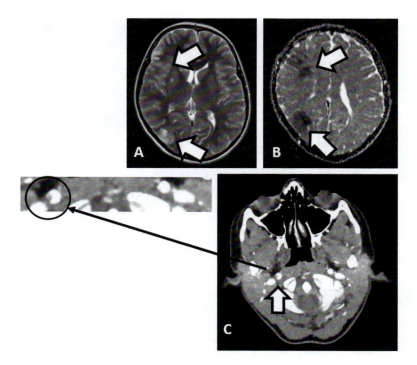

Figure 8.64 Craniocervical arterial dissection. A 14-year-old girl presents with right-sided headache and 30 minute episodes of left hand weakness and slurred speech. She was discharged from A&E with a diagnosis of stress-related hyperventilation. T2 (A) and apparent diffusion coefficient (B) intracranial, axial MRI sequences (performed following progressive symptoms) show areas of left hemispheric infarction in keeping with embolic stroke. Axial intracranial CTA (C) shows a crescent-shaped, hyperintense mural hematoma within the left ICA, consistent with arterial dissection.

mortality, seizures; cognitive, sensorimotor and visual impairments. Seizures, coma, and parenchymal infarction are predictors of adverse outcome.

HOMOCYSTINURIA

Homocystinuria (HCU) is an autosomal recessive condition of cystathionine beta synthase deficiency and disordered methionine metabolism. High homocysteine levels are procoagulant, presenting risk of arterial and venous thrombosis plus stroke. Additional features include ectopia lentis, learning and behavioural difficulties. Complications can be prevented with newborn screening and life-long treatment (pyridoxine, low protein diet, betaine). Those with vascular complications may need life-long anticoagulation.

IRON DEFICIENCY ANAEMIA (IDA)

IDA is an independent risk factor for AIS and CVST and is notable as common, preventable, and treatable. Dietary IDA is prominent. Contributory factors include lack of parental mixed feeding awareness and child defiance around eating a varied diet. Pathophysiology includes blood viscosity related to reactive thrombocytosis, reduced deformability and flow of microcytic red cells and exacerbation of regional brain hypoxia.

PERINATAL VASCULAR STROKE SYNDROMES

These conditions represent the earliest ischaemic and haemorrhagic insults to the developing brain. In-utero events ('presumed perinatal') have delayed presentation with early hand preference, motor delay and/or seizures in infancy. Acute neonatal vascular injury typically presents with seizures, apnoea, and encephalopathy. *Perinatal ischaemic stroke*, a focal arterial or venous

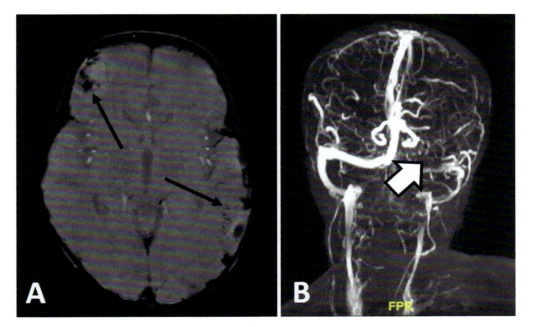

Figure 8.65 Cerebral venous sinus thrombosis (CVST). A 3-year-old girl presents with drowsiness, irritability, pallor and splenomegaly. There was associated bradycardia, hypertension, lower limb hypertonia, hyperreflexia and a left up-going plantar reflex. She had bilateral papilloedema and a CSF opening pressure of 29 cmH2O. Haemoglobin was 53 g/L with microcytosis, thrombocytosis, low ferritin and iron saturation. She drank 30 oz of milk/day and was Epstein-Barr virus IgM and PCR positive in blood. Axial intracranial MRI susceptibility weighted imaging (A) shows venous ischaemia and petechial haemorrhage in right frontal and left temporal lobes (black arrows). Head and neck MR venography (B) shows dural venous sinus thrombosis of the left transverse and sigmoid sinuses extending into the internal jugular vein (white arrows). There was also cortical vein thrombosis of the right anterior frontal lobe and left temporal convexity.

occlusion, occurs from 20 weeks gestation until 28 postnatal days. It includes acute *neonatal arterial ischaemic stroke* (NAIS), presenting in the first four weeks of life (Figure 8.66) or *presumed perinatal arterial ischaemic stroke* (PPAIS; Figure 8.67) and *periventricular venous infarction* (PVI; Figure 8.68), which present beyond the neonatal period. Rate of AIS recurrence is low, hence antithrombotic prophylaxis is generally not indicated. *Perinatal haemorrhagic stroke*, a focal intraparenchymal bleed in term/near term neonates, occurs in the first 28 days of life. As with their ischaemic counterparts, *neonatal haemorrhagic stroke* (NHS) manifests early, whilst *presumed perinatal haemorrhagic stroke* (PPHS) has delayed presentation. *COL4A1/2* mutations should be considered in perinatal HS, in particular where associated with congenital cataracts and white matter changes (Figure 8.69). Neonatal CVST is described elsewhere in this section.

FUNCTIONAL NEUROLOGICAL DISORDERS

WHAT ARE FUNCTIONAL NEUROLOGICAL DISORDERS?

Functional neurological disorders (FND) are a heterogenous group of conditions caused by disordered neurologic *function*. This gives rise to a host of neurological signs and symptoms (Table 8.22) which are not better accounted for by another diagnosis. Examination findings are generally inconsistent, contributing to clinician uncertainty and the patient is often embarked on a 'diagnostic odyssey'.

FND can be thought of as central nervous system dysfunction at the level of the brain. Other components of the nervous system (spinal cord, nerves and muscles) are intact, but the brain is unable to integrate output and input information, e.g. to and from a particular body part. Chronicity, levels of disability and impact on quality of life are generally high. Recognition is key

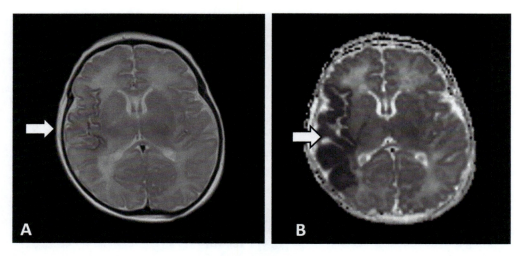

Figure 8.66 Neonatal AIS. A term infant develops hypoglycaemia and left focal motor seizures aged 18 hours, following delivery by emergency caesarean section for features of foetal distress, maternal hypertension, proteinuria and chorioamnionitis. Brain MRI on day seven of life shows recent right MCA infarction (A) with diffusion restriction (B). MRA demonstrated no proximal vessel stenosis or intravascular thrombus. She also had a PFO (left-to-right flow) and weakly positive anti-cardiolipin IgG.

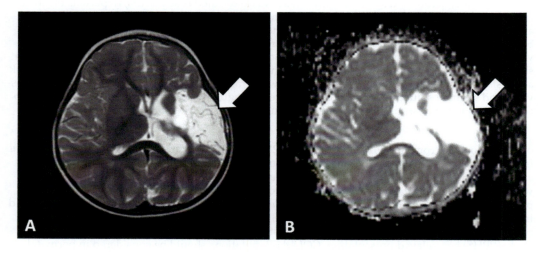

Figure 8.67 Presumed perinatal AIS. A 3-month-old infant presents with a paucity of right upper limb movements. She was born at term via an emergency caesarean section. There was history of first trimester bleeding. MRI brain scan aged 21 months shows mature left MCA infarct with cystic encephalomalacia (A). Diffusion weighted imaging shows no acute diffusion restriction (B). There was no evidence of focal arteriopathy.

so that a positive diagnosis can be given, exposure to unnecessary investigations and treatments avoided and appropriate management given as soon as possible.

Classification and Terminiology

Historically classification has been poor and terminology inaccurate, likely a reflection of proposed aetiologies at the time. Previously used terms include psychosomatic, psychogenic, somatising and conversion disorder; 'psycho-' implying origin of the disorder in the mind with emphasis on a mind-body divide. There was also sense of a lack of validity (e.g. 'non-organic') and some maintenance of diagnostic uncertainty (e.g. 'medically unexplained').

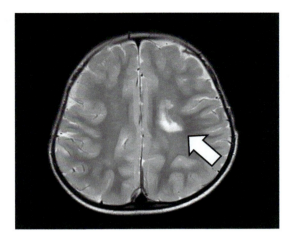

Figure 8.68 Periventricular venous infarction (PVI). A 2-year-old boy with early left hand preference from 6 months of age and frequent falls. Examination shows right lower limb circumduction gait and right upper limb posturing on running (stressed gait testing). He was born at term in good condition. There is history of maternal postpartum haemorrhage requiring blood transfusion. Axial intracranial MRI T2 sequence shows focal white matter hyperintensity and volume loss involving the left centrum semiovale and corona radiata (white arrow), consistent with PVI.

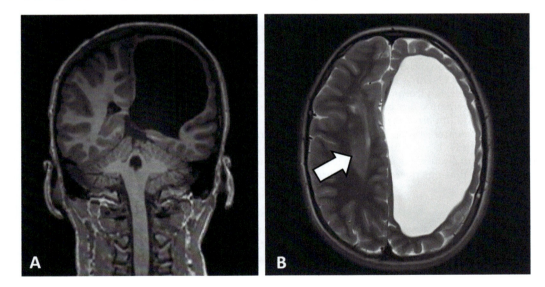

Figure 8.69 COL4A1-related HS. A 14-year-old boy with an antenatally detected porencephalic cyst (A; coronal intracranial MRI T1 sequence) develops early right-body hemiparesis and focal motor seizures. Axial intracranial MRI T2 image (B) shows associated right fronto-parietal white matter change (white arrow).

Recent decades have seen a shift in how the medical community think about and approach FND. It is no longer considered a diagnosis of exclusion, but one of inclusion based on hallmarks in history and positive 'rule-in' clinical signs. 'Functional neurological disorder' is now the term of choice for research and patient communities. FND has also replaced conversion disorder as a primary diagnostic label in the Diagnostic and Statistical Manual of Mental Disorders, Fifth Edition (March 2022).

In 2022 FND was identified as one of top ten UK research priorities for interventions in childhood neurological disorders (Childhood Neurological Conditions Priority Setting Partnership), in particular which psychological interventions are most effective.

Table 8.22: **Some Functional Neurological Symptoms**

- Limb weakness
- Movement disorder
- Tremor
- Dystonia
- Gait disorder
- Facial symptoms
- Tics
- Drop attacks
- Seizures
- Sensory symptoms
- Cognitive symptoms
- Speech and swallowing problems
- Dizziness
- Jerks and twitches
- Bladder symptoms
- Visual symptoms

Prevalence

Exact prevalence for FND in childhood is probably unknown as rates are challenging to determine. Current literature reports a likely underestimation for FND in general. Establishing prevalence would require further prospective population studies with accurate diagnosis and coding. In practice FND represents a common reason for referral to paediatric neurology services.

Cause

Historically a paradigm of psychological distress being converted into neurological symptoms was adopted. However, whilst adverse childhood experiences, stressors (academic, social) and certain personality traits (e.g. perfectionism) are common, FND also occurs in their absence. Prominent co-morbidities include mood disturbance (anxiety, depression), learning difficulties, attention deficit hyperactivity and autism spectrum disorders. These may be undiagnosed and should be assessed in their own right, but again are unlikely the singular cause.

Over decades FND has emerged as a disorder at the interface between neurology and psychiatry, with genetic, environmental and psychosocial factors likely at play. Recent concepts include disordered predictive processing (i.e. predicted sensorimotor experience and sensorimotor 'input' mismatch) and impaired sense of agency.

Imaging research studies have described structural and physiological differences in the brains of adults with FND, including differing hippocampal and amygdala volumes, oxygen consumption and brain circuitry dysfunction (e.g. limbic system). Whilst causality has not been established, these findings may provide information regarding mechanisms and possible targets for intervention.

Clinical Presentation

Presentation occurs across a wide range of healthcare settings; A&E attendance is prominent, mimicking neurological emergencies such as stroke, coma, status epilepticus and cauda equina syndrome. Female preponderance is notable. Affected children tend to be > 10 years, although patients as young as 5 have been reported. Associated symptoms of headache, pain and fatigue are common. FND concurrent with other diagnoses is also well recognised e.g. dissociative seizures and epilepsy, functional tics and Tourette syndrome. Presentation may be triggered (e.g. by an episode of infection, intercurrent illness, pain or physical injury) or spontaneous.

Tips for Clinical Assessment

- Note any hallmark features of FND, e.g. abrupt onset (may be in association with dissociative symptoms, e.g. panic), waxing and waning course (not specific).

- List all symptoms.

  - This gives the patient opportunity to report wholly and for the clinician to explore the evolution of the presentation. History of multiple symptoms and previous surgeries with negative pathology are highly suggestive of FND.

  - Understand what symptom(s) are most impactful. A patient referred for twitching may find pain their most intrusive symptom, which may require independent assessment.

Table 8.23: Some Positive Clinical Signs in FND

Functional Symptom	Sign/Test	Findings
Limb weakness	Collapsing weakness	• Limb collapses, e.g. with light touch • Worsening limb weakness with increasing attention/effort applied to complete a given task
Leg weakness	Hoover's sign	1. Perform in sitting or lying 2. Test hip extension in affected leg – hip extension is *weak* 3. Test contralateral hip flexion against resistance – hip extension in affected leg returns to *normal*
	Hip abductor sign	Hip abduction weakness that improves with contralateral hip abduction
Gait disturbance		Examination features include excessive truncal sway, veering and knee buckling. May improve with asking the child to walk with eyes closed, performing a dual task (e.g. 'count backwards') or 'skating' instead of walking
Tremor	Entrainment test	Paced volitional movements in another body part e.g. finger tapping in contralateral hand, stops or influences the rhythm of the functional tremor ('tremor entrainment')
Dystonia		Usually presents with fixed ankle inversion, flexion of fingers or; jaw deviation, platysma, orbicularis contraction +/– tongue deviation
Sensory disturbance		Midline splitting or feeling 'numb from the waist down' are commonly reported Look for inconsistencies in examination, e.g. patchy vs dermatomal sensory loss
Seizures (dissociative)	If not directly witnessed request mobile phone footage Consider video telemetry to capture onset, evolution and offset of event (i.e. not just to 'rule out epilepsy')	• Long duration • Eyes shut (often tight at the beginning of an attack) • Side-to-side head or body movements • Asynchronous movements • 'Stop/start' (fluctuation in course) • Pelvic thrusting • Urinary incontinence and physical injury are *not* distinguishing • May occur in recovery from general anaesthetic • High daily frequency/frequent hospital admissions prominent • May be mismanaged as status epilepticus
Visual loss	Suggest specialist ophthalmology assessment	Includes increasing visual constriction (spiralling visual fields on perimetry) the longer testing goes on

■ The patient may report feeling a body part is 'not own their own' or being disconnected.

■ Screen for co-morbid mood disorders, learning and social communication difficulties.

■ Consider whether there may be any safeguarding concerns.

■ Observe for evidence of inconsistency, e.g. voluntary actions getting in and out of a chair/bed vs performance in formal muscle power testing; semiological or motor patterns specific for FND.

■ Note positive clinical examination signs.

■ Muscle tone and deep tendon reflexes should be within normal limits.

■ A physio- and occupational-therapy assessment for motor presentations can be very helpful. These are often detailed, function focussed and findings can reinforce the diagnosis (Figure 8.70).

Common reasons for misdiagnosis include over reliance on:

■ Psychological factors.

■ Normal investigations – some forms of epilepsy have a normal ictal EEG, e.g. nocturnal frontal lobe epilepsy.

- 'Bizarre' appearance, e.g. the hypermotor movements of frontal lobe seizures can look quite peculiar, some dystonic gaits improve on walking backwards, hemisensory loss in thalamic lesions.

How to Give a Positive Diagnosis

This is essential in order to be able to progress with treatment. Patients and families often don't understand why they have FND. Explaining that it is a known condition, common and treatable helps.

- Be inclusive, i.e. share what the patient *has* versus what they *don't* have (FND is more than the absence of another disease).

- Acknowledge that symptoms are real.

- Showing the patient and their family their positive signs is very powerful. This reinforces that there is reversibility and the possibility to recover.

- Experts in the field often use the analogy of the brain as a computer, i.e. there is no hardware (physical brain) problem, but the computer software or operating system (the way the brain sends and receives information) isn't working properly.

Management

Whilst clinical FND services in adults are advancing, care pathways for children and adolescents remains somewhat fragmented. In general a multidisciplinary team approach is recommended, including the following:

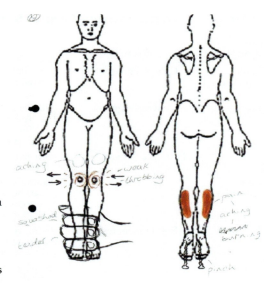

Figure 8.70 A 14-year-old girl who woke up with a 'squeezing' pain in her legs developed paraesthesia around her knees and dense paraparesis over hours. She was admitted as an emergency under the neurosurgical team for suspected cauda equina syndrome. There was no sphincter involvement. Sensory testing was normal throughout. MRI brain and spine was normal. She used her hands to move her lower limbs on and off the bed and muscle co-contraction could be felt. Physiotherapy colleagues obtained this drawing of her lower limb patchy sensory disturbance and pain.

- Paediatrician, neurologist, Child and Adolescent Mental Health specialist (CAMHS) plus allied therapy services (e.g. physio-, occupational therapy, speech and language). Such collaboration increases confidence, enhances engagement and improves patient experience.

- 'Re-training the brain' using physical and evidence based psychological therapies e.g. cognitive behavioural therapy.

- There may be a role for pharmacological interventions in some, mainly in the treatment of concurrent mood disturbance (CAMHS led).

- Online education and self-help (e.g. neurosymptoms.org, NHS inform). These are useful resources, but not a substitute for clinical care.

- Consider referral for placement in a specialist treatment rehabilitation service for complex, refractory cases.

Prognosis

Recovery is possible but variable. The factors influencing this are likely multifold. Most children and young people make a good recovery; a proportion don't and are no less impacted by associated disability than those with other neurological conditions. Affected children may go on to develop other symptoms.

REFERENCES

- Tan AP, Mankad K, Gonçalves FG, et al. Solving the diagnostic dilemma. *Top Magn Reson Imaging*. 2018 Aug;27(4):197–217. doi: 10.1097/RMR.0000000000000170. PMID: 30086108.
- Darwish AH. Posterior reversible encephalopathy syndrome in children: A prospective follow-up study. *J Child Neurol*. 2020 Jan;35(1):55–62. doi:10.1177/0883073819876470. Epub 2019 Sep 30. PMID: 31570037.
- Royal College of Paediatrics and Child Health. (2017). Stroke in childhood clinical guideline for diagnosis, management and rehabilitation. https://www.rcpch.ac.uk/resources/stroke-in-childhood-clinical-guideline
- Classification Committee of The International Headache Society. *The International Classification of Headache Disorders*, 3rd Edition. https://ichd-3.org/
- National Institute for Health and Care Excellence. (2021). Headaches in over 12s: Diagnosis and management [NICE Guideline CG150]. https://www.nice.org.uk/guidance/cg150
- The Brain Tumour Charity. *Better Safe Than Tumour*. https://www.headsmart.org.uk/ (Access 2023).
- The Migraine Trust. (2020). *The State of the Migraine Nation; Who is Living with Migraine in the UK?; Rapid Research Review.*

FURTHER READING

- Williams CA, Dagli A, Battaglia A. Genetic disorders associated with macrocephaly. *Am J Med Genet A*. 2008 Aug 1;146A(15):2023–2037. doi: 10.1002/ajmg.a.32434. PMID: 18629877.
- https://www.genomicseducation.hee.nhs.uk/genotes/in-the-clinic/presentation-child-with-macrocephaly/
- Children's Brain Tumour Research Centre. (2017). The brain pathways guideline: A guideline to assist healthcare professionals in the assessment of children who may have a brain tumour. https://bettersafethantumour.com/clinical/clinical-guideline/
- https://www.thebraintumourcharity.org/ (Access 2023).
- https://www.childrenwithcancer.org.uk/ (Access 2023).
- https://www.cancerresearchuk.org/ (Access 2023).
- Kanter J, Phillips S, Schlenz AM, et al. Successful implementation trial to improve stroke risk (TCD) screening in children with sickle cell anemia: A roadmap to care enhancement. *Blood* 2023;142(1).
- Bhate S, Ganesan V. A practical approach to acute hemiparesis in children. *Dev Med Child Neurol*. 2015 Aug;57:689e97.
- Eleftheriou D, Moraitis E, Hong Y, et al. Microparticle-mediated VZV propagation and endothelial activation: Mechanism of VZV vasculopathy. *Neurology*. 2020 Feb 4;94:e474e80.
- Keeling D, Tait RC, Watson H. Peri-operative management of anticoagulation and antiplatelet therapy. *Br J Haematol*. 2016;175:602e13.
- Mackay MT, Monagle P, Babl FE. Brain attacks and stroke in children. *J Paediatrics Child Health*. 2016;52:158e63.
- Markus HS, Levi C, King A, et al. Cervical artery dissection in stroke study (CADISS) investigators. Antiplatelet therapy vs anticoagulation therapy in cervical artery dissection: The cervical artery dissection in stroke study (CADISS) randomized clinical trial final results. *JAMA Neurol*. 2019 Jun 1;76:657e64.
- Munot P, De Vile C, Hemingway C, et al. Severe iron deficiency anaemia and ischaemic stroke in children. *Arch Dis Child*. 2011 Mar;96(3):276–279. doi:10.1136/adc.2010.189241. Epub 2010 Oct 27. PMID: 21030379.
- Parikh T, Goti A, Yashi K, et al. Pediatric sickle cell disease and stroke: A literature review. *Cureus*. 2023;15(1):e34003. DOI 10.7759/cureus.34003
- Alwis A, Ganesan V. 'Brain attacks' and acute stroke in childhood: A practical approach in a time of proposed thrombolysis. *Paediatr. Child Health*. 2021;31(5):181–188. ISSN 1751-7222. doi:10.1016/j.paed.2021.02.002.
- Royal College of Paediatrics and Child Health. (2015 Update, Revised 2019). *The Management of Children and Young People with an Acute Decrease in Conscious Level. A Nationally Developed Evidence-based Guideline for Practitioners*. https://www.rcpch.ac.uk/resources/management-children-young-people-acute-decrease-conscious-level-clinical-guideline

- Walker M. Treatment of non-convulsive status epilepticus. International League Against Epilepsy Lectures, 2015.
- Wells E, Hacohen Y, Waldman A, et al. Neuroimmune disorders of the central nervous system in children in the molecular era. *Nat Rev Neurol*. 2018 Jul;14(7):433–445. doi:10.1038/s41582-018-0024-9. Erratum in: *Nat Rev Neurol*. 2018 Dec;14(12):749. PMID: 29925924.
- Sabanathan S, Abdel-Mannan O, Mankad K, et al. Clinical features, investigations, and outcomes of pediatric limbic encephalitis: A multicenter study. *Ann Clin Transl Neurol*. 2022 Jan;9(1):67–78. doi:10.1002/acn3.51494. Epub 2022 Jan 11. PMID: 35015932; PMCID: PMC8791799.
- Nosadini M, Thomas T, Eyre M, et al International consensus recommendations for the treatment of pediatric NMDAR antibody encephalitis. *Neurol Neuroimmunol Neuroinflamm*. 2021 Jul 22;8(5):e1052. doi:10.1212/NXI.0000000000001052. PMID: 34301820; PMCID: PMC8299516.
- Stone J, Burton C, Carson A. Recognising and explaining functional neurological disorder. *BMJ*. 2020 Oct 21;371:m3745. doi:10.1136/bmj.m3745. PMID: 33087335.
- Bennett K, Diamond C, Hoeritzauer I, et al. A practical review of functional neurological disorder (FND) for the general physician. *Clin Med (Lond)*. 2021 Jan;21(1):28–36. doi:10.7861/clinmed.2020-0987. PMID: 33479065; PMCID: PMC7850207.
- Heyman I. Mind the gap: Integrating physical and mental healthcare for children with functional symptoms. *Arch Dis Child*. 2019 Dec;104(12):1127–1128. doi:10.1136/archdischild-2019-317854. Epub 2019 Sep 10. PMID: 31506259.
- Nonnekes J, Růžička E, Serranová T, et al. *Neurology*. Jun 2020;94(24):1093–1099. doi: 10.1212/WNL.0000000000009649.
- Perjoc RS, Roza E, Vladacenco OA, et al. Teleanu RI. Functional neurological disorder-old problem new perspective. *Int J Environ Res Public Health*. 2023 Jan 8;20(2):1099. doi:10.3390/ijerph20021099. PMID: 36673871; PMCID: PMC9859618.

9 Gastroenterology

Susan Hill, Keith Lindley and Edward Gaynor

PART 1: Presentation with Gastrointestinal Symptoms

ACUTE GASTROENTERITIS

Incidence

Common condition with 0.3–0.8 episodes/child/year worldwide. It is the commonest reason for hospitalisation in infants aged 6–24 months.

Aetiology/Pathogenesis

Acute usually viral infectious disease are common in developed countries although bacterial and protozoal pathogens do occur. Commonest viruses are norovirus, small round virus and rotavirus (Figure 9.1). Others include adenovirus, astrovirus and calicivirus (Figures 9.2 and 9.3). In children, 10–15% of coronavirus (SARS-CoV-2) episodes present with acute diarrhoea. Rotavirus traditionally affects children aged 6–24 months. Diarrhoeal mechanisms include small intestinal villus damage and direct (neurogenic) stimulation of water and electrolyte transport.

Clinical Presentation

Acute onset vomiting (usually) followed by diarrhoea, often with abdominal pain, anorexia and possible pyrexia. Incubation is about 2–10 days.

Diagnosis

History of frequency, volume and content of diarrhoea and vomitus with details of recent fluid intake, and urine output and colour, to indicate state of hydration. If dehydration suspected, record fluid intake and urine, vomit and stool output and examine clinically (see Table 9.1). Request stool virology, microscopy and culture. Exclude urinary tract infection.

Treatment

Oral rehydration solution (ORS), i.e. water/balanced electrolyte solution with low carbohydrate concentration to drive active electrolyte absorption; hypo-osmolar solutions are better absorbed. Offer ORS in small quantities frequently/every 15–30 minutes; absorbed best immediately after vomiting. After four hours of ORS restart normal feeding. If not drinking ORS, consider a nasogastric (NG) tube and intravenous (IV) fluids. If abnormal blood electrolyte levels occur adapt composition and speed of fluid administration. Commercially available ORS should be given

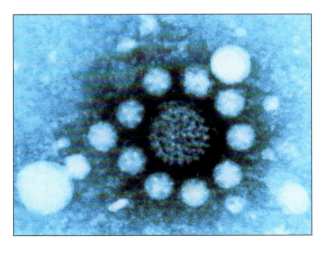

Figure 9.1   Acute gastroenteritis. Electron microscopy of enteric viruses: 9.1: Rotavirus (centre) and astrovirus (surrounding).

DOI: 10.1201/9781003175186-9

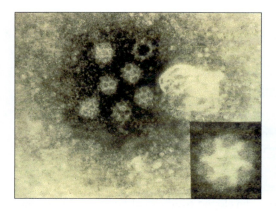

Figure 9.2 Calicivirus.

Figure 9.3 Small round virus.

Table 9.1: Clinical Features of Dehydration

Percentage weight loss	Severity	Clinical	Signs
< 5%	Mild	Not unwell	Dry mucous membranes, thirst
5–10%	Moderate	Unwell	Apathetic, Sunken eyes and fontanelle (infants)
			Reduced skin turgor, oliguria, tachypnoea
10–15%	Severe	Shocked	Poor peripheral circulation, hypotension, tachycardia
> 15%	Critical	Moribund	Severely shocked

and homemade preparations (1 tablespoon sugar, and 1 teaspoon of salt/1 pint of water) avoided. Encourage food reintroduction early, but consider lactose-free in first 72 hours and if profuse diarrhoea continues since transitory secondary lactose intolerance is common.

Rotavirus vaccine, a live attenuated two-dose oral monovalent vaccine is recommended by the World Health Organisation (WHO) in infants worldwide and is in the UK vaccination schedule by 4 months of age.

Prognosis

Full recovery usually < two days, but can persist for 10–14 days.

Viral infectivity can remain after clinical recovery.

Good handwashing is essential to prevent spread.

If immunocompromised, symptoms may persist > two weeks.

Rarely children develop post-enteritis syndrome, chronic diarrhoea, in which an acquired immunologically mediated sensitivity to dietary food proteins might be implicated.

■ Acquired immunity makes episodes clinically milder with increasing age.

FALTERING GROWTH/FAILURE TO THRIVE

Aetiology/Pathogenesis

Can be categorised as: 1. inadequate or inappropriate nutritional intake, 2. malabsorption (see Table 9.2 and 9.3). metabolic or endocrine disorders (see chapters 'Endocrinology' and 'Metabolic Diseases').

Clinical Presentation

Failure to gain weight and/or length/height at expected rates according to the WHO/UK centile charts (Table 9.2 and Figure 9.4), or weight > two centiles < height centile.

Diagnosis

Obtain history of feeding, diet, bowel motions, behaviour/activity/energy level and family and psychosocial background.

Table 9.2: Major Gastrointestinal Causes of Faltering Growth

1. **Inadequate calorie intake:**
- Protein-calorie mal/under-nutritionMajor organ failure
- Feeding problems
- Oro-motor dysfunction
- Neuromuscular disease
- Psychosocial deprivation
- Fabricated or induced illness
- Vomiting
- Gastro-oesophageal reflux
  2. **Malabsorption:**
- Small intestinal enteropathy
- Coeliac disease
- Food sensitive enteropathy
- Small intestinal Crohn disease
- Eosinophilic gastroenteropathy
- Autoimmune/enteropathy
- systemic immunodeficiency-related enteropathy
- Genetic/Autosomal recessive enteropathies e.g. tufting enteropathy, microvillous inclusion disease, tricho-hepato-enteric disease
- Protein-losing enteropathy
- Lymphangiectasia
- Pancreatic insufficiency
- Shwachmann–Bodian–Diamond syndrome
- Cystic fibrosis
- CHO intolerance
- Lactase deficiency
- Sucrase-isomaltase deficiency

Table 9.3: Artificial Feeding Devices

- nasogastric tube*
  - Gastrostomy** if support expected to be needed for > 2–3 months (**Figure 9.5**).
  - Naso-jejunal tube* if gastric feed not tolerated
  - Gastro-jejunostomy**
  - Jejunostomy** for longer-term small intestinal feeding if the gastro-jejunostomy frequently becomes displaced with the tip re-entering the stomach
    - *nasogastric and naso-jejunal tube tip can become displaced with risk of aspiration
    - ** gastrostomy or jejunostomy can develop irritation, granuloma and local skin infection at the insertion site.

Investigate as guided by history and clinical presentation.

Differential Diagnosis: 'Catch down' growth, i.e. slow, normal growth during infancy if birth weight centile >genetically defined centile. Over the first 12 months the infant's length and weight gradually adjusts to the genetically defined centile, i.e. large babies at birth usually gain weight more slowly and smaller babies more rapidly during the first year. Growth in a healthy, well-nourished infant is largely genetically determined.

Treatment and Prognosis

According to underlying diagnosis; please refer to individual disease section.

FEEDING DIFFICULTIES

Incidence/Aetiology

Common with aetiology ranging from poor feeding technique, incorrect feed concentration, and inappropriate type of feed, to major organ failure. Please see Table 9.2 for possible diagnoses.
If an infant is fed via an artificial feeding device (nasogastric tube, gastrostomy, central venous catheter) for a prolonged period and not offered oral feed s/he will not develop/lose oral feeding skills. Poor feeding can be a secondary behavioural problem, that may persist after the underlying disease has resolved/improved.

Diagnosis

Unable or unwilling to ingest sufficient food or nutrition for normal weight gain and growth. Affected children may gag on food or fluids and refuse food by turning head away when offered the spoon or teat. Vomiting and poor weight gain are common. Feeding observation and advice by an experienced nurse/professional, e.g. health visitor, preferably initially in the home may resolve the problem. If symptoms persist clinically examine for evidence of underlying disease and investigate according to findings. Investigations might include intestinal endoscopy, oesophageal pH-impedance study, intestinal radiological contrast studies and radio-nuclear gastric emptying study, swallowing videofluoroscopy (if unsafe swallow suspected) and/or high-resolution oesophageal impedance manometry. Urine culture is essential.

Treatment

1. Treat underlying disease.

2. Advice may include cautious stimulation to 'desensitise', initially just touching the face around the mouth, then introducing a variety of shapes and textures to suck, lick and mouth and offering mealtime food for 'messy play'.

3. If symptoms persist despite advice, refer to specialist feeding nurse, speech therapist or other professional with specialist feeding knowledge. A multidisciplinary feeding clinic is required in more resistant cases.

4. If unable to ingest sufficient calories despite appropriate treatment, a commercially available liquid dietary supplement/'sip feed' can be offered and if not tolerated orally, may need the supplement via gastrostomy or other artificial feeding device whilst feeding difficulties continue.

5. Feed may be given as daytime boluses, or if poorly tolerated continuously overnight.

Prognosis

- Dependent on aetiology.

- If a chronic underlying medical disorder the child may need artificial enteral feeding for months/years.

- 'wean' artificial feeding at earliest opportunity and remove artificial feeding device when the child thrives without using it for about six months.

- Psychological dependence on an artificial feeding device can develop.

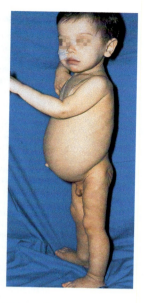

Figure 9.4 Faltering growth/Failure to thrive: severely undernourished appearance with distended abdomen, and buttock wasting.

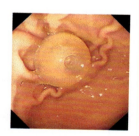

Figure 9.5 Endoscopic view of water inflated gastrostomy balloon *in situ.*

CONSTIPATION

Incidence/Genetics/Aetiology

Common condition and affets up to 20% children at some stage.

Usually functional, with subtypes with a physical basis. It can be due to slow intestinal transit, associated with colonic inertia (uncommon) or a defaecatory disorder with a rectal outlet problem.

If there is a difficulty in passing stool from birth with/without delayed passage of meconium, investigate physical/anatomical causes, e.g. Hirschsprung disease, anal stenosis, ano-rectal malformations (when the apparent anus is a fistula) and primary enteric neuromuscular diseases.

If difficult defaecation commences after normal passage of meconium and infant stool pattern for several weeks, consider atopy related anal spasm (dyschezia rather than constipation).

In older children with normal infant stool passage, functional faecal retention syndromes are prevalent, with primary causes including anal fissure and behavioural disturbances.

Allergy and inflammation can alter intestinal transit; gastrointestinal food allergy, coeliac and Crohn disease can present with constipation over a wide age range.

Onset of functional constipation maybe with a primary event, such as poor fluid and/or calorie intake resulting in a small amount of hard stool that is ultimately expelled with painful defaecation (possibly with an anal fissure enhancing pain), with subsequent efforts to hold stool in and avoid defaecation. Acquired megarectum with poor faecal sensation and retained faecal mass may ensue with eventual overflow faecal incontinence and soiling with psychological factors.

Clinical Presentation/Diagnosis/Differential Diagnosis

Infrequent passage of usually hard stool. Age and cause specific. Functional constipation may present with:

- Abnormally hard and often large stool with increased time between defaecation causing distress when opening bowels.

- Wilful faecal retention with young children adopting stereotypical postures to contract the pelvic floor to retain stool when they have the urge to defaecate.

- Soiling – escape of stool into underclothing.

Investigations include:

- Examine spine, sacrum and lower limb reflexes to exclude neuropathic bowel.

- Abdominal x-ray with radio-opaque markers:
  - swallow a different marker each day for three consecutive days and x-ray on the fourth day (Figure 9.6)
  - to estimate intestinal transit time and distinguish defaecatory disorders from slow transit constipation
  - more accurate if undertaken following complete faecal disimpaction.

- Blood tests to exclude hypothyroidism and coeliac disease.

- Rectal biopsy histology to investigate for increased mucosal acetylcholinesterase-positive nerve fibres and absence of submucosa ganglion cells seen in Hirschsprung disease (see the chapter 'Neonatal and General Paediatric Surgery').

- Blood specific IgE for foods (including milk, egg, wheat, soya).

- Colonoscopy with mucosal biopsy histology: in atopic children may demonstrate underlying eosinophilic/allergic/other inflammatory disorders.

- Further investigations if clinically indicated, e.g. sweat test, anorectal manometry.

Treatment

- According to underlying aetiology.

- Functional constipation management guidance is largely consensus rather than evidence based.

- Early treatment is important to break longer-term habit related to fear of painful defaecation.

Initial Medical Treatment

- Soften and evacuate retained stool with polyethylene glycol (PEG) and electrolyte solutions, lactulose and/or sodium docusate.

- If needed add a Prokinetic: Sennokot +/– sodium picosulphate or in older children bisacodyl (secretogogue and prokinetic), to ensure evacuation.

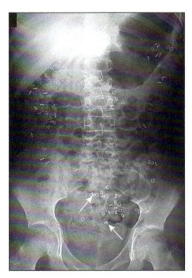

Figure 9.6 Plain abdominal x-ray demonstrating positions of three different shaped radio-opaque markers swallowed on three consecutive days and now situated in different parts of the left colon.

- Disimpact resistant cases with nasogastric PEG solution.

- Only use Micro or phosphate enemas to evacuate rectal masses if the child understands and co-operates or may heighten discomfort and defaecation fear.

Maintenance Drug Treatment

- Daily PEG/electrolyte solution

- If required simultaneous osmotic and stimulant laxatives (Table 9.4): lactulose (5–10 ml tds) or methylcellulose tablets for osmotic effect + senna (infants and older children).

- Once-daily senna to prevent re-accumulation of faeces (effect for 12–14 hours post dose).

- Rarely – regular rectal/colonic irrigation with large volumes of water (Peristeen).

- Parallel child and family psychological treatment needed in about 50% school age children.

- Appropriate dietary exclusions for atopic-related food allergic colitis.

Prognosis

- Stimulant laxatives usually required for > 12 months to prevent relapse.

- Patients' dependent on longer medical treatment require specialist assessment as some 'treatment failures' have generalised or segmental large intestinal intrinsic neuromuscular disease.

INFANTILE COLIC
Incidence/Aetiology
Common. Cows' milk and/or other dietary proteins are associated in some cases and transient lactose malabsorption is implicated in some others.

Clinical Presentation/Diagnosis
Excessive crying or fussing in an otherwise healthy, thriving infant, usually from 4 weeks to 3 months old. Episodic crying, usually in the evening, is defined as colic if persists > three hours/day for > three days/week for > three weeks. Other problems, such as overheating, too cold, inappropriate feeding or discomfort, should be discounted. The condition is likely to be stressful for the whole family.

Treatment
Reassure parents. Many infants improve with reduced stimulation. Exclusion of dietary cow's milk should be tried for a two-week period and symptoms reassessed:

- If breastfeeding, mother should exclude all cow's milk products from her own diet (ensuring adequate calcium intake if continued beyond trial period).

- If formula/bottle fed change to an extensively hydrolysed formula.

Supportive counselling and continuing reassurance may be needed.

Prognosis
Usually resolves spontaneously by 4–5 months of age.

Table 9.4: Laxatives

Osmotic	Stimulant
Lactulose	Sennokot
Polyethylene glycol	Docusate sodium
Methylcellulose	Sodium picosulphate
Phosphate enemas	Bisacodyl
Sodium citrate enemas	Microlax enema

RECURRENT ABDOMINAL PAIN

Incidence/Aetiology

Affects up to one in ten children. Improvement in gastrointestinal investigation techniques has led to more organic diagnoses although many cases remain 'functional'. Broad differential diagnosis includes congenital and acquired pancreatic and gall bladder disease and unusual aetiologies such as intermittent testicular torsion.

Diagnosis

More than three attacks of abdominal pain over > three months, sufficiently severe to interfere with normal activities. A careful, thorough clinical history and examination are essential to check for a wide range of disorders. When physical findings are inconsistent, e.g. extreme abdominal tenderness on superficial palpation yet able to move in an unrestricted pattern, consider a functional cause. A psychosocial history is important if functional disease suspected.

Initial investigations include urine culture, full blood count, C-reactive protein, blood urea and electrolytes, liver function tests, stool culture, faecal occult blood and further investigations according to symptoms. If possible, examine and investigate the patient during an attack. Abdominal ultrasound might demonstrate bowel wall thickening, pancreato-biliary, ovarian or urinary tract disease. If pain persists and is not resolving, upper and/or lower gastrointestinal endoscopy should be considered.

Treatment

According to underlying cause. Functional abdominal pain usually responds better to cognitive behavioural therapy and hypnotherapy with multidisciplinary team (MDT) support than to pharmacological approaches. Rehabilitation is key when pain has resulted in social withdrawal from school and peers.

Prognosis

Long-term follow-up indicates improvement with age, although many patients remain symptomatic into adult life.

TODDLER'S DIARRHOEA

Incidence/Genetics

Common, affecting males > females with familial predisposition; about 80% have an affected sibling or a parent with a history of irritable bowel

Aetiology

Clinical manifestations are related to fast intestinal transit, with adequate nutrient absorption. There is often rapid gastric emptying with failure to induce the postprandial motility pattern. Dietary fruit sugar, fructose is absorbed slowly and if incompletely absorbed may exacerbate symptoms by an osmotic effect and fermentation products within the colon. Immunological, usually non-IgE-mediated reactions to food protein allergens (food allergy) can also cause rapid transit.

Diagnosis

Loose, frequent, foul-smelling, daytime stool, usually with mucus, in children aged 1–6 years. Affected children frequently need to defaecate during a meal. Stool microscopy and culture should be performed. Upper intestinal endoscopy with mucosal biopsy histology is needed if inadequate weight gain and additional colonoscopy if nocturnal diarrhoea or blood in the stool. Eosinophilic gastrointestinal disease may be detected histologically.

Treatment

- limit fruit juices and/or fruit and fibre and increase fat intake.

- If positive food specific IgE/other suspicion of slow onset, non-IgE-mediated food allergy (e.g. personal/family atopy), a six to eight week trial of dietary exclusion of the suspected food is warranted and symptoms reassessed (see allergic colitis). The most common offending foods are cow's milk, egg and wheat.

- Some children benefit from Calogen (long-chain triglyceride, LCT) with meals to delay gastric emptying, or loperamide treatment.

Prognosis

Diarrhoea improves with age, although symptoms can persist into adulthood.

INFANTILE CHRONIC INTRACTABLE DIARRHOEA WITH FALTERING GROWTH
Incidence/Genetics

Rare genetic conditions most common in societies with consanguineous marriages since autosomal recessive or X-linked inheritance.

Aetiology

Small intestinal mucosal disorders either associated with normal systemic immunity or immunodeficiency:

1. Mucosal disorders with normal systemic immunity include:

   - Tufting enteropathy: EpCAM chromosome 2, SPINT2 chromosome 19

   - Tricho-hepato-enteric syndrome: TTC37, chromosome 5

   - Microvillous inclusion disease: MYO5B, chromosome 18 (Figure 9.7).

2. Mucosal disorders with systemic immunodeficiency include:

   - Certain autoimmune enteropathies e.g. immune dysregulation, polyendocrinopathy, enteropathy, X-linked (IPEX) syndrome: IPEX, FOXP3 gene on the X chromosome

   - Severe infantile or very early onset IBD, intestinal atresias: TTC7a deficiency

   - (see very early onset IBD – VEOIBD)

   - No specific diagnosis.

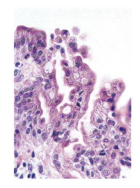

Figure 9.7 Tufting enteropathy. Histological appearance of small intestinal mucosa with 'grape-like' tufts at villus tip (×25).

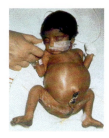

Figure 9.8 Neonate with severe, intractable, watery diarrhoea and faltering growth, with abdominal distention and perianal/nappy area excoriation.

Diagnosis

Loose stool > four times/day for > two weeks, with faltering growth.

(Figures 9.8 and 9.9) and > 3 negative stool cultures (MC&S, ova, cysts, parasites) and virology.

- Watery stool may be mistaken for urine.

- **Intractable if diarrhoea persists** even after extensive investigation and medical treatment. See Table 9.5 for investigations.

Treatment

- Stabilise the patient, restoring good fluid and electrolyte balance.

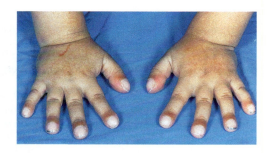

Figure 9.9 Anaemia and finger clubbing in intractable diarrhoea and malabsorption.

- Gradual oral/enteral feed re/introduction (see the section 'Intestinal Failure' section below).

- If enteral feed reintroduction fails urgently refer to specialist IF rehabilitation service for investigation and management.

- Specific treatment according to underlying disease (see appropriate section), e.g. immunomodulatory treatment for intestinal mucosal inflammation (see the section 'Irritable Bowel Disease').

- Plus supportive therapy with parenteral nutrition (PN).

Table 9.5: Chronic Intractable Diarrhoea Investigations

At general hospital	Specialist service
Stool m.c&s	Repeat Stool m.c&s + microscopy for fat globules
Stool virology*	blood immunoglobulin IgG, IgA, IgM, IgE, coeliac screen
Urine m.c&s	If watery diarrhoea, stool Na, reducing substances + sugar chromatography if positive
FBC, CRP	Stool alpha-1 antitrypsin
Blood urea, electrolytes, Ca, PO4, Mg, HCO3	genetic panel testing
Faecal calprotectin	blood immunological studies
Blood albumin, bilirubin, liver enzymes	Upper and lower intestinal endoscopy with mucosal biopsies for histology, periodic acid Schiff (PAS) staining, (Figures 9.10 and 9.11), electron microscopy (Figures 9.12 to 9.14)
Blood immunoglobulin levels coeliac screen specific IgE for foods	Upper intestinal radiological gastrointestinal contrast study
Stool elastase*	Stool and urine toxicology screen

* At specialist centre if unavailable

Prognosis

- Outcome varies according to diagnosis with and within each diagnosis, e.g. tufting enteropathy outcome ranges from gaining enteral autonomy in early/mid-childhood or early adult life to remaining parenteral nutrition dependent.

- When treatment fails long-term PN is needed (see chronic intestinal failure below).

- Many conditions improve with age and enteral autonomy is gained.

- Some conditions with systemic immunodeficiency may need bone marrow transplant.

INTESTINAL FAILURE (IF)

Reduction in gut function to below the minimum necessary for adequate absorption of macronutrients and/or water and electrolytes so that IV supplementation is required to maintain health and/or growth. It is classified as: Type 1 self-limiting, Type 2 prolonged and Type 3 long-term.

Aetiology/Pathogenesis

Underlying primary digestive disorder (PDD) or primary non-digestive disorder (PNDD), see Table 9.6 below.

Diagnosis

IF is prolonged or long-term when after appropriate management of the underlying disease it is not possible to absorb sufficient oral/enteral feed using the most appropriate type of feed administered in the best possible manner.

Please see the Table 9.5 for Essential investigations for chronic intractable diarrhoeal diseases (see the sections for SBS and for motility disorders).

Differential Diagnosis

A small minority of children presenting with IF have fabricated or induced illness. It is important to ensure urine/stool/other specimens are obtained by a professional. 24-hour one-to-one nursing care is often necessary to effectively assess the child.

Treatment

Patients should be investigated and managed by a specialist IF rehabilitation centre. The main aims are:

1. Maximise intestinal absorptive capacity by treating underlying disease.

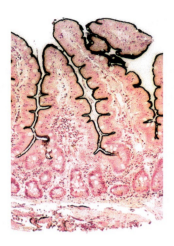

Figure 9.10 PAS Enterocyte Brush border staining of normal small intestine (×40).

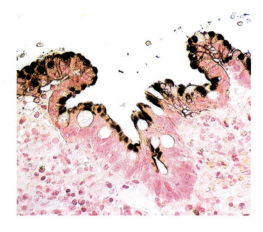

Figure 9.11 PAS Enterocyte Brush border staining in microvillous inclusion disease illustrating abnormal microvilli (×100).

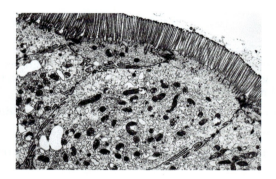

Figure 9.12 Electron microscope appearance of normal small intestinal enterocyte microvilli (×13,000).

2. Regularly re-trial gradual introduction of appropriate oral/enteral feed if at all possible.

- if oral intake is insufficient reduce it to the maximum that is not associated with symptoms and is enjoyed by the patient

- insert artificial feeding device (see Table 9.3)

- trial bolus and/or continuous feed

- In most cases hydrolysate or elemental commercial liquid feed or modular feed in a few cases.

- maintain normal weight gain and growth with PN support (see short bowel syndrome)

- PN should be prescribed and administered in an appropriate clinical setting with MDT support

3. Long-term care.

- If the underlying disease fails to respond to treatment the child should be discharged home on overnight PN enabling daytime school attendance and other activities.

- Parents/carers undergo a formal training programme to these abbreviations connect/disconnect PN and troubleshoot potential complications.

- Management should be by a specialist multidisciplinary IF rehabilitation team.

- Regularly monitor for and treat potentially life-threatening complications.

Table 9.6: Indications for PN

Primary digestive disorder	Primary non-digestive disorder
Post-operative abdominal surgery	Prematurity
Short bowel syndrome (SBS). Aetiologies include: necrotising enterocolitis (NEC) gastroschisis intestinal atresia congenital short bowel/antenatal volvulus total colonic + small intestinal aganglionosis	Major organ failure, e.g. Neuro-degenerative disorder
Chronic intractable diarrhoea with faltering growth (also see the section 'Very Early Onset Inflammatory Bowel Disease')	Chemotherapy Radiotherapy
	Severe trauma Extensive burns
Motility disorder: paediatric intestinal pseudo-obstruction (PIPO) -intestinal dysmotility	Bone marrow transplant Systemic immunodeficiencies
	Fabricated/induced illness

- Complications include inappropriate weight gain, metabolic, catheter-related bloodstream infections/CRBSI, intestinal failure-associated liver disease/IFALD and thrombotic disorders.

Prognosis

- Children on PN can grow and develop normally, attending school, and participate in other activities including swimming.

- > 50% wean off PN, developing enteral autonomy after months or years.

- PIPO/other dysmotility has the worst prognosis.

- In a few cases PN treatment fails and intestinal transplant (+/− liver) assessment is needed if

  - loss of most central venous access

  - Severe IFALD liver disease

  - Unpredictable high volume intestinal fluid losses

- Life expectancy for intestinal transplant is lower with home PN than managed by an IF rehabilitation service.

- Children can expect to survive throughout childhood and into adult life even with chronic IF.

PART 2: Gastrointestinal Diagnoses

COELIAC DISEASE

Incidence/Genetics

The worldwide incidence (in all ethnicities) is 0.5–1% and 2–3% in Caucasians with a high wheat intake. It is associated with ~3% risk, with one copy of HLA-DQ2 (DQ2.5 or DQ2.2) or DQ8 genotype and ~10% risk with two copies of either. Frequency is increased in Down's, Turner's and William's syndromes and selective IgA deficiency.

Aetiology

Chronic immune-mediated small intestinal enteropathy associated with ingestion of gluten in genetically predisposed individuals that resolves with dietary avoidance of gluten. Tissue transglutaminase (tTg) is the major autoantigen. Ingestion of wheat, barley or rye initiates immunologically mediated tissue injury in association with particular HLA and several non-HLA genes. An environmental trigger is necessary, identical twin concordance rates are approximately 70%. It is associated with other autoimmune diseases especially insulin-dependent diabetes and hypothyroidism.

Clinical Presentation/Diagnosis

Classically presents with anorexia, vomiting, abdominal distension, diarrhoea, irritability, faltering growth and buttock wasting in infant/young child on a wheat containing diet. Other

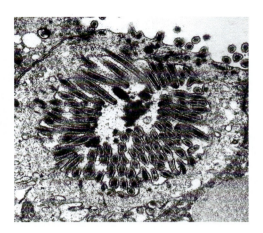

Figure 9.13 Electron microscope appearance of distorted enterocyte microvilli in microvillous inclusion disease (×13,000).

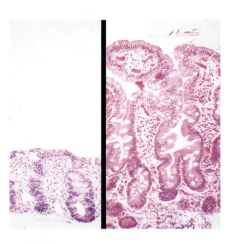

Figure 9.14 Histological appearance of subtotal villous atrophy compared with normal small intestine.

presentations include constipation, non-specific abdominal pain, anaemia, recurrent oral aphthous ulceration and rarely epilepsy with intracranial calcification and unexplained neurological conditions, e.g. palsies, neuropathies, migraine. Dermatitis herpetiformis and splenic atrophy more commonly present in adults. Many children and adults are asymptomatic (Figure 9.15).

Presents at any age throughout life, although most cases start in childhood.

The 2020 European Society of Paediatric Gastroenterology, Hepatology and Nutrition (ESPGHAN) criteria for coeliac disease diagnosis [REF] are:

- In symptomatic children measure IgA class transglutaminase 2 antibody (TTG-IgA) levels. If blood TTG-IgA level ≥ 10 times the upper limit of normal on two separate samples alongside positive endomysial antibodies (EMAIgA) can be diagnosed without intestinal histology.

- If low blood IgA level (low for age or < 0.2 g/L if > 3 years old), an IgG-based TTG test should be performed.

- HLA testing is unnecessary in a symptomatic child with positive serology.

- Children with lower positive TTG-IgA titres < 10 times the upper limit of normal, and asymptomatic children positive on screening, should undergo upper intestinal endoscopy with biopsies to reduce risk of false positive diagnosis.

- Endoscopy must be done on a gluten-containing diet with ≥ five biopsies from distal duodenum and ≥ 1 from the duodenal bulb. Where typical histological changes are seen (see pathology below) the diagnosis is secure (Figure 9.16).

- If atypical histology consider HLA-genotyping and/or repeat biopsy on a gluten free diet and repeat again following gluten rechallenge.

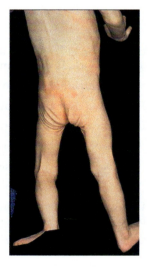

Figure 9.15 Coeliac disease, showing severe buttocks and thigh wasting.

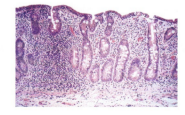

Figure 9.16 Coeliac disease. Proximal small intestine histology (×400). Subtotal villous atrophy with villous shortening, crypt hypertrophy, increased intraepithelial lymphocyte numbers and lamina propria plasma cells.

Coeliac disease abnormalities include iron-deficiency anaemia, low red cell and serum folate, low plasma albumin and prolonged prothrombin time. Stool elastase can be low due to secondary pancreatic exocrine insufficiency and there may be transient lactase deficiency on presentation.

Pathology

Typical duodenal histology is hyperplastic subtotal villous atrophy, with increased lamina propria plasma cells and increased ratio of intraepithelial lymphocytes to surface epithelial cells – Marsh Types 2 and 3 are supportive of the diagnosis. However, changes can be patchy with variable villus atrophy, crypt hyperplasia, lamina propria inflammation and surface epithelium. Immunological abnormalities include increased proportion of intraepithelial lymphocytes with gamma/delta T-cell receptors, reduced lamina propria suppressor cell numbers and increased antibody (including antigliadin antibody) production. Gluten-specific CD4 positive T-cells are restricted by the HLA-DQ2 heterodimer. There is aberrant HLA-DR expression by immature crypt enterocytes, reduced enterocyte survival time and increased intestinal permeability.

Differential Diagnosis

Wheat sensitive enteropathy and atopy-associated wheat allergy have different immunological aetiologies, can be transient and are commonest in infants and preschool children (see the section 'Food Sensitive Enteropathy').

Treatment

Dietary exclusion of wheat, rye, barley and initially oat avoidance. Trial reintroducing certified wheat free oats after one year if the child is well and tTG normalised, but exclude again if symptoms develop. Some children have a transient lactose intolerance. Easy access to paediatric dietitian(s) must be ensured. Advise families to join Coeliac UK: website www.coeliac.co.uk and/or other international support organisations.

Prognosis

- Coeliac disease is life-long but controlled with a gluten free diet.

- If patient fails to avoid gluten > infertility risk and reduced bone mineral density.

- Malignancy, in particular small intestinal T-cell lymphoma may rarely develop in later life, possibly more commonly if gluten ingestion continues.

GASTRO-OESOPHAGEAL REFLUX

Incidence/Aetiology

Gastroesophageal reflux, GOR is universal in infancy and mostly of no pathological significance. When pathological it is termed Gastroesophageal reflux disease, GORD. Disease mechanisms include transient lower oesophageal sphincter relaxations (TLESRs) un-associated with swallowing, hiatus hernia, lax lower oesophageal sphincter, chronic cough and increased transdiaphragmatic pressure gradient, e.g. with wheeze.

Diagnosis

Passive movement of gastric contents from the stomach into the oesophagus. Usually neonatal onset, with excessive posseting and regurgitation of milk after and/or between feeds often with feeding difficulties, poor weight gain or chronic cough. Children present with excessive regurgitation/posseting, oesophagitis or respiratory disease with possible apnoea. The refluxate is not bile-stained, but occasionally blood-stained if oesophageal excoriation. Older infants may be reluctant to ingest solid food and have gagging and choking episodes. Symptoms in older children include retrosternal and epigastric pain.

Investigations should be reserved for children who do not respond to initial medical treatment and include:

- Full Blood Count

- 24-hour oesophageal impedance/pH study

- Upper gastrointestinal radiological contrast study to exclude underlying structural disorder, e.g. intestinal malrotation

- Upper gastrointestinal endoscopy and mucosal biopsies sometimes indicated

- High-resolution oesophageal impedance/manometry, a highly specialised test, can be used to determine the reflux mechanism

- If aspiration suspected sputum or broncho-alveolar lavage fluid could be examined for fat laden macrophages.

Differential Diagnosis

Distinguish from vomiting (emesis) and rumination which have different aetiologies and treatments. In young infants consider hypertrophic pyloric stenosis or feeding mismanagement. Non-IgE-mediated cow's milk protein/other food allergy can sometimes be confused with GORD. Exclude urinary tract/other infection.

Treatment

In healthy thriving infants use symptomatic treatments such as:

- Placing the infant in left lateral position or with the head elevated.

- Thicken feeds with, e.g. Carobel or if growth faltering consider Vitaquik.

- Gaviscon.

More severe/complicated reflux may require:

- Proton pump inhibitor.

- Baclofen (inhibits TLESRs and accelerates gastric emptying).

- Manage associated disease, for example, exclude offending food(s) from diet (see 'Non-IgE-mediated food sensitive enteropathy').

- Trans-pyloric small intestinal tube feeding may be needed when symptoms persist despite treatment and if needed longer term a gastro-jejunostomy should be inserted.

- Surgical management with fundoplication if aspiration episodes or chronic oesophagitis despite maximal medical therapy or other complications, e.g. oesophageal stricture (see surgical section).

Prognosis

Infantile reflux usually becomes asymptomatic/resolves by second year of life. In some, more prolonged medical treatment is necessary.

CYCLIC VOMITING SYNDROME (CVS)

Incidence/Aetiology

Rare with variable estimates of incidence/prevalence. Episodes are commonly precipitated by infections, anxiety, excitement, tiredness, motion and menstrual periods. There is a personal, > 40%, or family history, about 30%, of migraine, and associated anxiety and depression in approximately 30%.

Diagnosis

Functional vomiting usually presents aged 3–7 years, affecting girls > boys, with ≥ three episodes/year (average 9.6 episodes/year) of intense nausea and vomiting usually lasting < one week (average 3.4 days) with return to baseline health between episodes.

CVS phases are: (i) baseline interictal health (ii) prodromal prior to vomiting onset when the patient experiences severe nausea and is usually extremely pale (iii) vomiting with up to six vomits/hour initially non-bilious but becoming bilious in association with prostration between vomits (iv) recovery phase with rapid return to baseline health. It may require several emergency presentations before being recognised.

Differential Diagnosis

Distinguish CVS from chronic vomiting. Consider and exclude urinary tract infections, brain space occupying lesion (with brain radiological imaging), intestinal malrotation with intermittent volvulus (with upper intestinal radiological contrast study to) or metabolic disorder.

Treatment

In interictal, phase 1:

- Lifestyle modifications to avoid specific triggers such as certain foods, tiredness, anxiety-provoking situations and particular types of motion.
- Prophylactic medications, e.g. antimigraine drugs (pizotifen, propranolol, amitriptyline, flunarizine and cyproheptadine), anticonvulsants (topiramate, levitaracetam and zonisamide) and anti-emetics (aprepitant).
- Dietary supplements, e.g. carnitine, coenzyme Q10 and riboflavin.

In prodromal phase 2, if sufficient time, treatments include:

- Antiemetics (5HT$_3$ antagonists, aprepitant/fosaprepitant, cyclizine), migraine treatments (sumatriptan), anxiolysis (benzodiazepines).

In established vomiting phase 3 about 50% require hospitalisation. Treatments include:

- IV fluids to resuscitate, replace ongoing losses and maintain normoglycaemia
- Anti-emetics (5HT$_3$ antagonists, fosaprepitant and cyclizine), anxiolysis (lorazepam), anti-hypertensives if severe hypertension (5% of cases)

FOOD SENSITIVE ENTEROPATHY

Incidence/Genetics

Gastrointestinal symptoms precipitated by cow's milk may affect 1 in 200 infants.

Aetiology/Pathogenesis

Non-IgE-mediated, slow onset food sensitive enteropathy occurs with ingestion of specific food antigens, most commonly cow's milk, also with egg, soya and wheat and has been described with almost any food, e.g. rice, chicken, fish. There may be associated family and/or personal history of atopic disease, or immunodeficiency, e.g. IgA deficiency. The enteropathy is usually a cell-mediated immunological reaction resulting in lack of tolerance of specific dietary antigen/s by the gut-associated lymphoid tissue, GALT. Some 'slow onset' food allergy may develop when intestinal immunity is compromised, e.g. post-enteritis syndrome or e.g. IgA deficiency that may predispose to excessive antigen absorption.

Diagnosis

Often presents with vomiting, diarrhoea, faltering growth, irritability and/or abdominal pain. Children may dislike the neat form of the offending food, e.g. children with cow's milk allergy may only ingest milk on cereal, in tea or milkshakes.

It is diagnosed when symptoms resolve on excluding the offending food from the diet for 6–8 weeks and recur when the food is reintroduced. If dietary exclusion fails or is inappropriate, upper intestinal endoscopy with duodenal mucosal biopsy maybe needed (Figure 9.17). Histologically, there is intestinal mucosal thinning with patchy, partial villous atrophy and increased lamina propria cellularity (Figure 9.18), possibly with an eosinophilic infiltration of small intestinal lamina propria.

Since cell-mediated or delayed allergic response, results of specific IgE antibodies and skin-prick test for dietary allergen is usually oflittle diagnostic relevance.

The definitive diagnosis is made when the enteropathy detected histologically on small intestinal biopsy has resolved on repeat biopsy (not usually clinically indicated) after a minimum of eight weeks dietary exclusion.

Differential Diagnosis

Distinguish from immediate hypersensitivity, IgE-mediated, allergic response to food, in which there is usually a reaction to the food within an hour and no underlying enteropathy. The enteropathy is histologically distinct and less severe than coeliac disease.

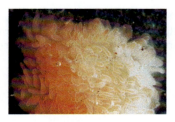

Figure 9.17   Food sensitive enteropathy. Dissecting microscope appearance of normal small intestinal villi when on an avoidance diet.

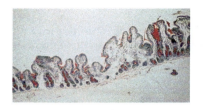

Figure 9.18   Food sensitive enteropathy. Small intestinal histology showing partial villous atrophy with mucosal thinning (×250).

Treatment

- dietary avoidance of the offending food for minimum trial period of 6–8 weeks, (with dietitian advice) simultaneously treats the patient and confirms the aetiology.

- Gradual food reintroduction can be attempted after several weeks or months of full health, e.g. using stepwise introduction of milk/dairy products.

- If symptoms recur, exclude the food again.

- Dietitian review on annual basis to ensure dietary adequacy and trial of food reintroduction at appropriate intervals if > 1 food avoided.

- Ensure calcium supplement/enriched plant-based milk cow's for long-term cow's milk avoidance.

Prognosis

Rapidly resolves when the offending food is excluded from the diet.

- Usually improves as GALT matures from about 18 months to 2 years of age but can persist throughout childhood and into adult life.

- Some children can tolerate a food in cooking, e.g. milk as cheese and yogurt, but not neat cow's milk, even in a cup of tea.

LACTOSE INTOLERANCE

Incidence/Aetiology

Common, associated with low/absent lactase enzyme of mature enterocytes on the tips of the small intestinal villi (Figures 9.19 and 9.20) due to:

1. Genetic reduction to 5–10% childhood level in non-Caucasians > 5 years old.

2. Secondary to acute gastroenteritis/other enteropathic disorder when villous atrophy occurs.

3. Primary hypolactasia, a rare genetic disorder of *LCT* Gene polymorphism. On chromosome 2q21-22.

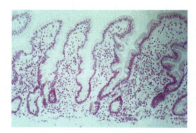

Figure 9.19   Absence of staining for lactase with normal small intestinal mucosal histology in child with alactasia.

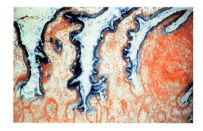

Figure 9.20   Normal small intestinal mucosa with positive brush border staining for lactase.

Diagnosis/Differential Diagnosis

- Loose, watery, frothy stools following ingestion of cow's milk with associated perianal excoriation.

- Stool sugar chromatography detects stool lactose.

- Chronic symptoms associated with cow's milk ingestion in Caucasians are most likely to be associated with a non-IgE-mediated/atopic-related cow's milk protein intolerance and not lactose.

Treatment/Prognosis

- Avoidance/low lactose diet.

- Congenital deficiencies are life-long, but asymptomatic if appropriate diet adhered to.

- Secondary post-acute gastroenteritis hypolactasia usually resolves within days/weeks.

EOSINOPHILIC GASTROINTESTINAL DISEASE

Spectrum of disorders grouped together as eosinophilic gastrointestinal diseases (EGID). They may be dependent or independent of allergic reaction to specific food proteins and be associated with a family history of atopy. Symptoms depend on the underlying disease:

- Mucosal with inflammation, malabsorption or gastrointestinal bleeding.

- Muscle layer affecting intestinal motility, typically with vomiting or constipation.

- Sub-serosal disease with eosinophilic ascites.

EOSINOPHILIC OESOPHAGITIS (EOE)

Incidence/Genetics

Incidence in resource rich countries is 0.95–1.28/10,000 and increasing, to about 7% in a positive family history. Susceptibility linkage in some families appears related to calpain-14 encoding gene upregulation in EoE oesophageal epithelial cells. Most children have atopic conditions.

Aetiology/Pathogenesis/Diagnosis

Chronic immunologically mediated reaction which causes oesophageal dysfunction primarily driven by eosinophilic inflammation. Multiple genes, host immune function and environmental triggers are suspected.

Diagnosed histologically with a minimum of 15 eosinophils/high-power field or $> 60/mm^2$ on oesophageal mucosal biopsy obtained during upper endoscopy with $\geq$ five biopsies from multiple oesophageal sites. Eosinophilic degranulation and epithelial infiltration may occur. Macroscopically, oesophageal ridging, furrowing or oesophageal rings (if multiple termed 'trachealised oesophagus') and, in some cases, a whitish oesophageal exudate may be seen (Figure 9.21).

Upper intestinal radiological contrast study may detect a 'ringed oesophagus'.

Diagnosis/Differential Diagnosis

Clinical features include feeding difficulties, dysphagia, food impaction, vomiting and abdominal pain. Associated problems include psoriasis, seborrheic dermatitis, asthma and allergic rhinitis.

In contrast to GORD, patients may not respond to proton pump inhibitor (PPI) treatment.

Treatment/Prognosis

- Approximately 15% respond to high dose PPI, e.g. lansoprazole 1 mg/kg/d.

- 15% respond to dietary exclusion, initially 1–2 food exclusions, then four, then six food eliminations and if refractory, consider an elemental diet.

- Approximately 15% respond to swallowed topical steroids e.g. oral viscous budesonide (OVB < 10 years 1 mg, > 10 years or 150 cm tall, 2 mg) or swallowed

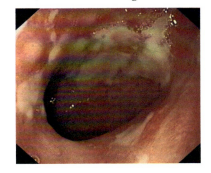

Figure 9.21 Reflux oesophagitis.

265

fluticasone. Mix OVB with a sucralose sugar-substitute using 10 teaspoons/0.5 mg budesonide (0.5 mg/2 ml).

- Oesophagitis may improve with age, but treatment required to manage symptoms and risk of progressive inflammation and oesophageal remodelling or stricturing.

- Endoscopic re-evaluation to assess histological response is advised, since symptoms poorly indicate treatment response.

EOSINOPHILIC GASTRITIS (EG), EOSINOPHILIC GASTROENTERITIS (EGE) AND EOSINOPHILIC ENTERITIS (EE)

Incidence/Genetics

Rare enteropathies which commonly involve stomach and duodenum.

Clinical Presentation/Diagnosis

Variable, including abdominal pain, nausea, vomiting, poor weight gain, diarrhoea and symptoms of intestinal pseudo-obstruction and there is ascites if significant small bowel disease, often with iron deficient anaemia. Essential investigations include gastrointestinal pan-endoscopy with mucosal biopsy of oesophagus, stomach, small intestine, ileum and colon.

Histological diagnosis with eosinophilic infiltration of intestinal mucosa/submucosa/muscle layer of intestinal biopsies. Often low blood albumin, globulins and haemoglobin with about 75% peripheral blood eosinophilia.

Differential Diagnosis

Food allergic and autoimmune enteropathy may present with similar symptoms and responds to similar treatment.

Treatment/Prognosis

- Exclusion of potentially offending dietary foods is often successful.

- 8–12 week course of enterally administered topical steroids, e.g. budesonide if severe symptoms.

- Systemic steroids, e.g. prednisolone maybe indicated, and if efficacious, transition to steroid-sparing agents, e.g. azathioprine.

- Endoscopic reassessment after 8–12 weeks is recommended.

- Prognosis is good if symptoms respond to treatment.

- As with other inflammatory gut conditions, functional symptoms may continue following successful treatment.

EOSINOPHILIC/ALLERGIC COLITIS (EC)

Incidence/Genetics

Commonest cause of non-infectious infantile diarrhoea with incidence 1.7–3.5/100,000 in United States with similar frequency in all ages. It is more common in males and often with a family history of atopy.

Diagnosis

Diarrhoea, often with blood and mucus in neonatal period or infancy in an otherwise healthy, thriving baby irrespective of breast or bottle feeding. It also presents as toddler's diarrhoea. Diagnosis is made on histological appearance of lamina propria inflammatory infiltrate ≥ 50 eosinophils per high powered field (HPF) in the right colon, and ≥ 30 in the left colon with plasma cells on colonoscopic mucosal biopsies. Macroscopically, there is typically patchy colonic erythema. Plasma immunoglobulin levels may demonstrate most commonly low IgA and/or reduced IgG subclass levels.

Treatment

- Dietary exclusion of offending foods, most commonly cow's milk, soya, egg and wheat in United Kingdom, but many other foods also implicated.

- If no response on endoscopic reassessment at 12 weeks, further dietary exclusion may be helpful.

- or trial a 5-aminosalicylate, 5-ASA.

- Refractory symptoms may require an elemental diet, topical steroids given enterally e.g. budesonide or course of systemic steroids, e.g. prednisolone 1.5 mg/kg/d for two weeks, then tapered.

Prognosis

Improves with age, but often persistent intolerance to ingestion of a large quantity of offending food. Offending foods maybe tolerated if the protein is denatured, such as with cooking.

INFLAMMATORY BOWEL DISEASE

Crohn disease (CD) and ulcerative colitis (UC) are chronic auto-inflammatory disorders primarily involving the gastrointestinal tract described as classical inflammatory bowel disease (IBD).

Features distinguishing UC from CD are site, type of inflammation and histology. Initial histological and clinical phenotype might be indeterminate, IBD-unclassified, IBD-U, then progress to CD or UC whilst around 15% remain IBD-U.

Genetic and environmental factors are important in IBD pathogenesis with > 200 genetic loci identified contributing to the risk of developing IBD although the relative risk with one mutation is generally marginal, (see UC and CD below). A combination of genetic polymorphisms appears to play a role, as first-degree relatives have approximately 3–20 times > BD risk.

Several single gene disorders associated with IBD are distinct from idiopathic IBD.

Ulcerative Colitis

Incidence/Genetics

Between 1 in 25,000–50,000 children with 15% monozygotic twin concordance and 15% with affected first-degree relative. UC is associated with HLA-DR2 and many genetic loci involved in microbial recognition, cytokine signalling, lymphocyte activation and intestinal epithelial defence that are also associated with CD.

Aetiology/Pathogenesis

Is unknown and multifactorial with immunological mechanisms including autoimmunity. In 80% there is an IgG1 antibody to a colonic polypeptide, specific to UC. Positive perinuclear anti-cytoplasmic antibody (p-ANCA) is associated with increased risk of primary sclerosing cholangitis and 'pouchitis' after surgery.

Inflammation usually confined to intestinal mucosa and becomes transmural in toxic dilatation of the colon when perforation is imminent. Whilst the colon is most severely affected, other gastrointestinal inflammation including the stomach and small intestine, can occur. Macroscopically, at colonoscopy the inflammation is continuous often with a granular haemorrhagic appearance, with friability and loss of vascular markings (Figure 9.22), although occasionally sparing the rectum. Histologically there is vascular congestion, crypt branching and abscesses, loss of goblet cells and Paneth cell metaplasia with mucosal inflammatory cell infiltration.

Diagnosis

Usually UC presents with frequent bloody diarrhoea and mucus often with colicky lower abdominal pain, anorexia, weight loss, and urgency of stool. A minority present with severe/fulminating colitis, often with toxic megacolon when vomiting pyrexia, tachycardia, severe abdominal pain, distension and tenderness may occur with reduced bowel sounds, bloody diarrhoea (> five stools/24 hours) and hypoalbuminaemia that should be viewed as a medical emergency. See Table 9.6 for extraintestinal manifestations.

Gastrointestinal pan-endoscopy is essential.

Paediatric UC activity Index (PUCAI) includes scoring of the presence and severity of abdominal pain, rectal bleeding, stool

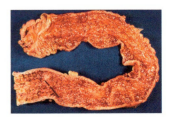

Figure 9.22 Ulcerative colitis showing extensive colonic involvement with inflammation and bleeding.

267

Table 9.6: Extra-Intestinal Manifestations of Classic Inflammatory Bowel Disease IBD

- Growth failure
- Arthritis and arthralgia: 20–25% UC, 11% Crohn
- Sacroiliitis and ankylosing spondylitis associated with HLA-B27
- Erythema nodosum in approximately 5% Crohn (> in Crohn)
- Pyoderma gangrenosum in 0.5–5% UC and 0.1% Crohn
- Liver disease:
- Sclerosing cholangitis
- Chronic active hepatitis and cholelithiasis: rare and can be severe
- Ocular manifestations:
- Uveitis < 3%
- Episcleritis and conjunctivitis
- Renal manifestations:
- Calcium oxalate stones < 5% children with Crohn (associated with ileal disease)

consistency and number/24 hours, nocturnal defaecation, and activity level. Please see the 2018 EPSGHAN guidance for management of acute UC.

Treatment

Aim to induce and maintain remission with:

- In mild disease an anti-inflammatory 5-aminosalicylate (5-ASA); generally two weeks to take effect.

- In more severe disease oral corticosteroids, reducing dose over 8–12 weeks, or primary monoclonal anti-TNFα therapy e.g. infliximab.

- If disease relapses when steroids are reduced/stopped consider azathioprine as a steroid-sparing agent after measuring thiopurine methyltransferase, TPMT activity to identify patients likely to be intolerant of regular azathioprine.

- Intravenous broad-spectrum antibiotics might be needed as an adjunct.

- Newer biologics, e.g. vedolizumab, ant-integrin $\alpha_4\beta_7$ are starting to be utilised in paediatric UC, and janus kinase (JAK) inhibitors such as tofacitinib are undergoing clinical trials.

There is no evidence that UC benefits from methotrexate administration.

- Surgical management with total colectomy and ileostomy formation is indicated for disease unresponsive to medical therapies, or refractory toxic megacolon. Subsequent ileo-anal pull-through with pouch formation may be undertaken.

- Up to 30% may develop antibodies to cow's milk; cow's milk avoidance might alleviate residual symptoms in some of these cases.

Prognosis

- Chronic relapsing disease course.

- Most children lead a normal lifestyle, but up to 20% have incapacitating disease.

- Risk of colonic malignancy increases if active pancolitis or left-sided colitis for > ten years. Colonoscopic surveillance is recommended ten years after diagnosis, with repeated surveillance at one, three or five years intervals depending on individual risk – NICE Clinical Guidelines (CG118).

- UC can be cured by total colectomy, but inflammation, pouchitis, of the surgically fashioned ileal pouch occurs in up to one-third of patients, usually those with ileitis pre-colectomy.

Crohn Disease
Incidence/Genetics

Increased since the 1950s to approximately 1 in 25,000 children, almost one-third of all cases presenting in late childhood with both sexes equally affected approximately 30% have a first-degree relative with IBD. Monozygotic twin concordance is 30%. Susceptibility is associated with MHC HLA-A2, HLA-DR1, and DQw5. There is an almost 20-fold increased CD risk with aberrant homozygous NOD2 gene (with 5% risk of ileal CD if homozygous).

Aetiology/Pathogenesis

The delicate pro- and anti-inflammatory balance managed by the GALT that tolerates normal bacterial commensals whilst enabling reactivity to intestinal pathogens is perturbed in CD with T helper (Th)1 cytokines and Th17 cytokines upregulated and impaired anti-inflammatory regulatory T-cell (Tregs) function. IL-23 is an important activator of Th17 cells and genes encoding proteins involved in IL-23 signalling and Th17 cell differentiation affect CD susceptibility, e.g. IL12B, CCR6, TNFSF15, and specific IL23R mutants (Arg381Gln) reduce risk approximately three-fold.

Clinical presentation is according to the predominant area/s of gut involved and presence or absence of stricturing and fistulae. Individuals with two disease-associated NOD2 mutations have more ileal disease and stricturing.

Diagnosis

Presents with insidious loss of appetite, weight loss, abdominal pain, diarrhoea and poor growth or short stature, delayed puberty, abdominal mass, perianal inflammation, aphthous mouth ulcers and extraintestinal problems, such as fever, arthritis, uveitis, erythema nodosum and liver disease. Disease is small intestinal alone in > 30% cases, colonic in 10–15% and ileocolitis in > 50% (Figures 9.23 and 9.24).

The definitive diagnosis is made on the histologically appearance of non-caseating epitheloid granulomata on intestinal mucosal biopsy. Investigate with upper intestinal endoscopy and colonoscopy with mucosal biopsies including terminal ileum. Macroscopically, CD appears as patchy inflammation with aphthous ulceration (Figure 9.25), sometimes with 'snail track' ulcers and 'cobblestone' appearance. Intestinal mucosal inflammatory infiltrate consists of monocytes, macrophages, lymphocytes and plasma cells and when acutely inflamed, neutrophils. Clinicopathological correlation is needed when pathology alone is not diagnostic.

Laboratory tests to monitor disease activity include blood platelets, haemoglobin, ESR/CRP, plasma albumin and faecal calprotectin. MRI enterographies (using contrast agents and medications, e.g. mannitol/lactulose for gut lumen distension) or small intestinal Barium contrast studies (Figure 9.26) in younger children, are undertaken to investigate for strictures, mucosal oedema/intestinal wall thickness and deep ulceration. Wireless video-capsule is becoming an additional standard of care.

Calculate Paediatric Crohn Disease Activity Index (PCDAI) at each clinic visit.

Treatment

Induce remission with induction of mucosal healing, not just clinical improvement, then continue therapy to maintain health. Treatments include:

- Exclusive liquid enteral nutrition (EN) with elemental or polymeric feed as sole nutritional source for 6–8 weeks is highly efficacious with full remission in > two-thirds of cases, especially if ileal disease. Inflammatory markers fall within few days of starting EEN. 'Nutritional' therapy also corrects nutritional deficiencies and facilitates 'catch up' weight gain and growth.

- Biological therapies including infliximab and adalimumab (monoclonal anti-TNF antibodies) are widely used. Anti-TNF therapies have an early role ('top-down') in fistulating disease or extensive small bowel disease, not responsive to EN. They are also effective in maintenance, although loss of response is seen with antibody formation. Co-administration with a thiopurine (dual therapy) is advised for infliximab. Newer therapies such as ustekinumab (targeting IL-12 and IL-23), are used for anti-TNF refractory disease.

- Azathioprine/mercaptopurine are used as disease modifying drugs. They are not useful in remission induction but once in remission they can help prevent recurrence.

- Antibiotics: metronidazole and ciprofloxacin often improve mucosal inflammation and perianal sepsis, but are not long-term therapies.

- Limited prednisolone use, e.g. symptomatic treatment of strictures whilst awaiting definitive therapy. Prednisolone is not used as first-line treatment since can induce clinical remission without mucosal healing and impairs bone density.

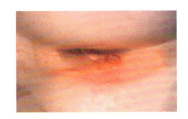

Figure 9.23 Crohn disease affecting perianal region.

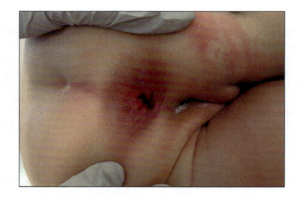

Figure 9.24   Crohn disease: perianal erythema and fissuring.

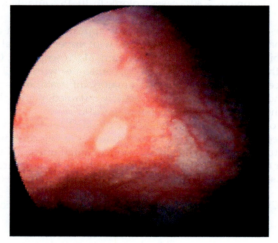

Figure 9.25   Crohn disease. Macroscopic appearance of colon, showing aphthous ulceration and loss of normal vascular pattern.

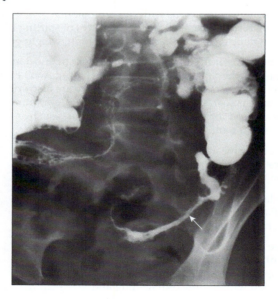

Figure 9.26   Crohn disease. radiological contrast studies demonstrating intestinal stricturing.

- Methotrexate can induce remission. It is used as a steroid-sparing agent and rarely as first-line treatment.

- Poor evidence for 5-aminosalicylate, 5-ASAs in colonic CD.

- Reserve surgery for chronic strictures or to de-function treatment resistant colonic disease, alongside other medications such as biological therapy.

Prognosis

- Usually chronic relapsing disease course.

- If well controlled with medical treatment, surgery is minimised.

- About 5% remain in remission after initial presentation, and another 5% have disease resistant to treatment, requiring aggressive medical treatment and possible surgery.

Very/Early Onset Inflammatory Bowel Disease (VEOIBD, EOIBD)
Incidence/Genetics

Rarely children develop IBD aged < 10 years, early onset IBD, EOIBD, often with > severity than in adolescents and adults. Onset < 6 years known as very early onset IBD, VEOIBD, has different underlying pathogenesis with approximately one-fifth (and one-third < 3 years old) with IBD-U. When onset is < 2 years old systemic immunodeficiencies are common. VEOIBD is associated with underlying monogenic disorders such as XIAP deficiency, chronic granulomatous disease, CGD, mutations in the β-polypeptide of cytochrome b-245, or other neutrophil defects.

Aetiology

Approximately 50 genetic disorders share IBD-immunology characteristics. Approximately 3–5% VEOIBD is monogenic, with incidence inversely associated with age of onset. Genetic defects present with IBD-like phenotype through several mechanisms:

1. Epithelial Barrier (e.g. TTC7A deficiency)

2. Phagocyte defects (e.g. glycogen storage disease type 1B [SLC37A4], congenital neutropenia [G6PC3])

3. Hyperinflammatory disorders (e.g. Mevalonate kinase deficiency [MVK])

4. Auto-inflammatory disorders (e.g. Familial Mediterranean Fever [MEFFV], X-linked lymphoproliferative syndrome 2 [XIAP])

5. T- and B-Cell defects (e.g. Agammaglobulinemia [BTK], SCID [IL2RG, CD3γ])

6. Immunoregulation (e.g. IPEX [FOXP3], IPEX-like [STAT1], IL-10 signalling defects [IL10RA, IL10RB, IL10])

Diagnosis

Children diagnosed aged < 6 years, should have EOIBD investigations (including targeted genetics and immunology) at a specialist centre with regular expertise in managing these disorders.

Treatment/Prognosis

- Many cases require PN support.

- Follows similar paradigms to CD and UC (please see above).

- If a monogenic disorder is identified appropriate treatment options, may include medical therapy, e.g. anti-TNF biologics, surgery, or allogeneic haematopoietic stem cell transplant.

- treatment response is poor in some conditions when long-term home PN is needed.

MULTISYSTEM INFLAMMATORY SYNDROME IN CHILDREN (MIS-C) – GI MANIFESTATIONS
Incidence/Genetics

MIS-C, also known as PIMS-TS (Paediatric inflammatory multisystem syndrome temporally associated with SARS-CoV-2) is a newly recognised condition associated with the SARS-CoV-2 virus.

During the COVID-19 pandemic, it was noted that although children were rarely affected severely with acute coronavirus, in very rare cases, children presented with symptoms similar to incomplete Kawasaki disease or toxic shock syndrome.

Aetiology

Strong association with SARS-CoV-2, with a three- to four-week lag between acute infection and MIS-C. It may represent a post-infectious complication of acquired immunity. The SARS-CoV-2 requires angiotensin converting enzyme-2 as a viral vector to enter cells. It is highly expressed in small intestinal enterocytes (as well as the lungs) – and may explain both symptoms.

Diagnosis

Diagnosis is clinical, with RCPCH consensus guidelines. Children present with fever and shock, often with respiratory distress or abnormal cardiac function and in 94% GI symptoms, such as vomiting, diarrhoea or abdominal pain. Check Coronavirus PCR and IgG serology to SARS-CoV-2. Routine blood tests show lymphocytopenia, neutrophilia, mild anaemia and thrombocytopenia. CRP, d-dimers and cytokines such as IL-6 are often raised. Faecal calprotectin is raised in approximately 20%, with distal ileum and caecum or liver abnormalities seen in 30% undergoing abdominal imaging.

Treatment

- Largely supportive, with targeted immunosuppressive therapy such as steroids, anti-TNF and anti-IL6 medications.
- Optimal treatment protocols continue to be evaluated – see the RECOVERY trial.
- any abnormal gastrointestinal and abdominal imaging should be followed-up; 95% GI tract, and 85% liver abnormalities resolved by 12 weeks.

LYMPHANGIECTASIA

Incidence/Genetics/Aetiology

Rare with pathological dilatation of an area of small intestinal lymphatic vessels and possible extraintestinal manifestation such as limb or lung involvement. Hennekam syndrome, an autosomal recessive condition, affects < 1 in 1,000,000 with characteristic facial appearance and developmental delay. Lymphangiectasia may develop secondary to elevated lymphatic pressure in congestive heart failure.

Diagnosis/Clinical Presentation

Macroscopic appearance of dilated lymphatics with diffusely swollen small intestinal mucosa seen on endoscopy, via video-capsule or enteroscopy. Small intestinal mucosal histology demonstrates dilated intestinal lymphatics with diffusely swollen mucosa and enlarged/distorted villi.

Diarrhoea, usually with oedema, develops when aged < 3 years, or in adolescence. There is faltering growth and increased frequency of infections with plasma lymphocytes < 1.5×10^9/l, low blood albumin, globulin and elevated stool alpha-1-antitrypsin level. If untreated chronic 'protein-losing enteropathy' with low blood cholesterol, calcium and fat-soluble vitamins develops.

Treatment and Prognosis

- Low-fat, high-protein, medium-chain triglyceride (MCT) diet, with fat-soluble vitamin supplements and regular albumin infusions if required.
- If severe PN may be needed.
- Consider surgical resection if affected area is limited.
- Severity is proportional to disease extent.

GASTRIC AND DUODENAL ULCERS

Incidence/Aetiology

Gastric ulcers are rare and usually secondary to other disorders, including burns, intracranial pathology, salicylates and other NSAIDs in children < 10 years.

Duodenal ulcers are associated with *Helicobacter pylori*.

Diagnosis

Neonatal peptic ulcers and secondary ulcers in older children commonly present with life-threatening haemorrhage or perforation. Abdominal pain may occur. Diagnosis is made on upper intestinal endoscopy (Figure 9.27).

Duodenal ulcers usually present with episodic epigastric pain, often awakening the child at night possibly with recurrent vomiting and haematemesis.

Diagnosis is made on macroscopic and histological appearance of mucosa obtained at upper intestinal endoscopy. Giemsa staining to detect *H. pylori* is essential.

Treatment/Prognosis

- PPI is first-line treatment for a Gastric ulcer.

- Secondary ulcers usually resolve completely after the acute episode.

- Treat duodenal ulcer as for *H. pylori* with recommended antibiotic combination.

- Excellent prognosis with lack of recurrence if *H. pylori* is eradicated.

PAEDIATRIC INTESTINAL PSEUDO-OBSTRUCTION (PIPO)

Incidence/Genetics/Aetiology

Rare, affecting < 1/40,000 live births with abnormal intestinal motility due to neuromuscular intestinal pathology. Up to 80% of cases are congenital, approximately 70% neuropathic and 30% myopathic.

Pathology of intestinal nerves, muscles or interstitial cells of Cajal:

- Additional intestinal muscle layer, X-linked FLNA mutations altering myocyte cytoskeleton filamin structure.

- Abnormal or deficient gamma-2 actin (smooth muscle contractile proteins) with ACTG2 gene mutation.

- Enteric nerve abnormalities including mitochondrial disorders (e.g. MNGIE see metabolic section).

- Infectious and autoimmune inflammatory pathologies.

- Syndromic forms with associated genetic mutations include filamin A (FLNA), L1CAM, actin G2 (ACTG2), thymidine phosphorylase (TYMP), polymerase γ (POLG), RAD21 and SGOL1.

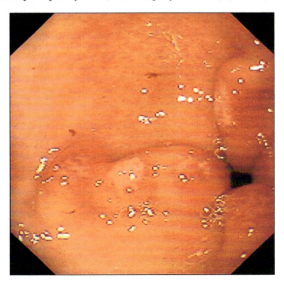

Figure 9.27 Endoscopic appearance of gastric ulcers and erosions adjacent to pylorus.

Diagnosis

Joint NASPGHAN/ESPGHAN consensus diagnostic criteria are >2 out of 4 of:

(i) Objective measure of small intestinal neuromuscular involvement (physiology, histopathology, transit studies).

(ii) Recurrent and/or persistently dilated loops of small intestine.

(iii) Genetic and/or metabolic abnormalities definitively associated with PIPO.

(iv) Inability to maintain adequate nutrition/growth on oral feeding.

80% present in infancy with 20% detected antenatally with non-obstructive megacystis. Childhood symptoms include abdominal distension, constipation, bilious vomiting and failure to thriv usually painless, severe pseudo-obstructive episodes may be continuous or intermittent. Malrotation occurs in > 30% with high risk of volvulus. Urological involvement in > 35% is commonly seen in hollow visceral myopathy and megacystis, microcolon hypoperistalsis syndrome (MMIHS), *ACTG2* gene associated conditions.

Diagnostic evaluation should be at a specialist centre with expertise in PIPO management.

Treatment/Prognosis

Supportive treatment with overnight continuous liquid enteral feeds to absorb sufficient nutrients and if not tolerated PN (Figures 9.28 and 9.29) with chronic IF in some cases.

There are many pharmacological treatment options, but response is generally poor. A potentially beneficial surgical procedure is decompressive ileostomy formation, which can result in improved feed tolerance in selected cases It is important to minimise surgery since adhesion-related complications are common. A few children on PN may require referral for intestinal transplant, usually late in the second decade of life.

SHORT BOWEL SYNDROME

Incidence/Aetiology

Short bowel syndrome (SBS) is a rare malabsorptive condition associated with a shortened small intestine resulting in failure of adequate weight gain and growth. The commonest aetiology in children is surgical resection of necrotising enterocolitis NEC and most cases present in the neonatal period. SBS incidence is increasing with improved premature birth survival.

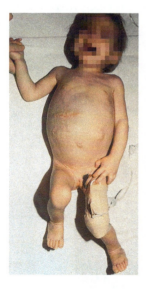

Figure 9.28 Intestinal pseudo-obstruction. abdominal distension and failure to thrive.

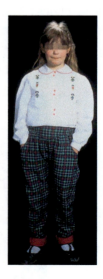

Figure 9.29 Intestinal pseudo-obstruction. The same child as in **9.28** growing and developing normally, solely on parenteral nutrition.

Mid-gut volvulus may present at any age with acute intestinal obstruction with/without bilious vomiting and if not diagnosed promptly and surgically treated without delay, extensive intestinal ischaemia occurs thus necessitating extensive but avoidable intestinal resection. Please see Table 9.6 for other aetiologies.

Infants with < 30–50 cm jejunum and ileum beyond the ligament of Treitz often have prolonged IF with dependence on PN > 27 days. Ultra-SBS refers to a small intestinal remnant < 10–20 cm.

Diagnosis

Diarrhoea and faltering growth with/without vomiting. Watery stool may be osmotic diarrhoea associated with sugar malabsorption. Symptoms are often worse if the ileo-caecal valve has been resected; the valve probably acts as an intestinal 'brake' and a barrier limiting colonic bacteria refluxing into the small intestine.

Investigations include:

- Upper intestinal radiological contrast study to exclude underlying anatomical abnormalities, e.g. strictures, excessive intestinal dilation.

- Oesophago-gastroduodenoscopy with colonoscopy if more severe diarrhoea and malabsorption than expected to exclude other pathology.

- Urine organic acids, blood D-lactate, stool and duodenal fluid m.c&s and/or hydrogen breath test to monitor for small intestinal bacterial overgrowth.

- Nutritional investigations include plasma electrolytes, urea, Ca, PO4, Mg, trace elements (zinc, copper, selenium), fat-soluble vitamins, A, D, E (most likely to be low) and K (prothrombin time), haemoglobin, ferritin and vitamin B12 (inevitable deficiency if terminal ileum resected, but may take several years to develop).

- Urine oxalate.

- Life-long annual monitoring of Vitamin B12, trace elements and fat-soluble vitamins if low levels detected in childhood.

Treatment

- Post-resection, PN is usually needed to ensure good electrolyte and fluid balance.

- Introduce oral/enteral feeds early to maintain entero-hepatic circulation and promote intestinal adaptation.

- Gradually reduce PN, with corresponding increase in enteral feeds as tolerated.

- Solid food usually tolerated > liquid enteral feed when aged > four to six months.

- If long-term PN needed, manage at home (see intestinal failure) by a specialist IF rehabilitation MDT team with > 10–20 home PN cases.

- GLP-2 treatment can assist enteral autonomy.

Prognosis

> 75% SBS patients who need home PN wean off within 4–5 years.

Adaptation is often sufficient for PN withdrawal if > 20 cm small intestine.

If ultra-SBS with < 20 cm small intestinal remnant, may depend on PN into adult life.

GLP-2 can promote intestinal autonomy in patients who would not have otherwise expected to gain it.

SBS children who have needed home PN are at risk of nutritional deficiencies and usually require life-long annual monitoring and supplements if deficiencies develop.

CONGENITAL INHERITED DIARRHOEAL DISORDERS
Congenital Chloride Diarrhoea

Aetiology/Incidence/Genetics

Autosomal recessive affecting 1 in 43,000 (Finnish data) with defective intestinal epithelial apical membrane chloride/bicarbonate exchanger molecule associated with mutations in *SLC26A3* gene, solute carrier family 26, chromosome 7.

Diagnosis

Secretory diarrhoea in utero leads to polyhydramnios premature birth, lack of meconium (watery stool mistaken for urine) and abdominal distension. Secretory diarrhoea persists even when nil by mouth. Rapid hyponatraemic, hypochloraemic dehydration with mild metabolic alkalosis, hypokalaemia and loss of > 10% birth weight in 24 hours with up to 300 ml/kg/d stool resulting in renal failure if unrecognised. Relevant investigations include plasma electrolytes and acid:base balance.

Treatment

- Intravenous fluid resuscitation with adequate sodium chloride replacement and
- Refer to specialist centre.
- Once stable, oral supplementation with sodium and potassium chloride, possibly requiring 6–10 mmol/kg/d chloride in infancy with <requirements with > age.
- Ratio Na:KCl typically 2:1 in infancy and 6:5 in older children.
- Butyrate therapy might reduce stool electrolyte losses by stimulating colonic chloride absorption.
- Consider gastrostomy in younger children.

Prognosis

- If diagnosed early and treated adequately, normal growth and development.
- Monitor blood electrolytes, urine sodium, blood pressure.
- Complications include secondary hyperaldosteronism and chronic renal failure.
- Acute diarrhoea episodes may require hospitalisation for IV fluids.

Glucose–Galactose Malabsorption
Incidence/Genetics/Aetiology

- Autosomal recessive, about 200 recognised cases worldwide.
- > 10% population has glucose intolerance, which maybe a milder form of the disease.
- Phenotype varies according to 'severity' of *SGLT1* gene mutation, chromosome 22.
- selective defect in intestinal sodium coupled glucose–galactose cotransporter.

Diagnosis

Severe osmotic diarrhoea from first glucose/galactose-containing feed, with positive faecal reducing substances. Diarrhoea stops when fasted. Stool sugar chromatography confirms diagnosis.

Treatment/Prognosis

Glucose and galactose free diet, substituting fructose-based feed. In older children/adults increasing amounts of glucose and galactose sometimes tolerated. If diagnosed and treated early, normal growth and development.

Sucrase–Isomaltase Deficiency

Incidence/Genetics Aetiology

Rare, autosomal recessive, *EC 3.2.1.48* gene, chromosome 3q25-q26, partial/total sucrase and reduced maltase levels on small intestinal brush border with wide phenotypic variation.

Diagnosis

Stool sugar chromatography positive for sucrose and low duodenal enterocyte sucrase level on frozen endoscopic duodenal biopsy assay. Frothy, watery diarrhoea starts when weaned onto sucrose/starch containing foods, possibly with secondary dehydration, faltering growth, vomiting and steatorrhoea.

Treatment/Prognosis

- Dietary sucrose and starch limited/avoided during first year of life.

- Variable starch tolerance from 2–3 years.

- Adult patients modify diet according to symptoms.

PANCREATIC DISEASE

Cystic Fibrosis – Intestinal
Incidence/Genetics/Aetiology

Commonest autosomal recessive disease affecting Caucasians, 1 in 2000–3000 live births with 5% carrier frequency. Abnormal epithelial cell chloride transport with mutations of transmembrane conductance regulator protein (*CFTR*) gene, chromosome 7, which encodes a cyclic-AMP regulated chloride and bicarbonate channel with > 400 recognised mutations. Familial concordance for disease severity since correlates with mutation type: severe ΔF508 mutation accounts for about 70% Caucasian cases. Patients with two 'severe' mutations have worse pancreatic failure.

Defective CFTR alters gastrointestinal and tracheobronchial epithelial cell electrolyte transport. Steatorrhoea secondary to reduced pancreatic exocrine secretions is the major gastrointestinal manifestation. Intestinal mucosal inflammation/enteropathy can also occur.

Clinical Presentation/Diagnosis

Abnormal sweat iontophoresis and genetics (please see the chapter 'Respiratory Medicine'). Presentation varies according to gene mutation; most UK cases are detected on neonatal screening. Gastrointestinal abnormalities involve the intestine, pancreas and liver:

- > 85% have fat malabsorption and faltering growth with some infants presenting with oedema, hypoalbuminaemia and anaemia and older children with large appetite and poor weight gain.

- Meconium ileus in about 10%.

- Rectal prolapse in < 20% usually from 1–2.5 years old and remits spontaneously by five years.

- Slow onset, non-IgE-mediated cow's milk protein intolerance in about 8% patients < 3 years old.

- Distal intestinal obstruction syndrome (DIOS) affects about 10% with intermittent intestinal obstruction with inspissated faecal contents (meconium ileus equivalent) in terminal ileum and right colon. Intussusception may occur. The aetiology is probably a secondary neuropathy consequent upon intestinal transmural lymphocytic inflammation.

  - 20–25% develop liver disease, progressing to cirrhosis in about 5%

  - Intrahepatic biliary epithelial cell damage predisposes to liver disease.

Intestinal investigations (please see the chapter 'Respiratory Medicine' for other investigations) include:

- Stool elastase: For pancreatic insufficiency.

- Plain abdominal x-ray in meconium ileus: Ground glass appearance (air bubbles trapped in meconium). Intraperitoneal calcification if meconium peritonitis.

- Barium enema in meconium ileus: Microcolon (Figure 9.30).

- Nutritional monitoring: Including serum fat-soluble vitamin and trace element levels, and urine Na.

Treatment

- hypertonic enema with intravenous fluid support for simple meconium ileus and if ineffective or 'meconium peritoneum' treat surgically.

Breast feeding is best and if unavailable give MCT-containing infant formula feeds (absorbed more efficiently)

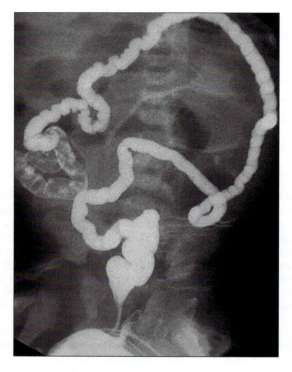

Figure 9.30   Cystic fibrosis. Barium study showing extensive microcolon in meconium ileus.

- Encourage high calorie, increased fat diet.
- Pancreatic enzyme (enteric-coated) replacement therapy (PERT) and fat-soluble vitamin supplements if stool elastase < 200µg/g. PERT dose usually < 10,000 IU/kg/d.
- If persistent steatorrhoea on this PERT dose exclude other causes of fat malabsorption, e.g. CF-related enteropathy.
- relieve DIOS with a mild laxative (if mild), oral N-acetylcysteine, gastrografin enema or intestinal lavage. Ensure appropriate dose of pancreatic supplements prescribed.

Prognosis

- If less severe genetic mutation with relatively good pancreatic function presentation is later and prognosis is better.

Shwachman–Bodian–Diamond Syndrome (SBDS)
Incidence/Aetiology/Genetics

Rare (1:80,000), autosomal recessive, SBDS gene mutations, chromosome 7, detected in > 90% cases. The SBDS protein is involved in key cellular functions including ribosomal function.

Diagnosis

- Feeding difficulties, faltering growth, diarrhoea and recurrent infections usually presenting in infancy.
- Haematological cytopenia of any lineage.
- exocrine pancreatic insufficiency.
- Supportive evidence includes bony abnormalities, short stature, hepatomegaly, learning and behavioural difficulties.

- Investigations include:
  - Stool elastase.
  - Ultrasound abdomen: possible small pancreas +/– lipomatosis.
  - Haematology: cyclical neutropenia and abnormal neutrophil mobility in > 90%, Cyclical thrombocytopenia in two-thirds and anaemia in 50%.
  - Bone marrow aspiration: possible fibrous tissue, fat or myeloid arrest.
  - Skeletal x-rays: abnormal femoral neck, short ribs with anterior flaring, vertebral wedging, clinodactyly and long bone changes.
  - Hepatomegaly with elevated transaminases.
  - Rarely, cardiac, respiratory, renal and/or testicular abnormalities.

Differential Diagnosis

Unlike cystic fibrosis, in SDS sweat electrolytes are normal. Food sensitive enteropathy and coeliac disease are excluded if histologically normal small intestinal mucosa. Consider other immunodeficiencies and bony abnormalities.

Treatment

- Specialist gastroenterology and haematology MDT service for diagnosis and shared care follow up.
- Ancreatic enzyme replacement starting dose 2000 units lipase/kg/d divided doses according to dietary fat intake.
- Monitor fat-soluble vitamin blood levels six-monthly and supplement if needed.
- Prophylactic antibiotics may reduce intercurrent infections.
- Iron-deficiency anaemia might require intravenous treatment.
- Neutropenia and recurrent invasive bacterial/fungal infections can benefit from granulocyte colony stimulating factor (G-CSF) therapy.
- If develop myelodysplastic syndrome, haematopoetic stem cell transplantation (HSCT) required.
- Regular dental surveillance.

Prognosis

- Most patients enjoy relatively good health.
- Poor growth persists, despite pancreatic enzyme replacement.
- Risk of myelodysplastic syndromes or leukaemia.

Acute Pancreatitis
Incidence/Genetics/Aetiology

About 30% associated with severe multi-system disease, e.g. sepsis, shock, systemic infection, collagen vascular diseases, IBD or Reye's syndrome. About 25% are related to trauma (blunt abdominal injury, including child abuse) or mechanical obstruction, others to metabolic disorders: hyperlipidaemia, hypercalcaemia, CF, renal disease, hypothermia, diabetes mellitus, organic acidaemias. Other pathologies include adverse reaction to medication, gallstones, congenital abnormalities of pancreaticobiliary drainage and post-ERCP. In up to 25% of cases there is no known predisposing factor.

Pancreatitis susceptibility genes include: *PRSS1* and *PRSS2* (cationic and anionic trypsinogens), *SPINK1* (serine protease inhibitor kazal Type 1), *CFTR* (cystic fibrosis conductance regulator), *CASR* (calcium sensing receptor), *CTRC* (chymotrypsin C), *CPA1* (chymotrypsinogen A1), *CEL* (carboxyl ester lipase)

Pathology

Pancreatic acinar cell injury leads to acute exocrine pancreatic inflammation then local and sometimes systemic inflammatory response. Experimental evidence has demonstrated intra-cellular acinar cell events at the initiation of cell injury.

Diagnosis

Sudden onset epigastric abdominal pain with severity increasing over several hours and persisting from hours-several weeks (average four days). Pain radiates usually through to the back in about 30% and episodes can be painless.

To diagnose, two-thirds of the following criteria is usually needed:

(i)   Characteristic pain

(ii) Pancreatic enzymes increased > 3x upper limit of normal

(iii) Imaging consistent with acute pancreatitis

Investigations include:

- Serum amylase: raised level for 2–5 days.

- Serum lipase elevated for longer since > half-life

- Early abdominal US and ALT level to exclude biliary pancreatitis.

- ALT > 150 IU/L < 48 hours after presentation = 85% predictive value for gallstone pancreatitis.

- Abdominal ultrasound: possible enlarged pancreas with reduced echogenicity.

- Contrast-enhanced CT scan – best on day four for evidence of pancreatic necrosis. Often normal in mild pancreatitis. Abnormalities include changes in pancreatic size and texture, pseudocyst, abscesses, calcification, duct enlargement, oedema, exudate and bowel distension.

- Measure CRP daily if CT evidence of pancreatic necrosis.

- Secretin stimulated MRCP – if recurrent acute pancreatitis to define ductular anatomy.

Differential Diagnosis

Other causes of abdominal pain and vomiting, e.g. biliary colic, intestinal malrotation, hepatitis.

Treatment

- Supportive, according to symptoms and complications.

- Severe acute pancreatitis needs intensive care.

- Initially stop oral intake and resuscitate early with IV lactated ringers' solution, shown to shorten hospital stay in children with acute pancreatitis.

- Analgesia.

- Octreotide is anecdotally helpful in reducing pain.

- Enteral nutrition with low-fat oral diet or liquid enteral feed once clinically stable.

- Predictive disease severity scores used in adults not validated in children. (Figures 9.31 and 9.32).

- Antibiotics not given routinely.

Prognosis

Varies from mild self-limiting abdominal discomfort to fulminant disease, progressing to multiorgan failure and, rarely, fatal outcome in hours or days.

Chronic Pancreatitis (Figure 9.33)

Incidence/Genetics

Idiopathic or autosomal dominant with 40–80% penetrance. Genetic associations include cationic trypsinogen (PRSS1), SPINK1, CFTR and chymotrypsinogen C (CTRC) mutations.

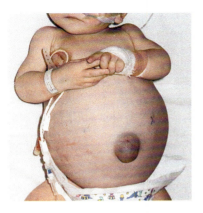

Figure 9.31 Acute pancreatitis: abdominal distension with blood-stained ascitic fluid, + positive Cullen's sign (peri-umbilical bruising).

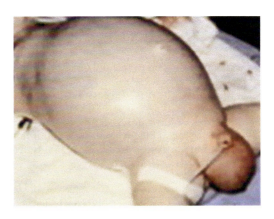

Figure 9.33 Severe abdominal distension with everted umbilicus and scrotal oedema in chronic pancreatitis.

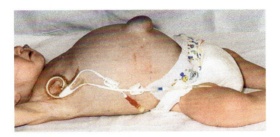

Figure 9.32 Management with PN and nasogastric drainage.

Diagnosis

- Onset from about 10 years but can present from 1 year.

- Episodic abdominal pain lasting two days–two weeks from monthly to yearly with < frequency with > age.
- Attacks maybe precipitated by large, fatty meals, alcohol and stress.
- Severe epigastric pain may radiate to the back and eased in fetal position.
- Epigastric tenderness with reduced bowel sounds and abdominal distension possible.
- Investigations include blood pancreatic enzyme levels, abdominal ultrasound, MRI.
- Endoscopic retrograde cholangiopancreatography (ERCP) when an anatomical cause suspected.

Treatment

Symptomatic and supportive. Pain relief difficult even with strong analgesics. Pancreatic enzyme replacement therapy occasionally needed with fat-soluble vitamin supplements

Prognosis

Long-term complications include pancreatic exocrine insufficiency and diabetes mellitus. If pancreatic duct dilated or pseudocyst or pancreatic ascites develop, pancreatico-jejunostomy maybe beneficial. Other patients lead normal lives without surgery.

INTESTINAL POLYPS

Solitary Juvenile Polyp

Incidence/Genetics

Sporadic affecting 1% preschool/school-aged children and up to 4% < 21 years. Male to female ratio is 3:2.

Aetiology/Clinical Presentation

Inflammatory colonic polyp, with over one in > 50% occurring proximal to sigmoid colon in about 60%. Painless rectal bleeding with/without faeces and/or mucus in 90%.

Abdominal pain after defaecation, polyp prolapse (dark beefy red mass) and/or sloughing of a larger polyp.

Diagnosis

Macroscopically a rounded polyp with slender stalk with hamartomatous histology (Figure 9.34).

Treatment/Prognosis

Colonoscopic polypectomy and histology. Low recurrence and no subsequent problems, e.g. malignancy.

Juvenile Polyposis Syndrome

Incidence/Genetics/Aetiology

Autosomal dominant, familial or sporadic with *BMPR1A*, *SMAD4* mutation of PTEN gene affecting 1:100,000–1:160,000 children.

Suspect when > five juvenile colonic and/or rectal polyps, multiple gastric and small intestinal juvenile polyps in addition to colonic, or > one polyp with family history of juvenile polyposis.

Diagnosis

Histologically hamartomatous polyp usually presenting with painless rectal bleeding (rarely life-threatening and maybe asymptomatic) and prolapse. Faltering growth, diarrhoea and intussusception are possible. Usually, symptomatic from 5 years when sporadic and 9 years when familial.

Treatment/Prognosis

Colonoscopic polypectomy and histology (Figure 9.35) followed by regular colonoscopic surveillance.

Risk of gastric and colonic malignancy (usually in adult life) if gastric involvement, but not if limited to colonic polyps.

Peutz–Jegher/Hereditary Intestinal Polyposis Syndrome

Incidence/Genetics /Aetiology

Autosomal dominant *STK11* gene, on chromosome 19, a possible tumour suppressor gene with incidence 1 in 50,000–200,000.

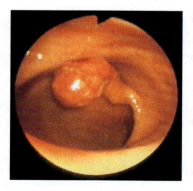

Figure 9.34 Isolated inflammatory/juvenile polyp.

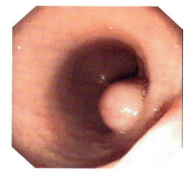

Figure 9.35 Juvenile polyposis syndrome: Polyp in duodenum.

Diagnosis

Hyperpigmented macules on lips and extending onto oral mucosa and facial skin (Figure 9.36). Commonly presents with abdominal pain with intussusception/mechanical intestinal polyp obstruction or iron-deficiency anaemia associated with bleeding polyp. Investigations include small intestinal radiological contrast study, upper intestinal endoscopy, video-capsule and colonoscopy with polypectomy (Figure 9.37). Diagnosis is histological finding of benign hamartomatous small intestinal and, in some cases, colonic polyps.

Differential Diagnosis

Oral hyperpigmentation also occurs with Addison disease and McCune–Albright syndrome.

Treatment/Prognosis

Endoscopic/laparoscopic polyp removal if causing excessive bleeding or intussusception.

Prognosis is usually good, but there is increased risk of intestinal and, rarely, gastric malignancy. Surveillance endoscopy needed.

PART 3: Infections and Infestations

HELICOBACTER PYLORI

(Please also see the section 'Duodenal Ulcer' above)

Incidence/Pathogenesis

Rare in children < 14 years in developed countries, but common in socio-economically deprived communities worldwide. *H. pylori* is a gram-negative, spiral, motile urease producing organism (Figure 9.38) that induces gastritis (often asymptomatic) by producing ammonia, probably toxic to gastric mucosa. Spread via person-to-person secretions.

Diagnosis

Gastric antral colonisation detected microscopically on Giemsa staining, urease testing and culture of mucosal biopsies obtained at upper gastrointestinal endoscopy.

Presents with epigastric pain, often nocturnal, and vomiting.

Screen stool for *Helicobacter* to diagnose and follow up post-eradication therapy.

Treatment/Prognosis

- Two-week course of triple therapy with a proton pump inhibitor plus antibiotics such as metronidazole and amoxicillin (or clarithromycin). Some regimes also include bismuth.

- Therapy is influenced by local antibiotic resistance patterns and whether the first or recurrent infection/treatment failure.

- Duodenal ulcers don't recur after *H. pylori* eradication.

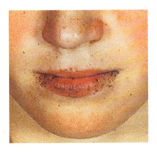

Figure 9.36 Brown pigmentation of lips and surrounds in Peutz–Jegher syndrome.

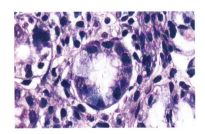

Figure 9.37 *Helicobacter*-like organisms within gastric glandular epithelium in sagittal cross-section.

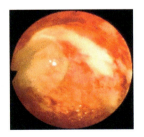

Figure 9.38 Colonic appearance of pseudomembranous colitis demonstrating severe erythema and yellow-white plaques.

BACTERIAL INFECTIONS OF THE SMALL AND LARGE INTESTINES

Campylobacter jejuni

Incidence/Aetiology

Usually sporadic with an unidentified source such as undercooked chicken/other meat or untreated water. It is the most frequently reported cause of acute bacterial diarrhoea in children worldwide, including the United Kingdom. Young children are most often affected.

Diagnosis

Malaise, headache, fever and within 24 hours, nausea, abdominal pain and mild to profuse watery, or bloody (especially young children) diarrhoea. Stool culture in low oxygen and high carbon-dioxyde environment detects gram-negative curvilinear rods. Infection can be associated wit,h Guillain–Barré syndrome.

Treatment

Usually self-limiting, but if systemically unwell and in patients < 2 years old treat with clarithromycin, azithromycin, erythromycin or occasionally ciprofloxacin.

Clostridium difficile

Aetiology

C. difficile is a gram-positive anaerobic bacterium that produces a cytotoxin and an enterotoxin. C. difficile toxin can be detected in healthy neonates, 10–50% of asymptomatic infants, and < 5% at 12 months.

Diagnosis

Diarrhoea varies from mild, acute, chronic, to severe if pseudomembranous colitis. Investigate stool for cytotoxin, toxigenic C. difficile or toxin A. Pseudomembranous colitis is characterised by macroscopic adherent yellow-white mucosal plaques on erythematous friable colonic mucosa (Figure 9.38).

Treatment

Any existing antibiotic treatment when diagnosed should be stopped and treatment with vancomycin or metronidazole commenced. Incidence can be reduced by probiotic treatment.

Salmonella

Incidence/Aetiology

Commonest in infancy and early childhood. Salmonella is a gram-negative, motile, aerobic bacillus, acquired from contaminated food or drink. Three types are Salmonella: enteritides (described here) choleraesius and typhi (typhoid fever).

Diagnosis

S. enteritides incubation usually 12–72 hours and longer in neonates. Usually presents with nausea and fever, then possibly watery or bloody diarrhoea. Complications including bacteraemia and systemic infection with meningitis, osteomyelitis and pneumonia are most common in infancy.

Treatment

ORS if possible and, if not, intravenous fluids. Antibiotics are not recommended, except in infants < 3 months old and bacteraemic children with signs of systemic infection.

Pathogenic Escherichia Coli

Incidence/Aetiology

E. coli are gram-negative motile bacilli that are some of the commonest healthy large intestinal flora. Pathogenic E. coli infection is one of the commonest causes of bacterial gastroenteritis worldwide. Transmission via faecal–oral contamination. Pathogenic mechanisms include:

1). Enterotoxin E. coli, ETEC produce heat labile (like cholera toxin) and heat stable toxins, resulting in profuse diarrhoea.

2). Enteroadherent *E. coli*, EPEC subdivided as tEPEC and aEPEC infection with attaching and effacing lesions cause infantile diarrhoea.

3). Enteroinvasive *E. coli*, EIEC produce the same shiga toxin as *Shigella dysenteriae*. Spread is through contaminated food and water and person to person.

4). Enterohaemorrhagic *E. coli*, EHEC, e.g. *E. coli* 0157 produce cytotoxin. They are transmitted from cattle and often acquired from undercooked fast food.

5). Enteroaggregative *E. coli*, EAEC have several virulence factors including adhesins, toxins and associated proteins.

6). Diffusely adherent DAEC.

Diagnosis

Presentation corresponds with the virulence mechanism (see Aetiology above):

- ETEC, 'traveller's diarrhoea' presents with nausea, vomiting, cramping abdominal pain and watery diarrhoea.

- Enteroadherent (EPEC) *E. coli* presents as above with additional fever and can persist for many weeks in children.

- EIEC presents with fever and bloody diarrhoea clinically indistinguishable from *Shigella* (Figure 9.39).

- EHEC causes bloody diarrhoea with haemolytic uraemic syndrome, HUS often developing about one week after onset, particularly in young children (Figure 9.40). Thrombocytopenic purpura may occur.

EAEC enteroaggregative *E. coli* can cause abdominal cramping pain and tenderness, watery, mucoid, or bloody diarrhoea, and sometimes nausea and vomiting.
Investigations include stool culture and antibiotic sensitivities.

Yersinia
Aetiology

A gram-negative bacillus spread via undercooked pork, contaminated milk and other food.

Diagnosis

Usually, acute self-limiting diarrhoea with possible fever, cramping abdominal pain, mimicking acute appendicitis and is the commonest bacterial aetiology of intussusception. Chronic diarrhoea may develop with erythema nodosum and arthritis. Infection can mimic Crohn disease with terminal ileal mucosal thickening, aphthous ulceration and nodularity. *Yersinia* isolation is difficult; a PCR-based assay may be feasible.

Treatment/Prognosis

Usually recover spontaneously in one to three weeks. Consider aminoglycoside or cephalosporin if treatment needed.

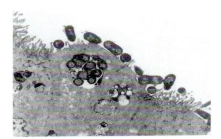

Figure 9.39 Electron microscopy of entero-pathogenic *Escherichia coli* with patchy micro-villous loss and cell invasion.

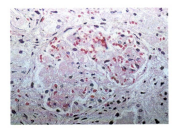

Figure 9.40 Renal biopsy of haemolytic uraemic syndrome, HUS showing micro-thrombi, swelling and destruction of glomerular capillaries.

INTESTINAL PARASITES

Giardia lamblia

Incidence/Pathogenesis

G. lamblia is a virtually worldwide flagellate protozoan, with infective cysts (that become motile
trophozoites) transmitted in food and water, faecal–
oral, person to person and by animals. Childhood
prevalence increases with age. It infects the small
intestine possibly causing an enteropathy of variable
severity.

Diagnosis

Usually chronic diarrhoea, nausea, foul-smelling flat-
ulence, poor appetite and steatorrhoea or occasionally acute watery diarrhoea, anorexia and abdominal
distension, or only minimal symptoms. Stool microscopy detects only 80%, even when several specimens
investigated. Organisms are visualised on duodenal
fluid microscopy and/or histologically on duodenal
mucosa (Figure 9.41). Symptoms may be suggestive
of coeliac disease, IBD or anorexia nervosa (anorexia
and weight loss).

Treatment/Prognosis

Single dose metronidazole, 30 mg/kg/day for three
days, or single dose tinidizole, 30 mg/kg/day.
Chronic infection is associated with immunoglobulin deficiency and poor growth.

Cryptosporidium

Incidence/Pathogenesis

Worldwide coccidian parasite that becomes incorporated in the small and/or large intestinal enterocytes,
external to the cytoplasm. Prevalence is > 10% in
undernourished iron deficient children in unhy-
gienic environments. Spread via water (sometimes in
UK tap water) and person to-person contact.

Pathogenesis may be related to microvillous membrane disruption resulting in enteropathy (Figures
9.42 and 9.43).

Diagnosis/Clinical Presentation

Acute, watery diarrhoea, fever, nausea, vomiting
and abdominal discomfort after 1–7 days incubation.
Prolonged symptoms occur in immunodeficiency,
including post-transplant. Oocytes can be detected
in stool, duodenal juices and sputum with suitable
staining techniques.

Treatment

Partial response to paromomycin, nitazoxanide
or azithromycin. Avoid by boiling tap water/
using bottled water if immunocompromised or
post-transplant.

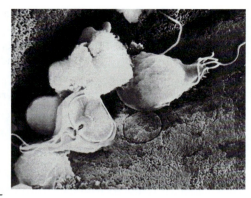

Figure 9.41 *Giardia lamblia*. Electron
micrograph of trophozoites in small
intestine.

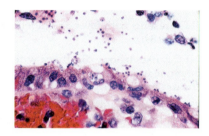

Figure 9.42 Cryptosporidiosos: intestinal specimen (×250).

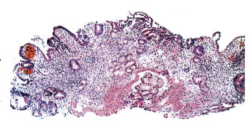

Figure 9.43 Cryptosporidiosos:
Cryptosporidium visible on small intestinal
mucosa (×16).

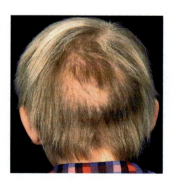

Figure 9.44 Menke disease: Pili torti.

Table 9.7: Trace Element Abnormalities

Mineral	Incidence/Genetics	Aetiology	Presentation/Diagnosis	Treatment/Prognosis
Copper Deficiency Cu	Rare	unsupplemented, long-term PN, severe malabsorption or – excessive zinc intake	Anaemia, neutropenia, bony abnormalities, skeletal fragility, skin depigmentation	Oral or IV copper
Menke's disease	X-linked recessive ATP7A Cu-transport protein Gene mutations 1 in 50,000–100,000.	Poor Cu absorption + metabolism with intracellular copper transport defect	As above + pili torti detected microscopically (Figure 9.44).	parenteral supplements
Copper Excess: Wilson Disease/ hepatolenticular degeneration	Rare autosomal recessive 1 in 30,000 worldwide. Carrier frequency 1 in 90 ATP7B gene mutations, chromosome 13.	inadequate biliary copper excretion	**Hepatic disease: from 5 years old,** ranging from acute self-limiting hepatitis to fulminant hepatic failure Chronic liver failure and cirrhosis in older patients . **Neurological:** motor disorder from about 6 years old, but usually in teens and 20s: tremor; incoordination, dystonia - later: drooling, dysarthria, gait disturbance . **Ophthalmological:** Kayser–Fleischer rings. **Psychiatric:** poor school performance, anxiety, depression, compulsive behaviour, psychosis. **Cardiac:** arrythmia, myocardial disease. **Renal:** proximal tubular dysfunction Renal calculi Penicillamine challenge: 24-hour urine Cu excretion (give 500 mg penicillamine, Urinary Cu excretion >1600 mcg/ > 25 micromol/24 hours probably Wilson's), usually low caeruloplasmin level (< 20 mg/dL or 200 mg/L) May need liver biopsies	Chelation therapy (see Chapter 8 Neurology). Normal life expectancy if diagnosed and treated early
Iron-Deficiency Fe please see Haematology Chapter 11	commonest in infancy and adolescence, particularly Asians, vegetarians and vegans	poor dietary intake: common in preschool children, particularly if high cow's milk intake Malabsorption: Coeliac disease/other Enteropathy, Excessive loss: gastrointestinal/ other blood loss e.g. severe GORD, gastritis, UC	Clinical: lethargy, poor exercise tolerance pica, poor appetite poor concentration span, lowered resistance to infection, poor thermoregulation anaemia. Investigations: haemoglobin; haematocrit; red blood cell indices to distinguish normocytic, or microcytic, hypochromic anaemia serum iron and total iron binding capacity (TIBC) plasma ferritin level. Rarely, bone marrow aspirate	Ensure adequate dietary intake - oral iron supplement or IV infusion if oral not absorbed - treat underlying disease
Selenium Deficiency Se		Rare: severe malabsorption unsupplemented long-term PN	Macrocytic anaemia, cardiomyopathy, myositis plasma glutathione peroxidase activity	Oral/enteral Se or IV supplements
Zinc Deficiency Zn	Rare minority of cases autosomal recessive acrodermatitis enteropathica selective defect in intestinal Zn absorption (see also the chapter 'Dermatology'). Most Zn excreted via gastrointestinal tract and some via kidneys	Inadequate nutritional intake: protein-energy malnutrition malabsorption, e.g. protracted diarrhoea, high- output fistula, SBS or acrodermatitis enteropathica	Scaly, erythematous skin rash with perioral and perianal bullae and pustules may occur symmetrically in interdigital areas and over buttocks, hands, feet and elbows (Figures 9.45 to 9.47) Alopecia, dystrophic nails, photophobia, conjunctivitis (Figures 9.60 to 9.63) diarrhoea with malabsorption, psychological and behavioural disturbances susceptibility to infection	Oral/enteral or parenteral supplement Treat underlying disease

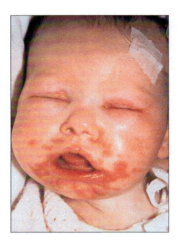

Figure 9.45 Zinc deficiency affecting peri-oral area and face.

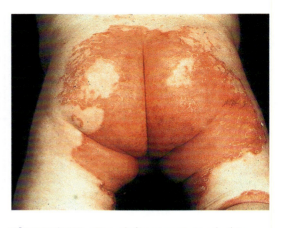

Figure 9.46 Zinc deficiency: Buttock skin rash.

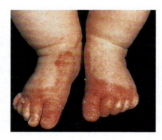

Figure 9.47 Zinc deficiency: Appearance of the feet.

Ascaris Lumbricoides (Roundworm)

Incidence/Aetiology

One of the commonest human parasitic infections worldwide, although uncommon in United Kingdom. Larvae hatch from ingested eggs, enter the venous system and migrate through the lungs to the oesophagus. Fertilised eggs from adult intestinal worms are passed with faeces to contaminate soil, with cycle recurrence when ingested.

Diagnosis

Usually asymptomatic, but cough, wheeze, fever and eosinophilia may occur during the pulmonary phase. Anorexia, abdominal cramps and intestinal obstruction can occur with heavy infestation. Migrating worms can cause jaundice with biliary obstruction, pancreatitis by blocking pancreatic ducts, appendicitis, and lead to volvulus, intussusception, intestinal perforation and peritonitis. Ova and adult worms can be detected with faecal microscopy and larvae in sputum and gastric washings.

Treatment

Mebendazole or piperazine. Endoscopic retrograde cholangiopancreatography, ERCP, to relieve biliary and/or pancreatic duct obstruction and surgery for intestinal obstruction.

Enterobius Vermicularis (Pinworm/Threadworm)

Incidence/Pathogenesis

E. vermicularis is most common in temperate and cold climates, but also occurs worldwide. Children, and household contacts of infected people are at highest infection risk.

Aetiology

Spread through human-to-human transmission, by ingesting eggs and/or by anal insertion.

Eggs are laid near the anus, and are readily transmitted through contamination of finger-nails, hands, night clothing and bed linen. They can remain viable for up to three weeks if moist environment.

Diagnosis

Anal pruritis, worst at night when adult females lay eggs perianally. Other symptoms include appendicitis and adult worms rarely migrate through the intestinal wall to invade other organs. The 'Sellotape test' involves placing clear adhesive tape over the perianal region at night, then removing and examining it for small white specks/ova in the morning.

Table 9.8: Vitamin Deficiencies

vitamin	Incidence/Aetiology	Diagnosis	Treatment/Prognosis	Dietary sources
Vitamin A Retinol	> 124 million deficient children worldwide Poor dietary intake or secondary to fat malabsorption	xerophthalmia: conjunctival xerosis Bitot spots, keratinisation, corneal necrosis (Figures 9.50 and 9.51). Vitamin A blood level < 200 µg/l	Oral supplement IM if severe deficiency Estimated 1–2 million deaths/year aged 1–4 years 250,000–500,000 blind/year – 50% < 12 months die after sight loss	yellow/orange fruit green/leafy vegetables, liver, milk, butter, cheese, eggs
Beriberi, Vitamin B₁/ Thiamin Deficiency it presents with	Beriberi manifests as: 'wet' beriberi: India and Far East breast-fed infants of mothers with polished rice diet 2. 'dry' beriberi/Wernicke's encephalopathy: Developed countries – sensory + motor neuropathy encephalopathy in children on total PN given > two weeks without B vitamins older children with polished rice based diet Presents with: drowsiness + meningism comatose	'wet' and 'dry' acute high output cardiac failure: coughing, choking, aphonia with laryngeal oedema Investigations: trial supplement blood transketolase activity	IM vitamin B (50–100 mg), then oral supplements	nuts, peas, beans, pulses brewer's yeast Polished rice should be enriched with thiamin
Riboflavin/Vitamin B₂ Deficiency	recurrent diarrhoea, malabsorption, haemo-/peritoneal-dialysis	Cheilosis, magenta coloured tongue (Figure 9.52), nasolabial seborrhoea If deficient, in vitro addition of flavin adenine dinucleotide increases erythrocyte glutathione reductase activity by > 30%.	Riboflavin 20 mg/d	Beef, pork, chicken, salmon, green vegetables, almonds
Vitamin B3 Deficiency Niacin	Pellagra: 1, Endemic in parts of Africa, where maize based diet. Poor bioavailability of nicotinic acid low tryptophan in maize. Pyridoxine deficiency: essential cofactor for nicotinic acid synthesis from trypyophan	Dementia,diarrhoea,dermatitis Skin: photosensitive dermatitis, scaling and pigmentation (Figure 9.53) Gut: angular stomatitis diarrhoea Neurological: depression, dementia, delirium, peripheral neuropathy Investigations: rapid response to supplements urinary levels of N1methyl nicotinamide and pyridone derivatives	Oral niacin or nicotinamide Or IV supplement four-hourly vitamin B (100 mg) preparation	Nutritional yeast Eggs Pulses, wholemeal cereals, meat, fish
Vitamin B6 Pyridoxine	iatrogenic when treated with pyridoxine antagonists: isoniazid, hydralazine, penicillamine, oestrogens – poor intake, malabsorption Autosomal recessive ALDH7A1 antiquitin gene, pyridoxine dependency	convulsions, depression, peripheral neuropathy, anorexia Investigations: 1. serum pyridoxal 5-phosphate; 2. in vitro > red cell AST and ALT in presence of pyridoxal 5-phosphate Rare: pyridoxine dependency; seizures from infancy	oral pyridoxine 10 mg/d High doses pyridoxine	Whole grain cereals bananas, liver, peanuts fish

(Continued)

Table 9.8: **Vitamin Deficiencies (Continued)**

vitamin	Incidence/Aetiology	Diagnosis	Treatment/Prognosis	Dietary sources
Cyanocobalamin/Vitamin B_{12} Deficiency	Vitamin B_{12} deficiency is common in: post-terminal ileal resection – vegan diet – intrinsic factor deficiency	Anaemia, yellow tinted skin, fatigue. glossitis, paraesthesia, ataxia and if severe, dementia. Investigations: blood B_{12}	IM hydroxycobalamin if post-terminal ileum resection or intrinsic factor deficiency. Oral supplement if deficient diet	derived solely from animal products: meat, fish, milk, cheese, eggs, some fortified foods
Vitamin C Ascorbic Acid Deficiency = Scurvy	Rarely in famines Severe autism with selective eating	bleeding of gums, hair follicles, capillaries irritability + painful limbs 'pseudoparalysis'. Investigations: 1. response to supplements; 2. plasma and white cell ascorbic acid level 3. bone x-ray: subperiosteal haematoma calcification with 'ground glass' metaphyses and 'smoke-ring' of epiphyseal cortical bone	Ascorbic acid 500 mg/day for 1 week treat immediately since risk of sudden death. rapid response to treatment, (bone remodelling takes months)	Citrus fruit green vegetables
Vitamin D	deficiency common in general population Incidence highest if avoid sunlight, pigmented skin, avoid dietary dairy products Fat malabsorption e.g. coeliac disease, Cystic Fibrosis, Crohn Disease vegan diet, obesity (Vitamin D taken up into fat cells). renal disease low 1,25 dihydroxy vitamin D (most active form), Anticonvulsants (induce hepatic enzymes) Rare autosomal recessive vitamin D-dependent rickets X-linked dominant hypophosphataemic rickets	• Rickets: genu valgum, epiphyseal swelling (especially distal radii) and growth retardation. • Skull: craniotabes, delayed closure of fontanelles and bossing of frontal and parietal bones. Chest: 'pectus carinatum', enlarged costochondral junctions, rib cage depression where the diaphragm is inserted (**Figure 9.52**). Delayed dentition, irritability, hypotonia, risk of severe asthma, respiratory failure, tetany, laryngospasm, convulsions, aminoaciduria. Investigations: blood alkaline phosphatase high phosphate and/or calcium low x-ray-wide metaphyseal plate and concave diaphyseal ends; plasma vitamin D level	10 µg/d of vitamin D Vitamin D 1000–5000 µg IV/d given until alkaline phosphatase normal, then 10 µg/d	Exposure to sunlight for ergocalciferol dietary source includes oily fish and fortified margarine. + 500 ml/d of milk for calcium requirements. important
Vitamin E/ Tocopherol	Rare: Fat malabsorption common vitamin E deficiency in children with long-term IF	steatorrhoea and haemolysis in premature neonates. Neurological changes: wide-based gait, spinocerebellar degeneration, ocular palsy Investigations: serum vitamin E level, red cell susceptibility to haemolysis by hydrogen peroxidase	oral or IM tocopherol	
Vitamin K	Rare: newborn infants, fat malabsorption	Coagulopathy, haemorrhagic disease of the newborn Deficiency: prolonged clotting and may affect bone formation. Intestinal flora can manufacture quinones with vitamin K activity. Antibiotics may lead to deficiency by supressing intestinal flora	Oral Vitamin K supplements	

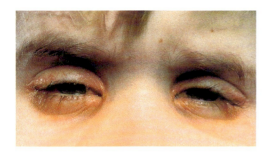

Figure 9.48 Vitamin A deficiency in child with SBS and steatorrhoea.

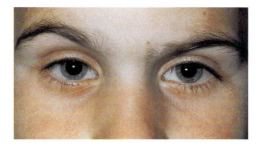

Figure 9.49 The child in 9.50 after treatment.

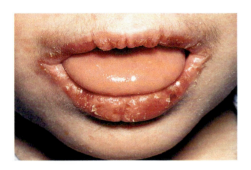

Figure 9.50 Angular stomatitis, cheilosis and magenta tongue with B-group vitamin deficiency.

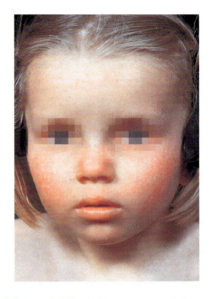

Figure 9.51 Pellagra associated dermatitis.

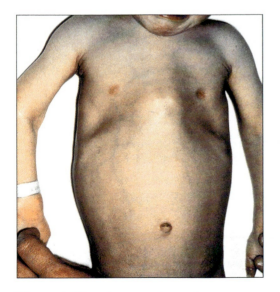

Figure 9.52 'Pectus carinatum', enlarged costochondral junctions, ribcage depression where the diaphragm is inserted.

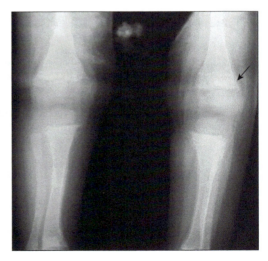

Figure 9.53 X-ray of femurs demonstrating wide metaphyseal plate and concave diaphyseal ends.

Treatment/Prognosis

Mebendazole and for infants, piperazine. Treat the whole family and repeat 2–4 weeks later to eradicate worms hatched since first treatment. Reinfection readily develops and should be prevented, by treating household contacts as above.

PART 4: Micronutrient Disorders (Deficiencies, Toxicity)

Micronutrient disorders may be related to inadequate or excessive dietary intake, malabsorption or abnormal metabolism. Children most at risk are those offered an inadequate diet, e.g. protein-calorie under-nutrition and children dependent on artificial nutrition, in particular PN. Please see Table 9.7 for details.

Plasma copper and zinc levels are inversely proportional.

VITAMIN DEFICIENCIES

Vitamins are organic food substances not synthesised by the body. Small amounts are essential for normal metabolism. The B-group vitamins and vitamin C are water soluble. Vitamins A, D, E and K are fat-soluble. If lipid is excluded from PN fat-soluble vitamins will not be given and enteral or IM supplements are needed. Please see Table 9.8 for details.

BIBLIOGRAPHY

General reading

- Guandalini, S. and Dhawan, A. (2022). *Textbook of pediatric gastroenterology, Hepatology and nutrition: A comprehensive guide to practice.* Cham: Springer.

Acute gastroenteritis

- Guarino A., Aguilar J., Berkley J. et al. (2022). Acute gastroenteritis in children of the world: What needs to be done? *J Pediatr Gastroenterol Nutr*, 70(5): 694-701. doi: 10.1097/MPG.0000000000002669. PMID: 32079974.

Faltering growth

- Derraik, J.G.B., Maessen, S.E., Gibbins, J.D. et al. (2020) Large-for-gestational-age phenotypes and obesity risk in adulthood: A study of 195,936 women. *Sci Rep* 10, 2157.

Constipation

- NICE. (2017). Constipation in children and young people: diagnosis and management. *NICE*. Available at: https://cks.nice.org.uk/topics/constipation-in-children

Recurrent abdominal pain

- Reust, C.E. and Williams, A. (2018). Recurrent abdominal pain in children. *Am Fam Physician*. 15:785–793. PMID: 30216016.

Cyclical vomiting

- Li, B.U.K. (2018). Managing cyclic vomiting syndrome in children: Beyond the guidelines. *Eur J Pediatr.* 177(10): 1435–1442. doi:10.1007/s00431-018-3218-7

Toddler's diarrhoea

- Giannattasio, A., Guarino, A., Lo Vecchio, A. (2016) Management of children with prolonged diarrhea. *F1000Res*, 5:F1000 Faculty Rev-206. doi:10.12688/f1000research.7469.1

Coeliac disease

- Husby, S. et al. (2020). European society paediatric gastroenterology, hepatology and nutrition guidelines for diagnosing coeliac disease 2020. *Journal of Pediatric Gastroenterology and Nutrition* 70(1) (2020): 141–156.
- ESPGHAN. (2020) New guidelines for the diagnosis of paediatric coeliac disease. *European Society for Pediatric Gastroenterology, Hepatology, and Nutrition*. Available at: New_Guidelines_for _the_diagnosis_of_paediatric_coeliac_disease.ESPGHAN_Advice_Guide.pdf

Gastro-oesophageal reflux

- Gonzalez Ayerbe, J.I., Hauser B., Salvatore S., et al. (2019). Diagnosis and management of gastro-esophageal reflux disease in infants and children: From guidelines to clinical practice. *Pediatr Gastroenterol Hepatol Nutr.*, 22(2): 107–121. doi:10.5223/pghn.2019.22.2.107

Food allergic gastrointestinal disease

- Jackman, L. and Moolenschot, K. (2021). Algorithm for dietary management of eosinophilic oesophagitis (EoE) in paediatrics on behalf of the BSPGHAN EoE working group Dietetic management of eosinophilic oesophagitis. *BSPGHAN*. Available at: https://bspghan.org.uk/wp-content/uploads/2021/11/Dietetic-management-of-EoE.pdf

Ulcerative colitis

- Turner, D., Ruemmele, F.M., Orlanski-Meyer. E. (2018). Management of paediatric ulcerative colitis, Part 1: Ambulatory care—An evidence-based guideline from European Crohn's and Colitis Organization and European Society of Paediatric Gastroenterology, Hepatology and Nutrition. *J Pediatr Gastroenterol Nutr*, 67: 257–291

Crohn disease

- Rheenen, P.F., Aloi, M., Assa, A. et al. (2021). The medical management of paediatric Crohn's disease: An ECCO-ESPGHAN guideline update. *Journal of Crohn's and* Colitis, 15: 171–194.

Very early onset IBD

- Holm, H. et al. (2014). The diagnostic approach to monogenic very early onset inflammatory bowel disease. *Gastroenterology*, 147: 990–1007. https://doi.org/10.1053/j.gastro.2014.07.023.

Helicobacter pylori

- National Institute for Health and Care Excellence. (2021). *Clostridioides difficile* infection: Antimicrobial prescribing. *NICE*. London: National Institute for Health and Care Excellence. Available from: https://www.ncbi.nlm.nih.gov/books/NBK573295/

Intestinal parasites

- Hodges, P. and Kelly, P. (2022). Intestinal parasites. In *Textbook of Pediatric Gastroenterology, Hepatology and Nutrition* (Editors: Guandalini, S. and Dhawan, A). Springer. 17–30

Cystic fibrosis

- National Institute for Health and Care Excellence. (2017). Cystic fibrosis: diagnosis and management. *NICE*. Available at: www.nice.org.uk/guidance/ng78

Pancreatitis

- Freeman, A.J., Maqbool, A., Bellin, M.D. et al. (2021). Medical management of chronic pancreatitis in children: A position paper by the North American Society for Pediatric Gastroenterology, Hepatology, and Nutrition Pancreas Committee. *JPGN*. 72: 324–340

Polyps

- Tripathi, P.R., Sen Sarma, M,. Yachha, S.K., Lal, R., Srivastava, A., and Poddar, U. (2021). Gastrointestinal polyps and polyposis in children: Experience of endoscopic and surgical outcomes. *Dig Dis*, 39(1): 25–32. doi: 10.1159/000508866. PMID: 32450557.

Infantile intractable diarrhoea

- Nocerino, A. and Guandalini, S. (2022). Microvillous inclusion disease and tufting enteropathy. In *Textbook of Pediatric Gastroenterology, Hepatology and Nutrition* (Editors: Guandalini, S. and Dhawan, A). Springer. 3–17.

Chronic intestinal failure

- Hill, S., Ksiazyk, J., Prell, C. et al. (2018). ESPGHAN/ESPEN/ESPR/CSPEN guidelines on pediatric parenteral nutrition: Home parenteral nutrition. *Clinical Nutrition*, 37(6): 2401–8.

Intestinal transplant

- Soltys, K.A., Bond, G., Sindhi R. et al. (2017). Pediatric intestinal transplantation. *Semin Pediatr Surg*. 26(4): 241–49. doi: 10.1053/j.sempedsurg.2017.07.007. PMID: 28964480

Micronutrient deficiencies

- Bronsky, J., Campoy C., and Braegger, C. (2018). ESPGHAN/ESPEN/ESPR/CSPEN guidelines on pediatric parenteral nutrition: Vitamins. *Clin Nutr*, 37(6B) 1–13.

10 Kidney Diseases

Stephen D. Marks

ACUTE KIDNEY INJURY

Incidence
Acute kidney injury (AKI) is a sudden decline in glomerular filtration rate (GFR) which is potentially reversible, with or without oliguria.

Aetiology
Pre-renal AKI is associated with decreased true intravascular volume or circulatory failure (Table 10.1). There is peripheral vasoconstriction, a low blood pressure and central venous pressure (CVP) and a fractional excretion of sodium of less than 1%. If AKI is due to renal causes, there is salt and water retention with blood, protein and casts in the urine, and symptoms specific to an accompanying disease (e.g. IgA vasculitis (previously called Henoch–Schönlein purpura) nephritis). AKI in a patient with undiagnosed chronic kidney disease (CKD) is suggested by a poorly grown child with long-standing symptoms of CKD.

Investigations
An ultrasound is the most important investigation, in order to identify hydro-ureteronephrosis caused by obstruction of the urinary tract that may require intervention, small kidneys of CKD, or large echobright kidneys with loss of cortico-medullary differentiation, typical of an acute process (Table 10.2). Percutaneous renal biopsy is indicated if the diagnosis is unclear, in order to exclude a crescentic nephritis that would require treatment with immunosuppression (Figure 10.1).

Table 10.1: Causes of Acute Kidney Injury

Pre-renal

Hypovolaemia and/or hypotension

(e.g. gastroenteritis, dehydration, sepsis, burns, cardiac failure, cardiac tamponade)

Renal

Arterial (e.g. haemolytic uraemic syndrome, arteritis, embolic)

Venous (e.g. renal venous thrombosis)

Glomerular (e.g. glomerulonephritis)

Interstitial (e.g. tubulointerstitial nephritis, pyelonephritis)

Tubular (e.g. acute tubular necrosis, ischaemic, toxic, obstructive)

Post-renal

Congenital obstruction

Acquired obstruction

Table 10.2: Investigation of Acute Kidney Injury

- Blood tests:
  - full blood count, blood film, coagulation screen
  - ESR, CRP and blood culture
  - sodium, potassium, chloride, bicarbonate, urea, creatinine, glucose, blood gas
  - calcium, phosphate, magnesium, albumin, ALP, liver function tests, CK, LDH, urate
  - ASO titre and antiDNase B
  - Complement C3, C4, serum immunoglobulins IgG, IgA and IgM
  - ANA, anti-dsDNA, ANCA and anti-GBM antibody
- Urine tests:
  - dipstick (blood and protein), microscopy and culture
  - sodium, urea, albumin, protein and creatinine
- Throat swab
- Stool culture
- Doppler renal ultrasound
- Percutaneous renal biopsy (if unknown cause of acute kidney injury)
- X-ray hand and wrist, chest x-ray, ECG, echocardiography and PTH if evidence of CKD

DOI: 10.1201/9781003175186-10

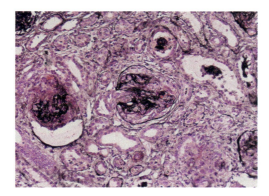

Figure 10.1 Histopathology of percutaneous renal biopsy showing a crescentic nephritis causing acute kidney injury with rapidly progressive glomerulonephritis.

Table 10.3: Indications for Dialysis

- Failure of conservative management
- Hyperkalaemia
- Severe hypo-or hypernatraemia
- Fluid overload resistant to medical therapy with pulmonary oedema and/or hypertension
- Severe acidosis
- Multiorgan failure

Treatment

Conservative management is by attention to fluid balance and diet (controlled protein, high calorie, low phosphate and potassium) and attention to fluid balance. Hypovolaemia should be corrected with normal saline or plasma. Fluid overload may respond to furosemide and fluid restriction to insensible losses, although some children may require kidney replacement therapy with dialysis (Table 10.3).

HAEMOLYTIC URAEMIC SYNDROME

Incidence/Aetiology

Haemolytic uraemic syndrome (HUS) is one of the commonest causes of AKI in childhood. The commonest cause is STEC-HUS caused by Shiga toxin or Verocytotoxin *Escherichia coli* (STEC or VTEC) which typically results in bloody diarrhoea.

- STEC-HUS occurs mainly in childhood but also in the elderly population, sporadically in summer months or in epidemics. Infective causes vary in different countries across the world, but Shigatoxin producing STEC 0157 H7 and other serotypes and *Shigella dysenteriae* Type 1 are the commonest aetiological organisms. Infections have been isolated from various sources from ingestion of unpasteurised milk and apple juice, unwashed vegetables, uncooked meat to contaminated water supplies.

- Atypical HUS accounts for 10% of cases, affects all ages without seasonal pattern. Infective causes are neuraminidase-producing *Streptococcus pneumoniae* and HIV. Inherited forms of this life-threatening disease, characterised by chronic uncontrolled complement activation, may have identifiable complement gene mutations (such as factor H and factor I mutations) in 60–70% of patients. Our genetics knowledge is evolving with autosomal dominant or recessive forms as well as neonatal presentation of inborn errors of cobalamin metabolism. The incidence is approximately two per million population, of which nearly 60% present in children, although the oldest patient has presented at age of 83 years, and can be associated with relapses with worsening hypertension, proteinuria and/or renal dysfunction. Deficiency of complement factor H-related (CFHR) proteins and CFH autoantibody positive HUS (DEAP-HUS) represents a unique subgroup of complement-mediated atypical HUS. CFH autoantibodies are found in 10 to 15% of atypical HUS patients and occur almost exclusively in patients with CFHR1 or CFHR3/CFHR1 deletions.

Drug-induced causes of HUS have been reported with calcineurin inhibitors (ciclosporin and tacrolimus), chemotherapeutic agents, antiplatelet agents and oral contraceptive pills. Other causes include bone marrow and solid organ transplantation, malignancy, pregnancy, systemic lupus erythematosus (SLE) and glomerulonephritis.

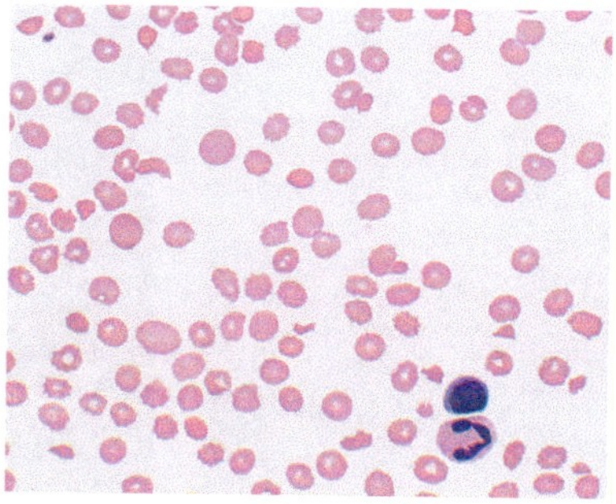

Clinical Presentation

HUS should always be considered in children who present with diarrhoea (often bloody), vomiting and severe abdominal pain with associated pallor, lethargy, jaundice, petechiae, bleeding, oligo-anuria, fluid overload, oedema, hypertension, convulsions, coma, pancreatitis and pneumonia.

Differential Diagnosis

There is an overlap with thrombotic thrombocytopenic purpura (TTP), which is also characterised by thrombocytopenia, microangiopathic haemolytic anaemia and abnormalities in renal function. However, neurological symptoms and signs, and associated fever, are much more prominent in TTP.

Figure 10.2 May Grünwald–Giemsa stained peripheral blood smear showing a reactive lymphocyte above a neutrophil (arrow) with evidence of microangiopathic haemolytic anaemia. There are numerous red blood cell fragments, thrombocytopenia, few spherocytes and polychromasia in a case of diarrhoea-associated haemolytic uraemic syndrome.

Diagnosis

A triad of Coombs' negative microangiopathic haemolytic anaemia (Figure 10.2) with fragmented red cells, thrombocytopenia and acute kidney injury is found. Investigations include: full blood count; differential white cell count; blood film; reticulocyte count; ferritin; Coombs' tests; group and save; urea; creatinine; serum electrolytes; glucose; amylase; lipase; lactate dehydrogenase; haptoglobin; liver function tests; serology; Thomsen–Friedenreich antigen (T-Ag); antistreptolysin O titre (ASOT); urine dipstick and urine albumin to creatinine ratio; stool culture and PCR; and Doppler renal ultrasound. Percutaneous renal biopsy is not routinely indicated in D+ HUS but may show predominant glomerular or arteriolar involvement and acute cortical necrosis.

Treatment

Overall treatment of HUS is similar to any cause of AKI therapy, with optimal fluid and electrolyte management, diuretic therapy, other antihypertensive agents and dialysis. There is no role for antibiotics which may exacerbate HUS, except when there is proven streptococcal infection. Unregulated complement leads to progression of symptoms so there should be consideration for plasma infusions and/or exchange in patients with atypical HUS (Figure 10.3). Eculizumab is a humanised anti-C5 monoclonal antibody that may overcome the lack of complement regulation and subsequently reduce the symptoms of C5 activation. Eculizumab blocks terminal complement activation and binds with high affinity to C5 so the proximal functions of complement remain intact (Figure 10.4). Eculizumab has superseded previous treatments of corticosteroids, intravenous immunoglobulin, vincristine and splenectomy for poorly responsive or resistant forms of atypical HUS, although patients may now be treated with the longer acting ravulizumab. Fluid overload with severe hypertension can exacerbate the clinical situation and kidney replacement therapy with peritoneal and haemodialysis may be required. However, early initiation with therapeutic eculizumab which can be long-term therapy to reduce requirement for kidney transplantation.

Prognosis

STEC-HUS results in complete recovery in the majority of cases without relapses, but can lead to CKD. There is reduced morbidity and mortality during epidemics by prompt recognition, identification and isolation of individuals to prevent spread, and elimination of the source with removal of contaminated food and water. The prognosis in atypical HUS is worse, with a progressive course and 25% relapse rate, with potentially improved clinical outcomes now with new therapeutic interventions.

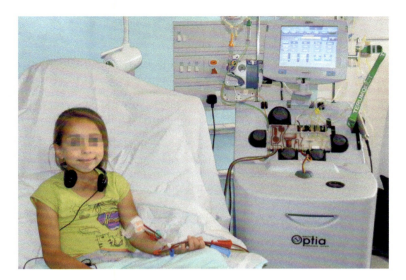

Figure 10.3 This patient is receiving treatment with immunoadsorption prior to ABO incompatible living related kidney transplantation for atypical haemolytic uraemic syndrome. Plasmapheresis has also been advocated for the glomerulonephritides (either primary renal diseases such as C3 glomerulopathy and rapidly progressive glomerulonephritis, or secondary to vasculitis or systemic lupus erythematosus).

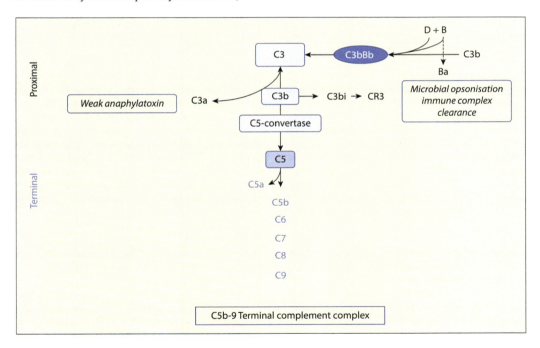

Figure 10.4 Eculizumab is a humanised anti-C5 monoclonal antibody that may overcome the lack of complement regulation and subsequently reduce the symptoms of C5 activation. Eculizumab blocks terminal complement activation and binds with high affinity to C5 so the proximal functions of complement remain intact.

GLOMERULONEPHRITIS

Introduction

The commonest cause of glomerulonephritis is a post-infectious glomerulonephritis where patients develop AKI after having an infection (typically streptococcal throat or skin infection) associated with bacterial growth on throat or skin swab, positive ASO titre and anti-DNase B with evidence of hypocomplementaemia (with low complement C3). Clinically, children present with features of nephritic syndrome (with haematuria, proteinuria, fluid overload, hypertension and oliguric AKI) with or without features of nephrotic syndrome.

Some children present with features of systemic disease, suggestive of SLE (with American College of Rheumatology and/or Systemic Lupus International Collaborating Clinics classification criteria [see also the chapter 'Rheumatology') with lupus nephritis. The International Society of Nephrology and Renal Pathology Society working groups published the histopathological classification of lupus nephritis (Figure 10.5).

Other patients may present with vasculitis. The Chapel Hill consensus criteria nomenclature update on the classification of vasculitis from 2012 distinguishes large vessel vasculitis from medium vessel vasculitis and immune complex and anti-neutrophil cytoplasmic antibody (ANCA)-associated small vessel vasculitis (Figure 10.6).

IGA VASCULITIS

Incidence/Aetiology

IgA vasculitis is the new term for Henoch–Schönlein purpura, a relatively common small vessel vasculitis, often preceded by upper respiratory tract infection, peaking at 4 to 6 years of age. Its cause is unknown; it is rarely associated with underlying C2 or C4 deficiency but an infectious trigger of genetically susceptible individuals is likely. Skin and renal histopathology reveal a leucocytoclastic vasculitis with IgA deposition and the same features as IgA nephropathy respectively.

Clinical Presentation

All patients develop a rash (required for diagnosis), typically symmetric and gravity dependent, especially on upper and lower limbs and buttocks (Figure 10.7). The rash is petechial or purpuric in nature, often palpable and non-blanching, although some children have macular or urticarial rashes initially. They may have oedema, especially of hands, feet, face and/or scrotum. Gastrointestinal tract involvement is present in 65% of cases, with bowel wall haemorrhage causing peri-umbilical abdominal pain, vomiting, and tenderness, but also melaena or intussusception with typical 'thumb-printing' on barium enema. Transient arthritis is present in 65% of cases in multiple joints, especially knees and ankles (see also the chapter 'Rheumatology'). Renal involvement is present in 50% of cases, which varies from microscopic or macroscopic haematuria to nephrotic syndrome, hypertension or rapidly progressive crescentic glomerulonephritis. Patients may have non-specific symptoms of malaise, fever and headaches.

Differential Diagnosis

Consider causes of thrombocytopenia (sepsis, leukaemia, idiopathic thrombocytopenic purpura, HUS) and vasculitis (SLE, microscopic polyangiitis, polyangiitis nodosa, post-infectious glomerulonephritis).

Diagnosis

FBC and clotting screen (to exclude thrombocytopenia and coagulation abnormalities); urea; creatinine; electrolytes; urinalysis (to detect significant renal involvement). If renal involvement is severe, consider complement C3, C4, antinuclear antibody (ANA), ANCA, ASOT and anti-DNase B, renal ultrasound and percutaneous renal biopsy. If intussusception is suspected, abdominal ultrasound should be performed.

Treatment

General treatment is with symptomatic pain relief, explanation and reassurance although nutritional supplementation may be required for prolonged episodes. Oral prednisolone 1–2 mg/kg/day may be given for severe gastrointestinal involvement (this has also been suggested for severe joint or skin involvement), and NSAIDs for joint pain. Consider intravenous methylprednisolone

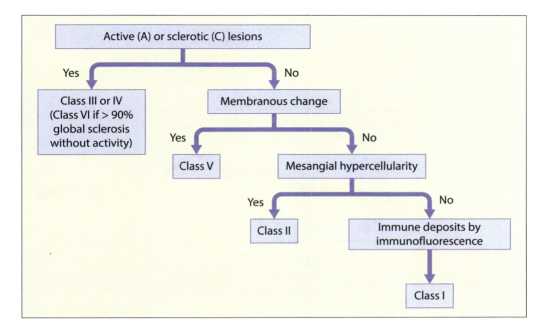

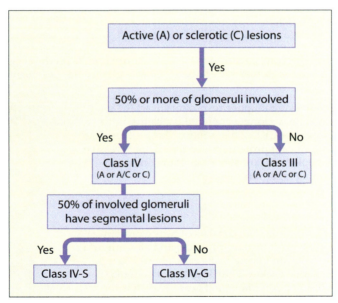

Figure 10.5 International Society of Nephrology/Renal pathology Society working group classification of lupus nephritis (modified from original source *JASN* 2004 *and Kidney Int* 2004 and 2018).

then oral prednisolone and mycophenolate mofetil with plasma exchange for severe vasculitis and consideration of cyclophosphamide for rapidly progressive glomerulonephritis. Follow-up for renal dysfunction, hypertension and proteinuria for at least one year after last recurrence of disease activity, or longer if these problems persist.

Prognosis

The prognosis is very good as it is usually self-limited with complete resolution by a mean of one month, but can recur, more rarely after years. Microscopic haematuria may persist, or macroscopic

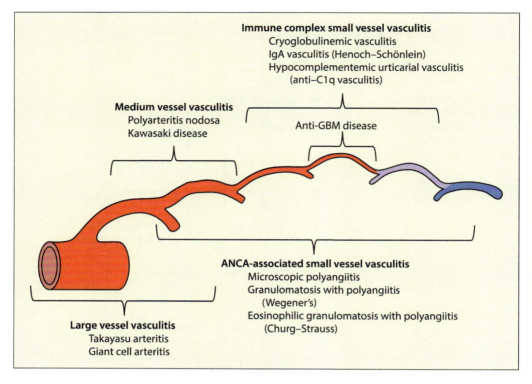

Figure 10.6 Chapel Hill consensus criteria nomenclature update on the classification of vasculitis from 2012. ANCA – anti-cytoplasmic antibody; GBM – glomerular basement membrane.

episodes occur after subsequent upper respiratory tract infections. One to five percent have long-term renal problems, with hypertension, proteinuria or CKD. This is more likely if there has been hypertension, significant proteinuria, or rapidly progressive crescentic glomerulonephritis at presentation. It uncommonly recurs after kidney transplantation.

NEPHROTIC SYNDROME

Incidence

Idiopathic nephrotic syndrome (NS) consists of heavy proteinuria (at least 3+ proteinuria on urinary dipstick) and albuminuria (early morning urine albumin to creatinine ratio above 200 mg/mmol), hypoalbuminaemia (below 25 to 30 g/l) and oedema, usually associated with hyperlipidaemia (Figure 10.8). It is the commonest chronic glomerular disease in children with an incidence of 2–4 cases per 100,000 children in the United Kingdom. It may be primary or secondary to an overt systemic disorder and is associated with atopy. The commonest type of NS in children is characterised by minimal histological changes in the glomeruli. This is called minimal change nephrotic syndrome (MCNS) (Figure 10.9) and is mostly responsive to corticosteroid therapy (steroid-sensitive nephrotic syndrome [SSNS]) (Table 10.4).

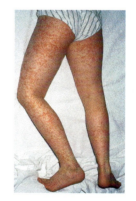

Figure 10.7 Classical purpuric rash on bilateral lower limbs of patient with IgA vasculitis.

Incidence of MCNS

MCNS usually presents in children aged 2–6 (median age of onset of 2.5) years, is commoner in boys and has greater prevalence in Asian children. There is heavy, highly selective proteinuria that responds to corticosteroid therapy. Microscopic (usually not macroscopic) haematuria may be present in up to 25% of cases (Table 10.5).

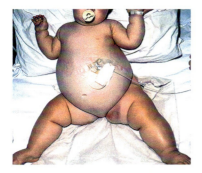

Figure 10.8 An infant aged 3.5 years with evidence of oedema due to nephrotic syndrome. The oedema is dependent in nephrotic syndrome, accumulating in low pressure areas around the eyes, in the legs and as ascites.

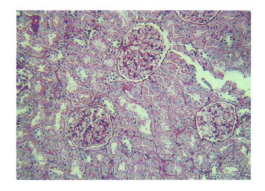

Figure 10.9 Minimal histological changes in the glomeruli from a percutaneous renal biopsy of a child with minimal change nephrotic syndrome.

Table 10.4: Glomerular Histology and Corticosteroid Responsiveness in Primary Nephrotic Syndrome in Children

Glomerular histology	% Children	% Steroid sensitive
Minimal change	78	95
Focal and segmental glomerulosclerosis	8	2
C3 glomerulopathy/membranoproliferative glomerulonephritis (MPGN)	6	1
Diffuse mesangial sclerosis	4	4
Glomerulonephritis	2	0
Membranous nephropathy	2	0

Table 10.5: Clinical and Laboratory Features in Children with Primary Nephrotic Syndrome

Percentage of cases	MCNS	FSGS	MPGN
Total	78	8	6
Age under 8 years	80	50	3
Male	60	69	36
Hypertension[a]	21	49	36
Microscopic haematuria[b]	23	48	51
Hypocomplementaemia[c]	1	4	74
Renal dysfunction[d]	33	41	50

[a] Hypertension is defined as systolic blood pressure above the 95th centile for age, sex and height centile and/or requiring antihypertensive agents.
[b] Microscopic haematuria is defined as the presence of red blood cells in the urine ($\geq$ three red blood cells per high power field) on urine microscopy.
[c] Hypocomplementaemia is defined as low complement C3 level (below the normal laboratory reference range).
[d] Renal dysfunction is defined as plasma creatinine above the 98th centile for age and sex.

DEFINITIONS

Diagnosis

Hypoalbuminaemia causes oedema and rapid albumin loss results in hypovolaemia with abdominal pain, shock and risk of thrombosis.

Venous thrombosis is multifactorial, with sluggish peripheral circulation, relative polycythaemia, hyperlipidaemia, platelet hyperaggregability, hyperfibrinogenaemia and loss of control proteins such as antithrombin-III, all contributing to the procoagulant state. Loss of IgG and complement components, particularly factor B of the alternative pathway, predisposes to infection, typically pneumococcal septicaemia and peritonitis.

Treatment

The primary treatment objective is to achieve remission, alleviate symptoms and prevent and treat acute risks such as infection, thrombosis and hypovolaemia with minimisation of long-term complications, such as bone disease, hypertension, Cushing syndrome, obesity, growth retardation, striae, cataracts and a variety of psychological, social and behavioural disturbances. The initial treatment is corticosteroids prior to the use of other immunosuppressive agents (Table 10.6). Percutaneous renal biopsy should be considered in atypical presentations (in infants under 12 months or adolescents over 12 years of age). Familial nephrotic syndrome, macroscopic haematuria, significant renal dysfunction or hypertension and steroid resistant nephrotic syndrome after four weeks of high-dose corticosteroids without response to intravenous methylprednisolone pulses are also an indication for genetics testing and/or percutaneous renal biopsy (Table 10.7). If the child is steroid sensitive, minimal change histology can be presumed and does not need to be confirmed by biopsy. Prophylactic penicillin should be prescribed when young patients are clinically nephrotic.

Prognosis

Children presenting with initial onset of NS have a 24-month sustained remission rate of 49% with a frequent relapse rate of 29%. One-third of children with MCNS have only a single episode, one-third relapse occasionally and one-third become steroid-dependent frequent relapsers. Relapses eventually cease and the development of steroid resistance is unusual; end-stage kidney disease almost never occurs (unless MCNS on initial biopsy is focal and segmental glomerulosclerosis [FSGS] on subsequent biopsies).

Table 10.6: Modern Treatment of Primary Nephrotic Syndrome

Level	Relapse	Treatment
1	Initial episode	Prednisolone 60 mg/m^2/d for 28 days with subsequent 40 mg/m^2 alternate days for 28 days
2	Subsequent relapses	Prednisolone 30–60 mg/m^2/d until remission pending severity with subsequent alternate day regimen for 3–4 weeks
4	Steroid sparing agents	Levamisole 2.5 mg/kg alternate days Cyclophosphamide 3 mg/kg/day for eight weeks Calcineurin inhibitor (ciclosporin/tacrolimus) Mycophenolate mofetil Intravenous rituximab

Table 10.7: Definitions

1. Nephrotic syndrome	Proteinuria > 40 mg/m^2/h, hypoalbuminaemia < 25 to 30 g/l and oedema
2. Remission	Proteinuria < 4 mg/m^2/h or no or trace of proteinuria on urine dipstick testing for three consecutive days irrespective of loss of oedema
3. Relapse	Proteinuria > 40 mg/m^2/h or at least 3+ proteinuria on urine dipstick testing for three consecutive days
4. Frequent relapses	Two relapses within six months of initial response or four or more relapses within any 12 month period
5. Steroid sensitive	Remission achieved within 28 days of corticosteroid therapy
6. Steroid resistance	Failure to achieve remission despite at least four weeks of high-dose corticosteroids (prednisolone 60 mg/m^2/d) and three pulses of intravenous methylprednisolone
7. Steroid dependence	Relapse on or within two weeks of corticosteroid therapy discontinuation or as tapering of corticosteroid therapy

CHRONIC KIDNEY DISEASE

Introduction

The commonest cause of irreversible kidney failure or CKD in childhood is congenital anomalies of the kidney and urinary tract. CKD is divided into the severity from Stage I, II, III, IV and V, corresponding to kidney function (%) or GFR of > 90, 60–89, 30–59, 15–29 and < 15 mls/min/1.73 m^2, respectively. Kidney replacement therapy is usually required for Stage V CKD and the gold standard therapy is pre-emptive living related kidney transplantation prior to the requirement of dialysis (assuming patients present before requiring kidney replacement therapy with dialysis or underlying condition does not require native nephrectomies).

Pathogenesis

Renal osteodystrophy is the term used to describe the disturbance of bone formation in CKD, secondary to abnormalities of vitamin D metabolism and secondary hyperparathyroidism. Reduced activity of the renal 1-α hydroxylase enzyme, with progressive renal failure, causes decreased production of the active hormone 1,25-dihydroxyvitamin D$_3$. This results in increased bone resorption (i.e. osteitis fibrosa due to secondary hyperparathyroidism) and impaired mineralisation of osteoid (i.e. rickets). Parathyroid hormone (PTH) secretion is stimulated by a fall in ionised calcium due to reduced calcium absorption mediated by 1,25-dihydroxyvitamin D$_3$ and hyperphosphataemia secondary to phosphate retention.

Diagnosis

Children with early changes of renal osteodystrophy are usually asymptomatic but if untreated they may develop bone pain with or without fractures or slipped epiphyses, skeletal deformities and weakness secondary to proximal myopathy (Figure 10.10).

A raised level of intact PTH is indicative of active bone disease. Measurements of intact PTH can be used to monitor treatment in conjunction with measurement of plasma phosphate, total calcium and ionised calcium. Indirect assessments of PTH activity (i.e. alkaline phosphatase, bone radiographs and biopsies and tubular resorption of phosphate) are less reliable.

Treatment

The principles of management of renal osteodystrophy are:

- Correction of acidosis using sodium bicarbonate.

- Phosphate restriction by control of dietary intake and the use of a phosphate binder (e.g. calcium carbonate to maintain plasma phosphate within the normal range for age).

- Supplements of oral 1-α-hydroxycholecalciferol or 1,25 dihydroxycholecalciferol to maintain the PTH within normal range, if not achieved by control of plasma phosphate. This may require the total calcium to be maintained at the upper end of the normal range.

Prognosis

With medical management and adherence to medications, this can be controlled with linear growth maintained, but progression may occur with deteriorating renal function.

CYSTIC KIDNEY DISEASES

Classification and Genetics

- Autosomal recessive polycystic kidney disease (ARPKD). Caused by mutations in *PKHD1* on 6p21.

- Autosomal dominant polycystic kidney diseases (ADPKD). Commonest mutation is in *PKD1* on 16p13. The gene codes for a cell signalling molecule. A minority of ADPKD cases are caused by *PKD2* on 4q, which encodes a calcium channel.

- Nephronophthisis. Caused by homozygous or compound heterozygous mutation in or deletion of the gene encoding nephrocystin on chromosome 2q13 (e.g. *NPHP1* with subsequent multiple identified genes).

- Renal cysts and diabetes syndrome (RCAD) caused by mutations and deletions in hepatocyte nuclear factor-1-beta (*HNF1B*) gene, which maps to chromosome 17q12.

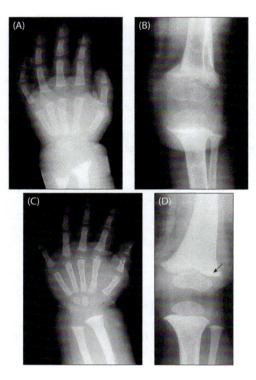

Figure 10.10 Bone radiographs of wrist and knee in a boy who presented aged 10 months with severe CKD secondary to posterior urethral valves and bilateral renal dysplasia. (A and B): pre-treatment. Coarse trabecular pattern with wide irregular metaphyseal plates and subperiosteal bone resorption, with periosteal reaction in the lower femur; (C and D): post-treatment. resolution of bone changes with the appearance of a dense white line indicating normal bone formation at the zone of provisional calcification (arrow).

- Glomerulocystic disease. Autosomal dominant with increasing understanding on underlying genetics (including *HNF1B*).

- Tuberous sclerosis. Autosomal dominant, with mutations of *TSC2* on 16pl3 (adjacent to *PKD1*).

- Von Hippel–Lindau disease. Autosomal dominant inheritance with mutation of gene on 3p25-26.

- Orofaciodigital syndrome Type 1. X-linked dominant.

- Acquired cystic kidney disease. Secondary to chronic hypokalaemia or uraemia.

Incidence

The incidence of ARPKD and ADPKD is 1 in 10,000 and 1000, respectively, in paediatric and adult populations together. The former accounts for the majority of cases in childhood but it is increasingly recognised that ADPKD is not uncommon in paediatric practice. Nephronophthisis is an autosomal recessive cystic kidney disease that is the most frequent genetic cause of CKD in childhood and adolescence. There are genetics advances in the other, rare causes that are listed above.

Clinical Presentation

ARPKD may present antenatally, with abnormal renal ultrasound (including enlarged, echogenic kidneys), or neonatally with nephromegaly, hypertension and/or renal dysfunction. Less severe cases have hypertension and renal dysfunction in infancy whereas, in later childhood, mild renal disease can coexist with liver fibrosis and portal hypertension. ADPKD can present with loin pain, urinary tract infections (UTI), mild renal dysfunction or hypertension in childhood but is generally clinically silent until adulthood. Some patients with ADPKD are diagnosed in childhood due to incidental findings on abdominal ultrasound or familial requests for ultrasound screening. This can be debated ethically, although some asymptomatic children may be recruited to clinical trials. There is a rare and severe early onset variety of ADPKD with tuberous sclerosis due to contiguous mutations of *PKD1* and *TSC2*. Nephronophthisis can be combined with extra-renal manifestations, including situs inversus, cardiac malformations, hepatic fibrosis, cerebellar vermis hypoplasia (Joubert syndrome), retinitis pigmentosa (Senior–Loken syndrome) and multiple developmental and neurological abnormalities (Meckel–Gruber syndrome).

Diagnosis

Prenatal genetic diagnosis of ADPKD or ARPKD is feasible, especially if DNA from affected relatives is available. Severe ARPKD may be detected in the last trimester by ultrasound scan showing enlarging kidneys and oligohydramnios.

Abdominal ultrasound scans (Figure 10.11) may not always reliably distinguish between ARPKD and early ADPKD, with cysts enlarging considerably in the course of ADPKD. Although renal cysts are seen well on CT scanning, this form of imaging is not routinely advocated in paediatric practice due to the radiation burden and as this is not superior to the less costly and less invasive ultrasound (Figure 10.12). It is always prudent to investigate the parents with renal ultrasound scans as they may be affected in ADPKD as new mutations are unusual. Liver cysts may be present in ADPKD and periportal liver fibrosis in ARPKD can be diagnosed by fibroscan, biopsy or suggested by isotope Tc-hepatobiliary iminodiacetic acid (HIDA) scans.

Pathology

Many cystic diseases are caused by ciliopathies, which are genetic disorders of the cellular cilia or the cilia anchoring structures. The basal bodies of ciliary function *PKHD1* and *PKD182* are expressed in the primary cilium, whereas OFD1 protein is expressed in the centrosome/basal body of the primary cilium. ARPKD cysts arise from collecting ducts while ADPKD cysts arise from all nephron segments. There are aberrations of cell proliferation, apoptosis, epithelial cell polarity and the extracellular matrix.

Treatment

Controlled trials in adults with ADPKD show that low protein diets, control of hypertension and cyst surgery have little, if any, significant influence on progression to renal failure. However, hypertension in PKD should be vigorously treated with ACE inhibitors or angiotensin receptor blockers to reduce cardiovascular damage and possibly slow progression. Tolvaptan is now licensed to slow down the growth of renal cysts, reduce overall renal growth and preserve renal function for longer. Kidney transplantation is effective, although native nephrectomy may be required for nephromegaly or recurrent UTI. Some children with ARPKD develop hepatic fibrosis

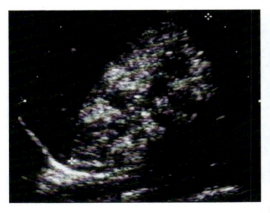

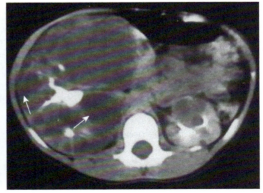

Figure 10.11 Ultrasound scan image demonstrating the large bright kidney of autosomal recessive polycystic kidney disease (ARPKD).

Figure 10.12 Computerised tomography scan of autosomal dominant polycystic kidney diseases (ADPKD). Note the asymmetrical involvement with visible cysts (arrows).

and portal hypertension, which may require sequential or combined liver–kidney transplantation. Hepatic cysts and Berry aneurysms in patients with ADPKD may also require treatment.

Prognosis

A significant proportion of ARPKD patients develop renal failure soon after birth and a small subset of ADPKD patients have a severe infantile presentation. Half of ARPKD patients develop end-stage kidney disease (ESKD) by adolescence, whereas only half of ADPKD patients develop uraemia in a lifetime. The rate of disease progression is highly variable even in single PKD kindreds.

CONGENITAL ANOMALIES OF THE KIDNEY AND URINARY TRACT (CAKUT)
Classification/Genetics

Renal agenesis and dysplasia represent malformations in which the foetal organs have failed to undergo a normal pattern of differentiation. In renal agenesis, no renal tissue can be detected. Dysplastic kidneys contain undifferentiated and metaplastic elements, while multi-cystic dysplastic kidneys are non-functioning kidneys containing large cysts; their excretory function is often absent or considerably reduced. Most are sporadic, although some are associated with other defects in multiple organs (e.g. CHARGE and VACTERL associations).

Rarely, families have been reported with definite inheritance of agenesis or dysplasia. These can occur in isolation or be syndromal (e.g. X-linked Kallmann syndrome with renal agenesis and infertility; autosomal dominant branchio-oto-renal syndrome with renal dysplasia and deafness; renal cysts and diabetes syndrome).

Incidence

The incidence of bilateral renal agenesis is highly variable, with unilateral disease often clinically silent and the estimated incidence is 1 in 1000 to 10,000. The incidence of multi-cystic dysplastic and renal hypoplasia/dysplasia is about 1 in 5000.

Clinical Presentation

Unilateral multi-cystic dysplastic kidneys may present as an abdominal mass in infancy although, these malformations are usually detected by antenatal ultrasound scanning. About 20–30% of such children have contralateral abnormalities, including pelvi-ureteric or vesico-ureteric junction obstruction. Bilateral renal malformations can result in oligohydramnios, premature delivery and the Potter sequence (oligohydramnios, oliguria, pulmonary hypoplasia and limb deformities). Renal dysplasia is very commonly associated with abnormalities of the lower urinary tract including obstructive lesions (e.g. posterior urethral valves in boys and ureterocoeles in girls).

Diagnosis

Renal dysplasia is suggested on ultrasound scanning by the visualisation of irregular-shaped organs with loss of cortico-medullary differentiation (Figure 10.13). Cysts, where present, can be identified but these cases need to be distinguished from PKD or hydronephrosis.

Technically, the diagnosis of dysplasia can only be made by histology but this is rarely clinically indicated. If ultrasound suggests unilateral agenesis, a dimercaptosuccinic acid (DMSA) isotope renogram can be performed to exclude the possibility of ectopic kidney tissue.

Pathology

Dysplastic kidneys contain immature ducts that are considered to be branches of the ureteric bud surrounded by fibromuscular and undifferentiated cells (Figure 10.14). There may also be metaplastic tissue includ-ing cartilage.

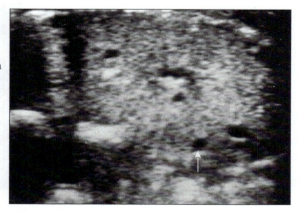

Figure 10.13 Renal ultrasound scan shows loss of cortico-medullary differentiation in a dysplastic kidney. Note the small subcortical cysts (arrow).

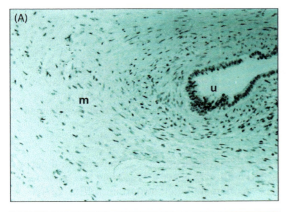

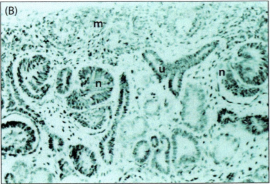

Figure 10.14 (A) Histology of a dysplastic kidney: note the lack of tissue differentiation versus a human foetal kidney (B), which contains primitive nephrons (n) in addition to mesenchyme (m) and branches of the ureteric bud (u).

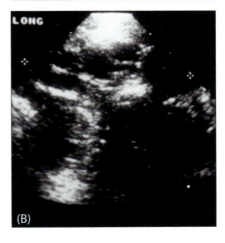

Figure 10.15 Renal ultrasound demonstrating multi-cystic dysplastic kidney, which partially involuted over two years.

Treatment

When bilateral malformations are associated with severe oligohydramnios, termination may be considered due to the poor prognosis associated with pulmonary hypoplasia. A subgroup with large bladders and urinary obstruction have been treated with vesico-amniotic shunts. Although this procedure may increase the amount of liquor, it is unproven whether lung growth is accelerated. Those with bilateral renal dysplasia require lifetime follow-up for the detection and treatment of CKD.

Unilateral multi-cystic dysplastic kidneys do not require any specific treatment. There is evidence that many of these involute spontaneously over months or years (Figure 10.15). There is no evidence now to recommend nephrectomy due to (disputed) risk of renal malignancy and hypertension.

Prognosis

Bilateral renal agenesis or severe dysplasia may cause neonatal death if associated with pulmonary hypoplasia. With advances in dialysis and transplantation, renal failure can be adequately treated although some of these children die in the first year from malformations of other organs (e.g. lung, heart, brain and gut). Unilateral renal agenesis may be clinically silent throughout life and has minimal increased morbidity if the contralateral kidney is normal, although deterioration in renal function may occur with age if there is associated contralateral renal dysplasia. Vesico-ureteric reflux (VUR) and contralateral kidney abnormalities occur in 30–50% of patients with unilateral dysplasia.

VESICO-URETERIC REFLUX

See also the chapter 'Urology'.

Classification

VUR is the retrograde passage of urine from the bladder into the ureter and/or the renal pelvis, calyces and collecting ducts. It can be secondary to high bladder pressure due either to anatomical lesions of the urethra (e.g. posterior urethral valves) or to neuromuscular incoordination of bladder emptying (e.g. neurogenic bladder). It can occur in children who have either normal or abnormal kidneys with CAKUT (e.g. bilateral renal dysplasia with VUR).

Genetics

Isolated primary VUR is an autosomal dominant disorder with incomplete penetrance and variable expression. Rarely primary VUR can be inherited (although several candidate loci have been defined) as part of a syndrome (e.g. with optic nerve colobomata when mutations of *PAX2* have been described).

Incidence

Estimates of the incidence of VUR in children range between 1 in 50 to 200. The risk of primary VUR in a sibling approaches 50% when screened with micturating cystourethrography (MCUG) before the age of 2.

Clinical Presentation

When VUR is associated with other abnormalities the clinical presentation is determined by the primary disease (e.g. poor urinary stream with posterior urethral valves). Primary VUR may be clinically silent and many of the milder cases regress over years. The commonest presentation is with UTI and indeed VUR is frequently diagnosed when investigating children for UTI. Recurrent pyelonephritis in the first years of life may lead to hypertension or CKD in later childhood or adulthood.

Diagnosis

Severe antenatal VUR can be detected as hydronephrosis on ultrasound scanning in the second and third trimester. In this case, a MCUG soon after birth will confirm the presence and define the extent of VUR, and will also diagnose any co-existing urethral pathology. It is important to exclude posterior urethral valves in boys as they require surgical resection. In younger children with UTI, MCUG is the investigation of choice to detect VUR (Figure 10.16), while in older toilet-trained children VUR can be diagnosed by indirect radionucleotide cystography (Figure 10.17). In addition, the kidneys should always be imaged to assess the presence of co-existing renal malformations (by ultrasound scan) or scarring (by DMSA isotope renography; Figure 10.18). Given the high familial incidence of primary VUR, screening of young siblings of index cases should be considered, especially if symptomatic febrile UTIs.

Pathology

There is an anatomical defect in primary VUR at the vesico-ureteric junction. Renal histopathology can demonstrate either immature tissues (dysplasia) or scarring (chronic interstitial fibrosis).

Treatment

All neonates with severe antenatal hydronephrosis should be commenced on prophylactic antibiotics pending definitive diagnosis. Posterior urethral valves should be resected and other associated defects treated. Management of primary VUR

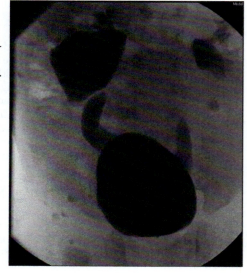

Figure 10.16 Micturating cystourethrography demonstrating bilateral vesico-ureteric reflux.

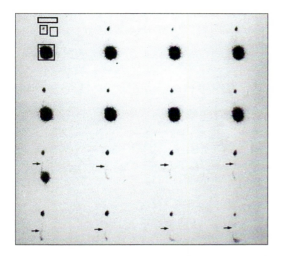

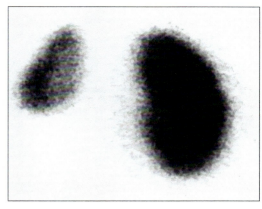

Figure 10.18 DMSA isotope is taken up by functional kidney tubules. In this posterior view, the left kidney is small after scarring from pyelonephritis.

Figure 10.17 Indirect radionucleotide cystography shows a small amount of isotope in the left kidney after injection of MAG3, which is filtered by the glomerulus. On sequential views, the urinary bladder empties upon voiding with reflux of isotope up the left ureter (arrows).

involves prompt diagnosis and management of febrile UTI to prevent renal damage caused by recurrent pyelonephritis. There is controversy regarding the effectiveness of either medical (long-term antibiotic prophylaxis) or surgical interventions (anti-reflux surgery) in affected children.

Prognosis

The long-term prognosis of primary VUR depends on the presence and severity of the associated nephropathy.

RENOVASCULAR HYPERTENSION

Introduction

The incidence of hypertension is increasing in children due to screening programmes, earlier detection of hypertension and the obesity epidemic. However, it is important to distinguish those patients with secondary forms of hypertension, such as renovascular hypertension.

Incidence

Renovascular disease accounts for 10% of children with hypertension and is often due to fibromuscular dysplasia. In some patients, this may be associated with mid-aortic syndrome, neurofibromatosis, William syndrome, Marfan syndrome and Klippel–Trenaunay–Weber and Feuerstein–Mims syndromes. The prevalence is estimated to be approximately 1 in 10,000 children.

Diagnosis

One-quarter of patients are diagnosed on routine blood pressure screening. Many have symptoms such as headache (50%), lethargy (39%), cardiac failure, failure to thrive, and weight loss at presentation. A significant number (10–15%) present with neurological features alone, such as facial palsy, hemiplegia and convulsions. Patients should have full examination to exclude coarctation of the aorta (COA), neurocutaneous stigmata and evidence of hypertensive retinopathy with fundoscopy.

Investigations

Patients require 24-hour ambulatory blood pressure monitoring (unless present with severe or malignant hypertension when this is required to monitor response to therapy as opposed to confirming hypertension). The most useful diagnostic tests include blood and urine tests (to see

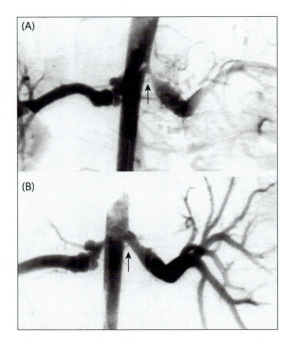

Figure 10.19 Digital subtraction renal angiography demonstrating left renal artery stenosis before (A) and after angioplasty (B).

if hypokalaemic metabolic alkalosis and evidence of hyper-reninaemic hyperaldosteronism, renal dysfunction, haematuria and/or proteinuria), echocardiography (to exclude target organ damage with left ventricular hypertrophy and exclusion of COA), Doppler renal ultrasound, DMSA scan prior to proceeding with renal vein renin measurements and digital subtraction angiography. However, the vascular disease may involve intra-renal vessels and other organs (particularly the brain). Therefore, investigations should also be directed to identify these, especially if there are cerebral symptoms.

Treatment

Children in hypertensive crisis should be treated with an intravenous anti-hypertensive agent such as labetalol or sodium nitroprusside initially, with very careful and slow reduction of blood pressure over 48 to 72 hours. Calcium channel blockers and beta-blockers are the most useful oral pharmacological agents in the treatment of renovascular hypertension. Furosemide can be used if there is evidence of fluid overload. ACE inhibitors are normally contraindicated; however, they may be necessary in the management of patients with difficult to control blood pressure or in subjects with severe intra-renal vascular disease.

Digital subtraction renal angiography and angioplasty (Figure 10.19) is the treatment of choice for cases with unilateral, main or branch artery stenoses. Some patients may need vascular reconstructive procedures. Approximately one-third of these achieve complete cure and most of the others show a reduction in drug therapy requirement after surgery.

Prognosis

Children require follow-up to ensure that their blood pressure is treated to reduce longer-term complications.

RENAL FANCONI SYNDROME

Incidence

The renal Fanconi syndrome consists of generalised proximal tubular dysfunction (aminoaciduria, glycosuria, bicarbonaturia, phosphaturia) and rickets or osteomalacia. Most cases occur as part of a metabolic disorder or are secondary to drugs/toxins, renal or other diseases (Table 10.8).

Table 10.8: Causes of Renal Fanconi Syndrome

Inherited (specific investigation or features)

Cystinosis (leucocyte cystine concentration)

Tyrosinaemia (plasma amino acids, urine organic acids)

Galactosaemia (galactose 1-phosphate uridyl transferase)

Fructosaemia (fructose-1-phosphate aldolase B)

Lowe syndrome (X-linked, cataracts, hypotonia)

Mitochondrial disorders (lactate, pyruvate)

Wilson disease (copper, caeruloplasmin)

Glycogen storage disease (hepatomegaly, hypoglycaemia)

Dent disease (X-linked, hypercalciuria, nephrocalcinosis)

Idiopathic: autosomal dominant/recessive/X-linked

Acquired

Drugs: ifosfamide, aminoglycosides, sodium valproate, cisplatin, azathioprine

Heavy metals: lead, cadmium, mercury

Nephrotic syndrome (rare)

Kidney transplantation

Tubulointerstitial nephritis

Amyloidosis

Myeloma

Diagnosis

Children present with both symptoms of the underlying cause and features of proximal tubular dysfunction: polyuria, polydipsia, recurrent dehydration, poor growth, vomiting and rickets. Children with cystinosis (the commonest inherited cause of Fanconi syndrome) often have a characteristic appearance with sparse, blond hair and a pale complexion, but the condition can occur in any racial group and non-Caucasian patients have a complexion appropriate to their racial group.

Investigations

Urinalysis may reveal glycosuria and proteinuria but this is not invariable. Plasma biochemistry usually shows hypokalaemia, hypophosphataemia, a hyperchloraemic metabolic acidosis (e.g. normal anion gap) and sometimes hyponatraemia and hypocalcaemia. The urine is usually alkaline but will acidify in the presence of severe acidosis (bicarbonate < 15 mmol/l) since it is a proximal renal tubular acidosis. Generalised aminoaciduria together with a low tubular reabsorption of phosphate confirm a Fanconi syndrome. Radiographs may demonstrate rickets. Specific investigations to determine the cause are listed in Table 10.8.

Treatment

In the acute situation, patients need rehydration with 0.9% saline usually with added potassium. Supplements of bicarbonate, potassium and phosphate are required. Vitamin D is used to treat rickets. Specific treatments are required for the causative metabolic conditions.

Prognosis

The outlook depends on the cause of the Fanconi syndrome. In addition, several of the causes lead to CKD (especially cystinosis, Lowe syndrome, tyrosinaemia and 'idiopathic' cases), although this occurs at a variable rate.

FURTHER READING

GENERAL

- Emma F, Goldstein S, Bagga A, et al. *Pediatric Nephrology,* 8th edition. Berlin, Heidelberg; Springer-Verlag, 2022.
- Rees L, Bockenhauer D, Webb NJA, et al. *Oxford Specialist Handbooks in Paediatrics: Paediatric Nephrology,* 2nd edition. Oxford; Oxford University Press, 2019.
- Schaefer F, Greenbaum L. *Pediatric Kidney Disease,* 3rd edition. Berlin, Heidelberg; Springer-Verlag, 2023.
- Wallace D, Shenoy M, Sinha MD. *Clinical Paediatric Nephrology,* 4th edition. Oxford; Oxford University Press, 2023.
- Haemolytic uraemic syndrome
- Jenkins C, Byrne L, Vishram B, et al. Shiga toxin-producing *Escherichia coli* haemolytic uraemic syndrome (STEC-HUS): Diagnosis, surveillance and public-health management in England. *J Med Microbiol* 2020;69(7):1034–1036.
- Loirat C, Fakhouri F, Ariceta G, et al. An international consensus approach to the management of atypical haemolytic uraemic syndrome in children. *Pediatric Nephrol* 2016;31(1):15–39.
- Walsh PR, Johnson S. Treatment and management of children with haemolytic uraemic syndrome. *Arch Dis Child* 2018;103(3):285–291.
- Chronic kidney disease
- Bacchetta J, Schmitt CP, Bakkaloglu SA, et al. Diagnosis and management of mineral and bone disorders in infants with CKD: Clinical practice points from the ESPN CKD-MBD and Dialysis working groups and the Pediatric Renal Nutrition Taskforce. *Pediatr Nephrol* 2023;38(9):3163–3181.
- McAlister L, Pugh P, Greenbaum L, et al. The dietary management of calcium and phosphate in children with CKD stages 2-5 and on dialysis-clinical practice recommendation from the Pediatric Renal Nutrition Taskforce. *Pediatr Nephrol* 2020;35(3):501–518.
- Rees L. Nutritional management in children with chronic kidney disease. *World Rev Nutr Diet* 2022;124:389–393.
- Cystic kidney diseases
- Gimpel C, Avni FE, Bergmann C, et al. Perinatal diagnosis, management, and follow-up of cystic renal diseases: A clinical practice recommendation with systematic literature reviews. *JAMA Pediatr* 2018;172(1):74–86.
- Gimpel C, Bergmann C, Bockenhauer D, et al. International consensus statement on the diagnosis and management of autosomal dominant polycystic kidney disease in children and young people. *Nat Rev Nephrol* 2019;15(11):713–726.
- McConnachie DJ, Stow JL, Mallett AJ. Ciliopathies and the kidney: A review. *Am J Kidney Dis* 2021;77(3):410–419.
- Congenital anomalies of the kidney and urinary tract
- Chevalier R. CAKUT: A pediatric and evolutionary perspective on the leading cause of CKD in childhood. *Pediatr Rep* 2023;15(1):143–153.
- Stein D, McNamara E. Congenital anomalies of the kidneys and urinary tract. *Clin Perinatol* 2022;49(3):791–798.
- Walawender L, Becknell B, Matsell DG. Congenital anomalies of the kidney and urinary tract: Defining risk factors of disease progression and determinants of outcomes. *Pediatr Nephrol* 2023;38(12):3963–3973.
- Vesico-ureteric reflux
- Hewitt IK, Montini G, Marks SD. Vesico-ureteric reflux in children and young people undergoing kidney transplantation. *Pediatr Nephrol* 2022;38(9):2987–2993.
- Landau Z, Cherniavsky E, Abofreha S, et al. Epidemiologic, microbiologic and imaging characteristics of urinary tract infections in hospitalized children < 2 years of age diagnosed with anatomic abnormalities of the urinary tract. *Pediatr Neonatol* 2022;63(4):402–409.
- Mattoo TK, Mohammad D. Primary vesicoureteral reflux and renal scarring. *Pediatr Clin North Am* 2022;69(6):1115–1129.
- Glomerulonephritis
- Bajema IM, Wilhelmus S, Alpers CE, et al. Revision of the International Society of Nephrology/Renal Pathology Society classification for lupus nephritis: Clarification of definitions, and modified National Institutes of Health activity and chronicity indices. *Kidney Int* 2018;93(4):789–796.

- Balasubramanian R, Marks SD. Post-infectious glomerulonephritis. *Pediatr Int Child Health* 2017;37(4):240–247.
- de Graeff N, Groot N, Brogan P, et al. European consensus-based recommendation for the diagnosis and treatment of rare paediatric vasculitides - The SHARE initiative. *Rheumatology (Oxford)* 2019;59(4):919.
- Fanouriakis A, Kostopoulou M, Cheema K, et al. 2019 Update of the Joint European League against Rheumatism and European Renal Association-European Dialysis and Transplant Association (EULAR/ERA-EDTA) recommendations for the management of lupus nephritis. *Ann Rheum Dis* 2020;79(6):713–723.
- Oni L, Wright RD, Marks SD, et al. Kidney outcomes for children with lupus nephritis. *Pediatr Nephrol* 2021;36(6):1377–1385.
- Nephrotic syndrome
- Boyer O, Trautmann A, Haffner D, et al. Steroid-sensitive nephrotic syndrome in children. *Nephrol Dial Transplant* 2022;gfac314.
- Mattoo TK, Sanjad S. Current understanding of nephrotic syndrome in children. *Pediatr Clin North Am* 2022;69(6):1079–1098.
- Trautmann A, Seide S, Lipska-Zietkiewicz BS, et al. Outcomes of steroid-resistant nephrotic syndrome in children not treated with intensified immunosuppression. *Pediatr Nephrol* 2023;38(5):1499–1511.
- Renovascular hypertension
- Inamura N, Sato M. Neonatal renovascular hypertension. *Pediatr Int* 2018;60(5):501.
- Kurt-Sukur ED, Brennan E, Davis M, et al. Presentation, treatment, and outcome of renovascular hypertension below 2 years of age. *Eur J Pediatr* 2022;181(9):3367–3375.
- Trautmann A, Roebuck DJ, McLaren CA, et al. Non-invasive imaging cannot replace formal angiography in the diagnosis of renovascular hypertension. *Pediatr Nephrol* 2017;32(3):495–502.

11 Haematology

Keith Sibson, Jack Bartram, Sara Ghorashian and Ajay Vora

INTRODUCTION

UK haematologists are responsible not only for the clinical care of malignant and non-malignant haematological disorders but also the reporting and interpretation of haemato-pathology, coagulation and transfusion laboratory results. The laboratory aspects of haematology are beyond the scope of this chapter. The focus here will be on clinical aspects of malignant and non-malignant haematological disorders in children.

LEUKAEMIA AND LYMPHOMA

Acute leukaemia is the most common form of cancer in children accounting for 30% of new diagnoses with around 85% with acute lymphoblastic leukaemia (ALL) and 15% acute myeloid leukaemia (AML). Chronic myeloid leukaemia (CML) is rare and chronic lymphocytic leukaemia (CLL) does not occur in children. Juvenile myelomonocytic leukaemia (JMML) is a rare myeloproliferative disorder that only occurs in children. Non-Hodgkin lymphomas (NHL) re-present around 20% of cancers in children and young adults. Hodgkin lymphoma is rare in young children, but the incidence rises in young adults.

NON-HODGKIN LYMPHOMA
Clinical Presentation

These lymphomas tend to spread along lymphoid tissue distributions, namely: lymph nodes, thymus, Waldeyer ring, Peyer's patches and bone marrow. Abdominal and intrathoracic disease presentations occur in approximately 35% and 25% of cases, respectively.

Common Subtypes

The majority of childhood and adolescents NHL are high-grade and clinically aggressive. There are three subgroups: (i) precursor lymphoid neoplasms (T-cell lymphoblastic lymphoma [15 to 20%] and B-cell lymphoblastic lymphoma [3%]); (ii) mature B-cell neoplasms (Burkitt lymphoma [35 to 40%], diffuse large B-cell lymphoma [15–20%] and primary mediastinal B-cell lymphoma [1 to 2%]); and (iii) mature T-cell neoplasms (anaplastic large cell lymphoma, ALK positive [15 to 20%]).

BURKITT LYMPHOMA

In Western countries the commonest presentation of the sporadic form of Burkitt lymphoma (BL) is with abdominal, bone marrow, lymph nodes (especially head and neck/nasopharyngeal) and ovaries, whilst in the endemic form seen in Equatorial Africa, New Guinea, Amazonian Brazil and Turkey, the jaw, abdomen, CNS and cerebrospinal fluid (CSF) have a higher frequency of involvement. In both types of BL, the MYC oncogene locus on chromosome 8q24 is deregulated as it is juxtaposed to one of the immunoglobulin gene loci, the commonest translocation being t(8;14) (q24;q32), which involves the immunoglobulin heavy chain gene locus in 80% of cases. Sporadic and endemic BL show similar typical morphological features

LYMPHOBLASTIC LYMPHOMA

Up to 70% of children with T-cell lymphoblastic lymphoma (T-LL) present with mediastinal involvement and respiratory symptoms, cervical and supraclavicular adenopathy or superior vena cava (SVC) syndrome. Lymphoblastic lymphoma is distinguished from ALL on the percentage of blasts in the marrow: ALL being diagnosed if there are greater than 25% blasts.

Diagnosis and Staging

NHL often presents with a rapidly growing tumour with potential life-threatening complications. Tissue procurement using the least invasive procedure and staging evaluation should be carried out as soon as possible. Staging is according to Murphy with treatment intensity based on stage and CNS/CSF disease.

DOI: 10.1201/9781003175186-11

Treatment

Surgery and radiotherapy have a very limited role in modern treatment strategies. NHL should be considered a systemic malignancy even when the disease is localised and multiagent chemotherapy is the treatment of choice. In general, children and adolescents with localised disease have an excellent outcome with approximately 90 to 95% long-term survival. Those with disseminated NHL have slightly worse but still relatively good outcome with > 80% chance of cure. Lymphoblastic lymphoma is treated on ALL protocols.

LEUKAEMIA

Clinical Features

Children with leukaemia frequently present with symptoms and signs of pancytopenia due to marrow failure. Fever, often due to leukaemia rather than infection, is present in 60% of patients. Young children with bone pain may present with a limp or refusal to bear weight. Bulky extramedullary disease, especially overt CNS disease, mediastinal mass and renal infiltrates are more common in T-lineage ALL. CNS involvement is usually lepto-meningeal rather than parenchymal and may present with symptoms of meningism or cranial nerve palsies. Painless enlargement of the scrotum may be due to a testicular infiltrate or hydrocele resulting from lymphatic obstruction. Rarely, the diagnosis is made in a child who has a blood count for minor, non-specific, symptoms.

Differential Diagnosis

Immune thrombocytopenic purpura (ITP) is the most common benign condition associated with symptoms that raise concern about leukaemia. Severe skin haemorrhage in an otherwise well child with isolated severe thrombocytopenia and normal blood film without circulating blasts distinguishes the condition from leukaemia. Pancytopenia due to aplastic anaemia is difficult to distinguish from 'aleukaemic leukaemia' without marrow examination. Rare cases of ALL present with an aplastic marrow without blasts, often accompanying severe sepsis, with spontaneous reconstitution of normal haemopoiesis on recovery from the infection. They re-present later with low counts and circulating lymphoblasts. Bone pain, arthralgia and occasionally arthritis may mimic juvenile arthritis in a minority of patients.

Laboratory Work-Up

A blood count at diagnosis shows varying degrees of pancytopenia which is more severe in AML and B-lineage than T-lineage ALL. Most patients have circulating blasts, but they may be difficult to detect in those with leucopenia without careful scrutiny of a blood film ('aleukaemic leukaemia'). Reactive hypereosinophilia with pulmonary infiltration and cardiomyopathy is a feature of a rare sub-type of B-lineage ALL with $t(5;14)(q31;q32)$/*IGH-IL3*. Coagulopathy is more common in AML, and invariably present in the promyelocytic subtype (APML). Patients with very high white cell counts are at risk of CNS haemorrhage due to leucostasis. Elevated uric acid and phosphorus levels may be seen due to rapid tumour proliferation in patients with high tumour burden. Leukaemic blast cells are identified morphologically at diagnosis in a cytospin of CSF in one-third of ALL and 5% of AML, most of whom have no neurological symptoms.

A bone marrow aspirate or trephine is usually heavily infiltrated with leukaemia blasts which are classified by flow cytometry into various subtypes of AML and ALL. Cytogenetic and molecular genetic profiling of the leukaemic blasts are essential for prognostication and treatment stratification. Traditional cytogenetic methods such as karyotyping and Fluorescence In Situ Hybridization (FISH) are being replaced by higher resolution methods such as single nucleotide polymorphism (SNP) arrays, large DNA panels, whole genome sequencing and RNA sequencing.

ACUTE LYMPHOBLASTIC LEUKAEMIA

Acute Lymphoblastic Leukaemia (ALL) has a high cure rate after treatment stratified by phenotype, genotype and early treatment response combined with incorporation of more effective formulations of existing drugs into treatment protocols and better supportive care. These have contributed to the improved survival rates observed in the last few decades (Figure 11.1). Treatment is for two years and modern protocols incorporate complex risk stratification models to target patients for more or less intensive chemotherapy or immune therapy approaches. Very few patients need haemopoietic stem cell transplant (HSCT) in first remission. Toxicity, immediate and late, remains a concern and innovative agents, including immune based approaches, are delivering

Improvements in overall survival for successive UK childhood ALL trials

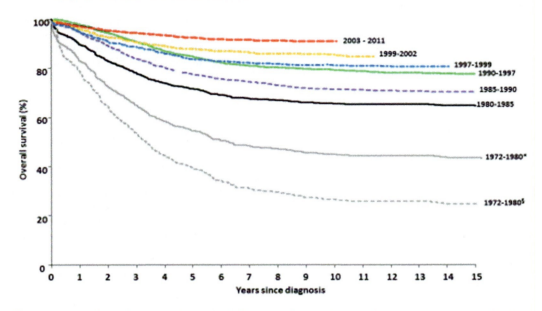

Figure 11.1 Overall survival among children with acute lymphoblastic leukaemia (ALL) who were enrolled in UKALL clinical trials, 1972–2011. Note: *standard treatment §non-standard treatment. Adapted from Bartram et al. Br J Haematol. 2020 Nov;191(4):562-567. doi: 10.1111/bjh.17162. PMID: 33190256.

improvements in efficacy whilst reducing the burden of therapy by replacing toxic elements of current treatment protocols.

ACUTE MYELOID LEUKAEMIA

Rarely, leukaemia can present in the newborn period (congenital leukaemia) and, if so, it usually presents as a monocytic variety of leukaemia with leukaemia cutis 'blueberry muffins' in two-thirds of patients (Figure 11.2.). They have marked hepatosplenomegaly and lymphadenopathy and CNS involvement is seen 50% of cases. Monocytic/myelomonocytic leukaemia can present with skin lesions, gum infiltration and involvement of other extramedullary sites in older children (Figures 11.3 and 11.4).

Diagnosis

The bone marrow in AML shows mixtures of myeloblasts and monoblasts (Figures 11.5 and 11.6). The current WHO classification incorporates cytogenetic and molecular genetic abnormalities which are or diagnostic and prognostic importance. A significant proportion of the neonatal leukaemias have 11q23 (*KMT2A* previously known as *MLL* gene) chromosomal abnormalities.

Treatment

Treatment of all types of AML involves risk directed intensive combination chemotherapy based on underlying leukaemia genetics and minimal residual disease assessment, with or without an allogeneic HSCT. Infants and neonates should receive size adjusted doses, as treatment-related mortality (specifically infection and cardiotoxicity) is a significant contributor to failure in this group of patients.

ACUTE PROMYELOCYTIC LEUKAEMIA

Acute promyelocytic leukaemia (APL/APML) (Figure 11.7) re-presents 5% of cases with characteristic blast morphology (plentiful Auer rods) (M3 in the FAB classification of AML) and the presence of t(15;17) translocation, creating the *PML-RARα* fusion gene. A coagulopathy (mostly

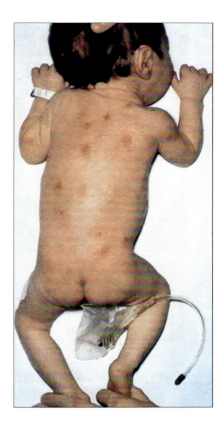

Figure 11.2 Congenital leukaemia: neonate with 'blueberry muffin' appearance.

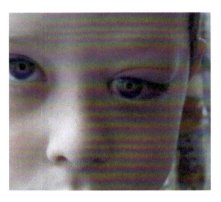

Figure 11.3 Proptosis secondary to granulocytic sarcoma.

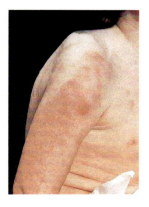

Figure 11.4 Leukaemia cutis in an older child.

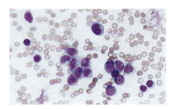

Figure 11.5 Myelomonocytic leukaemia (FaB M4 subtype).

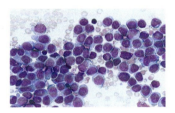

Figure 11.6 Monocytic leukaemia (FaB M5 subtype).

haemorrhagic) occurs in most patients and can be life threatening, hence should be treated as a medical emergency with blood components. Recently, chemotherapy-free regimens consisting of ATRA and arsenic trioxide have obtained > 90% cure rates with reduced toxicity compared with chemotherapy-containing regimens.

JUVENILE MYELOMONOCYTIC LEUKAEMIA

Juvenile myelomonocytic leukaemia (JMML) is a rare (1 per 1 million children per year) disorder of early childhood (median age of 2 years; range 0.1–11.4) characterised by uncontrolled proliferation of monocytes, as well as myelodysplastic features of anaemia and thrombocytopenia. The usual clinical presentation is splenomegaly, maculopapular rash (Figure 11.8), lymphadenopathy, fever, high WCC (Figure 11.9) and an absolute monocytosis (> 1×10^9/l) (Table 11.1). *Café-au-lait* spots (Figure 11.10) may be present due to underlying neurofibromatosis-1 (NF1) and other congenital syndromes such as Noonan should be excluded. Allogeneic HSCT is the only curative therapy in the majority of children, with overall survival rates of 50%.

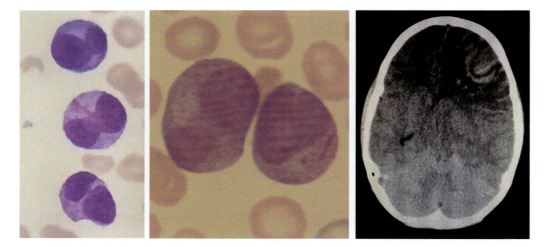

Figure 11.7 Acute promyelocytic leukaemia.

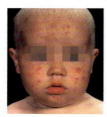

Figure 11.8 Juvenile myelomonocytic leukaemia: erythematous maculopapules on the face.

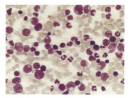

Figure 11.9 Juvenile myelomonocytic leukaemia: bone marrow morphology showing dysplastic change in the myeloid lineage.

PAEDIATRIC MYELODYSPLASTIC SYNDROMES

Clinical Presentation

Myelodysplastic syndrome (MDS) is rare in childhood and associated with ineffective haematopoiesis, characterised by abnormal dysplastic cells and cytopenias. They are clonal myeloid stem cell disorders with a high risk of progression to AML. MDS can be primary (*de novo* or idiopathic) or secondary, associated with syndromes such as DS, Fanconi anaemia, Shawachman–Diamond or due to previous chemotherapy.

Diagnosis

The marrow often shows cytogenetic and molecular genetic abnormalities of prognostic importance and which distinguish hypocellular MDS from severe aplastic anaemia.

The blood smear may be helpful (Figure 11.11) and monosomy 7 (Figure 11.12) is present in approximately 30% of primary childhood MDS and approximately 50% of therapy-related MDS. Allogeneic HSCT is the only curative option.

Haematological Disorders and Down Syndrome

Down syndrome (DS) is associated with a number of distinct haematological disorders occurring at different ages.

TRANSIENT ABNORMAL MYELOPOIESIS

Children with DS have a predilection to develop transient myelopoiesis (TAM), occurring in up to 10%. This is a rare clonal 'pre-leukaemic' condition that is characterised by circulating megakaryoblasts (Figure 11.13) and spontaneous resolution within 3–6 months of life in the majority of cases.

Table 11.1: World Health Organisation Criteria of Juvenile Myelomonocytic Leukaemia

1. Clinical and haematological features (all four mandatory)
 – Peripheral monocytosis (> 1 ×10⁹/l)
 -Absence of t(9;22) or BCR-ABL (not CML)
 -Bone marrow or blood with < 20% blasts (not AML)
 -Splenomegaly

2. Oncogenetic studies (1 find sufficient)
 – Somatic mutation in PTPN11, K-RAS or N-RAS
 -Clinical diagnosis of NF-1 or germline NF1 mutation
 -Germline CBL mutation and loss of heterozygosity of CBL

3. Only for those patients without oncogenetic parameters, besides the clinical and haematologic features listed under one at at least two of the following:
 Monosomy 7 or any other chromosomal abnormality
 -Myeloid precursors in the blood
 -Increased haemoglobin F for age
 -GM-CSF hypersensitivity in colony assay
 -Hyperphosphorylation of STAT5

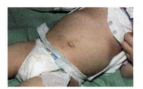

Figure 11.10   Juvenile myelomonocytic leukaemia: cafe-au-lait spots.

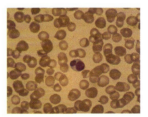

Figure 11.11   Myelodysplasia: dysplastic neutrophil, so called pseudo pelger–huet form.

Clinical Presentation and Molecular Pathogenesis

Presentation is in first month of life with hepatosplenomegaly, leucocytosis, preserved haemo-globin, moderate thrombocytopenia and circulating blasts. (Figure 11.14). A minority die in utero or are born in extremis from severe hydrops, massive hepatosplenomegaly, liver failure, ascites, severe coagulopathy, pericardial/pleural effusions and cardiac failure due to platelet derived growth factor released from megakaryoblasts. Acquired somatic mutations in exon 2 of the haema-topoietic transcription factor gene *GATA1* are diagnostic of the condition.

Follow-Up and Treatment

The majority do not require treatment. Low-dose cytarabine is effective in those with hepatic, renal and cardiac involvement. Follow-up to age 4 years as up to 20% of cases will develop Myeloid Leukaemia of Down's Syndrome (MLDS).

MYELOID LEUKAEMIA OF DOWN SYNDROME (MLDS)

MLDS develops in approximately 1% of children with DS. Many have a relatively indolent course characterised by a period of thrombocytopenia (commonest presenting cytopenia) and MDS in association with marrow fibrosis and blasts (Figure 11.15). MLDS has a superior outcome (> 80% cure) compared to non-DS children with AML (~60%).

ACUTE LYMPHOBLASTIC LEUKAEMIA AND DS

The incidence of ALL in children with DS is approximately 30-fold higher than in the general population and accounts for approximately 3% of all cases of ALL. ALL has an inferior outcomes compared with children with non-DS ALL.

ALLOGENEIC HAEMOPOISTIC STEM CELL TRANSPLANTATION (ALLO-HSCT) AND CELLULAR THERAPY

Allo-HSCT (replacement of recipient haemopoiesis and immune system with that of an allogeneic donor) and cellular therapies such as donor leucocyte infusions and other adoptive T-cell therapies

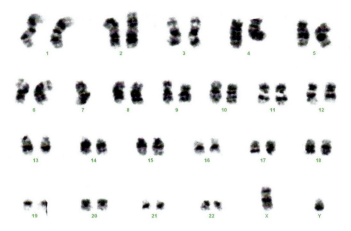

Figure 11.12   Myelodysplasia: G-banded karyotype of bone marrow from a patient with raeB1 showing the abnormality: 45,XY,-7 (monosomy 7).

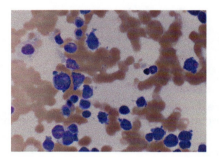

Figure 11.13   Transient myeloproliferative disorder: circulating megakaryoblast with classic cytoplasmic blebbing.

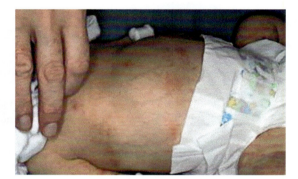

Figure 11.14   Transient myeloproliferative disorder: tMD cutis.

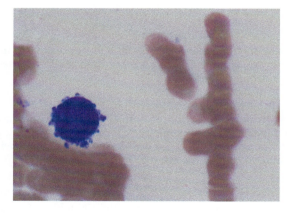

Figure 11.15   Down syndrome myeloid leukaemia: leukaemic blast cells of megakaryocytic-erythroid origin.

are curative for a range of malignant and non-malignant haematological disorders, primary immune deficiency, and metabolic disorders.

The procedure requires conditioning treatment (either chemotherapy, radiotherapy or both) to ablate recipient haemopoiesis and eliminate host T lymphocytes and antigen presenting cells which would otherwise reject incoming donor haemopoietic stem cells (HSC). The donor is generally selected to provide a close match for major histocompatibility complex (MHC) genes with the recipient. Once engrafted, the donor HSC reconstitutes the patient's haemopoiesis and immune system through a process of differentiation and subsequent education in the bone marrow and thymus, in the case of B and T-cells, respectively. Conditioning regimes differ in degree of bone marrow (or myelo-) ablation. In children, myeloablative conditioning is used for patients with leukaemia and is associated with early therapy-related complications such as mucositis, sinusoidal obstruction syndrome, pulmonary fibrosis and late effects (growth, puberty, loss of fertility, secondary malignancies and late cardiac dysfunction). Reduced intensity/toxicity regimens are used for patients with poor performance status or high risk of toxicity (Fanconi anaemia) and incorporate more intensive immune suppression to prevent rejection with associated higher risk of viral reactivations and relapse. Recipient–donor chimerism is tracked in the peripheral blood or bone marrow after transplant to monitor engraftment status.

Donor-derived immune cells can cause graft-vs-host disease (GVHD) which can affect multiple organs and has early (acute) and late (chronic) phases. Hence post-transplant immune suppression such as ciclosporin is given for 3–6 months following HSC infusion after which the donor immune system usually becomes tolerant of host antigens. By contrast, donor-derived immune cells can drive graft-versus-leukaemia (GVL) responses which reduce the risk of relapse of malignant disorders by eliminating emergent malignant cells of host origin.

One way to redirect the host immune system to recognise malignant cells is to genetically engineer T-cells with a novel immune-receptor. This can be a native T-cell receptor, or a synthetic receptor such as a chimeric antigen receptor (CAR) Figure 11.16. Recipient-derived CAR-engineered T-cells have recently gained prominence due to studies demonstrating remarkable outcomes in relapsed/ refractory disease particularly in patients with relapse of ALL post allo-HSCT for whom there otherwise are few curative options.

Introduction to Anaemias

Anaemia is common in children and it may be acute and transient or chronic and life-long (Table 11.2). A full blood count, reticulocyte count, bilirubin/LDH and blood film can help direct further investigations. The reticulocyte count distinguishes increased red cell breakdown (haemolysis) or blood loss (high) from reduced production (low). The commonest cause is iron deficiency which is associated with a low mean cell volume (MCV) (microcytic) and mean cell haemoglobin concentration (MCH) (hypochromic) anaemia whereas B12/folate deficiency are much less common and associated with raised MCV (macrocytosis). Reticulocytosis can also be associated with macrocytosis as young red cells are larger, as can MDS or bone marrow failure. Hence, bone marrow investigations should be undertaken in patients with persistent macrocytic anaemia with normal reticulocyte count and B12/folate levels. Microcytosis is also seen in thalassaemias, some membrane disorders (hereditary pyropoikilocytosis, HPP, and sometimes hereditary spherocytosis (HS) and one form of congenital sideroblastic anaemia (CSA). Iron studies and Hb HPLC (haemoglobin high performance liquid chromatography including measurement of the HbA2 level which is raised in beta-thalassaemia trait) will distinguish iron deficiency from thalassaemia. Blood counts should be interpreted in the context of the age-specific normal ranges, especially in the first six months of life when the physiological switch from fetal to adult haemoglobin occurs.

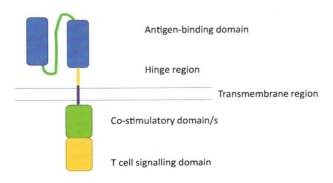

Figure 11.16 Anatomy of a chimeric antigen receptor (CAR).

Table 11.2: Causes of Anaemia in Children.

Underproduction	Increased destruction
Congenital Bone marrow failure syndromes *Diamond Blackfan Anaemia* *Shwachman Diamond Syndrome* *Fanconi Anaemia* Congenital sideroblastic anaemia *X linked (ALAS2, ABCB7)* *AR (SLC25A38, GLRX5, PUS1, YARS2)* *Maternal (Pearson's syndrome)* Congenital dyserythropoietic anaemia *Types I–III (& IV–VII)* *With thrombocytopenia (GATA1)*	**Inside the red cell** Haemoglobin disorders *Sickle cell disease* *Thalassemias* Enzyme deficiencies *G6PD, PK, others*
Acquired Bone marrow infiltration *Leukaemia/lymphoma* *Other malignancy* Bone marrow dysfunction *Myelodysplastic syndrome* *Haematinic deficiency (B12, folate, iron)* *Poisoning (drugs)* Bone marrow shut down *Aplastic anaemia* *Transient erythroblastopenia* *Parvovirus*	**Red cell membrane** Structural defects *Hereditary spherocytosis,* *elliptocytosis and pyropoikilocytosis* Antibody-mediated *Haemolytic disease of the newborn* *Autoimmune haemolytic anaemia* *Haemolytic transfusion reactions* **Outside the red cell** Haemorrhage Mechanical haemolysis *AV malformations* *Prosthetic valves* *DIC, TTP*

Iron Deficiency

Iron deficiency in children is most often due to inadequate diet, particularly in toddlers who have not weaned and are still largely dependent on milk. Malabsorption and bleeding are uncommon causes but coeliac disease should be excluded in a patient who fails to respond to iron supplementation. Rare mutations in genes regulating iron absorption genes should be excluded if malabsorption and blood loss has been excluded in a child who has not responded to adequate courses of iron supplementation. The diagnosis is made on the basis of a microcytic hypochromic anaemia with low serum iron, ferritin and raised total iron binding capacity, (TIBC). The differential is thalassemia trait which should have a normal ferritin and iron profile.

Iron deficiency may be an incidental finding, or children can present with pallor and fatigue. When severe and chronic, it can also cause developmental delay and, rarely, cerebral venous thrombosis. The mainstay of treatment is oral iron supplementation (continued until the haemoglobin and MCV have normalised and then for a further three months to fully replenish iron stores) whilst resolving underlying cause. Intravenous iron infusions should be reserved for patients who are unable to absorb oral iron or the rare genetic condition IRIDA (iron refractory iron deficiency anaemia).

Vitamin B12 and Folate Deficiency

Vitamin B12 and folate deficiency lead to a macrocytic anaemia with a low reticulocyte count, and sometimes other cytopenias. There may be a raised LDH and typical findings on the blood film (hypersegmented neutrophils, teardrop cells and red cell fragments). The diagnosis is confirmed by a low serum B12 or red cell folate.

Although restricted diet can cause B12/folate deficiency in strict vegans who do not take vitamin supplementation, malabsorption should be excluded in patients with apparently normal diet and no history of surgery such as gastrectomy or small bowel resection. Folic acid is absorbed in the proximal small intestine and B12 in the terminal ileum, so malabsorptive states affecting these areas can cause the corresponding deficiencies. B12 deficiency can also be caused by pernicious anaemia (an autoimmune condition causing antibodies to intrinsic factor, which is required for B12 absorption) as well as rare genetic disorders affecting B12 absorption and transport. Neonates can also be affected by untreated maternal B12 deficiency, particularly if the baby is solely breast fed for a prolonged period. An important but very rare autosomal recessive condition, transcobalamin II deficiency, causes functional B12 deficiency, in which serum B12 levels are normal, but

B12 cannot be transported into cells. It should be suspected in infants with developmental regression within 6 to 12 months of age, diarrhoea and pancytopenia. A raised serum homocysteine and methylmalonic acid and genetic testing will provide confirmation of the diagnosis.

Management is with supplementation and treatment of the underlying cause where possible. Transcobalamin II deficiency is treated with supraphysiological doses of intramuscular B12 several times a week. Neurological recovery is rapid and complete if treated early.

G6PD and Other Enzyme Deficiencies

Deficiency of a number of intracellular red cell enzymes can cause haemolytic anaemia. The most common is glucose 6 phosphate dehydrogenase (G6PD) deficiency, in which red blood cells are susceptible to oxidative damage due to infection or exposure to fava (broad) beans and certain drugs. Inheritance is X-linked, however carrier girls can be mildly affected, and more rarely can present like boys due to extreme lyonisation or double heterozygotes. Haemolysis manifests as acute pallor, jaundice and haemoglobinuria and requires urgent red cell transfusion if severe. Reticulocytes have a higher G6PD content than mature red cells giving a false normal G6PD level in the acute phase, hence the level should be checked when the reticulocyte count is normal and at least three months after red cell transfusion. Families should be advised to avoid fava beans, naphthalene, henna tattoos and a list of drugs known to precipitate a crisis.

Hereditary Spherocytosis and Other Membrane Disorders

Abnormalities in red cell membrane proteins due to genetic mutations result in a change in their shape and deformability. The most common, HS, is caused by variants in the ankyrin-spectrin complex, band 3 or protein 4.2 genes which result in an abnormal cytoskeleton and spherical red cells. Inheritance is usually dominant but some cases are recessive. The chronic haemolysis may present in the neonatal period, with early onset, severe or prolonged jaundice. Milder cases can go undetected for many years, sometimes being picked up as an incidental finding or presenting with an exacerbation of the condition due to an infection or cholecystitis due to pigment gall bladder calculi. Parvovirus infection can cause a precipitous fall in Hb due to infection of red cell precursors causing transient red cell aplasia requiring urgent transfusion. The diagnosis is suspected on the basis of a haemolytic anaemia, spherocytes on the blood film and a negative direct antiglobulin test (DAT). It is confirmed by a positive family history or by analysis of eosin-5 maleimide (EMA) binding on flow cytometry of red cells. Management is with folic acid during steady state and transfusions as required for acute exacerbations. Splenectomy is usually curative but reserved for patients with severe haemolysis.

Hereditary pyropoikilocytosis (HPP) is due to homozygous or compound heterozygous mutations in the alpha and beta spectrin genes. This leads to the red cells adopting a variety of bizarre shapes and sizes and a severe chronic haemolytic anaemia. Management is the same as for severe HS.

Hereditary elliptocyosis, on the other hand, is due to heterozygous mutations in the alpha spectrin or protein 4.1 genes and usually only causes mild haemolysis. Diagnosis is often incidental, when a blood film is examined for some reason and the typical elliptoid shape of the red cells is seen.

Haemoglobinopathies

Haemoglobin comprises four globin chains wrapped around an iron-containing haem group, and an inherited abnormality of one or more of these globin chains cause haemoglobinopathies. Babies are born predominantly with HbF (consisting of two alpha and two delta chains) which is gradually replaced by HbA (two alpha and two beta chains) over the first few months of life. Therefore, alpha globin disorders can present at birth, whereas beta globin disorders do not present until at least 4 to 6 months of age.

Sickle Cell Disease (SCD)

SCD is one of the most common single gene disorders in the United Kingdom, affecting around 1 in 2500 live births. It is caused by a mutation in codon 6 of the beta globin gene (situated on chromosome 11), leading to glutamic acid being replaced by valine as the 6th amino acid in the beta globin chain. HbS carriers are asymptomatic and partially protected against malaria, hence individuals with ancestral links to areas where malaria is endemic (Africa, Eastern Mediterranean, South Asia and the Middle East) are at risk. There is an antenatal and neonatal screening programme in the United Kingdom to identify newborns with SCD.

Patients with homozygous (HbSS) or compound heterozygous HbSC, HbSD[Punjab], HbSO[Arab], HbSE or HbSβ thalassaemia mutations develop acute and chronic complications of the disease.

Polymerisation of HbS in the deoxygenated state alters the shape of the red cells, leading to impaired circulation. This is manifest by acute painful vaso-occlusive crises, chest syndrome, splenic or hepatic sequestration and priapism. Chronic tissue damage can lead to stroke, hyposplenism (with resultant risk of infection with encapsulated bacteria), renal and liver impairment and cardiopulmonary failure.

Patients with SCD should be managed by specialist haemoglobinopathy teams. The management includes pneumococcal vaccination and penicillin prophylaxis from 3 months of age, good hydration and avoidance of exposure to extreme temperatures to prevent vaso-occlusive crises. Milder crises can be managed at home with oral fluids and simple analgesia but severe symptoms require hospitalisation for intravenous analgesia, fluids and broad spectrum antibiotics as necessary. Urgent red cell exchange transfusion is indicated for acute chest syndrome and stroke to reduce HbS to below 30%. Surgery should be carefully planned in advance and follow guidelines for pre-operative top-up or exchange transfusion.

Longer-term management includes treatment with hydroxycarbamide which reduces the frequency and severity of crises by increasing HbF levels and screening for cerebrovascular disease by transcranial Doppler ultrasonography from the age of 2 years to identify patients at increased risk of stroke for regular transfusions and iron chelation. HSCT is curative but reserved for patients with severe disease with a matched family donor and gene therapy is an attractive potential option for the future.

Thalassaemia

In the commonest form, beta-thalassaemia, production of beta globin chains is absent (β^0 thalassemia) or reduced (β^+ thalassaemia), leading to an excess of free alpha chains in red blood cells following the switch from HbF to HbA in early infancy. This leads to ineffective red cell production, severe anaemia and compensatory extramedullary haematopoiesis. It is inherited in an autosomal recessive fashion, with carriers being clinically unaffected (except for having a mild microcytic anaemia, called thalassaemia trait). The inheritance of alpha thalassaemia is more complicated, as two alpha globin genes are inherited from each parent. Children with one or two affected genes are asymptomatic (thalassaemia trait), those with three affected genes have an intermediate condition called HbH (manifest by a moderate chronic haemolytic anaemia) and those with all four genes affected have a very severe anaemia which is usually fatal antenatally (Barts hydrops fetalis). Thalassaemia is common in families originating from the Mediterranean, the Middle East, South Asia, South East Asia and the Far East. There is an antenatal screening programme in the United Kingdom.

Most patients require transfusions by 6 to 9 months of age but the exact timing should depend on feeding, growth and development. Once transfusions are initiated, the Hb should be maintained above 90 g/l, with the aim of optimising growth, energy levels and quality of life, as well as inhibiting extramedullary haematopoiesis. The main complication of regular red cell transfusions is iron overload. Untreated, this leads to the gradual development of liver fibrosis, cardiac failure, diabetes mellitus, poor growth, delay or absence of puberty and other endocrine abnormalities. Hence, an appropriate iron chelator should be started after the first 10 to 12 red cell transfusions. HSCT is an option and families should be given a chance to discuss this at an early stage. Gene therapy studies are showing promising results.

Autoimmune Haemolytic Anaemia (AIHA)

This is an uncommon condition, affecting approximately 1 in 100,000 per year. It can occur as an isolated condition, often following a viral infection, as part of a primary disorder of immune dysregulation, such as severe combined immunodeficiency (SCID) or autoimmune lymphoproliferative syndrome (ALPS), or as the presenting feature of a rheumatological condition.

Patients present with sudden onset fatigue, pallor and jaundice due to severe anaemia, reticulocytosis, unconjugated hyperbilirubinaemia and a positive direct antiglobulin test (DAT). In warm AIHA (majority of paediatric cases), the DAT is positive to IgG and C3d, the blood film shows numerous spherocytes and the haemolysis is predominantly extravascular. In cold AIHA it is typically positive to C3d +/– IgM, although in paroxysmal cold haemoglobinuria (PCH), a condition peculiar to young children, the DAT is actually positive for IgG and is identified in the transfusion laboratory by the Donath Landsteiner test (demonstrating the antibody binding to red cells at 4°C and causing haemolysis at 37°C).

Management is with red cells transfusions and prednisolone 2 mg/kg/day until there is consistent improvement in the haemoglobin and other markers of haemolysis followed by a slow wean over many months. Refractory or relapse cases may respond to rituximab or mycophenolate mofetil. PCH does not respond to corticosteroids and the mainstay of treatment is keeping the patient warm, as well as warming any blood that is transfused. Folic acid should be given to all patients until full resolution.

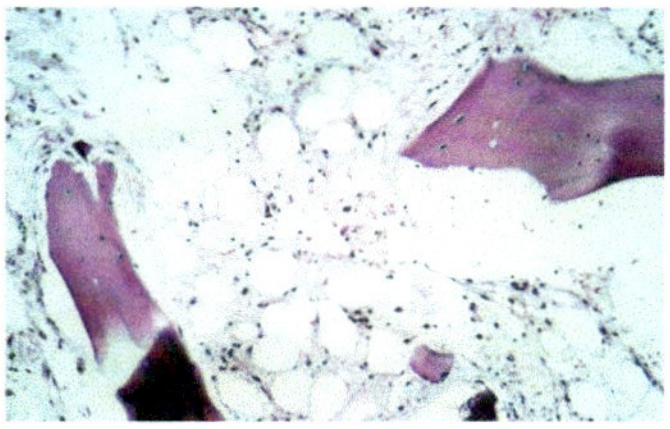

APLASTIC ANAEMIA AND BONE MARROW FAILURE SYNDROMES (BMFS)

These conditions are characterised by a reduction in haematopoiesis affecting one or more lineages manifested as a reduction in bone marrow cellularity (Figure 11.17).

Figure 11.17 Severe aplastic anaemia: bone marrow biopsy showing hypocellular marrow with less that 5% cellularity, so called 'empty' marrow.

Inherited Bone Marrow Failure Syndromes

Patients present with cytopenias and/or associated somatic features and have a variable predisposition to malignancy or immune deficiency. Some patients can present with subtle or atypical clinical features such as isolated bone marrow without somatic features or vice versa. Atypical presentation may also be contributed to by compartment-specific genetic reversion and mosaicism. All patients presenting with aplastic anaemia, MDS, AML, and chronic unexplained cytopenias, excess haematologic or other toxicities during treatment of a malignancy which can be associated with bone marrow failure syndromes should be investigated. A few specific conditions are considered below.

Fanconi Anaemia (FA)

This usually presents towards the end of the first decade of life, but can present in adulthood. A third of cases will not have associated somatic features. It is characterised by genomic instability caused by spontaneous chromosomal breakage and sensitivity to agents which cross-link DNA as a result of a diverse range of mutations interfering with DNA repair mechanisms. As a result, there are diverse inheritance patterns.

Dyskeratosis Congenita (DKC)

This condition arises due to mutations in genes involved with maintenance of telomere length. Bone marrow failure arises due to short telomere length in haematopoietic stem cells (HSCs). There are associated mucocutaneous somatic abnormalities, particularly nail dystrophy, oral leucoplakia and abnormal skin pigmentation as well as hepatic cirrhosis and pulmonary fibrosis. Since telomeres below the first centile can be documented in rare patients with other inherited bone marrow failure syndromes and acquired aplastic anaemia, screening tests for telomere length should be followed by genetic confirmation where possible.

Diamond Blackfan Anaemia (DBA)

The most common manifestations include macrocytic anaemia with short stature, thumb anomalies and congenital heart disease. This often presents in early infancy, sometimes at birth with profound anaemia and absent reticulocyte response.

Acquired Bone Marrow Failure Disorders

These include acquired aplastic anaemia, paroxysmal nocturnal haemoglobinuria (PNH, rare in children) and hypoplastic myelodysplastic syndromes (MDS), Rarely drugs (chloramphenicol) and environmental exposure to benzenes or radiation can also cause aplastic anaemia but it is a diagnosis of exclusion with severity classified on the basis of degree of cytopenia and marrow cellularity in the absence of myelofibrosis or an infiltrate. PNH occurs when a clone of HSC develops an acquired mutation of the PIGA gene resulting in a loss of glycosylphosphatidylinositol (GPI)-anchored proteins on cell membranes which renders red cells susceptible to complement-mediated intravascular haemolysis. Overlap between features of these syndromes can lead to diagnostic complexity. For example, patients with aplastic anaemia may have features of dysplasia and a low level PNH clone.

Therapy of Bone Marrow Failure Disorders

Supportive care is essential including blood product support and prevention of infection with antibiotic and antifungal prophylaxis. HSCT is definitive therapy for both inherited and acquired severe aplastic anaemia (SAA) but some FA and DKC patients respond well to danazol as temporising treatment prior to transplantation. Acquired SAA is an auto-immune disorder which responds to immunosuppression (IS) with horse anti-thymocyte globulin and ciclosporin. IS is given to children without a fully matched family or unrelated donor.

THROMBOCYTOPENIAS

Thrombocytopenia is common, particularly in hospitalised neonates and is either due to under-production or increased consumption. Platelet transfusions give good increments in the former whereas they are poor in the latter. Bone marrow failure due to infiltration, chemotherapy or disorders referred to above (including rare inherited conditions such as congenital amegakaryo-cytic thrombocytopenia (CAMT) or thrombocytopoenia absent radii (TAR) syndromes that present with isolated thrombocytopenia) affect production; the most common causes of consumption are sepsis, hypersplenism, idiopathic thrombocytopenic purpura or immune thrombocytopenia (ITP) and neonatal alloimmune thrombocytopenia (NAIT). The cause is usually apparent from the history, pattern of the thrombocytopenia, examination of the patient and thorough analysis of the blood count and blood film, although specific diagnosis may require more detailed investigations.

Immune Thrombocytopenia (ITP)

ITP affects around 4 per 100,000 children, with a peak age of onset between 2 and 5 years old. It typically presents with sudden onset widespread bruising and petechiae and an isolated severe thrombocytopenia. Often there is a recent history of a viral illness and rarely a new drug or recent vaccination, but sometimes there is no apparent trigger. Most cases occur in otherwise healthy children, but a small percentage will be part of a broader immunological or rheumatological condition, as with AIHA. There is no specific test for ITP and it remains a diagnosis of exclusion made on the basis of the typical clinical presentation, isolated thrombocytopenia and normal blood film. Atypical features warrant further investigations.

ITP spontaneously resolves in 70–80% of children within a year of presentation, with most of these improving in the first few weeks. The remainder are classified as having chronic ITP, which is still likely to improve or resolve completely at some point, although it is impossible to predict when this will occur. ITP is more likely to become chronic if the ANA or DAT is positive, or the child is over the age of 10 years at presentation.

Children without bleeding can be managed on a watch and wait approach, but families require support and education, a point of contact for advice and open access in an emergency. Patients presenting with bleeding should be treated with one of the rescue therapies, either intravenous immunoglobulin (IVIg) or a short course of prednisolone. Life-threatening (such as intra-cranial) bleeding is rare (< 1% of cases) but should be treated aggressively with IVIg, high dose methyl-prednisolone and platelet transfusions. Tranexamic acid is a useful adjunct. Children who have required repeated courses of rescue therapy over many months, or who have had a single life-threatening bleed, should be offered one of the second line treatments.

Inherited Thrombocytopenias

As well as the inherited bone marrow failure syndromes and genetic syndromes in which thrombocytopenia frequently occurs (e.g. 22q11 deletion, Wiskott–Aldrich and Noonan syndromes) there are an increasing number of genetic disorders in which thrombocytopenia is the main or sole abnormality. Such conditions should be considered in children with chronic thrombocytopenia, particularly if they present in infancy, with a pattern which is not suggestive of another condition (many of them have a very stable mild to moderate thrombocytopenia) or if the degree of bleeding seems excessive for the platelet count (as some of them have an associated platelet dysfunction). The blood film may show large size or reduced granulation of platelets.

THROMBOCYTOSIS

Most cases of thrombocytosis in children are secondary to iron deficiency, acute infections or surgery. Platelet counts in young children can reach very high levels during the recovery phase of serious infections, even up to $2000 \times 10^9/l$. This is not associated with thrombotic events and no treatment is required. Thrombocytosis persisting more than a few months after an infection or surgery – or after iron deficiency has been adequately treated – should prompt a search for an occult infection or inflammatory condition. An ultrasound should also be performed to exclude a congenitally absent spleen.

If no cause is identified, then essential thrombocytosis (ET) should be considered. This bone marrow disorder is extremely rare in children and is due to either inherited variants in *THPO* or *MPL* (the genes for thrombopoietin and the thrombopoietin receptor) or occasionally acquired variants in *JAK2*, *CALR* or *MPL*. Patients with ET have a long-term increased risk of thrombosis and transformation to leukaemia. They require monitoring and follow up and should be considered for treatment with aspirin and hydroxycarbamide as they get older.

NEUTROPENIA

Neutropenia is also common in children, being seen transiently in neonates with bacterial sepsis, in older children with viral infections and in some metabolic conditions during periods of decompensation.

Severe Neutropenias

Persistent severe neutropenia in a neonate or young infant can be due to neonatal alloimmune neutropenia (NAIN) or severe congenital neutropenia (SCN). Both conditions can lead to severe bacterial infections, but the former recovers within the first few months when the maternal antibodies disappear, whereas the latter is due to inherited mutations in *ELANE*, *G6PC3*, *HAX1* or *GATA2* and is therefore permanent. Patients with SCN require antibiotic prophylaxis and treatment with GCSF, as well as careful monitoring due to the risk of transformation to leukaemia. Cyclical neutropenia is another genetic condition caused by mutations in *ELANE*, but unlike SCN, does not transform to leukaemia. Patients with this condition typically present with an intermittent neutropenia, often on a roughly three-week cycle, with corresponding episodic mouth ulcers and infections. Neutropenia is often the first haematological abnormality in Shwachman–Diamond Syndrome.

Autoimmune Neutropenia

This typically presents in young children (aged 6 months to 2 years) as an isolated neutropenia. Diagnosis is made by identifying antibodies to mature neutrophils on serum samples. The degree of neutropenia is variable, but even when numerically severe (< 0.2×10^9/l) the condition is still relatively benign. This is because neutrophil production is unaffected and patients can usually mount a decent neutrophil response during infections. Autoimmune neutropenia of infancy and early childhood has a very good prognosis, with spontaneous resolution occurring in the vast majority within two years of diagnosis.

Benign Ethnic Neutropenia

This is extremely common in families of African, Middle Eastern and West Indian descent. Neutrophil counts can be as low as 0.5×10^9/l in infancy and down to 1.0×10^9/l in older children, but there is no increased risk of infection. The pathophysiology is not entirely clear, but seems to be due to either a defect in release of mature neutrophils from the bone marrow or an increase in migration of neutrophils from the circulation into tissues. No investigations are required if the blood count is otherwise normal and there is no atypical history of infections.

DISORDERS OF COAGULATION

Severe inherited bleeding disorders may cause symptoms at birth, but more commonly present after children become mobile or following a surgical challenge. Acquired bleeding disorders can present at any age. An understanding of coagulation tests is important when assessing patients.

Activated partial thromboplastin time (APTT) assesses levels of intrinsic pathway clotting factors (VIII, IX, XI and XII) plus common pathway factors (X, V, II and fibrinogen). The prothrombin time (PT) assesses the extrinsic pathway (factor VII) and the common pathway (X, V, II and fibrinogen).

Some bleeding disorders will not be identified on standard clotting tests, as the PT and APTT will be normal. These include mild von Willebrand disease, FXIII deficiency and platelet function disorders (many of which also have a normal platelet count).

Haemophilia

This is an X-linked disorder affecting boys, although carrier girls can be mildly affected. Haemophilia A, due to factor VIII deficiency is more common, affecting 1 in 5000 male births. Haemophilia B affects 1 in 25,000 males and is due to factor IX deficiency. Both lead to an isolated prolonged APTT. The severity is classified according to baseline factor level: severe < 1 iu/dl, moderate 1–5 iu/dl, mild > 5 iu/dl. Children with severe (and some with moderate) haemophilia present with lumpy bruises as they start to mobilise, and are then at risk of recurrent bleeds into muscles and joints. A small percentage present with intracranial haemorrhage, either related to birth or spontaneously in early infancy. Children with mild haemophilia also bruise easily, although these tend not to be lumpy, and they usually only experience bleeding at mucosal sites.

Patients with severe (and some with moderate) disease require regular treatment with recombinant factor VIII or IX concentrate (called prophylaxis) to protect them from recurrent bleeds. Patients can develop inhibitors to this treatment, rendering it ineffective and necessitating the use of alternative bypassing agents which may be less effective.

Patients with mild disease do not require regular prophylaxis, but occasionally require treatment following a traumatic bleed or to cover surgery. DDAVP can also be used for short periods in mild Haemophilia A, as it stimulates transient release of endogenous factor VIII. The anti-fibrinolytic drug, tranexamic acid, is useful as an adjunctive treatment, and also on its own for minor bleeds.

Von Willebrand Disease (vWD)

This is the commonest inherited bleeding disorder, affecting around 1% of the population. Patients either have a reduced level of von Willebrand factor (vWF, Type 1), dysfunctional vWF (Type 2) or absent vWF (Type 3). VWF is essential for primary haemostasis and stabilising factor VIII. Patients with vWD often have a low factor VIII, and this may lead to a prolonged APTT (but this is not universal). Inheritance is autosomal dominant, except types 2N and 3, which are recessive. VWD can also rarely be acquired, particularly in relation to Wilms tumours.

Patients with Type 1 vWD present with easy bruising, with or without abnormal mucosal bleeding (particularly epistaxis and menorrhagia). Type 3 vWD has a similar clinical presentation to severe haemophilia, whereas Type 2 disease is variable, depending on the subtype and the levels of vWF activity. The vast majority of patients have Type 1 disease and do not require regular treatment. DDAVP leads to a three to fivefold increase in the vWF and factor VIII levels temporarily, so can be very useful for bleeds and minor surgical procedures in mild Type 1 (and some Type 2) disease. Most patients with Type 3 disease require regular prophylaxis with intravenous vWF concentrate.

PLATELET FUNCTION DEFECTS

Individually these are all rare, but collectively they are quite common. Some are isolated inherited conditions (e.g. Bernard Soulier), some are part of a broader genetic syndrome (e.g. Noonan or Hermansky–Pudlak syndromes) and others are secondary to drugs or acquired conditions (e.g. uraemia). They can be associated with thrombocytopenia (e.g. grey platelet syndrome) but the majority have a normal platelet count, and they should have a normal clotting screen.

The most severe platelet function disorder is Glanzmann thrombasthenia. This is an autosomal recessive condition caused by absent expression of the platelet glycoprotein IIbIIIa. This glycoprotein is crucial in enabling platelets to bind fibrinogen and adhere to each other during the development of the platelet plug in primary haemostasis. Patients usually present in early infancy with widespread bruising, petechiae and mucosal bleeding. Treatment of bleeds is with platelet transfusions, recombinant factor VIIa and tranexamic acid. HSCT is the only potential cure and should be considered in patients with frequent or severe bleeds.

Disseminated Intravascular Coagulation (DIC)

DIC describes systemic activation of coagulation, leading to enhanced fibrin formation (with the risk of organ failure) and consumption of platelets and clotting factors (with the risk of bleeding). It is triggered by an underlying disorder, most commonly sepsis. Bloods show a prolonged PT and APTT, reduced fibrinogen and thrombocytopenia. Appropriate management is treatment of the underlying disorder, rather than the coagulation results, but if there is associated bleeding, then blood product support may be required. In patients presenting with some forms of leukaemia, bleeding from DIC can be severe, and aggressive blood product support is necessary.

Vitamin K Deficiency

Vitamin K is essential for activation of clotting factors II, VII, IX and X. Deficiency can therefore cause a prolonged PT and APTT, although in mild or early cases, an isolated prolonged PT may be the only finding, as factor VII has the shortest half-life. Severe deficiency in neonates and young infants (if vitamin K has not been administered at birth) can lead to gastrointestinal or intracranial haemorrhage. Treatment is with oral or intravenous vitamin K, and patients who are bleeding should also be given plasma or prothrombin complex concentrate.

THROMBOSIS

Thromboembolic disease is uncommon in paediatrics and is very rare in otherwise healthy children. Most cases of thrombosis are seen in patients admitted to intensive care units, particularly in relation to indwelling central lines. Other risk factors include cancer, sepsis, COVID-19, inflammatory conditions, some drugs (combined oral contraceptive, asparaginase), severe dehydration, obesity and immobility. Inherited thrombophilias (e.g. antithrombin, protein C and protein S deficiencies, factor V Leiden and prothrombin gene mutations) can contribute to the risk, but rarely lead to a thrombotic event in childhood without additional acquired risk factors.

Treatment of thrombosis is initially with heparin for at least the first five days, which is then either continued or switched to an oral anticoagulant to complete 3–6 months of treatment. Direct oral anticoagulants (such as rivaroxaban) are becoming the oral treatments of choice in this setting, but warfarin is still indicated in the context of antiphospholipid syndrome or mechanical heart valves. Life or limb-threatening thrombosis requires urgent thrombolysis (using tissue plasminogen activator).

Purpura Fulminans

This is a rare, but very serious manifestation of severe protein C or S deficiency. Children present with purpuric lesions, which rapidly spread to cover large areas of skin, becoming necrotic and threatening viability of fingers and toes. It can occur in neonates born with inherited severe protein C deficiency, who are also invariably blind due to retinal vein occlusion, and rarely following chicken pox due to acquired protein S deficiency. Both scenarios are medical emergencies, requiring urgent treatment with plasma infusions (to replace the missing protein C or S) as well as plasma exchange and immunosuppression in the acquired cases.

FURTHER READING

- Arceci R, Hann I, Smith O, Hoffbrand AV. *Pediatric Hematology*, 3rd Edin. Wiley, 2008
- Orkin S, Nathan D, Ginsburg D, Look AT, Fisher D, Lux S. Nathan and Oski's Haematology of Infancy and Childhood, 7th edn. Saunders, 2009
- Vora A. *Childhood Acute Lymphoblastic Leukemia.* Springer, 2017
- Maude S, Laetsch T, Buechner J, et al. Tisagenlecleucel in Children and Young Adults with B-Cell Lymphoblastic Leukemia. *N Engl J Med* 2018; 378:439-448

12 Oncology

Darren Hargrave, Tanzina Chowdhury and Olga Slater

INTRODUCTION

Cancer affects about 1 in 600 children worldwide. Leukaemia is the most common form (30–35% of all cancer in childhood), followed by brain tumours (20–25%), lymphomas including Hodgkin disease (10%), soft tissue sarcomas, particularly rhabdomyosarcoma (7%), neuroblastoma (7%) and Wilms tumour (5.5%). Leukaemia and lymphoma are covered in the chapter 'Haematology'.

Survival in childhood cancer has significantly improved over the past few decades, with over 75% of all children in developed countries now being cured. This resulted from sequential national and international clinical trials that have optimised a multi-modality treatment approach, which, depending on the type of cancer, includes surgery, chemotherapy, radiotherapy, and biological therapies. However, survival rates for many childhood cancers are now plateauing and for some aggressive malignancies, e.g. high-risk brain tumours and bone sarcomas there has been little improvement in survival over the past decade and new approaches are necessary (Table 12.1).

The success of multi-modality treatments means that, around one in 750 young people in their 20s are long-term survivors of childhood cancer, but many will have significant long-term side effects because of their primary treatment. Therefore, specialist survivorship programmes are in place to anticipate, screen for and address these issues.

Over the past decade there has been a huge increase in the understanding of the molecular basis of childhood cancer, which are driven by abnormalities of cellular pathways that are often involved in normal development. This has led to a revision and refinement of tumour classifications, better risk stratification and identification of new targets for potential novel therapies using small molecules and monoclonal antibodies. In addition, immunotherapies are being developed that harness the body's own immune system to target cancer cells. It is hoped that these new-targeted therapies will not only help to improve survival further in childhood cancer but also potentially reduce late side effects.

TUMOURS OF THE CENTRAL NERVOUS SYSTEM

Primary malignancies of the CNS account for 25% of all cancers in childhood. There has been a fundamental paradigm shift in the WHO 2021 Fifth Edition CNS Tumour Classification (WHO CNS5) by integrating histology with molecular diagnostics to form an integrated diagnosis. There is now a recognition of the specific differences between adult and paediatric CNS tumours.

MEDULLOBLASTOMA/CNS EMBRYONAL TUMOURS
Incidence, Aetiology, Classification and Genetics

CNS Embryonal tumours are a heterogenous group, previously classified as either medulloblastoma (MB) or supratentorial primitive neuroectodermal tumours (PNETs). The advent of advanced molecular sequencing has allowed the identification of new molecular defined for both MB and other CNS embryonal tumours (WHO CNS5). MB arise in the cerebellum and are the most common malignant childhood brain tumour, affecting 6.6 children per million per year with a median age at diagnosis of 5 years. The histological variants of MB (i.e. desmoplastic/nodular, with extensive nodularity, large cell, and anaplastic) have been combined with the molecular classification to in an integrated approach with a consensus of four distinct molecular subgroups; 10% are WNT (Wingless) activated, 25% are SHH (Sonic Hedgehog) activated (either TP53-wild-type or mutant) and 65% are non-WNT/non-SHH (often referred to as groups 3 and 4). MB is associated with several cancer predisposition syndromes including Gorlin syndrome (PTCH/ SUFU mutations – SHH-MB subgroup), Li–Fraumeni syndrome (loss of TP53 function), Turcot syndrome (mismatch repair gene and APC mutations) and Rubenstein–Taybi syndrome (CREEBP and EP300 mutations).

Other embryonal tumours include atypical teratoid rhabdoid tumours (ATRT), embryonal tumour with multi-layered rosettes (ETMR), cribriform neuroepithelial tumour, CNS neuroblastoma, FOXR2-activated and CNS tumour with BCOR internal tandem duplication all very rare, are finally grouped into the category of embryonal tumours 'not otherwise specified' (NOS). ATRT, occurs at a median age below 20 months, with the genomic hallmark of an extremely stable

DOI: 10.1201/9781003175186-12

Table 12.1: **Types of Childhood Cancer and Cure Rates**

Type of cancer	Percentage of childhood cancers	Average cure rate (%)
Acute lymphoblastic leukaemia	25	80–85
Brain tumours	25	Depends on the type of the brain tumour
Hodgkin disease	4	90
Non-Hodgkin lymphoma	6	80
Soft tissue sarcoma	7	70
Acute myeloid leukaemia	5	70
Neuroblastoma	7	Depends on the type and the risk category
Wilms tumour	5.5	85
Osteosarcoma	2.5	65
Ewing sarcoma	1.5	65
Malignant germ cell tumours	3.5	80–90
Retinoblastoma	3	98
Hepatoblastoma	1	90

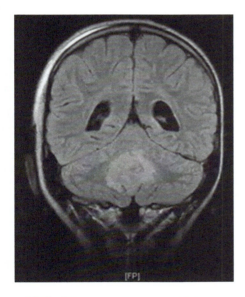

Figure 12.1 T2-weighted coronal MRI scan: Posterior fossa mass, which proved to be medulloblastoma. This patient did not present with obstructive hydrocephalus.

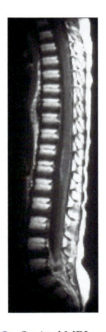

Figure 12.2 Sagittal MRI scan of spine showing enhancing spinal deposits.

genome with classically bi-allelic loss of function of SMARCB1 which can be present as a germline mutation in up to a third of the patients

Clinical Presentation

Cerebellar tumours present with ataxia and signs of raised ICP. Patients with tumours in the pineal region (pineoblastoma) may have Parinaud syndrome (failure of upward gaze, dilated pupils that react to convergence but not light, nystagmus and lid retraction).

Diagnosis and Investigations

MRI or CT scanning will reveal the presence of the tumour (Figure 12.1). Spinal imaging (with MRI) is mandatory to exclude spinal metastases (Figure 12.2). Post-operative imaging to report the degree of surgical resection and CSF staging to check for the presence of malignant cells is required. Complex risk stratification for MB consisting or clinical, imaging, histology and molecular profiling have evolved both as prognostic factors and to direct therapy. Similar criteria are being developed for other CNS embryonal tumours.

Treatment/Prognosis

Overall survival rates for patients with medulloblastoma have reached 70–80% using treatment protocols that include a combination of surgery, craniospinal radiotherapy and chemotherapy. As with all brain tumours there is a need to balance survival with the neurological side effects of the treatment, and age at onset plus risk stratification guides management decisions. This is most developed in MB with low, standard, high and very high risk in addition to young/ infant groups, directing the use or not of radiotherapy (local or craniospinal) and dose applied as well the intensity of chemotherapy. With current risk stratification and treatments, five-year survival rates are 90% or better (low-risk WNT and SHH-MB), standard (70–80%) and very high-risk groups with survival of lower than 60% (high-risk SHH and group 3 and 4). Attempts to delay or avoid radiotherapy, in infant/ young (< 3 years) using intensive high-dose chemotherapy regimens with peripheral stem cell rescue have had some success dependent on the underlying biology. Management of ATRT is often similar to those employed in young/ infant MB protocols including intrathecal administered chemotherapy. Relapses are local or disseminated through the craniospinal axis. Salvage therapy for children who have been irradiated as part of their primary therapy is rarely curative.

PAEDIATRIC GLIOMAS, GLIONEURONAL AND NEURONAL TUMOURS
Incidence, Aetiology, Classification and Genetics

The recent WHO CNS5 classification has divided diffuse gliomas into adult-type and paediatric types which primarily (but not always) occur within these age groups. This is refined in to paediatric-type low-grade and high-grade diffuse gliomas. The low-grade group includes four entities: Diffuse astrocytoma, MYB- or MYBL1-altered; Angiocentric glioma; Polymorphous low-grade neuroepithelial tumour of the young (PLNTY) and Diffuse low-grade glioma, MAPK pathway-altered. The high-grade family also comprises four types: diffuse midline glioma, H3 K27-altered; diffuse hemispheric glioma, H3 G34-mutant, diffuse paediatric-type high-grade glioma, H3-wildtype and IDH-wildtype; and infant-type hemispheric glioma. Diffuse midline glioma (DMG) includes the previous entity described as diffuse pontine glioma (DIPG) but now defined by presence of H3 K27 mutations or EZHIP protein over-expression and occur in other midline locations in the brain and spine. In addition, new groups of 'circumscribed astrocytic gliomas' including, the most common childhood brain tumour Pilocytic astrocytoma (PA), as well as less frequent Pleomorphic xanthoastrocytoma (PXA), Subependymal giant cell astrocytoma (SEGA) and Astroblastoma, MN1-altered and 'Neuronal and glioneuronal tumours' were designated in WHO CNS5.

However, paediatric gliomas are still mainly treated according to the previous groupings of low-grade and high-grade gliomas.

LOW-GRADE GLIOMA

Paediatric low-grade gliomas (PLGG) represent 25–30% of all childhood CNS tumours and has a peak incidence in the first decade of life. They can occur in all locations including cerebellum, brainstem, supratentorial and spinal. Patients with neurofibromatosis Type 1 (NF1) are predisposed to PLGG particularly in the optic pathways and patients with tuberous sclerosis have a predilection to the SEGA type of PLGG. Sporadic PLGG are characterised by genomic alterations involving activation of BRAF and the ERK/MAPK pathway such as the BRAF-KIAA1549 gene fusion, or BRAF V600E point mutations. Other less common mutations have also been found in FGFR1, PTPN11 and NTRK2 fusion genes. Angiocentric gliomas which typically arise in children and young adults as cerebral tumours presenting with seizures, have MYB gene alterations present in almost all cases often with QKI being the primary fusion partner.

Clinical Presentation

Cerebellar astrocytomas present with raised ICP and ataxia. Optic pathway tumours (Figure 12.3) lead to squint, proptosis or visual loss. Hypothalamic involvement can produce growth disturbance, precocious or delayed puberty and changes in mood. Diabetes insipidus is rare in

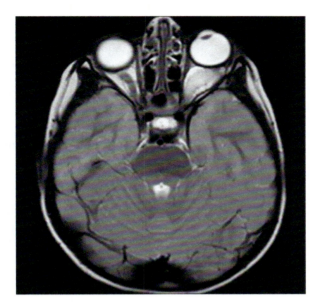

Figure 12.3 T2-weighted axial MRI showing left-sided optic pathway glioma with proptosis. There is no sign of neurofibromatosis-1.

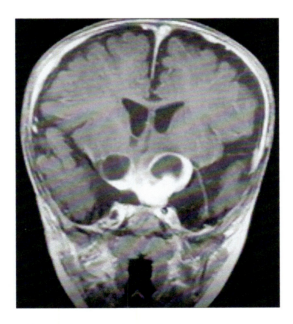

Figure 12.4 Coronal MRI scan showing chiasmatic glioma with cyst formation.

hypothalamic low-grade astroctyomas and its presence should raise the question of whether the tumour is a craniopharyngioma or a germ cell tumour.

Diagnosis and Investigations

MRI ophthalmology scan (Figure 12.4) and routine spinal imaging is recommended but the incidence of neuroaxis dissemination at diagnosis is under 5%. Ophthalmological and endocrine assessments are mandatory in optic pathway tumours. A biopsy is increasingly required, except in NF1, to elucidate the exact type of PLGG and driving mutation.

Treatment/Prognosis

Over 90% of children with cerebellar astrocytoma are cured by surgery alone. Surgery has a role in unilateral optic nerve tumours with total visual loss, but most optic pathway tumours can be managed with chemotherapy or radiotherapy treatment being instituted for tumour growth or an increase in symptoms. Children with NF1 have a better prognosis and should only be treated with chemotherapy if there is 'threat' to vision or clinical/radiological evidence of tumour growth. Radiotherapy should be avoided in children with NF1 due to the increased incidence of vasculopathy and second malignancy in later life. The long-term overall survival for PLGG is high with > 90% at ten years plus but many patients have a chronic natural history of multiple progressions before the tumour stops growing with resulting and often significant morbidity and high burden from treatments. The most widely used chemotherapy for PLGG is carboplatin with vincristine. Radiation therapy is usually reserved until progressive disease following failure of chemotherapy and if required highly conformal techniques such as proton beam therapy are preferred to reduce late side effects. The increased knowledge of the underlying biology of PLGG has led to the use of targeted therapies for PLGG such as mammalian target of rapamycin (mTOR) inhibitors, e.g. everolimus for the treatment of SEGA and oral small molecule inhibitors such as BRAF (e.g. dabrafenib) and MEK (e.g. selumetinib and trametinib) inhibitors for BRAF altered PLGG.

HIGH-GRADE GLIOMA

Paediatric high-grade glioma (PHGG) comprise around 20–25% of childhood brain tumours and the incidence increases with age. Forty percent occur in the cerebral hemispheres, 10% arise in the pons and the remainder in the thalami, hypothalamic regions, basal ganglia or spine. PHGG is a heterogenous group comprising with differing molecular drivers; DMG (H3 K27M altered either H3 K27 mutations or EZHIP protein overexpression), diffuse hemispheric glioma, (H3 G34-mutations), diffuse paediatric-type high-grade glioma, (H3-wildtype and IDH-wildtype); and Infant-type hemispheric glioma (NTRK family, ALK, ROS, MET gene fusions). Patients with the following cancer predisposition syndromes are at an increased risk of PHGG, biallelic mismatch repair deficiency, Li–Fraumeni and NF1 plus PLGG can develop following treatment for a prior CNS tumour usually after irradiation.

Clinical Presentation

Aa with all CNS tumours, location and the presence or absence of raised ICP. Weakness, visual disturbances, cranial nerve palsies and hemiplegia are found in around 50% of cases for supratentorial PHGG, whereas those arising from the pons (previously called DIPG) presenting with a brief classical triad of cranial nerve deficits, long tract signs and ataxia and have a peak incidence at 5–8 years of age.

Diagnosis and Investigations

MRI scanning of brain and spine is required used for diagnosis, although spread within the neuroaxis is uncommon but can occur. Brainstem PHGG show classical appearances on MRI (Figure 12.5). Even with the new WHO CNS5 and DMG is based on specific molecular alterations the role of biopsy as standard of care remains of debate due to the current poor prognosis of DIPG and is often reserved for cases with an atypical history/imaging or as part of a clinical trial.

Treatment/Prognosis

The completeness of surgical resection in PHGG is an important prognostic variable but a complete resection is usually impossible due to the diffuse infiltrative nature and location of the tumour. Pons centred PHGG are not amenable to surgery current standard treatment in children older than 3 years of age is combined

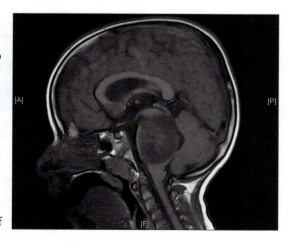

Figure 12.5 T1-weighted sagittal MRI showing diffuse intrinsic pontine glioma.

chemo–radiotherapy with temozolomide, but the majority of patients still die from their disease, with less than 20% surviving five years. For DIPG tumours radiotherapy is useful in controlling symptoms and extends survival but is essentially palliative with a dismal median survival of 9–13 months. New insights into the molecular biology of paediatric high-grade glioma may lead to new-targeted therapies for, e.g. targeting BRAFV600E mutated PHGG, NTRK, ALK, ROS, MET gene fusions in infant-type hemispheric glioma or the use of immune checkpoint inhibitors in PHGG associated with biallelic mismatch repair deficiency.

EPENDYMOMA

Incidence, Aetiology, Classification and Genetics

Ependymomas comprise 10% of all CNS tumours of childhood; 70% arise in the posterior fossa (Group A and B subtypes) and 30% supratentorially (ZFTA fusion and YAP1 fusion–positive subtypes). The mean age at diagnosis is 5 years but the peak age of incidence is 2 years. Ependymomas account for 25% of primary spinal cord tumours (MYCN-amplified and myxopapillary subtypes) but present later.

Clinical Presentation

Posterior fossa tumours present with raised intracranial pressure (ICP) and ataxia. Cranial nerve palsies and vomiting are more common than in medulloblastoma due to adherence of the tumour to the floor of the fourth ventricle. Patients with supratentorial tumours present with seizures, focal neurological deficits or raised ICP.

Diagnosis and Investigations

As with all CNS tumours, initial CT or MRI scans will reveal the primary tumour (Figure 12.6) but full neuroaxis MR imaging is required for staging. Metastases within the CNS can occur but are infrequent at diagnosis (10%). The prognostic value of histological grading is unclear.

Treatment/Prognosis

Complete surgical resection is prognostically important but sometimes difficult to achieve due to adherence of tumour to the vital structures. Staged or second-look surgery should always be considered for residual disease. Involved field focal radiotherapy, rather than craniospinal radiation, is recommended, as most relapses are at the site of the primary tumour. Modern conformal techniques (e.g. proton radiotherapy) are now the standard allowing radiotherapy to be considered for younger patients. Chemotherapy is used in infants but its role in older children continues to be investigated. Current five-year survival ranges from 50% to 75%.

RHABDOMYOSARCOMA, OTHER SOFT TISSUE SARCOMAS AND FIBROMATOSIS

Incidence, Aetiology, Classification and Genetics

Rhabdomyosarcoma (RMS) is the commonest soft tissue sarcoma (STS) in children, representing 7% of all childhood cancers. Incidence is four million per year. Majority of RMS are sporadic but 5–10% can be explained by inheritance of a 'cancer predisposition gene', mutated *TP53* gene on chromosome 17p, causing the Li–Fraumeni syndrome, which can also be feature in brain tumours, adrenal tumours and early developing breast cancer. Genetic counselling and clinical and imaging surveillance is available for family members with *TP53* mutations. Two main subtypes off rhabdomyosarcoma occurs in children: the alveolar (ARMS), which has pathognomonic fusion gene (PAX3 or PAX7/FOXO1), rendering it more aggressive, more difficult to treat and more frequently metastatic than embryonal variety (ERMS). Small proportion of alveolar subtype do not have the fusion and there are hence fusion positive and fusion negative ARMS. RMS are stratified for treatment purposes according to the recognised risk factors: postsurgical stage, molecular pathology (fusion negative or fusion positive), size, age, nodal involvement and localisation.

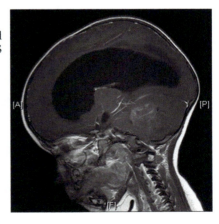

Figure 12.6 T1-weighted MRI scan showing a posterior fossa mass with obstructive hydrocephalus. The histopathology was in keeping with ependymoma.

Clinical Presentation

Around 40% of RMS arises in the head or neck, 20–25% in the pelvis and 25–30% in the trunk and limbs. The orbit is the commonest head and neck site. Painless proptosis (Figures 12.7 and 12.8) is usual and the differential diagnosis includes orbital cellulitis, LCH and other cancers, especially acute leukaemia, secondary neuroblastoma and optic nerve glioma. Middle ear or paranasal sinus tumours may present with aural pain or chronic discharge and delay in diagnosis is common because the problem is often first regarded as 'inflammatory'.

Genitourinary and pelvic primary tumours present either as a visible mass with or without bleeding and discharge, for example at the vaginal introitus (Figure 12.9) or by causing symptoms of pelvic outlet obstruction, most often retention of urine. Tumours arising under mucosa often have a tell-tale 'botryoid' appearance (Figure 12.9).

Limb and trunk primaries arise as painless swellings, if they grow 'outwards' or with one or more of a variety of symptoms (spinal stiffness or pain, pleural effusion, intestinal obstruction) if they grow internally. Some 'primaries' can be tiny, and hard to identify, while others reach 15–20 cm or more in diameter. Back pain is serious symptom in children.

Diagnosis and Investigations

The primary tumour is usually best imaged by MRI, including draining lymph nodes. CT of the chest, whole body FDG PET/CT and bone marrow aspirates (BMA) and trephine biopsy are routine

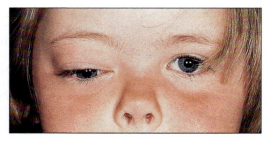

Figure 12.7 Orbital rhabdomyosarcoma of the right eye showing downward and outward displacement of the globe. Occasionally, the swelling looks 'inflammatory' (see text).

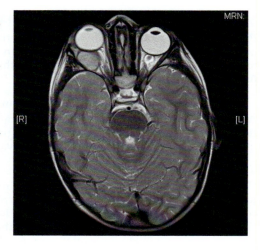

Figure 12.8 T2 MRI of the right orbital rhabdomyosarcoma involving lateral orbital muscles; the patient responded only partially to chemotherapy and required radiotherapy.

part of the staging. Biopsy, with molecular pathology studies, can be performed percutaneously or endoscopically. The biopsy position should be clearly marked and included in the final surgical resection. Draining lymph nodes should be biopsied if the tumour arises in the limbs, or in any location if the lymph nodes are abnormal on imaging. CSF examination is indicated if the tumour is parameningeal.

Treatment/Prognosis

Multi-modality treatment is required. Patients receive primary chemotherapy, 'IVA' (ifosfamide, vincristine and actinomycin D) forms backbone of chemotherapy. Other drugs, such as doxorubicin, irinotecan or topotecan are also used. Local control may involve radiotherapy and/or surgery. Radiotherapy is effective in RMS and well tolerated by young patients but affects bony and soft tissue growth, sometimes with disastrous

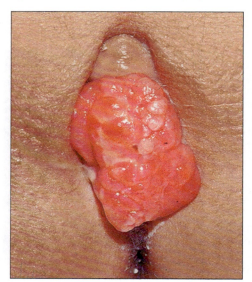

Figure 12.9 Vaginal submucosal embryonal rhabdomyomsarcoma with characteristic 'botryoid' appearance.

cosmetic results. New radiotherapy approaches as proton beam radiotherapy, brachytherapy or intensity modulated radiotherapy are used in an attempt to minimise long-term effects. Primary surgery is only used for easily resected 'peripheral' tumours, such as paratesticular primaries, to reduce morbidity, but less extensive surgery may be used after chemotherapy. For high-risk tumours prolonged low dose maintenance chemotherapy with cyclophosphamide and vinorelbine is used.

Response is best monitored with MRI and is usually good initially. After induction chemotherapy, depending on the response and the group stratification the patient might be treated with surgery and or RT, followed by further chemotherapy. Many children still need surgery and RT for cure, but a proportion can be spared the 'late effects' of these treatments (Figure 12.10).

Embryonal tumours have significantly better prognosis than alveolar. Up to 25–30% of tumours recur, most usually locally which emphasises the value of local control. The recurrence usually happens within the first three years from diagnosis and is treated with second-line chemotherapy, further surgery and RT (if not given first time round). The prognosis depends on the time and type of the relapse, previous treatment given and biology of the tumour.

Metastatic disease presents in 15–20% of patients at diagnosis and has the worst outcome, which depends on the number of the involved sites and biology of the tumour.

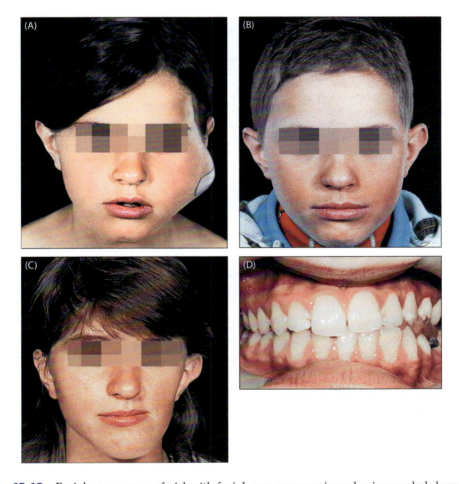

Figure 12.10   Facial appearance of girl with facial, non-parameningeal primary rhabdomyosarcoma. (A) at diagnosis, aged 7 years; (B) at the end of treatment with chemotherapy ('VAC' combination) and external beam radiotherapy; (C) showing marked facial hemiatropy due to radiotherapy; (D) she also had severe dental caries on the side of the radiotherapy. Multiple plastic surgical and orthodontic procedures were needed, but she married and gave birth to two normal sons, despite a high cumulative dose of cyclophosphamide.

OTHER SOFT TISSUE SARCOMAS

Other STS subtypes, more commonly seen in adolescents and young adults are synovial sarcoma, desmoplastic small round cell tumour and other entities. Two types of STS are seen in children.

INFANTILE FIBROSARCOMA

This entity occurs in young children affecting the limbs, especially legs, and has low metastatic potential (Figures 12.11). A high proportion of the tumours have recurring t(12;15) translocation leading to a fusion gene *ETV6-NTRK3* abnormality not found in other STSs. Surgical resection is the mainstay of treatment, but to prevent mutilation, chemotherapy with vincristine and actinomycin D is advocated, followed by surgical resection. If surgery is not possible and chemotherapy not applicable or effective targeted therapy with NTRK inhibitors (Larotrectinib, Entrectinib) could be utilised.

AGGRESSIVE FIBROMATOSIS

Aggressive/infantile fibromatosis occurs in young children and is different from adult desmoid fibromatosis. Infantile fibromatosis can occur at any site and presents like isolated, slowly growing, hard lump. Intra-abdominal desmoids are more common in adults and could be a feature of the familial adenomatous polyposis (FAP) gene. Following biopsy to establish diagnosis, the initial management is observation provided there are no functional deficits, pain or threat to organs. If treatment is required chemotherapy with vinblastine and methotrexate if the first line of treatment. Vinorelbine, imatinib or other tyrosine kinase inhibitors could be used in resistant cases.

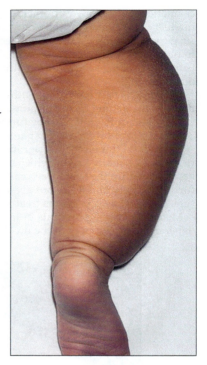

Figure 12.11 Infantile fibrosarcoma of the right calf at diagnosis (posterior view) in an infant. She received six months of chemotherapy with vincristine and actinomycin D, which initiated tumour regression.

EWING SARCOMA/PERIPHERAL PRIMITIVE NEUROECTODERMAL TUMOUR

Incidence, Aetiology, Classification and Genetics

Ewing sarcoma classically occurs in the second decade of life, affecting fewer than three in every 1 million children under 15 years of age. Their distinction from other small round blue cell tumours of childhood could be difficult. Both Ewing sarcoma and pPNET share the same characteristic chromosome translocation, most commonly t(11;22) with corresponding fusion genes *EWS/FLI1* or *EWS/FLI2*.

Clinical Presentation

Ewing sarcoma of bone presents as pain and swelling. Pelvis, femur, tibia and fibula are most commonly affected. The soft tissue Ewing tumours or peripheral primitive neuroectodermal tumours (pPNET) present with intrathoracic disease, or as paravertebral or retroperitoneal masses. Children can also have systemic symptoms such as tiredness and weight loss.

Diagnosis and Investigations

Plain radiographs may reveal 'moth-eaten' bone with periosteal elevation. MRI scans define the extent of soft tissue involvement (Figure 12.12). Metastatic disease should be sought in the lungs (CT chest) (Figure 12.13), bones (whole-body MRI or FDG PET/CT) and bone marrow (aspirate). Samples of the tumour should be analysed histopathologically (characteristically CD99 is positive on immunohistochemistry) with molecular pathology analysis for translocation.

Treatment/Prognosis

Aggressive chemotherapy with alkylating agents and anthracyclines delivered in a compressed schedule reduces disease bulk and treats micrometastatic disease. Good local control with surgery and/or radiotherapy is essential but difficult to achieve in pelvic sites. Intensification

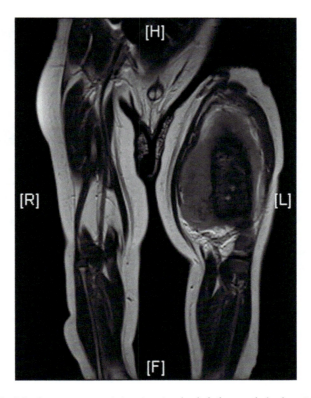

Figure 12.12 MRI of the large mass originating in the left femoral shaft, with associated expansion of the bone, cortical irregularity and periosteal reaction and large soft tissue mass. The patient was 9 months old and had further metastatic disease in the lungs and bones.

of chemotherapy and high-dose chemotherapy with autologous stem cell transfer could be used in refractory, recurrent or metastatic disease (Figure 12.14).

The tumour volume (> 200 ml), poor response to chemotherapy (< 90% necrosis) and the presence of metastatic disease are poor prognostic factors. With aggressive therapy, around 65% of patients with localised disease can be cured.

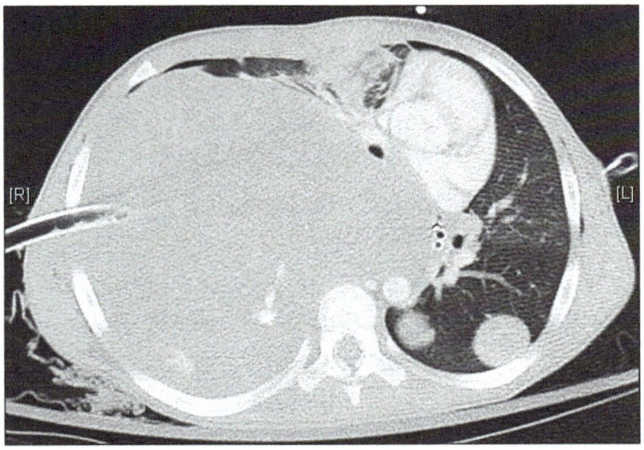

OSTEOSARCOMA
Incidence/Aetiology

Osteosarcoma accounts for 2.5% of paediatric cancers under the age of 15 years, as the peak age coincides with a period of rapid bone growth at the time of puberty. Male to female ratio is 2:1. Several genetic conditions are associated with development of osteosarcoma: Li–Fraumeni syndrome, Rothmud–Thomson, Werner and Bloom syndromes.

Figure 12.13 CT scan of a peripheral primitive neuroectodermal tumour (Askin tumour) of the right chest with pulmonary metastases and rib involvement. The patient had a long history of asthma and presented with cardiac arrest in her school.

Clinical Presentation

Osteosarcoma presents with bone pain, swelling and loss of function in adjacent joints. Symptoms are often attributed to sports injuries in active adolescents. Night pain, systemic symptoms, weight loss or failure of symptoms to resolve with conservative management should alert the clinician.

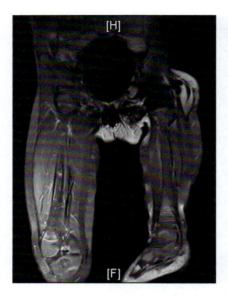

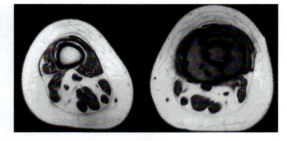

Figure 12.15 T1-weighted axial MRI of the distal femora, showing swelling of the left thigh caused by a tumour of the femur, which both involves the intramedullary region and extends into the soft tissues around the cortex.

Figure 12.14 The same patient as in 12.12 two years after treatment with chemotherapy, surgery with rotationplasty and high-dose chemotherapy with autologous stem cell rescue.

The presenting sites of the disease in the order of frequency are: distal femur, proximal tibia and proximal humerus. Axial tumours constitute 10% of all osteosarcomas.

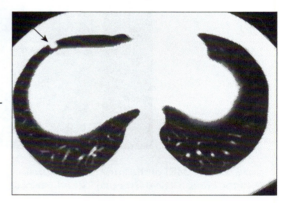

Diagnosis and Investigations

- **Plain radiographs** show a partly lytic, partly sclerotic lesion affecting the metaphysis of a long bone, eroding the cortex, elevating the periosteum to cause a Codman's triangle, with 'sunburst' calcification extending into soft tissues.

Figure 12.16 Thoracic CT scan showing small solitary pulmonary metastasis at the right lung base anteriorly.

- **MRI** of the primary site will show the extent of intramedullary tumour and spread into surrounding soft tissues including neurovascular bundles (Figures 12.15).

- **CT** of the primary site may show calcification in extraosseous tumour. CT of the lungs is mandatory to identify pulmonary metastases in 10–15% at presentation (Figure 12.16).

- Whole body MRI or FDG PET/CT will show the primary tumour and any bone metastases. The biopsy needle tract or incision should be placed in such a way that it can be incorporated into the final surgical excision.

Treatment/Prognosis

Chemotherapy has improved the prognosis of operable osteosarcoma from approximately 20% to about 65%. It is given both prior (neoadjuvant) to and after definitive surgery (adjuvant). The standard chemotherapy regimen includes doxorubicin, cisplatin and high-dose methotrexate. Chemotherapy is also used for inoperable and metastatic osteosarcoma, but survival rates are poor and only 25–50% of patients survive five years. Prognostic factors obtained from large international multi-institutional studies are tumour site and size, presence of metastases, surgical remission and tumour necrosis after neoadjuvant chemotherapy.

Wide surgical excision remains the mainstay of surgical treatment. Advances in surgical techniques and implants have dramatically reduced the need for amputation. Most tumours arise in the metaphyseal region and abut or involve the growth plate; surgical resection will lead to limb length discrepancy. Extendible prostheses have been developed to allow *in vivo* lengthening (triggered by an external magnetic field) as the child grows (Figure 12.17). The other innovative approaches use intercalary allografts and joint sparing reconstructions. In some patient's limb salvage techniques called rotation-plasty can be used. This involves resection of the tumour with the amputation of the knee region, with reunion of the rotated distal limb. For responding tumours, thoracotomy and resection of pulmonary metastases is undertaken.

Radiotherapy has limited role in osteosarcoma, but it may be a useful means of achieving local control of inoperable tumours with new radiation techniques offering some further benefits.

In cases of osteosarcoma arising as a second malignancy, their prognosis may approach that of otherwise comparable patients with primary osteosarcoma if treated by an appropriate multi-modality approach.

NEUROBLASTOMA

Incidence, Aetiology, Classification and Genetics

Neuroblastoma is the commonest extracranial solid tumour, accounting for 7% of all childhood cancer. Neuroblastoma is a disease of the very young: 40% is diagnosed in infants, 35% are patients of 1–2 years and 25% are > 2 years, with the disease becoming rare after the age of 10.

It arises from neural crest cells; primary tumours are located in the adrenal glands or sympathetic ganglia of thoracic or abdominal chain. The clinical behaviour of neuroblastoma is very variable, with some tumours undergoing spontaneous regression and others progressing rapidly with a poor prognosis, in spite of aggressive multi-modality therapy.

There is an internationally accepted neuroblastoma risk group classification by the International Neuroblastoma Risk Group (INRG), using criteria such as age, histology, image defined risk factors and the genomic profile, where neuroblastoma can be divided into very low risk, low risk, intermediate risk and high risk depending on outcome (Table 12.2). In the literature reference will also be made to an earlier surgical staging developed by the International Neuroblastoma Staging Study group (INSS). There are more recent and detailed classifications which are beyond the scope of this text.

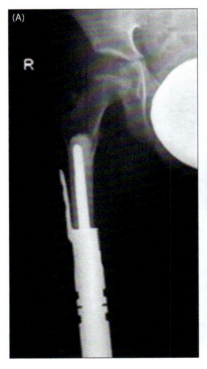
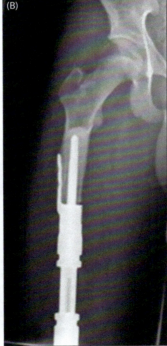

Figure 12.17 Radiograph of extendable growing prosthesis in a child (A) at the end of treatment and (B) several years later.

341

Table 12.2: International Neuroblastoma Risk Group (INRG) Consensus Pretreatment Classification Schema

INRG Stage	Age (months)	Histologic Category	Grade of Tumour Differentiation	MYCN	11q Aberration	Ploidy	Pretreatment Risk Group
L1/L2		GN maturing; GNB intermixed					A Very low
L1		Any, except GN maturing or GNB intermixed		NA			B Very low
				Amp			K High
L2	< 18	Any, except GN maturing or GNB intermixed		NA	No		D Low
					Yes		G Intermediate
	≥ 18	GNB nodular; neuroblastoma	Differentiating	NA	No		E Low
					Yes		H Intermediate
			Poorly differenciated or undifferenciated	NA			
				Amp			N High
M	< 18			NA		Hyperdiploid	F Low
	< 12			NA		Diploid	I Intermediate
	12 to < 18			NA		Diploid	J Intermediate
	< 18			Amp			O High
	≥ 18						P High
MS	< 18			NA	No		C Very low
					Yes		Q High
				Amp			R High

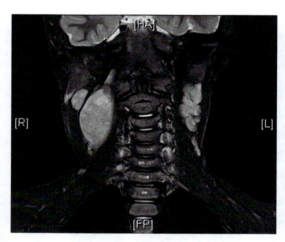

Figure 12.18 MRI: neuroblastoma image defined risk factors. L1, no involvement of the vital organs and structures.

Familial cases are very rare. The tumours can have acquired genetic mutations in MYCN and ALK oncogenes, segmental chromosomal abnormalities (SCA) in 1p,11q and 17q, as well as loss of function of the tumour suppressor PHOX2B.

Diagnosis and Investigations

Urinary catecholamine metabolites (HVA and VMA) are usually raised. MRI scans of the primary tumour will show the extent of the disease locally and allow identification of image defined risk factors L1 or L2 (Figures 12.18, 12.19). Tumours may be calcified. Most tumours are positive on radio-iodine labelled metaiodobenzylguanidine (MIBG) scan, which is essential to exclude distant disease (Figure 12.20). If MIBG is negative at the primary site, then 18F-FDG PET CT will

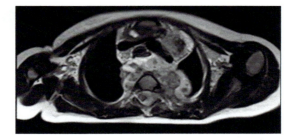

Figure 12.19 MRI: neuroblastoma image defined risk factors. L2, tumour compressing the trachea, extending intraspinally and encasing the aorta.

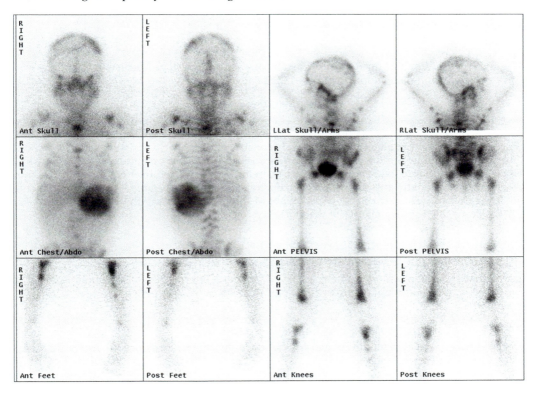

Figure 12.20 MIBG scan of disseminated neuroblastoma – there is avid uptake in the left abdominal tumour with diffuse metastatic disease in the bones. From Cohn S.L. et al.: The International Neuroblastoma Risk Group Classification System. An INRG Task Force Report. *J Clin Oncol* 2009; 27: 289–297.

need to be done to exclude bony and soft tissue metastases. A biopsy of the primary tumour or a metastatic site is mandatory for histology, biology, and the genomic profile, which also predicts outcome. Any tumour with amplification of the MYCN oncongene (MYCNA) is high risk. BMA and trephine biopsies are essential to exclude bone marrow disease.

VERY LOW AND LOW-RISK NEUROBLASTOMA
Incidence, Aetiology, Classification and Genetics

The true incidence of low-risk disease is unknown. Screening all infants for urinary catecholamine metabolites detects those with low-risk disease but unfortunately not those who would go on to develop high-risk disease. Low-risk tumours occur mainly in children < 18 months of age, have favourable histology, may express TrkA protein and be hyperdiploid. Tumours may show SCAs but no *MYCNA*.

Clinical Presentation

Congenital localised neuroblastoma, presenting within the first 3 months of life, is very low risk and can regress spontaneously. Full staging does not have to be done immediately and these infants can be monitored clinically. Infants with stage Ms (special) disease present with rapidly increasing hepatomegaly may have skin deposits (Figure 12.21). Other tumours, local groups L1 or L2 may be detected incidentally. Most children with low-risk disease are diagnosed < 18 months and even if there are metastases will be treated with standard chemotherapy and surgery as long as there as there is no *MYCN amplification*.

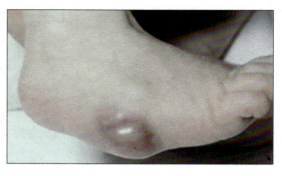

Figure 12.21 Metastatic neuroblastoma in a baby (stage Ms) – deposit in the skin.

Diagnosis and Investigations

BMA and trephines will be positive in metastatic disease though stage Ms disease may show < 10% of nucleated non-haematopoietic cells in the bone marrow.

Treatment/Prognosis

There are different low-risk treatment groups depending on whether life-threatening symptoms are present or SCAs are found in the tumour. Most children will get a combination of chemotherapy and surgery. The chemotherapy mainly consists of carboplatin and etoposide. Resection of the primary tumour is often performed at diagnosis in L1 disease and after chemotherapy in L2 disease. Stage Ms can regress spontaneously but, in infants with rapid liver enlargement, chemotherapy and occasionally low dose RT or even embolisation may be needed. Over 95% of patients with low-risk disease survive. Seventy percent of Ms patients survive, with uncontrolled hepatic growth accounting for the majority of the mortality.

INTERMEDIATE-RISK NEUROBLASTOMA

Incidence, Aetiology, Classification and Genetics

Approximately 30% present with intermediate-risk disease. Intermediate-risk tumours can have both favourable and unfavourable histology, often show SCAs but do not have *MYCN* amplification.

Clinical Presentation

Most patients present > 18 months of age and have a large primary tumour with image defined risk factors L2 and no metastases.

Diagnosis and Investigations

The diagnosis is made by biopsy and grouping by full staging.

Treatment/Prognosis

Treatment includes chemotherapy and surgery. Additional RT to the site of the primary and/ or 13-cis-retinoic acid therapy may be indicated. In older children and adults, a more high-risk approach to treatment may be advised. The five-year event free survival is > 70%.

HIGH-RISK NEUROBLASTOMA

Incidence, Aetiology, Classification and Genetics

Approximately 50% of all patients present with high-risk disease. Histology is unfavourable, poorly differentiated neuroblastoma. No characteristic chromosomal translocations have been identified but several genetic changes occur in tumour cells. The following are associated with a poor prognosis: *MYCNA*, 1p or 11q deletion, 17q gain, reduced expression of the high affinity nerve growth factor receptor (TrKA) and diploid DNA index. *MYCN* amplification is used to stratify for high-risk therapy in patients with localised disease.

Clinical Presentation

The 'classic' presentation is with a hard abdominal mass in a sweaty, hypertensive, irritable child with black eyes and a limp, but many will present without any of these features, for example simply with bone pain.

Diagnosis and Investigation

Grouping should be performed according to INRG (Table 12.2).

Treatment/Prognosis

The majority of high-risk neuroblastoma are sensitive to both chemotherapy and radiation. Dose intense chemotherapy aims to reduce the size of the primary tumour and clear metastatic disease. Further therapy involves resection of the primary tumour and high-dose chemotherapy with autologous peripheral blood stem cell rescue. Oral 13-cis-retinoic acid to 'differentiate' residual tumour and the addition of GD2 directed immunotherapy should further improve outcome. The more recent approaches aim to intensify treatment using tandem high-dose chemotherapy, therapeutic MIBG and their combination. CAR-T-cells for refractory disease is in an experimental phase.

Survival is improving; however, although 50% of patients with high-risk disease survive greater than five years the ten-year survival rate is still only around 30%. In high-risk disease young children fare better than older patients, age being a continuous parameter.

Children can present with signs of spinal cord compression and need to be treated as a medical emergency. They should be started on oral dexamethasone, have an immediate MRI of the spine and if neuroblastoma is suspected should start chemotherapy treatment the same day. Discussion with the neurosurgeons should always take place urgently and where appropriate an intervention should be planned before the blood count drops following chemotherapy.

RENAL TUMOURS

Incidence, Aetiology, Classification and Genetics

Renal malignancy accounts for 6–7% of childhood cancer. Wilms' tumour (WT) comprises 90% of tumours with around 80 new cases in the United Kingdom each year. The highest incidence of WT is found in children of African descent (ten cases/million) and the lowest in Asian populations (three cases/million). The remaining heterogenous group of non-Wilms tumours includes rhabdoid tumour of the kidney, clear cell sarcoma of the kidney, renal medullary carcinoma, and renal cell carcinoma where the prognosis is significantly less favourable. Mesoblastic nephroma generally presents in infants under 6 months of age and has an excellent prognosis with surgery only.

Table 12.3: Renal Tumours of Childhood

Tumour type	Comments
Wilms tumour	80% present < 5 years 5% bilateral
Clear cell sarcoma	3–5% of renal tumours Can metastasise to bone and/or brain Overall survival 75%
Rhabdoid tumour	1% of renal tumours with 65% presenting < 12 months Poor survival rates ~20% Associated with brain ATRT
Neuroblastoma	Rarely intrarenal
Soft tissue sarcoma	Desmoplastic small round cell tumours (DSRCT), rhabdomyosarcoma
Carcinoma	1.7% renal cell In adolescents, associated with Von Hippel–Lindau syndrome, medullary carcinoma
Non-Hodgkin lymphoma	Usually bilateral, diffuse involvement
Mesoblastic nephroma	Presents usually < 12 months Usually benign although the cellular type can metastasise
Cystic partially differentiated nephroblastoma	Benign
Angiomyolipoma	Benign, in association with tuberous sclerosis

ATRT: atypical teratoid/rhabdoid

The genetic changes that underlie WT are diverse and are driven by an array of over 40 cancer genes, many of which are involved in foetal nephrogenesis. Abnormalities of a) the *WT1* gene, (associated with glomerulosclerosis and disorders of sexual development DSD, and WAGR Wilms tumour, aniridia, genitourinary anomalies and range of developmental delays), b) WNT pathway (Simpson–Golabi–Behmel syndrome) and c) IGF signalling (Beckwith Weidemann spectrum) all have central roles in tumourigenesis in patients with these cancer predisposition syndromes (CPS). WT susceptibility is noted in germline mutations in *DIS3L2* (Perlman syndrome), *TP53* (Li-Fraumeni) and *PALB2/BRCA2* (Fanconi anaemia), as well as in *REST, CHEK2* and *PALB2* in non-syndromic patients. Familial Wilms tumour pedigrees account for 1–2% of cases and are known to involve several different heritable mutations including *DICER1, CTR9* and the *FWT1* and *FWT2* loci involving *TRIM28*. Mutations in microRNA processing genes, transcription factor homeobox genes *SIX1* and *SIX2*, genes encoding histone modification proteins BCOR and MAP3K4, transcriptional co-repressors, and MYCN-interacting proteins are all implicated in WT pathogenesis.

Surveillance with three monthly abdominal pelvic ultrasound is recommend for all CPS described above associated with a 5% increased risk of WT development, to be initiated at birth or as soon as a CPS is diagnosed and continued until 7 years of age regardless of the underlying CPS diagnosis.

Clinical Presentation

WT typically presents as an incidental finding of a symptomless abdominal mass. One-third of patients present with associated abdominal pain, a third with haematuria and a quarter with hypertension. Most children with WT are between 1 and 5 years of age with the majority under 2 years of age. Children rarely present with significant systemic ill-health, but may present with fever, weight loss and anorexia in cases of stage 4 disease where chest metastases are present, or in a large tumour causing local invasion. Such symptoms in an older child with a renal mass may point to a diagnosis of non-WT such as renal cell carcinoma or clear cell sarcoma of the kidney. Congenital anomalies are seen in 9% of patients presenting with WT.

Diagnosis and Investigations

Laboratory investigations should exclude neuroblastoma, and identify any anaemia, or coagulopathy caused by the presence of transient von Willebrand factor deficiency. Imaging should include ultrasound, and abdomen/pelvis MRI as gold standard (with CT also satisfactory) to demonstrate the renal origin of the primary tumour(s), exclude bilateral disease (Figure 12.22) and determine the presence of inferior vena cava involvement (Figures 12.23 and 12.24). Chest x-ray and chest CT is required metastatic staging, and those with suspected or established CCSK or rhabdoid tumour of the kidney (RTK) should also have isotope bone scan and MRI scan of the brain.

Biopsy is no longer required in the United Kingdom if imaging features are consistent with Wilms tumour, age criteria are fulfilled, and other diagnoses satisfactorily excluded. Where biopsy

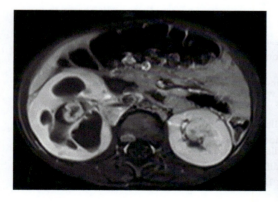

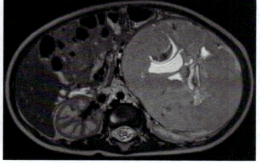

Figure 12.22 MRI STIR sequence of bilateral renal tumours in a child with ambiguous genitalia. histopathology and subsequent surgery confirmed bilateral high-risk Wilms tumour.

Figure 12.23 Large left-sided renal mass, with typical claw-like residue of normal kidney and patent left renal vein and inferior vena cava.

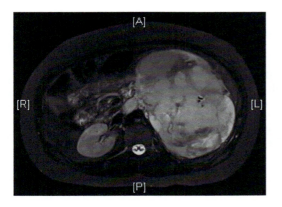

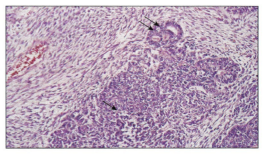

Figure 12.25 'Typical' triphasic Wilms tumour (favourable histology, Fh) showing blastema (single arrow), epithelial structures (double arrow) and stroma.

Figure 12.24 Large left-sided Wilms tumour with extension into the left renal vein abutting the inferior vena cava. The mass is heterogenous, suggesting internal haemorrhage.

is performed, WT histology mimics the developing kidney with triphasic components of stromal, epithelial and blastemal tissue (Figure 12.25). In Europe WT are classified, after a short course of preoperative chemotherapy, into low-/intermediate-/high-risk groups depending on the degree of necrosis, blastema content and presence of anaplasia. This histopathological classification along with the stage of the resected tumour determines the post-operative treatment regimen.

Persistence of nephrogenic blastema beyond 36 weeks of gestation results in what has been labelled a nephrogenic rest (NR) and can occur throughout the kidney with varied histologic and radiological appearances, and may be isolated, multiple, or diffuse, and may coexist with clearly imaged WT lesions. Their presence raises a concern for evolution of Wilms tumour in the future and will require careful management depending on the individual case.

Treatment and Prognosis

The timing of surgery differs for children treated in Europe compared to the United States. Primary nephrectomy followed by chemotherapy and possible radiotherapy is the standard of care in North America, except for bilateral tumours which as in Europe, are treated with six weeks of preoperative chemotherapy. In the United Kingdom and Europe, preoperative chemotherapy prior to tumour nephrectomy is the standard approach to minimise surgical morbidity, reduce surgical stage and hence post-operative treatment intensity, and particularly to assess the tumour response to chemotherapy to allow levels of anticipated risk of relapse to be assigned to the disease and thus tailor the intensity of post-operative treatment. The current focus of both North American and European groups is on using molecular and other biomarkers to risk stratify patients at diagnosis to optimise treatment and outcome.

Overall outcome has historically been similar for both European and North American approaches. Five-year overall survival for WT is 80%, 90% in localised non-high-risk disease, falling to 60% in diffuse anaplastic disease. Approximately half can be salvaged at relapse, particularly if they have received only one or two chemotherapy drugs and no radiotherapy at initial treatment.

RENAL CELL CARCINOMA

Clinical Presentation/Treatment

Renal cell carcinoma (RCC) presents with an abdominal mass and haematuria. The tumour may metastasise to the abdominal lymph nodes, liver, lungs and bone. The differences emerging between childhood and adulthood RCC prevent generalised application of therapies to children that are validated for adults. Forty percent of RCC in childhood are characterised by translocation involving transcription factor E3 (TFE3) family members (involving Xp11.2 or 6p21). This emphasises the importance of prospective classification of RCCs in children using molecular pathology. The treatment for RCC in children and adolescents remains radical nephrectomy, but the systemic therapy (especially in metastatic disease) is with targeted agents such as sunitinib, rather than conventional cytotoxic chemotherapy, which is largely ineffective, although large international studies are needed to validate this approach.

LIVER TUMOURS

Incidence, Aetiology, Classification and Genetics

In sharp contrast to adults, primary liver tumours in children are more common than secondary tumours. Both benign and malignant types occur (Table 12.4). Overall, they represent about 1% of all children's cancers. Males are more commonly affected than females.

Hepatoblastoma usually occurs *de novo*, CTNNB1 mutations have been reported in more than 80% of cases but may be associated with FAP and with Beckwith–Wiedemann syndrome. Hepatocellular carcinoma often arises in a liver previously damaged by the hepatitis B or C virus, or by metabolic liver disease, especially glycogen storage disease (GSD) type I and tyrosinosis. Enormous progress has been made in reducing the incidence of hepatocellular carcinoma worldwide through perinatal hepatitis B vaccination programmes.

Clinical Presentation

Liver tumours usually present with upper abdominal distension (Figure 12.26), while pain is unusual. In very young children a differential diagnosis of stage Ms neuroblastoma with diffuse metastatic spread to the liver can usually be made by identifying an adrenal primary tumour by ultrasound. Besides increased levels of alpha-fetoprotein (AFP), which must be interpreted in the light of normal values for the patient's age, thrombocytosis (due to release of a thrombopoietin) is characteristic of hepatoblastoma and hepatocellular carcinoma.

Diagnosis and Investigations

MRI alongside Doppler ultrasound is better than CT at displaying the anatomy and focality of the primary tumour and is used to identify the pre-treatment extent of disease or PRETEXT (Figure 12.27). The lungs are by far the most frequent site for metastatic hepatoblastoma and hepatocellular carcinoma, so chest x-ray and CT scan of the lungs are mandatory.

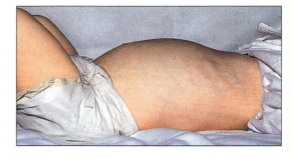

Treatment/Monitoring/Prognosis

Benign tumours are usually treated by surgery alone. Exceptions are haemangiomas, especially infantile haemangioma when

Figure 12.26 Distended upper abdomen in a child with hepatoblastoma. Note that there is no jaundice.

Table 12.4: Types of Liver Tumour and Relationship to Level[a] of Serum Alpha-Fetoprotein (AFP) at Diagnosis

	Undetectable	Slight elevation	Very high
Benign			
Adenoma	50%	50%	–
Haemangioma	All	–	–
Haemangioendothelioma	All	–	–
Mesenchymal hamartoma	50%	50%	–
Malignant			
Hepatoblastoma	< 5%	< 5%	> 95%
Hepatocellular carcinoma[b]	25%	25%	50%
Sarcoma	All	–	–
Malignant germ cell tumour[c]	< 5%	< 5%	> 95%*
Non-Hodgkin's lymphoma[d]	All	–	–

[a] Account must be taken of the child's age in interpreting values.
[b] Fibrolamellar variant associated with normal serum AFP but elevated serum Vit B12 and TCII (transcobolamin II) levels.
[c] Can also have elevated serum β-hCG.
[d] In Non-Hodgkin's lymphoma, liver enlargement is usually diffuse.

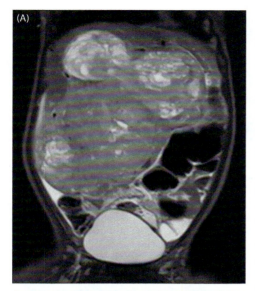

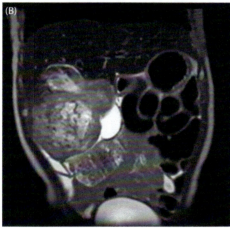

Figure 12.27   MRI: coronal STIR (A) and t2 (B) of a patient with hepatoblastoma at diagnosis and after six weeks of chemotherapy.

medical treatment (in the form of propranolol) alongside careful observation with serial imaging is preferred. Sometimes congenital haemangiomas may present with high output cardiac failure due to the intralesional A–V shunting, in which case transarterial embolisation is preferred to surgery. Malignant tumours are treated with chemotherapy to destroy metastases and shrink the primary tumour, followed by delayed surgical resection and then further chemotherapy. Chemotherapy is cisplatin based, including an anthracycline for high-risk hepatoblastoma and hepatocellular carcinoma. Treatment is usually dictated by international studies. Monitoring is by serial imaging with serum AFP, ultrasound, MRI and chest x-rays in the case of hepatoblastoma/hepatocellular carcinoma. It is essential to monitor serum AFP 1–2 weekly during the treatment and three monthly for three years off treatment. The prognosis has much improved in recent years. Hepatoblastoma is a surgical disease – patient require complete surgical resection for improved outcome. Overall, the cure of hepatoblastoma is now over 90% for standard risk disease and 75% for metastatic disease. Liver transplant from either living related or unknown donor is necessary for PRETEXT IV tumours responding to chemotherapy, without evidence of extrahepatic spread after completion of chemotherapy.

The main side effect of cisplatin chemotherapy is risk of reduced hearing. STS (sodium thiosulphate) has been proven to significantly protect the hearing without any detrimental effects on cure.

For hepatocellular carcinoma, prognosis is still relatively poor because tumours are often multifocal and/or metastatic at diagnosis; however, unifocal tumours are curable in at least 50% of cases.

LANGERHANS CELL HISTIOCYTOSIS

Incidence, Aetiology, Classification and Genetics

Langerhans cell histiocytosis (LCH) is a rare disorder characterised by lesions with an accumulation of Langerhans cells with other immune cells, resulting in tissue damage. LCH occurs at all ages from the neonatal period through childhood to adulthood. The UK childhood incidence is approximately 4.1 per million children under 14 years per year with a 2:1 predominance in males. The median age at presentation is 6 years. LCH lesions, show the pathognomonic CD1a+ve Langerhans cell with macrophages, eosinophils, multi-nucleated giant cells and T-cells. Studies support the universal activation of ERK in LCH; ERK activation in most cases is explained by BRAF (usually V600E) and MAP2K1 alterations.

Clinical Presentation

The disease may involve any organ of the body apart from kidneys and gonads. Single system disease, which occurs in approximately 70% of cases, involves one organ or system, most commonly the skeleton (Figure 12.28), skin or lymph nodes and presents with a bone or soft tissue lump in otherwise well child. Skin rash waxes and wanes, but never clears up completely. Persistent cradle cap is typical as well as the rash in the nappy area and axillae. Craniofacial involvement with proptosis or mastoiditis may result in diabetes insipidus due to involvement of the posterior pituitary and loss of hearing due to damage to the inner ear. Multi-system disease (Figures

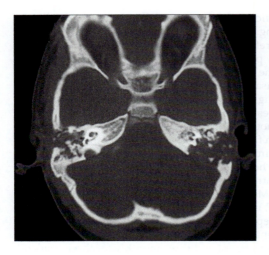

Figure 12.28 High-resolution CT scan of skull, showing a soft-tissue mass in the middle ear with adjacent destruction of the petrous temporal bone and invasion of the structures of the middle and inner ear. The patient, a 5-year-old female, presented with an aural polyp and deafness. Only the skeleton was involved in this patient ('single system disease').

12.29 and 12.30) involves two or more organs or systems. Involvement of the 'risk' organs – liver, spleen and bone marrow – causes fever, failure to thrive, widespread rash, anaemia and organomegaly represents risk to life and requires aggressive therapy.

Congenital LCH may occur at, or soon after birth, with skin nodules, diffuse rash and occasionally purpuric lesions. Isolated lesions can be treated with topical therapy, but the infant must be closely monitored for symptoms of other organ involvement.

Diabetes insipidus or neurodegenerative

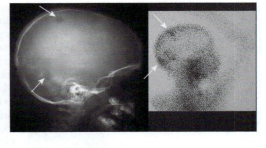

Figure 12.29 Skull radiograph showing 'punchedout' lytic deposits in the skull table of a 5-year-old male with 'multi-system' Langerhans cell histiocytosis. The inset shows the corresponding radionuclide scan after injection of an ^{111}In radiolabelled mouse anti-CD1a antibody. There is increased uptake in the skull lesions and in Waldeyer's ring.

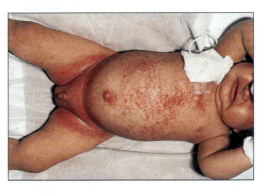

Figure 12.30 Widespread, confluent central truncal rash and petechiae in an infant with multisystem Langerhans cell histiocytosis (LCH) and thrombocytopenia due to 'haemopoietic failure' despite treatment. This 14-month-old male died 6 months later, from progressive LCH.

LCH might occur as a complication of LCH many years after therapy. Diabetes insipidus (presenting with increased fluid intake (up to 5–6 litres/day and, excessive micturition and enuresis) occurs more commonly in patients who had the involvement of the facial or base of the skull bones and requires lifelong therapy with desmopressin replacement. Neurodegenerative LCH presents with ataxia, tremor, dysarthria, cognitive or behavioural problems and should be thought of in children treated for LCH who present with these problems.

Diagnosis and Investigations

The complete evaluation of any patient presenting with LCH includes complete history and detailed physical examination with special attention to the skin, lymph nodes, ears, oral cavity, bones, lungs, thyroid, liver and spleen size, bone abnormalities, growth velocity, and history of excessive thirst and urination. Investigations include comprehensive blood tests, abdominal ultrasound, skeletal survey and chest x-ray. CT scan of the head may be indicated if orbital, mastoid, or other maxillofacial involvement, lung CT if abnormal x-ray or symptoms. Contrast MRI scan of brain/ spine for patients with diabetes insipidus or suspected brain or vertebral involvement. Biopsy of an appropriate site is required to make a definitive diagnosis. Tissue should be analysed for presence off BRAF mutation. Bone marrow aspirate is indicated for patient with abnormal blood count.

Treatment/Prognosis

Single system disease often needs minimal treatment. Isolated bone disease may respond to biopsy and curettage alone, or additional intralesional steroid, and lymph node involvement might need excision alone. Skin disease may respond to topical agents. Multi-focal bone involvement and multi-system disease are treated with systemic therapy to induce an early response and to minimise the immediate and longer-term effects of tissue destruction by the disease, using agents that would not cause long-term morbidity. The most commonly used systemic chemotherapy regimen is the combination of vinblastine and prednisone, but more intensive regimens using cladribine, cytarabine in patients with multisystem high-risk organ involvement that is refractory to chemotherapy. More recently targeted therapy with oral small molecule inhibitors such as BRAF (e.g. dabrafenib, vemurafenib) and MEK (e.g. trametinib) inhibitors have shown promising preliminary activity.

Overall, five-year survival of patients with single system disease is close to 100%, while for those with low-risk multi-system disease; this reduces to approximately 80%. Survival is closely linked to the extent of disease at presentation when high-risk organs (liver, spleen, and/or bone marrow) are involved, as well as the response to initial treatment. Many studies have confirmed the high mortality rate (35%) in high-risk multisystem patients who do not respond well to therapy in the first six weeks. Because of treatment advances, including early implementation of additional therapy for poor responders, the outcome for children with LCH involving high-risk organs has improved, overall survival (OS) rate of 84% for patients treated for 12-months with systemic chemotherapy.

RETINOBLASTOMA

Incidence, Aetiology, Classification and Genetics

Retinoblastoma affects 1 in 20,000 children, which is equivalent to about 45 cases per year in the United Kingdom, accounting for 3% of the cancers occurring in children younger than 15 years. More than 90% of cases are diagnosed before 5 years of age, with two-thirds before age 2 years.

Retinoblastoma occurs in a heritable (25–30%) and non-heritable form (70–75%). Tumours arise following loss of function of both copies of the *RB1* tumour suppressor gene. In non-heritable cases, both copies of the gene are mutated in a single cell by random genetic events, whereas in heritable cases there is a germline mutation in one copy of the gene and then a single somatic event results in tumorigenesis (Knudson hypothesis). Patients with heritable retinoblastoma are predisposed to tumours in later life, osteosarcoma, STS and melanoma being the most prevalent.

Clinical Presentation

Children with bilateral retinoblastoma present earlier (median age 8 months) than the unilateral form (median age 28 months). Presenting signs include leukocoria (Figure 12.31), strabismus, red eye and reduced vision. Tumours are bilateral in 30% of cases. All newly diagnosed children undergo molecular analysis of the *RB1* gene and when a germline mutation is identified, first-degree relatives are offered mutation screening. Preimplantation diagnosis can be offered to parents when their mutation is known.

Diagnosis and Investigations

Skilled ocular examination is mandatory to define the extent of intraocular disease (Figure 12.32). Eyes are classified from A–E depending on the extent of the intraocular disease. Ultrasound examination of the globe is helpful. MR head scanning is reserved for suspected extraocular disease and to exclude trilateral retinoblastoma. CSF cytology and bone marrow examinations are undertaken in patients with adverse histological features at risk of metastatic disease.

Treatment/Prognosis

Treatment of intraocular tumours is dependent on tumour size and location. Focal therapies, laser therapy and cryotherapy are used for

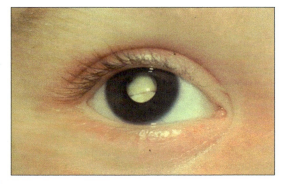

Figure 12.31 Lack of the red eye reflex (leucocoria) in a child with retinoblastoma.

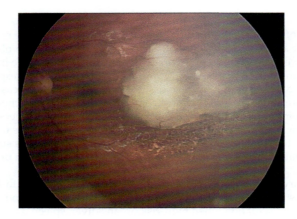

Figure 12.32 Retinoblastoma – fundal photograph of multi-focal tumour. (Courtesy of Dr A. Reddy, Barts and the London NHS Trust.)

small, localised tumours. Enucleation of the eye is the treatment of choice for E eyes and the most common treatment for unilateral disease, with 80% of unilateral children undergoing primary surgery. Children with bilateral tumours usually receive primary chemotherapy with focal consolidation therapies as indicated.

Salvage therapies include intra-arterial chemotherapy for multi-focal relapses with radioactive scleral plaques for localised relapses. External beam radiation is now only rarely used but remains an effective salvage treatment in bilateral cases where chemotherapy and focal treatments have failed.

Retinoblastoma has an excellent prognosis with a 98% five-year survival rate. Deaths from second cancers are now a greater risk for patients with heritable retinoblastoma than the primary tumour itself.

EXTRACRANIAL MALIGNANT GERM CELL TUMOURS
Incidence, Aetiology, Classification and Genetics
Malignant germ cell tumours, derived from primordial germ cells, occur in gonadal and extragonadal sites and account for 3% of cancers in children younger than 15 years. In the foetal/neonatal age group, most extracranial GCTs are benign teratomas occurring at midline locations, including the head and neck, sacrococcyx, and retroperitoneum. The incidence of malignant extracranial GCTs increases with the onset of puberty, such that they represent approximately 15% of cancers in male adolescents aged 15 to 19 years and 4% of cancers in female adolescents aged 15 to 19 years.

Clinical Presentation
Sites affected include sacrococcygeal (Figure 12.33), gonadal, mediastinal, vaginal, uterine and abdominal. Malignant tumours may develop in patients who have had previously 'benign' tumours resected.

Diagnosis and Investigations
The measurement of tumour markers AFP and beta-human choriogonadotrophin (β-hCG) helps in diagnosis and follow-up. Teratomas and germinomas secrete neither AFP nor β-hCG. Yolk-sac tumours and endodermal sinus tumours secrete AFP, choriocarcinomas secrete β-hCG, and embryonal carcinomas secrete both markers. Individual tumours may have a mixture of histopathological types within them. Accurate imaging of the primary site and evaluation for metastatic disease with a CT scan of the chest and a bone scan are important.

Treatment/Prognosis
Chemotherapy, in particular platinum agents have revolutionised treatment efficacy in germ cell tumours. Surgery and radiotherapy are also used as a part of multi-modality approach. Cisplatin or carboplatin are used in combination with etoposide, ifosfamide or bleomycin in various combinations. Secreting tumours produce serum markers, which are excellent predictors of response, but need to be interpreted with caution in young babies whose AFP might be physiologically

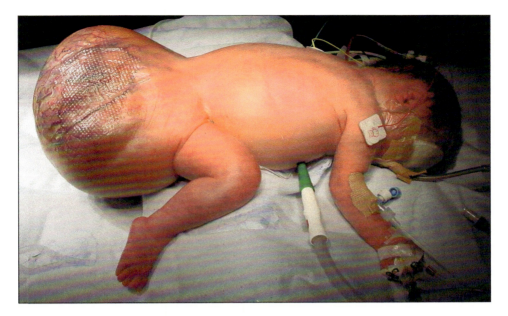

Figure 12.33   Sacrococcygeal teratoma in a newborn baby. Treatment is primary resection, which involves tumour mass and coccyx.

raised. Delayed tumour resection is the mainstay of treatment, but radiation is avoided, when possible, especially in younger children.

The outcomes are excellent with overall survival reaching 80%. Most relapses occur in the primary site within the first two years of diagnosis and careful follow-up with serum tumour markers is mandatory as early recognition of a relapse and appropriate treatment yield good outcome. Chemotherapy, together with rigorous local control with surgery and radiotherapy are essential for cure of the relapse, which is still achievable.

RARE TUMOURS

Rarer cancer types encountered in children may be truly rare paediatric cancers, or rare instances of 'adult cancers' affecting children. These tumours may pose particular problems for clinicians because there is often no standard approach to their treatment. The formation of a rare tumour group within the national (CCLG) and international (SIOP) children cancer groups aims to help alleviate this problem. Once the diagnosis is confirmed, a careful family history is mandatory, as rare tumours may be associated with an underlying genetic predisposition.

LATE EFFECTS OF CANCER TREATMENT

The present-day multi-modality treatment has improved overall five-year survival, so that more than 80% of childhood cancer sufferers can expect to live to adulthood. Unfortunately, this comes at a cost, as most current treatments are not specific to tumour cells and therefore damage to normal tissue can occur. This translates into a three-fold risk of premature death after 45 years and increased morbidity compared with their peers. Long-term follow-up studies have identified that 67% of survivors suffer long-term conditions, with one-quarter of those being severe. The degree of damage depends upon the organ characteristics (cell turnover, treatment sensitivity), age and development of the patient, gender, genetic predisposition and the synergistic effects of the treatments. Furthermore, psychosocial problems can occur in both patients and their families following the cancer diagnosis and its treatment. The late sequelae can be very diverse, presenting during treatment (cisplatin induced hearing loss, neurological deficiency after brain tumour surgery), or many decades later (second malignant neoplasms, cardiovascular disease). In certain cases, the functional damage can remain static, progress or improve over time.

The most frequent fatal adverse effects are the development of second malignant neoplasms and cardiovascular disease. Important consequences that affect quality of life are endocrine dysfunction and infertility. Table 12.5 gives examples of the consequences of treatment.

Table 12.5: Consequences of Childhood Cancer Treatment

Treatment	Organ/tissue affected	Outcome
Surgery	Brain	Neurological deficit
Radiotherapy	Organ within radiation field	Disturbance of growth and development, e.g. hypoplasia of soft tissue/bone
		Second malignant neoplasm presenting often many years after treatment.
	Brain	Pituitary dysfunction, degree dependant on dose
	Heart	Cardiovascular disease
Chemotherapy		
Anthracyclines	Heart	Cardiomyopathy, dose dependant
Alkylating agents	Gonadal dysfunction	Predominantly in males, dose dependant
Epidophyloxins	Bone marrow	Leukaemia
Cisplatin/carboplatin	Hearing	Hearing dysfunction occurs during treatment
	Kidney	Renal impairment occurs during treatment

It is very important to be aware of these problems and take responsibility to provide an effective follow-up programme tailored to the needs of the survivor. Care may range from multidisciplinary input to regular surveillance (breast cancer surveillance for survivors who received chest radiotherapy) to minimal self-care managed by the survivor. To assist this aim, all survivors and their health care providers should have treatment summaries and care plans. Effective aftercare should provide surveillance and management for late effects, support for psychosocial issues and education regarding risks of adverse effects and lifestyle, employment and financial issues with the aim of reducing mortality, morbidity and improving quality of life.

REFERENCES/FURTHER READING

General reading
- Pfister SM, Reyes-Múgica M, et al. Alaggio R. A summary of the inaugural WHO classification of pediatric tumors: Transitioning from the optical into the molecular era. *Cancer Discov.* 2022 Feb;12(2):331–355. doi:10.1158/2159-8290.CD-21-1094. Epub 2021 Dec 17. PMID: 34921008; PMCID: PMC9401511.
- Grant CN, Rhee D, Tracy ET, et al. Pediatric solid tumors and associated cancer predisposition syndromes: Workup, management, and surveillance. A summary from the APSA Cancer Committee. *J Pediatr Surg.* 2022 Mar;57(3):430–442. doi:10.1016/j.jpedsurg.2021.08.008. Epub 2021 Aug 24. PMID: 34503817.

Tumours of the central nervous system
- Horbinski C, Berger T, Packer RJ, et al. Clinical implications of the 2021 edition of the WHO classification of central nervous system tumours. *Nat Rev Neurol.* 2022 Sep;18(9):515–529. doi:10.1038/s41582-022-00679-w. Epub 2022 Jun 21. PMID: 35729337.

Sarcomas
- Ferrari A, Brennan B, Casanova M, et al. Pediatric non-rhabdomyosarcoma soft tissue sarcomas: Standard of care and treatment recommendations from the European Paediatric Soft Tissue Sarcoma Study Group (EpSSG). *Cancer Manag Res.* 2022 Sep 23;14:2885–2902. doi:10.2147/CMAR.S368381. PMID: 36176694; PMCID: PMC9514781.
- Strauss SJ, Frezza AM, Abecassis N, et al. ESMO Guidelines Committee, EURACAN, GENTURIS and ERN PaedCan. Electronic address: clinicalguidelines@esmo.org. Bone sarcomas: ESMO-EURACAN-GENTURIS-ERN PaedCan Clinical Practice Guideline for diagnosis, treatment and follow-up. *Ann Oncol.* 2021 Dec;32(12):1520–1536. doi:10.1016/j.annonc.2021.08.1995. Epub 2021 Sep 6. PMID: 34500044.

Neuroblastoma
- Qiu B, Matthay KK. Advancing therapy for neuroblastoma. *Nat Rev Clin Oncol.* 2022 Aug;19(8):515–533. doi:10.1038/s41571-022-00643-z. Epub 2022 May 25. PMID: 35614230.

- Tolbert VP, Matthay KK. Neuroblastoma: Clinical and biological approach to risk stratification and treatment. *Cell Tissue Res*. 2018 May;372(2):195–209. doi:10.1007/s00441-018-2821-2. Epub 2018 Mar 23. PMID: 29572647; PMCID: PMC5918153.

Renal tumours
- Jackson TJ, Brisse HJ, Pritchard-Jones K, et al. SIOP RTSG Biopsy Working Group. How we approach paediatric renal tumour core needle biopsy in the setting of preoperative chemo-therapy: A Review from the SIOP Renal Tumour Study Group. *Pediatr Blood Cancer*. 2022 Sep;69(9):e29702. doi:10.1002/pbc.29702. Epub 2022 May 19. PMID: 35587187.
- Michel G, Mulder RL, van der Pal HJH, Skinner R, Bárdi E, Brown MC, Vetsch J, Frey E, Windsor R, Kremer LCM, Levitt G. Evidence-based recommendations for the organization of long-term follow-up care for childhood and adolescent cancer survivors: A report from the PanCareSurFup Guidelines Working Group. *J Cancer Surviv*. 2019 Oct;13(5):759–772. doi:10.1007/s11764-019-00795-5. Epub 2019 Aug 8. PMID: 31396878.

13 Endocrinology

Mehul Dattani and Catherine Peters

THE SHORT CHILD

This is the commonest reason for referral of a child to an endocrinologist, and the algorithm (Figure 13.1) gives an approach to the management of this condition. See following pages for a description of some of these conditions in more detail.

DISORDERS OF THE GROWTH HORMONE AXIS

Before investigating the growth hormone (GH) axis, it is important to exclude other causes of short stature and investigations should be performed to exclude non-endocrine pathology (e.g. renal and coeliac disease). Disorders of the GH axis occur when there is disruption to the production of hormones or to their receptors (Figure 13.2).

GROWTH HORMONE DEFICIENCY/INSUFFICIENCY

Incidence/Genetics

The incidence of GH deficiency/insufficiency (GHD/GHI) in its classical form is 1 in 3000. Hereditary forms of GH deficiency arising as a result of *GH1* gene mutations or GHRH receptor mutations are rare, accounting for 5 to 10% of cases (Table 13.1).

Diagnosis

Children with GH deficiency typically have normal birth weight and may rarely present with neonatal hypoglycaemia. The height velocity slows from around the end of the first year of life. Later presentation is classically with short stature with a poor growth velocity (Figure 13.3a) and a round, immature face with frontal bossing (Figure 13.3b). Micropenis may be a feature.

GH insufficiency may be associated with other pituitary hormone deficiencies as part of an evolving endocrinopathy. There may be evidence of associated disorders (e.g. midline cleft palate, optic nerve hypoplasia, agenesis of the corpus callosum, absence of the septum pellucidum and Fanconi's anaemia). The bone age is usually delayed, as is the dentition. The concentration of insulin-like growth factor (IGF1) and its binding protein (IGF-BP3) may be low in GHD/GHI as these are GH-dependent factors, but the sensitivities and specificities of these tests in isolation are poor.

If the diagnosis of GHD or GHI is suspected, further evaluation in the form of provocative biochemical tests of GH secretion may be indicated. Insulin-induced hypoglycaemia or glucagon provocation are most widely used. Alternative tests include arginine, clonidine and growth hormone-releasing hormone stimulation tests. These tests can be dangerous and should be performed by experienced operators in tertiary referral centres. The results are dependent on the assay in use, and so the test results for any one centre need to be carefully evaluated. Physiological tests of GH secretion may be of greater relevance, but they require sampling of blood for GH concentrations at 20 minute intervals over a 12 to 24 hour period and are therefore expensive and time-consuming, with a lack of reproducibility.

MRI of the brain and pituitary may reveal anterior pituitary hypoplasia, often in association with an undescended / ectopic posterior pituitary and an absent infundibulum (known as the pituitary stalk interruption syndrome, PSIS) (Figures 13.4A and 13.4B).

Treatment

Replacement with a daily subcutaneous dose rhGH (0.02 to 0.05 mg/kg/day) restores normal growth velocity after a period of catch-up growth and is associated with minimal side effects in replacement doses. The most severely GH-insufficient children will respond best and often to low doses. Monitoring of IGF1/IGF-BP3 concentrations aid in dosage optimisation.

Prognosis

The prognosis for final height in GHD/GHI is excellent, provided that treatment is commenced at an early age to allow time for catch up.

DOI: 10.1201/9781003175186-13

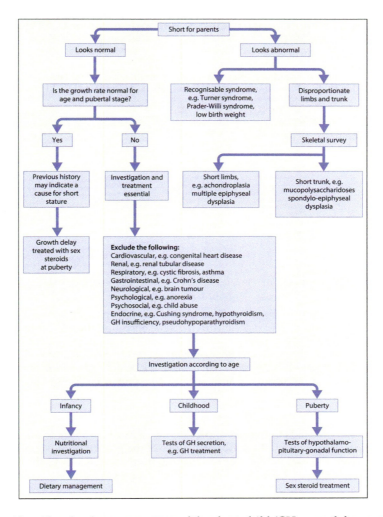

Figure 13.1 Algorithm for the management of the short child (GH, growth hormone).

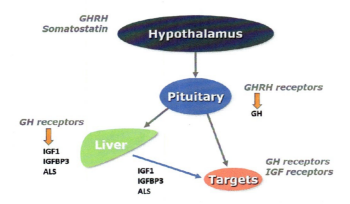

Figure 13.2 The GH axis. Each hormone also applied negative feedback to the hypothalamus and pituitary (not shown).

Table 13.1: GH Deficiency/insufficiency Pathogenesis and Aetiology

Congenital
Hereditary – gene deletion/mutation
- Idiopathic GHRH deficiency
- Developmental abnormalities – pituitary aplasia, hypoplasia, midline brain and facial defects, many of which are associated with mutations in transcription factors such as HESX1, LHX3, LHX4, PROP1 and PIT1/POU1F1.

Acquired
Perinatal trauma
- Hypothalamic/pituitary tumours

Secondary to
Cranial irradiation
- Head injury
- Infection
- Sarcoidosis
- Histiocytosis

Transient due to
Low sex hormone concentration
- Psychosocial deprivation
- Hypothyroidism

GH INSENSITIVITY

Incidence/Genetics

Classic GH insensitivity (Laron-type dwarfism) is an extremely rare autosomal recessive condition caused by molecular mutations and deletions in the gene encoding the GH receptor gene which leads to severe GH insensitivity. Milder mutations in the GH receptor gene have been described in some cases of idiopathic short stature. Recessive mutations in *STAT5B*, the *IGF1* gene, the *IGFR* Type 1, and Acid-labile subunit (ALS) have also been described in association with GH insensitivity phenotypes. Recently, heterozygous dominant negative mutations in STAT5B have been associated with GH insensitivity.

Pathogenesis/Aetiology

The abnormal GH receptor fails to interact appropriately with GH, leading to an inability to generate IGF1 and subsequent growth failure. Abnormalities of the post-receptor signalling pathway including STAT5B can also lead to GH insensitivity and immune deficiency which can manifest as interstitial pneumonia. IGF1 circulates bound to binding proteins and the ALS. Defects in the

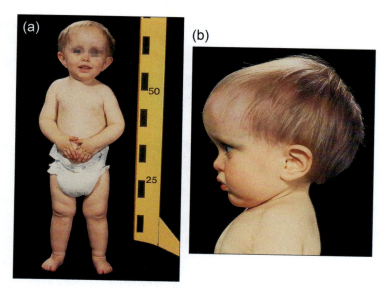

Figure 13.3a,b GH deficiency: The classic appearance in a child presenting with (a) short stature and (b) midfacial hypoplasia with frontal bossing.

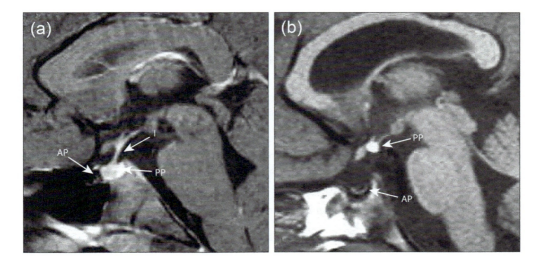

Figure 13.4a,b (a) MRI showing a normal anterior pituitary (AP) with the posterior pituitary (PP) locate normally in the sella turcica. The the infundibulum (I) connecting the pituitary to the hypothalamus. (b) MRI of a child with congenital growth hormone deficiency (GHD) showing deVere hypoplasia of the anterior pituitary (AP) with an undescended posterior pituitary (PP) at the level of the ruber cinereum. Note the absence of the pituitary stalk. This appearance reflects a developmental abnormality and is commonly observed in patients with isolated GHD and combined pituitary hormone deficiency.

synthesis of ALS also lead to IGF1 deficiency. IGF1 gene deletions have been associated with deafness, microcephaly and learning deficit.

Diagnosis

GH insensitivity may present with hypoglycaemia in the neonatal period, and the birth weight may be low. In childhood, clinical presentation resembles GH deficient children but with more severe short stature (Figure 13.5) and an extremely poor growth rate. Bone age is delayed with respect to chronological age, but advanced with respect to height age. Other features include micropenis, small hands and feet, craniofacial anomalies such as a saddle nose (Figure 13.6), excess subcutaneous fat, sparse hair growth, delayed closure of anterior fontanelles, and a prominent forehead. Hip dysplasia and a chubby appearance are other associated features. Pubertal delay may be a feature. More recently, partial insensitivity to GH has been described in children who present with idiopathic short stature. Immune deficits and arthritis have been associated with STAT5B mutations.

Essential investigations are as for GHD/GHI. Unlike GHD/GHI, the basal concentration of GH in serum is normal or elevated, with an exaggerated peak GH in response to provocation and low basal IGF1 and IGF-BP3 concentrations. Additionally, an IGF1 generation test fails to demonstrate an increase in the IGF1 concentration following the administration of rhGH. GH-binding protein may be present or absent, depending on the underlying molecular lesion. In children with short stature secondary to partial GH insensitivity, GH-binding protein concentrations are low. GH concentrations are normal or high, with low IGF1 concentrations.

Treatment

Children with Laron-type dwarfism and other forms of GH insensitivity are treated using recombinant IGF1 treatment. Height velocity is increased, but close monitoring of patients is essential as the treatment is not without side effects (including hypoglycaemia, hypokalaemia and papilloedema). In children with partial GH insensitivity, it is possible to treat with high doses of GH to improve the height velocity, but final height data are not available to date.

Prognosis

The height prognosis without treatment is extremely poor. The role of recombinant IGF1 treatment with respect to an increase in final height remains to be established.

THE SMALL FOR GESTATIONAL AGE CHILD

Incidence

Infants born with a weight and/or length less than −2 standard deviation score (SDS) for gestational age at birth are considered small for gestational age. Rarely, children will have an underlying syndrome of which Russell–Silver syndrome is well described with an incidence between 1 in 30,000 to 100,000.

Pathogenesis/Aetiology

80% of low birth weight children will catch up in the first two years of life. Others may have chromosomal disorders, dysmorphic syndromes such as 3M syndrome, recognised environmental insult in utero (e.g. rubella, cytomegalovirus, alcohol, maternal smoking, anticonvulsants, placental dysfunction) and imprinting defects, as in Russell–Silver syndrome.

Diagnosis

SGA infants have a birth weight that is inappropriately low for gestation and in relation to the birth weights of other siblings. They may present with neonatal hypoglycaemia and, if so, investigations should be performed to exclude other pathology (e.g. congenital hyperinsulinism, β-oxidation defect). Feeding problems in the first year of life are common in this group of children, and children who do not demonstrate catch-up growth are usually short and very slim. If a reduced growth velocity is documented, investigations should be carried out to exclude coincident pathology (e.g. GH insufficiency). A karyotype may be indicated if a genetic syndrome is suspected.

In Russell–Silver syndrome, children fail to demonstrate significant catch-up growth and have a very poor appetite, feeding difficulties and low BMI. Additionally, clinical features include relative macrocephaly at birth, protruding forehead, asymmetry of the face (Figure 13.7A) and limbs, clinodactyly (Figure 13.7B), a small triangular facies, genital anomalies, and excessive sweating.

Treatment

Growth hormone treatment is approved for children who are born small for gestational age and fail to catch up by the age of 4 years. Additionally, treatment may be required for complications such as hypoglycaemia (frequent feeds), effects of hemi-hypertrophy and dental crowding.

Prognosis

The prognosis for height is highly variable, and a significant proportion (~40%) will have final heights that fall considerably short of their mid-parental target height. Growth hormone treatment has been demonstrated to improve height in the short term, but effects on final height are variable.

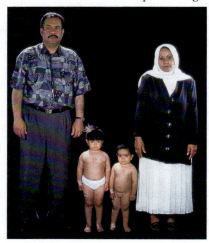

Figure 13.5 Classic GH insensitivity (Laron-type dwarfism): extreme short stature in two siblings, shown here with their parents.

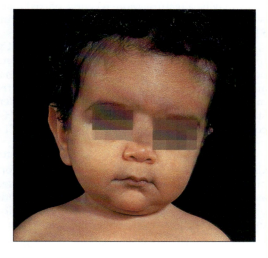

Figure 13.6 Laron-type dwarfism: typical facial features.

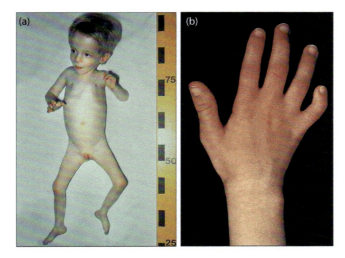

Figure 13.7A, B Russell–Silver syndrome with (A) poor subcutaneous fat and (B) fifth finger clinodactyly.

Early puberty may further limit final height. Learning difficulties may be associated.

The relationship between in utero growth restriction and adult cardiovascular disease risk (Barker hypothesis) suggest an increased risk of cardiovascular and metabolic disease in adulthood particularly hypertension, diabetes and obesity.

TURNER SYNDROME AND SHOX DEFICIENCY

Incidence/Genetics

See also the chapter 'Genetics'.

Short stature in Turner syndrome occurs due to loss of one copy of the *SHOX* gene located on the pseudo-autosomal regions of the X and Y chromosome. Abnormalities of this gene may also lead to short stature in children without evidence of Turners syndrome and should be considered as part of the short stature investigation screen. Loss of both *SHOX* genes leads to Leri–Weill syndrome with severe skeletal abnormalities, including a Madelung deformity of the forearm (Figure 13.8).

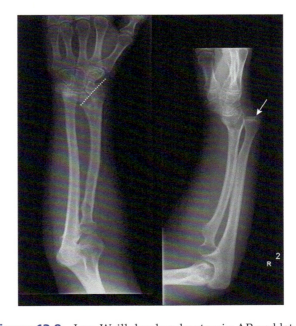

Figure 13.8 Len–Weill dyschondrosteosis: AP and lateral radiographs of the right forearm in a teenage girl with heterozygous *SHOX* mutation. The radius is shortened, with a growth disturbance of the medial aspect of the distal radial physis, producing an increased tilt to the distal radius – the Madelung deformity (dotted line). In this case, the distal ulnar is dislocated due to the radial shortening.

Diagnosis

Turner syndrome may present in the neonatal period with lymphoedema of the hands and feet (Figure 13.9A) or coarctation of the aorta. Birth weight may be low (≤ 1 SDS). Other clinical signs which may be present include widely-spaced nipples, anomalous auricles, epicanthic folds, micrognathia, low posterior hairline, webbed neck, cubitus valgus, osteoporosis, scoliosis narrow hyperconvex nails (Figure 13.9B), excessive pigmented naevi, idiopathic

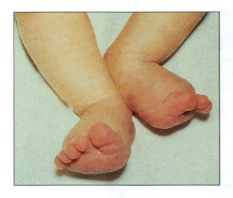

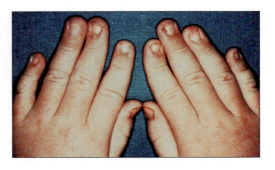

Figure 13.9B Dysplastic nails in a child with Turner syndrome.

Figure 13.9A Lymphoedema of the feet.

hypertension, and aortic stenosis. Diagnosis in childhood is often made in the investigation of progressive short stature due to a poor height velocity around the 25th centile.

Ovarian failure with streak gonads is observed in the vast majority of patients. Recurrent middle ear infections and autoimmune thyroiditis are common and sensorineural deafness, specific learning abnormalities, diabetes mellitus, and coeliac disease are associated. Renal anomalies (particularly horseshoe kidney) and cardiac anomalies (bicuspid aortic valve) are frequently identified in these patients. Essential investigations are karyotype, echocardiogram, cardiac MRI, renal and pelvic ultrasound scans, gonadotrophins and thyroid function noting liver dysfunction is a later feature.

Treatment

Appropriate treatment of any cardiac and renal abnormalities and blood pressure monitoring. Growth promotion may be achieved with the use of low-dose anabolic steroids (oxandrolone), growth hormone and oestrogen. Pubertal induction with oestrogens and the later addition of progestogens is required in the majority of cases at the appropriate age. Ten percent of girls with Turner syndrome have a spontaneous onset of puberty but very few go on to achieve menarche (5–10%) and fertility (1%). Complications such as hypothyroidism are treated as they arise. If a Y chromosomal cell line has been demonstrated, the dysgenetic gonads should be removed because of the possibility of malignant change. Psychological support is also recommended as associated anxiety related disorders are well recognised.

Prognosis

The prognosis for final height is determined to a large extent by the parental heights. In the Western world, the mean final height of women with Turner syndrome is in the region of 143 to 146 cm, which is approximately 20 cm less than the average final height for normal adult females. The use of *in vitro* fertilisation and embryo implantation techniques have improved the prospects for childbearing.

PRADER–WILLI SYNDROME

Incidence/Genetics

See also the chapter 'Genetics'.

Diagnosis

Prader–Willi syndrome (PWS) usually presents in the neonatal period with hypotonia and feeding difficulties. Birth weight may be low or normal. Characteristic facial features include a narrow forehead, almond-shaped eyes, strabismus and micrognathia. Small hands and feet are a feature of the condition, with tapering fingers and clinodactyly. Scoliosis, congenital dislocation of the hips, neurodevelopmental delay and hypogonadism with a micropenis, hypoplastic scrotum and bilateral cryptorchidism are other features of the condition.

Insatiable appetite from the age of one to two years leads to gross obesity (Figure 13.10) with the ensuing complications of genu valgum, cellulitis, intertrigo, obesity, hypoventilation syndrome and diabetes mellitus. Endocrine features relate to hypothalamic defects. These include hypogonadotrophic hypogonadism leading to poor secondary sexual development and delayed menarche

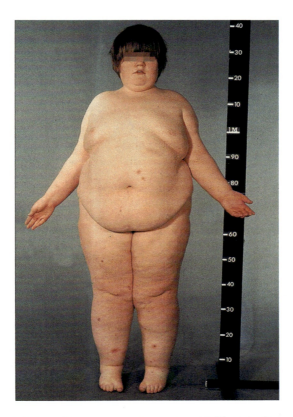

Figure 13.10 Prader–Willi syndrome: gross obesity in a child. Note the small hands and feet.

and growth hormone deficiency. Short stature is a feature in a significant proportion of cases, with the development of adrenarche and a poor pubertal growth spurt.

Treatment

The mainstay of treatment is severe dietary restriction. Energy requirements for growth are low, and these should be calculated and calorie intake appropriately restricted. Neurodevelopmental delay and behavioural difficulties in some children compound the difficulties inherent in dietary restriction. In boys, bilateral orchidopexies may be required and hypogonadotrophic hypogonadism requires testosterone treatment. In girls, menarche may be delayed and oestrogen treatment may be required.

Growth hormone treatment is licenced for use in PWS children with poor growth. It has been demonstrated to improve the hypotonia and motor development associated with PWS. However, there is a risk of lymphoid tissue overgrowth and airway obstruction necessitating ENT and sleep study assessment prior to commencing GH treatment. Central adrenal insufficiency is less common, but adrenal function should also be assessed prior to commencement of GH therapy.

Prognosis

Dietary restriction and weight gain are often managed well in childhood, but become increasingly difficult in the young adult, with the consequence of gross obesity. Premature death due to bronchopneumonia or cardiorespiratory failure and Pickwickian syndrome with hypoventilation is usual. Additionally, the stress on the family is considerable.

SKELETAL DYSPLASIAS

Several of these exist but only the commoner forms are described here; namely, achondroplasia, hypochondroplasia, spondylo-epiphyseal dysplasia and multiple epiphyseal dysplasia.

Incidence/Genetics

Achondroplasia occurs in 1 in 10,000 to 15,000. Inherited as an autosomal dominant condition with a fresh mutation rate of 90% and associated with older paternal age. It is caused by an activating mutation in the transmembrane domain of the fibroblast growth factor receptor-3 (FGFR3).

Hypochondroplasia is also inherited as an autosomal dominant trait and is due to activating mutations in the intracellular tyrosine kinase domain FGFR3 receptor.

Spondylo-epiphyseal dysplasia/mutiple epiphyseal dysplasia are rare with autosomal dominant inheritance.

Diagnosis

Achondroplasia (Figure 13.11) presents in the neonatal period with short-limbs and characteristic craniofacial features including a large head with marked frontal bossing, a low nasal bridge and mild mid-facial hypoplasia. Skeletal abnormalities include small cuboid vertebral bodies with short pedicles and progressive narrowing of lumbar interpedicular distance. Lumbar lordosis, mild thoraco-lumbar kyphosis, small iliac wings, short tubular bones and a short trident hand are other features of the condition (see Figure 13.11). Mild hypotonia with some early motor delay is an occasional feature. Hydrocephalus secondary to a narrow foramen magnum is an associated feature. Spinal cord and/or root compression can occur as a consequence of kyphosis, spinal canal stenosis or disc lesions. Associated features include upper airways obstruction and recurrent otitis media. Pseudoachondroplasia resembles achondroplasia clinically.

Hypochondroplasia patients usually present with short stature in relation to mid-parental target height centile. The growth rate is initially normal, with a compromised pubertal growth spurt. Skeletal abnormalities are characteristic. Disproportion may only be apparent in puberty, although more severe cases may present earlier with disproportion. Family history often reveals disproportionate short stature in one or both parents.

Spondylo-epiphyseal dysplasia is characterised by prenatal onset growth deficiency, malar hypoplasia, cleft palate, severely shortened spine, lumbar lordosis, kyphoscoliosis, decreased arm span, weakness, talipes varus and developmental dysplasia of the hip.

Multiple epiphyseal dysplasia is characterised by short stature, with short metacarpals and phalanges, ovoid, flattened vertebral bodies, waddling gait, slow growth and early osteoarthritis. These features are by no means invariable.

Essential investigations include a skeletal survey, especially an antero-posterior view of the spine to show diagnostic radiological features. In hypochondroplasia, there is loss of the normal widening of the interpedicular distance proceeding down the lumbar spine. In achondroplasia, neuroradiological imaging may be indicated if hydrocephalus is suspected.

Treatment

Correction of hydrocephalus and orthopaedic abnormalities. The use of growth hormone (GH) to treat achondroplastic and hypochondroplastic children has limited effect on final height. More promising is the use of the C-type natriuretic peptide analogue, vosoritide in achondroplasia. Limb lengthening may be an option in achondroplasia and severe cases of hypochondroplasia. The gain in height needs to be balanced against the time and discomfort involved in these procedures.

Prognosis

Without intervention, the height prognosis can be poor in achondroplasia with a mean final height of 100 to 140 cm. It is more variable in hypochondroplasia. While in the short term it can promote growth, the long-term benefits of vosoritide need to be established.

THE TALL CHILD

A height attained which is greater than one might expect for the family, a growth rate which is constantly around the 90th centile, and an increasing height prediction are all reasons to investigate the tall child. Figure 13.12 suggests a plan of management for children with tall stature.

Some of the conditions leading to tall stature will be further discussed in the next sections.

MARFAN SYNDROME

Incidence/Genetics

See also the chapter 'Genetics'.

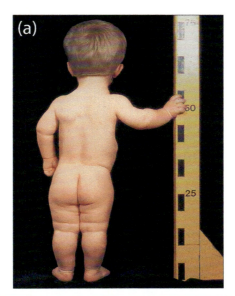

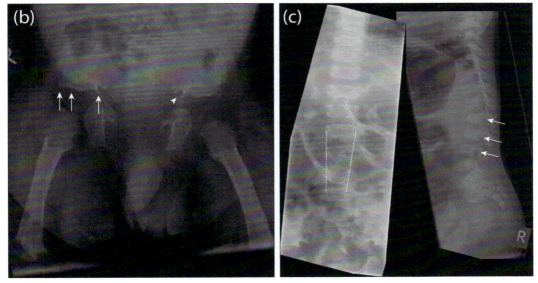

Figure 13.11a–c (a) Achondroplasia: typical childhood proportions. (b) Pelvic radiograph in a 6-month-old male with achondroplasia. The iliac bones are small and squared off, being no wider than the acetabulum. The sacrosciatic notch (arrow head) is markedly narrowed. The acetabulum is almost horizontal and shows 'spikes' medially, centrally, and laterally (white arrows) – the 'trident' appearance. Note the apparent oval radiolucency in the upper femora, a typical feature at this age, due to sloping and foreshortening of the upper femoral metaphysis. (c) AP and lateral spinal radiographs in a 6-month-old male with achondroplasia. On the AP view the distance between the pedicles becomes narrower in the lower lumbar spine (dotted white lines); on the lateral view the vertebral bodies are smaller, with a bullet shape and scalloping of their posterior borders (white arrows).

Pathogenesis/Aetiology

Heterozygous mutations in the fibrillin gene *FBN1* on chromosome 15q lead to widespread connective tissue abnormalities, and the characteristic skeletal, ocular and cardiovascular manifestations of Marfan syndrome.

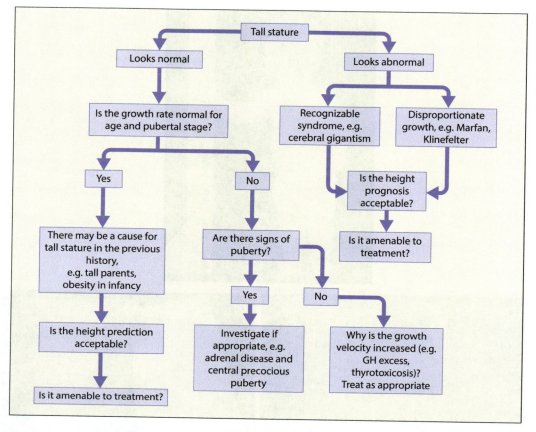

Figure 13.12 Algorithm for the management of the tall child (GH, growth hormone). Some of the conditions leading to tall stature will be discussed in the following sections.

Diagnosis

Patients present with tall stature. Other features include arachnodactyly (Figure 13.13), wide arm span, joint laxity, kyphoscoliosis, narrow face, high-arched palate, bluish sclerae, upward lenticular dislocation, aortic incompetence, dissecting aneurysm of aorta, mitral valve prolapse and inguinal or femoral herniae. The diagnosis is clinical and is often delayed until a cardiac presentation in adulthood. Investigations should include an echocardiogram, chromosomal analysis, and measurement of urinary homocystine to exclude homocystinuria, the main differential diagnosis.

Treatment

Tall stature may be limited by early induction of puberty. Cardiac lesions may need surgical intervention.

Prognosis

This is dictated by the cardiac anomalies.

PITUITARY GIGANTISM

Incidence/Genetics

This is extremely rare. Activating Gsα mutations in signal-transducing G-proteins may account for up to 40% of adult somatotroph adenomas. Mutations in the Aryl Hydrocarbon Interacting Protein (AIP) can lead to dominantly inherited familial isolated pituitary adenomas (FIPA). Recently,

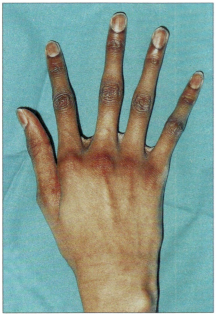

Figure 13.13 Clinical appearance of arachnodactyly in a child with Marfan syndrome.

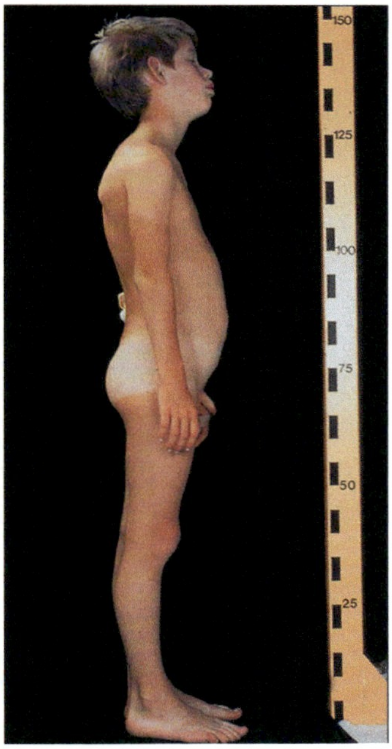

Figure 13.14 Pituitary gigantism in a child: note the large feet.

early-onset pituitary gigantism has been associated with microduplications of Xq26.3 including the gene encoding the orphan G-protein coupled receptor *GPR101* (known as XLAG).

Pathogenesis/Aetiology

The underlying lesion is usually a somatotroph adenoma. These lesions are associated with McCune–Albright syndrome, Multiple endocrine neoplasia I (MEN I), and Carney complex.

Diagnosis

Usually presents with tall stature, irrespective of the mid-parental target centile (Figure 13.14). The height velocity is generally greater than the 75th to 98th centiles. Bone age is not advanced and precocious puberty should be excluded by clinical examination. Visual fields may reveal a deficit, although it is unlikely that a GH-secreting adenoma will be large enough to lead to such a deficit. A 24-hour GH secretory profile with measurement of serum GH concentrations at 20-minute intervals is characterised by an inability of GH concentrations to achieve undetectable baseline concentrations (i.e. there are no troughs of GH secretion). The IGF-1 and BP3 concentrations are elevated. Failure to suppress GH secretion following an oral glucose load is often characteristic.

MRI of the pituitary gland is the first line investigation. The paradoxical increase in GH secretion seen in adults in response to an oral glucose or thyrotrophin-releasing hormone (TRH), is more complex in childhood as this response can be seen in normal children during puberty.

Treatment

Definitive treatment is trans-sphenoidal surgical removal of the adenoma. Medical treatment includes somatostatin analogues (octreotide), dopamine agonists (bromocriptine, cabergoline) or a growth hormone receptor antagonist (pegvisomant). Pegvisomant is the most effective medical treatment and can reduce IGF1 concentrations into the normal range, although it will have no effect on circulating GH concentrations or tumour size. Radiotherapy has limited effect, but may be used as second line treatment.

Prognosis

The overall prognosis in cases of isolated pituitary adenoma post-surgical removal is good, although there is a possibility that the lesion will recur. In McCune-Albright syndrome and MEN I, the prognosis must be guarded, due to other complications associated with these conditions.

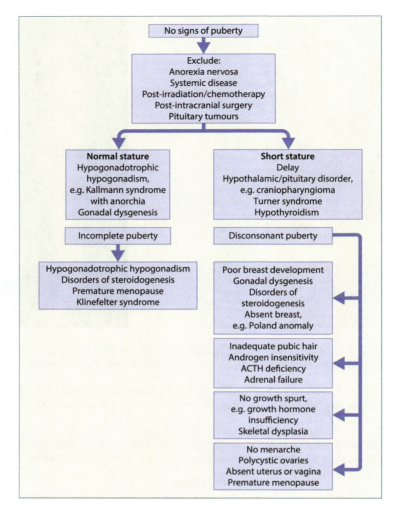

Figure 13.15 Algorithm for the diagnosis of late puberty (ACTH, adrenocorticotrhophic hormone).

LATE PUBERTY

The algorithm offers an approach to the diagnosis of conditions leading to late puberty (Figure 13.15).

KLINEFELTER SYNDROME

Incidence/Genetics

The incidence is 1 in 500 male births. Chromosomal analysis reveals at least one extra X chromosome added to the normal XY karyotype, most commonly 47 XXY.

Pathogenesis/Aetiology

Tall stature results not only from the presence of additional chromosomal material but also from inadequate sexual development, which allows growth to continue at a normal rate far beyond its usual age of cessation.

Diagnosis

This condition usually presents with tall stature and disproportionate long legs (Figure 13.16). The patients tend to be slim initially, but can be obese as adults. Other features include hypogonadism with small testes and inadequate virilisation, infertility and gynaecomastia. More severe disorders of sex development have been reported, including complete sex reversal. Children with this condition can have a low IQ with poor school performance. Investigations should include a karyotype and serum LH and FSH which are usually elevated (hypergonadotrophic hypogonadism). The serum testosterone is consequently low. A pelvic USS is indicated if cryptorchidism is a feature.

Treatment

Pubertal induction and treatment with testosterone. Some Klinefelter children enter a spontaneous puberty, but this may arrest. Earlier treatment with testosterone can prevent and improve gynaecomastia and can limit the tall stature associated with this condition.

Prognosis

Pubertal development is completed with the addition of testosterone therapy. However, patients are generally infertile and have an increased susceptibility to autoimmune disorders, breast cancer and extragonadal germ cell tumours

EARLY PUBERTY

The algorithm in Figure 13.17 gives an approach to the diagnosis of early puberty. Subsequent sections will discuss some of these conditions in more detail. Of essence to the diagnosis is the clinical assessment as to whether puberty is consonant or not (i.e. whether the sequence of pubertal development is normal or not), with enlargement of testicular size in boys and breast development in girls being the first signs of gonadotrophin-dependent precocious puberty.

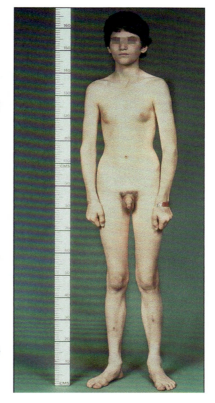

Figure 13.16 Klinefelter syndrome: tall stature and slim build with eunuchoid appearance in a boy.

PREMATURE THELARCHE/THELARCHE VARIANT OR 'BENIGN' PRECOCIOUS PUBERTY

Incidence/Genetics

Premature thelarche is a sporadic condition which is commonly observed, particularly in neonates. Thelarche variant is less common and is likely to be a form of slowly progressing precocious puberty.

Pathogenesis/Aetiology

Ovarian cyst development due to isolated pulsatile FSH secretion results in the secretion of oestrogen and isolated breast development.

Diagnosis

In premature thelarche, girls usually present with isolated early breast development (Figure 13.18). The age of onset is usually below two years and frequently continues as an extension of the neonatal breast enlargement caused by placental transmission of maternal oestrogens. Over 80% of girls have cyclical breast development which waxes and wanes at intervals of four to six weeks. Such development is usually associated with isolated ovarian cyst development, which is due to premature but isolated pulsatile FSH secretion. The uterus is of an appropriate size and shape for age, with no endometrial echo and only exceptionally is there a vaginal bleed. Growth is at a normal rate, and the bone age is not advanced. There are no other signs of puberty.

In thelarche variant, breast development may be associated with increased stature, advanced bone age, a small uterus, and an ovarian morphology which is between that for premature thelarche and precocious puberty. Investigations should include a bone age in children over the age of 3 years (advanced in thelarche variant, but not in premature thelarche) and a pelvic ultrasound scan

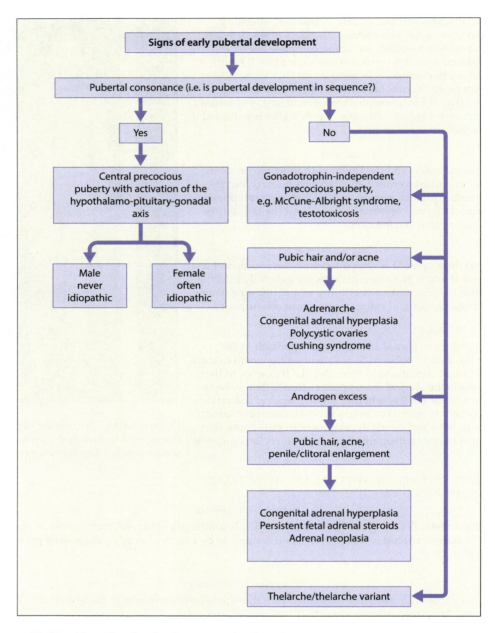

Figure 13.17 Algorithm for the diagnosis of early puberty.

(Figure 13.19). FSH concentrations are raised, with a pulsatile secretory pattern, and the response of FSH to GnRH (gonadotrophin-releasing hormone) is brisk. Thyroid function should be tested, since in primary hypothyroidism, isolated breast development may occur due to elevated FSH concentrations.

Treatment
No treatment is required for these conditions.

Prognosis
Both conditions are benign with no effect on the growth prognosis. The conditions may continue largely unchanged with waxing and waning of breast size in parallel to ovarian cyst size until puberty.

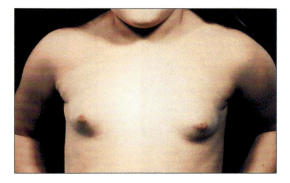

Figure 13.18 Thelarche in a 5-year-old girl.

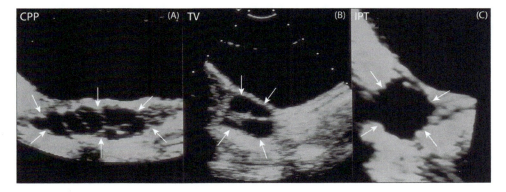

Figure 13.19 (A) Pelvic ultrasound in central precocious puberty, (B) compared with thelarche variant, (C) and isolated premature thelarche.

GONADOTROPHIN-DEPENDENT (CENTRAL) PRECOCIOUS PUBERTY

Incidence/Genetics

The condition is relatively common in girls (Male:Female ratio of 1:10) and most cases are sporadic. In a few cases, mutations in the maternally imprinted gene *MKRN3*, have been implicated in the aetiology of central precocious puberty. The condition has autosomal dominant inheritance and is exclusively paternally transmitted.

Pathogenesis/Aetiology

Premature activation of the hypothalamic-pituitary gonadal axis leads to a sequence of sexual maturation that is identical to that of normal puberty. In girls, often no underlying cause can be demonstrated. In boys, pineal and other intracranial tumours and hamartomata may be present. Other causes of secondary central precocious puberty include hydrocephalus and neurofibromatosis and previous cranial irradiation.

Hypothalamic hamartomata (Figure 13.20) present with early puberty in both sexes and are congenital tumours containing GnRH neurones which secrete GnRH to induce puberty. They are otherwise benign but are associated with gelastic seizures and developmental delay in some cases.

Diagnosis

In girls, breast development is the first sign (Figure 13.21). In boys, testicular enlargement is the first sign and the aetiology is rarely idiopathic. Signs of an underlying condition may be present (e.g. neurological abnormalities secondary to a brain tumour, hydrocephalus, neurofibromatosis). Neuroradiological imaging of the brain is indicated in all boys with precocious puberty, and in all girls with neurological signs and symptoms.

Tall stature with an increased height velocity is a feature of central precocious puberty in both boys and girls. Behavioural disturbances may also be evident, with an inappropriate degree of

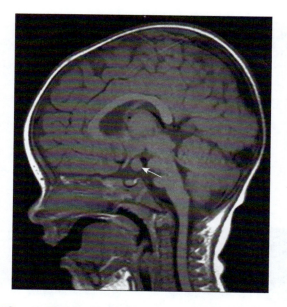

Figure 13.20 Hypothalamic hamartoma (arrow).

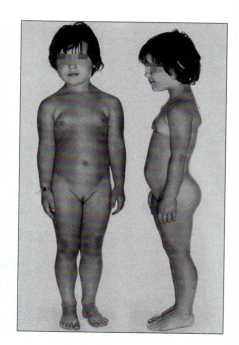

Figure 13.21 Idiopathic gonadotropin dependent precocious puberty in a 6-year-old girl.

sexualisation. A pelvic ultrasound scan in girls will reveal a multicystic ovarian morphology in response to pulsatile gonadotrophin secretion. Demonstration of a physiological pulsatile pattern of gonadotrophin secretion over a 24-hour period is expensive and time-consuming. An LHRH test shows a brisk pubertal LH and FSH response to LHRH (luteinising hormone-releasing hormone) with LH predominance and often a detectable LH at baseline. The bone age will be advanced.

Treatment

Treatment is indicated if puberty occurs at an early age with consequent implications for final height and psychological disturbance. Masturbation and sexualised behaviour can lead to major problems for the family, particularly in boys. Additionally, the onset of menarche at primary school may be a cause of distress. Treatment can alter the final height prognosis in the younger child; the use of growth hormone has not been shown to improve the height prognosis.

Gonadotrophin-releasing hormone analogues are used in the treatment of this complex condition when there is likely to be compromise to final height or where there are significant psychological considerations.

Prognosis

Although pubertal development can be arrested, the final height of these children may be unaffected by treatment if not started early. Early sexual maturation is associated with the early growth acceleration of puberty, and rapid epiphyseal maturation occurs in response to increased sex steroid secretion, which ultimately limits growth. Although children with early puberty tend to be tall when they are young, their final height prognosis is compromised. The earlier the onset of puberty and the shorter the parental heights, the shorter the child's final height will be. Polycystic ovarian syndrome can be a late problem.

MCCUNE–ALBRIGHT SYNDROME

Incidence/Genetics

McCune–Albright syndrome is a rare condition caused by an activating mutation in the gene encoding the α-subunit of Gs, the G-protein that stimulates cAMP formation. The mutation is found to a variable extent in different affected endocrine and non-endocrine tissues, consistent with the mosaic distribution of abnormal cells generated by a somatic cell mutation early in embryogenesis.

Diagnosis

Presentation is varied, and clinical features include the presence of large irregular pigmented lesions (unilateral in 50%) (Figure 13.22), polyostotic fibrous dysplasia, gonadotrophin independent precocious puberty (Figure 13.22) and other endocrinopathies (e.g. Cushing syndrome, excessive GH secretion by pituitary somatotroph adenomata, and thyrotoxicosis). Patients with this condition can present at any age, including the neonatal period. Non-endocrine abnormalities include chronic hepatic disease, thymic hyperplasia, and cardiopulmonary disease.

A skeletal survey and a bone scan show the characteristic bony abnormalities of polyostotic fibrous dysplasia (Figure 13.22). Precocious puberty is caused by autonomously functioning follicular cysts and therefore GnRH stimulation fails to increase gonadotrophin levels. Gonadotrophin-dependent puberty occurs later. Appropriate investigations for Cushing syndrome, thyrotoxicosis and pituitary adenomata leading to GH excess are performed as and when necessary. Other investigations should include liver function tests and an echocardiogram.

Treatment

The precocious puberty can be difficult to control. Agents used include cyproterone acetate, medroxyprogesterone and aromatase inhibitors (testolactone, letrozole, anastrozole), but they are all of limited efficacy. Abnormalities of other endocrine glands are treated as and when the problems arise (e.g. bilateral adrenalectomy for Cushing syndrome, carbimazole for thyrotoxicosis).

Prognosis

This is variable. The prognosis is much poorer for early-onset McCune–Albright syndrome with multi-organ involvement. Sudden death can occur due to cardiopulmonary involvement.

POLYCYSTIC OVARIAN DISEASE

Incidence/Genetics

The incidence shows a familial predisposition, although the genes implicated have not been identified to date. Polycystic ovaries can be found in 6% of 6-year-old girls and this increases to 25% of the female adult population on pelvic ultrasound scanning.

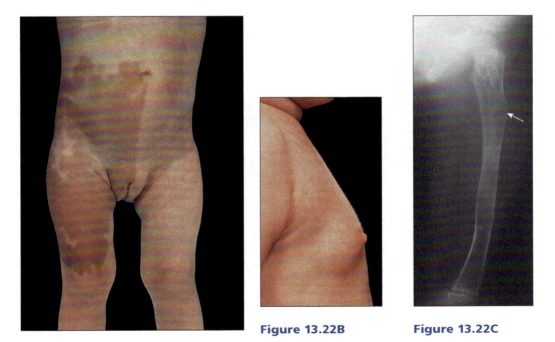

Figure 13.22B　　**Figure 13.22C**

Figure 13.22A McCune–Albright syndrome. (A) Typical café-au-lait pigmented area with an irregular margin in a child; (B) precocious puberty (gonadotropin-independent) in a 2-year-old girl; and (C) polyostotic fibrous dysplasia in a child.

Pathogenesis/Aetiology

Predisposing factors include hyperandrogenism (e.g. congenital adrenal hyperplasia), insulin insensitivity, tall stature and obesity. Treatment with growth hormone is also associated with PCO, as is diabetes mellitus.

Diagnosis

This condition usually presents with late menarche and menstrual irregularities, and accounts for 87% of irregular menstrual cycles in unselected adult females. The polycystic ovarian syndrome (PCOS) is characterised by hyperandrogenism, oligo-anovulation and evidence of polycystic ovaries on ultrasound. Patients may present with oligomenorrhea, acne, hirsutism, obesity, acanthosis nigricans or insulin-insensitivity

Pelvic ultrasound scan (USS) shows the classical appearance of large ovaries with increased stroma and a characteristic arrangement of 12 or more follicles around the periphery of the ovary (Figure 13.23). Other investigations include serum LH (elevated in 70% of PCOS patients), raised concentrations of androgens, reduced SHBG, an elevated fasting glucose and measurement of elevated insulin concentrations during an oral glucose tolerance test. Raised IGF1 concentrations due to suppressed IGF binding proteins lead to further androgen stimulation. The diagnosis of late-onset congenital adrenal hyperplasia (see below) and other causes of hyperandrogenism need to be excluded in children who present predominantly with hirsutism.

Treatment

Irregularities of the menstrual cycles can be controlled with oral contraceptive pills containing an anti-androgenic progesterone. Other anti-androgens (cyproterone acetate, spironolactone and flutamide) can also be used to alleviate the effects of hyperandrogenism. Insulin sensitisers, including metformin, and dermatological treatments may also be considered.

Prognosis

Fertility can be impaired in up to 25% of women. However, in the vast majority of individuals fertility is normal. The long-term outlook is also determined by the presence of obesity, hypertension and diabetes mellitus.

THYROID DISORDERS

CONGENITAL HYPOTHYROIDISM

Incidence/Genetics

Primary congenital hypothyroidism is due to dysgenesis of the thyroid gland or dyshormonogenesis. The incidence is 1 in 3000 newborn infants. Those cases due to an inborn error of

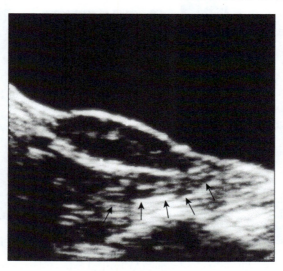

Figure 13.23 Polycystic ovary syndrome: classic ovarian ultrasound appearance, with a 'necklace' of cysts around the periphery of the ovary.

hormonogenesis are inherited in an autosomal recessive fashion (e.g. *TSHR*, *TG*, *TPO*), while those due to a dysgenetic gland have a low recurrence rate. Mutations in genes encoding transcription factors including PAX8, TTF1 and TTF2, as well as Borealin and TUBB1, are associated with the latter. Central congenital hypothyroidism due to TSH deficiency has an incidence of 1:18,000 and may be isolated or associated with other pituitary hormone deficiencies. Recently identified genetic causes of congenital central hypothyroidism include *IGSF1*, *TSH*, *TRHR*, and *TBLX1*.

Pathogenesis/Aetiology

The thyroid gland develops from endoderm in the midline of the pharyngeal floor at the base of the developing tongue. As the thyroid descends to the final position in the neck, it is connected to the tongue by the thyroglossal duct, which later obliterates. Incomplete obliteration can predispose to the formation of a thyroglossal cyst (Figure 13.24). Failure of descent of the thyroid can lead to ectopia and dysgenesis (Figure 13.25).

Diagnosis

In the United Kingdom, newborn screening for primary congenital hypothyroidism is based on TSH bloodspot screening at 5 to 7 days of age and has almost eliminated the severe clinical manifestations of prolonged thyroxine deficiency (cretinism). Clinical features, may include umbilical hernia, macroglossia, constipation, feeding problems, lethargy, prolonged jaundice, hoarse cry, hypotonia, coarse facies (Figure 13.26), growth failure, delayed closure of fontanelles, hypothermia and a dry, mottled skin. Other congenital malformations are present in 7% of cases.

Investigations include serum fT4 concentration (low) and TSH (elevated). A thyroid radioisotope scan may differentiate between dygenesis, ectopia and gland in situ. Audiological assessment is also recommended.

Transient hypothyroidism occurs in some children and may be due to milder forms of dyshormonogenesis (such as seen with some *DUOX2* mutations), maternal antibody transmission, drugs or iodine imbalance. Children with low thyroxine requirements, should be considered for a trial off thyroxine treatment at 3 years of age to establish if the hypothyroidism is permanent or transient.

If the hypothyroidism is secondary (due to congenital TRH or TSH deficiency), assessment of pituitary/hypothalamic function including measurement of GH, cortisol, prolactin and gonadotrophin secretion may be indicated. A TRH test may be appropriate in some instances.

Treatment

Treatment is with thyroxine at a starting dose of 8 to 10 μg/kg/day (maximum 50 μg) with frequent initial

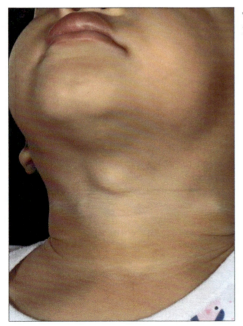

Figure 13.24 Thyroglossal cyst.

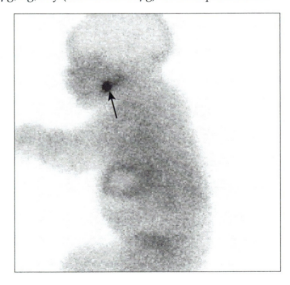

Figure 13.25 Sublingual thyroid gland demonstrated on technetium scan.

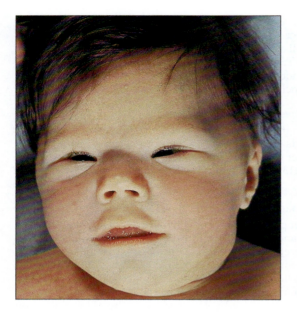

Figure 13.26 Congenital hypothyroidism: Typical coarse facies of a child.

clinical and biochemical follow up, particularly in the first year of life. Subsequent monitoring includes documentation of the growth rate, which is a sensitive measure of thyroid function.

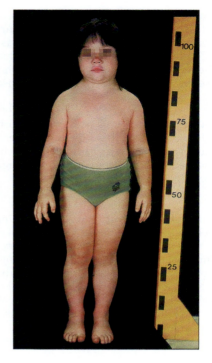

Figure 13.27 Acquired hypothyroidism: typical appearance of a child. Note the disproportion between height and weight.

Prognosis

The severe neurodevelopmental sequelae of delayed treatment of congenital hypothyroidism are rarely seen. Nevertheless, the intelligence quotient (IQ) of these patients may be impaired compared with control groups and this appears to be related to the severity and duration of thyroxine deficiency in utero and after birth.

ACQUIRED HYPOTHYROIDISM

Incidence/Genetics

Autoimmune hypothyroidism is associated with a family history in 30 to 40% of cases and is one of the commonest forms of acquired hypothyroidism.

Pathogenesis/Aetiology

Worldwide, iodine deficiency is the commonest cause of hypothyroidism. Causes of acquired hypothyroidism include goitrogenic agents, thyroid dysgenesis, auto-immune thyroiditis, pituitary TSH deficiency (e.g. post-cranial irradiation and craniopharyngioma), endemic iodine deficiency and cystinosis. Chromosomal disorders (i.e. Turner, Down's and Klinefelter syndromes) are associated with an increased incidence of hypothyroidism, which is probably autoimmune in origin.

Diagnosis

This can present at any age, usually with a gradual onset. The most important sign in childhood is growth failure, and a goitre may be present. There is a modest weight gain, with disproportion between weight and height gain (Figure 13.27). Isolated breast development or testicular enlargement, without other signs of puberty or an increase in height velocity may be associated. In contrast, pubertal delay or arrest can also be a feature. Other signs of classical hypothyroidism are slow to develop (e.g. lethargy, cold intolerance, constipation, bradycardia, dry skin, coarse facies, proximal myopathy). Classically, tendon reflex relaxation is slow and the bone age is delayed.

There may be features of other autoimmune conditions (e.g. Addison's disease, myasthenia gravis, insulin-dependent diabetes mellitus, pernicious anaemia, malabsorption and vitiligo) as thyroid disease may be a component of polyglandular autoimmune disease.

Investigations should include free thyroxine, serum TSH, thyroid peroxidase autoantibodies, thyroglobulin, FSH and prolactin (may be elevated in primary hypothyroidism). Family members are at increased risk of autoimmune hypothyroidism and should be screened where appropriate.

Treatment

Treatment with thyroxine should be commenced cautiously, at a dosage of 50 μg/m²/day initially, with a subsequent increase to 100 μg/m²/day, depending on the TSH level. There is an initial catch-up growth phase and subsequent return to a normal height velocity.

Commencement of treatment can lead to behavioural changes due to normalisation of serum fT4 and adjustment as the child returns to normal activity. The family and teachers should be warned of potential initial behavioural disruption.

Prognosis

The prognosis for final height, fertility and general health is excellent, provided treatment is commenced early and adherence is good.

GRAVES' DISEASE

Incidence/Genetics

Autoimmune thyrotoxicosis is six to eight times more common in girls. Often, a family history of autoimmune thyroid disease can be elicited.

Pathogenesis/Aetiology

Thyroid-stimulating antibodies are present in the serum of these patients and are responsible for the clinical picture observed. Autonomous functioning thyroid nodules are rare in children, as is autonomous TSH production from the thyrotroph or pituitary tumours.

Diagnosis

This can occur in preschool children, but there is a sharp increase in incidence in adolescence. The onset may be abrupt or insidious. Presenting features may include nervousness, palpitations, tremor, excessive perspiration, an increased appetite, muscle weakness, marked weight loss and behavioural abnormalities. Tachycardia, a widened pulse pressure, an overactive praecordium and heart failure may dominate the clinical picture. A goitre is the most frequent clinical sign, the size being variable (Figure 13.28). A bruit and a thrill may be features of the goitre.

Eye signs of Graves disease are variable and are usually parasympathetic signs including lid retraction, lid lag and associated conjunctival irritation. Severe Graves ophthalmopathy with exophthalmos, proptosis, ophthalmoplegia caused by inflammation and swelling of periorbital muscles, is uncommon in children. Graves dermopathy, with accumulation of mucopolysaccharides in skin and subcutaneous tissues is rare.

There may be evidence of other autoimmune conditions (e.g. vitiligo, Addison's disease, myasthenia gravis, pernicious anaemia and insulin-dependent diabetes mellitus). Measurement of fT4, fT3 (raised) and TSH concentrations (suppressed) are mandatory. Thyroid receptor antibodies (TRAb) are the most useful in diagnosis and tracking of the disease. A thyroid ultrasound scan may be required if a solitary nodule is suspected.

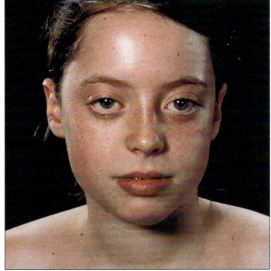

Figure 13.28   Graves' disease: Thyroid goitre.

Treatment

Treatment with anti-thyroid medication such as carbimazole or methimazole. Propranolol to block the peripheral thyroxine effects can be a useful initial adjunct. Carbimazole is associated with agranulocytosis and Propylthiouracil (PTU) is no longer recommended as a first line treatment due to hepatotoxic side effects. The condition may relapse once the medication is stopped; remission rates are low in children and may be < 50% after four years. In the long-term, definitive treatment in the form of a thyroidectomy or radioactive iodine may be indicated.

Complications of surgery include hypoparathyroidism and recurrent laryngeal nerve damage. Alternatively, radioactive iodine is easy to administer and cheap. To date, concern about radiation oncogenesis and genetic damage has limited its use to adolescents, although anxieties regarding the former have largely been alleviated in adults. It is contraindicated in children with Grave's eye disease. Post-treatment hypothyroidism needs to be treated with thyroxine.

Prognosis

Once definitive treatment has been performed, life-long thyroxine treatment is indicated. The course of the eye manifestations and the thyroid disease may differ, and exophthalmos may persist in spite of satisfactory treatment of the hyperthyroidism.

ADRENAL DISORDERS

CUSHING SYNDROME

Incidence/Genetics

Iatrogenic Cushing syndrome is relatively common. Endogenous Cushing syndrome is rare and the underlying lesion is usually a pituitary adenoma (Cushing disease). Adrenal tumours predominate in female infants under 2 years of age, in whom the underlying diagnosis may be that of the McCune–Albright syndrome. Ectopic ACTH production in children leading to Cushing syndrome is extremely rare. Cushing syndrome is sporadic, although very rare forms of familial hypercortisolism have been described. A number of genetic mutations have been identified in association with Cushing syndrome (e.g. PDE8B, PRKAR1A, PDE11A).

Pathogenesis/Aetiology

Cushing syndrome can be iatrogenic, due to a CRH- or ACTH-secreting tumour (either in the pituitary gland or due to ectopic secretion of the stimulating hormone), ACTH-independent Cushing syndrome due to adrenal neoplasms, or nodular adrenal hyperplasia. This may be familial, as in the Carney complex (bilateral micronodular adrenal hyperplasia, pigmented lentigines, atrial myxomas and other tumours). Up to 50% of cases of the Carney complex are caused by mutations in the *PRKAR1A* gene. McCune–Albright syndrome can also lead to primary adrenal Cushing syndrome.

Diagnosis

Children with this syndrome present with excessive weight gain leading to rapidly progressing obesity that is mainly truncal in nature (Figure 13.29). Other features include round facies (Figure 13.30), a mid-scapular fat pad, hypertension, purple striae (Figure 13.31), hirsutism, osteoporosis, hypogonadism, proximal myopathy, susceptibility to bruising and infection, cataracts, pubertal arrest, amenorrhoea, emotional lability and growth arrest, although, initially, androgen secretion may lead to acceleration of the height velocity.

In Cushing disease (due to a pituitary adenoma), headaches and visual disturbance may be a feature, with impaired visual fields, and even papilloedema. Diagnosis can be extremely difficult, and is based upon elevated plasma cortisol concentrations with a loss of circadian rhythm and elevated 24-hour urinary free cortisol. In pituitary-dependent Cushing disease, ACTH concentrations are detectable in the face of raised cortisol concentrations. In primary adrenal Cushing syndrome, ACTH concentrations will be suppressed in the face of elevated cortisol concentrations.

In ectopic Cushing syndrome, both cortisol and ACTH concentrations are extremely high. Once the diagnosis is established, the source of the excess cortisol production needs to be established. Dexamethasone suppresses cortisol production in normal individuals. In pituitary-dependent Cushing disease, low-dose dexamethasone will not suppress cortisol secretion, but high-dose dexamethasone will suppress it in approximately 80% of cases.

Adrenal and ectopic Cushing syndrome will not suppress with any dose of dexamethasone. Administration of CRH (corticotrophin-releasing hormone) can be helpful in differentiating

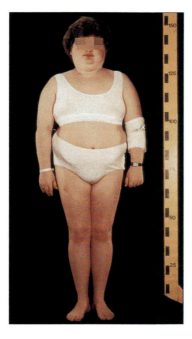

Figure 13.29   Cushing syndrome: Central obesity.

an adrenal and pituitary cause of the syndrome. Imaging of the pituitary and adrenals using an MRI scanner is usually indicated in order to locate the tumour, although the sensitivity is poor (70%). Inferior petrosal sinus sampling has a similar sensitivity and can be performed to locate a pituitary lesion and to lateralise a pituitary adenoma.

Treatment

Pituitary-dependent Cushing disease is usually treated by trans-sphenoidal removal of the adenoma by an experienced neurosurgeon. Where an adrenal tumour is defined, surgical removal of the tumour is indicated. Medical treatment with metyrapone or ketoconazole may be required to suppress cortisol production but is not without its own problems and is generally used as a temporary measure. Adrenalectomy is usually indicated in cases of adrenal neoplasms or multinodular adrenal hyperplasia, although subtotal resection may be an option in certain cases.

Prognosis

In untreated patients, the mortality and morbidity (osteoporosis, glucose intolerance and hypertension) from this condition is high. Following surgical treatment of Cushing disease, there is a strong possibility that the condition either does not remit, or relapses. Further exploration of the pituitary with a possible total hypophysectomy may be indicated. Radiotherapy can be used as a second line treatment. These treatments lead to panhypopituitarism and will need replacement hydrocortisone, thyroxine, gonadotrophins or sex steroids, growth hormone and DDAVP treatment. However, the outlook is better than bilateral adrenalectomy with consequent Nelson's syndrome. If the Cushing syndrome is due to an adrenal carcinoma or an ectopic source (usually a lung carcinoid), the prognosis is much worse.

PRIMARY ADRENAL INSUFFICIENCY

Incidence/Genetics

Primary adrenal insufficiency may be congenital or acquired. Congenital forms include congenital

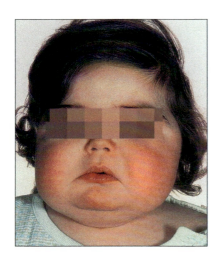

Figure 13.30   Cushing syndrome: 'Moonlike' facies in a child.

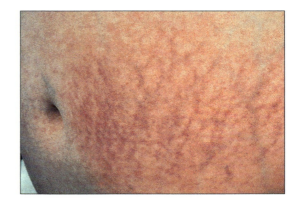

Figure 13.31   Cushing syndrome: Purple abdominal striae in a child.

adrenal hyperplasia which has an incidence of 1 in 15,000 and is discussed below. Congenital adrenal hypoplasia is reported in 1 in 12,500 births. Inheritance is either as an autosomal or X-linked recessive condition. Mutations in *DAX1* are associated with the X-linked form of the disease. Mutations in *WNT4* (SERKAL syndrome), *SAMD9* (MIRAGE syndrome) and *CDKN1C* (IMAGE syndrome).

Autoimmune adrenal insufficiency is associated with the two types of polyglandular autoimmune syndrome (Table 13.2). Type I is associated with mutations in the *AIRE* (Autoimmune Regulator) gene on chromosome 21. Familial glucocorticoid deficiency (FGD) and Triple A syndrome are characterised by an insensitivity to ACTH concentrations. FGD is caused by mutations in the ACTH receptor (*MC2R*), or mutations in the MC2R accessory protein *MRAP*. More recently, mutations in the genes encoding Nicotinamide Nucleotide Transhydrogenase (NNT) and Minichromosome maintenance-deficient 4 (MCM4) have also been associated with FGD. Triple A syndrome is autosomal dominant and secondary to mutations in the *ALADIN* gene.

Pathogenesis/Aetiology

Causes of primary adrenal insufficiency include congenital adrenal hypoplasia, defects of adrenal steroid biosynthesis, adrenal haemorrhage, autoimmune adrenalitis, multiple endocrinopathy, infections (e.g. tuberculosis and Waterhouse–Friederichsen syndrome), adrenoleukodystrophy (see also the chapter 'Metabolic Diseases') and iatrogenic (chemical or surgical) causes.

Diagnosis

Congenital adrenal insufficiency usually presents in the neonatal period with hypoglycaemia, salt loss, apnoeic episodes, dehydration, poor feeding, failure to thrive, vomiting and hyperpigmentation. In Addison's disease, presentation is usually later and symptoms and signs include lethargy, anorexia, vomiting, weight loss, irritability, salt-losing adrenal crisis, hypoglycaemia, syncope and hyperpigmentation of the skin and mucosal surfaces.

In adrenoleukodystrophy, neurological symptoms and signs may develop first, with features of adrenal insufficiency developing between the ages of 4 and 5 years. In the polyglandular autoimmune syndrome, features of other autoimmune conditions such as hypoparathyroidism, diabetes mellitus, vitiligo, autoimmune gastrointestinal disease, arthritis, myasthenia gravis, coeliac disease and pernicious anaemia may also be present. Mucocutaneous candidiasis is a feature of Type 1 polyglandular autoimmune syndrome.

FGD may present as acute or chronic glucocorticoid insufficiency in childhood. Production of aldosterone is generally maintained because the adrenal zona glomerulosa is regulated by the renin-angiotensin system, although rarely FGD is associated with early mineralocorticoid deficiency. Although glucocorticoid insufficiency is seen in around 80% of patients with Triple A syndrome (Adrenal deficiency, Achalasia of the cardia and Alacrima), the condition rarely presents in

Table 13.2: Polyglandular Autoimmune Syndrome

	Type 1	Type 2
Inheritance (autosomal)	Recessive (due to mutations in AIRE)	Dominant
Age at onset	Childhood (< 12 years)	Adulthood (> 30 years)
Female: male ratio	1.5:1	1.8:1
HLA association	None	B6, -Dw3, -DR3
Disease components:		
Addison disease	65%	100%
Hypoparathyroidism	80%	None
Mucocutaneous candidiasis	75%	None
Alopecia	25%	< 1%
Malabsorption	22%	None
Gonadal failure	20%	20%
Pernicious anaemia	13%	<1%
Autoimmune thyroid disease	10%	70%
Chronic active hepatitis	10%	None
Diabetes mellitus	8%	5%
Vitiligo	8%	5%

this manner. It is also associated with progressive neurological symptoms, sensorineural deafness, peripheral neuropathies and autonomic dysfunction.

Investigations should include plasma urea and electrolytes (hyponatraemia, hyperkalaemia), cortisol profile (low cortisol), synacthen test (no cortisol response to exogenous ACTH), plasma ACTH concentration (elevated), plasma renin activity and aldosterone concentration (renin raised with low aldosterone if mineralocorticoid deficient), auto-antibody screen, thyroid function, plasma calcium. Fasting glucose will be low in Addison disease, but elevated if associated with diabetes mellitus). Plasma very long-chain fatty acids (VLCFA) levels are useful in excluding a diagnosis of adrenoleukodystrophy.

Treatment

Hypovolaemia should be corrected with adequate fluid and sodium replacement. Maintenance treatment includes replacement doses of glucocorticoids with hydrocortisone, and mineralocorticoid treatment with 9α-fludrocortisone if mineralocorticoid deficiency is confirmed. When hypothyroidism is present in a child with chronic adrenal insufficiency, adequate glucocorticoid therapy should be established before commencing thyroxine therapy, to avoid precipitation of an adrenal crisis. Children with ACTH insensitivity require treatment with physiological replacement doses of glucocorticoids. The use of higher doses of glucocorticoids to suppress the ACTH concentration into the normal range should be avoided.

Prognosis

Given correct treatment and adequate parental support, patients with congenital adrenal hypoplasia and Addison disease can lead a normal life with a normal lifespan. Growth and pubertal development need careful monitoring. Hypogonadotrophic hypogonadism is associated with congenital adrenal hypoplasia and puberty may need to be induced. The prognosis in polyglandular autoimmune disease is poor if chronic active hepatitis is also present. The prognosis in adrenoleukodystrophy is that of the underlying neurological disorder, which progresses inexorably. MIRAGE, SERKAL and IMAGE syndromes are complex multidisciplinary disorders with multiple abnormalities.

AMBIGUOUS GENITALIA

See also the chapter 'Urology'.

Incidence Genetics

The causes of undervirilisation and overvirilisation leading to ambiguity of genitalia are listed in Table 13.3. Congenital adrenal hyperplasia and 5α-reductase deficiency (Figures 13.32 and 13.33) are inherited as autosomal recessive disorders. Mutations of the genes encoding 5α-reductase, 21-hydroxylase, steroidogenic factor 1 (SF1), Wilms' tumour (WT) and the androgen receptor have been described. The incidence of CAH is 1 in 15,000, while 5α-reductase deficiency and androgen insensitivity are much rarer.

Diagnosis

Usually present at birth. The gender of the child should not be assigned without confirmation. Early referral to an expert Disorders of Sex Development (DSD) team should be made. Note should be made of presence or absence of palpable gonads and their position if felt. External genitalia in virilised 46XX females can be described with Prader staging and the external masculinisation

Table 13.3: Aetiology of Ambiguous Genitalia

Inadequate masculinisation
Leydig cell hypoplasia
Inborn errors of testosterone biosynthesis in adrenals, testes or both
5a-reductase deficiency
Defect in target tissues, e.g. androgen insensitivity
Associated with dysmorphic syndromes – e.g. Smith–Lemli–Opitz, Dubowitz, Aniridia–Wilms, etc.

Virilised female
Virilisation by androgens of fetal origin – e.g. congenital adrenal hyperplasia
Virilisation by androgens of maternal origin – e.g. anabolic steroids, danazol, virilising maternal tumour
Dysmorphic syndromes – e.g. Seckel, Zellweger Presence of testicular tissue – e.g. ovotestis

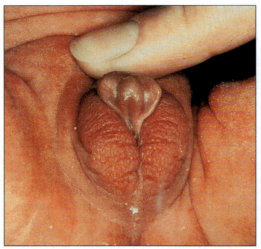

Figure 13.32 Virilisation in a newborn baby (karyotype 46XX) due to 21-hydroxylase deficiency.

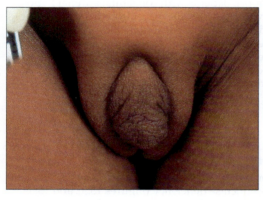

Figure 13.33 5α-reductase deficiency in a 9-year-old 46XY male.

score may also be useful. There may be associated dysmorphic features.

Investigations

Karyotype (or QF PCR for Y chromosome) should be sent immediately. Further investigations should include plasma electrolytes, serum 17-hydroxy progesterone, urinary steroid profile, plasma ACTH, testosterone, dihydro-testosterone, adrenal androgens, LH, FSH, plasma renin activity, aldosterone, and DNA analysis. Pelvic ultrasound scans may be helpful, An examination under anaesthesia by an expert DSD urologist can help to determine diagnosis and management by identification of gonads, internal anatomy and biopsy if indicated.

Treatment

The primary initial aim is to determine sex of rearing. Medical treatment is the mainstay of treatment (e.g. steroid hormone replacement in congenital adrenal hyperplasia, androgens for micropenis treatment). Gonadectomy should be considered for patients with dysgenetic or non-functional gonads, especially those with Y-bearing cell lines, which have an increased risk of malignant change in the gonad. Psychological support is essential. Hypospadias repair may be required. Currently there is a broad principle of delaying other surgical procedures until the child gains competence to consent.

Prognosis

Dependent on underlying condition and appropriateness of gender assignment.

CONGENITAL ADRENAL HYPERPLASIA

Incidence/Genetics

The inheritance for all forms of CAH is autosomal recessive; 21-hydroxylase deficiency is the commonest cause of CAH, with a frequency of between 1 in 5000 to 23,000 for the homozygous affected state, depending on the population studied. At the molecular level, the inheritance is best understood for 21-hydroxylase deficiency, where the gene encoding the microsomal cytochrome P450 21-hydroxylase enzyme system (CYP21B) and a pseudogene (CYP21A) are located in the HLA complex. Mutations and deletions in the CYP21B gene are associated with the variable phenotype seen in this condition. Rarer forms include CAH due to deficiencies of 11-beta hydroxylase (CYP11B1 deficiency) or 17-alpha hydroxylase (CYP17A1 deficiency); the former can present with hypertension and virilisation, and the latter with lack of virilisation and hypertension. Some forms of CAH are due to mutations in the gene encoding P450 oxidoreductase (POR). POR is an electron donor enzyme to cytochrome P450 (CYP) enzymes and deficiency leads to impairment of several enzymes involved in glucocorticoid and sex steroid synthesis, with a biochemical pattern indicating both CYP21B and CYP17A1 deficiencies. See Table 13.4.

Pathogenesis/Aetiology

These autosomal recessive conditions result in enzyme deficiencies in the adrenal glands, preventing synthesis of vital steroids, and resulting in accumulation of the substrate steroid preceding the block. The loss of feedback leads to ongoing excessive ACTH drive and further exacerbates the

Table 13.4: Phenotypes Associated with Congenital Adrenal Hyperplasia

Enzyme defect	Ambiguous genitalia		Salt loss	Hypertension	Puberty
	Male	Female			
CYP11A/StAR (Steroidogenic Acute Regulatory Protein)	+	−	+	−	Absent
3β-hydroxy-steroid dehydrogenase	+	+	+	−	Absent
17-hydroxylase (P450c17)	+	−	−	+	Absent
21-hydroxylase (P450c21)	−	+	+	−	Precocious
11-hydroxylase (P450c11ß)	−	+	−	+	Precocious
Oxidoreductase	+/−	+	−	+/−	Normal/incomplete

condition with promotion of cholesterol incorporation into the adrenal cortex giving rise to the adrenal hyperplasia. Early genotype-phenotype studies have already shown that the correlation between clinical, biochemical and molecular genetic findings in patients with classical 21-hydroxylase deficiency is not absolute.

Diagnosis

Children with congenital adrenal hyperplasia may present with ambiguous genitalia at birth, a salt-losing crisis in the newborn period, hypertension, precocious puberty in males, virilisation in females and 'bilateral cryptorchidism' with breast development in puberty (i.e. females raised inappropriately as males) (Figure 13.34). Hypoglycaemia is a rare feature of the condition. Clinical manifestations of POR deficiency include adrenal insufficiency without salt loss or with disorders of sex development in both sexes.

In non-classical 21-hydroxylase deficiency, females are born with normal external genitalia. Clinical manifestations from increased androgen production can appear later in childhood or adolescence, and include hirsutism, temporal baldness, acne, delayed menarche, menstrual irregularities, clitoro-

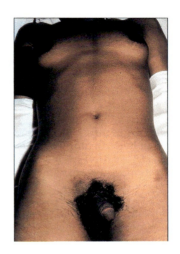

Figure 13.34 Congenital adrenal hyperplasia: Excessive virilisation in a female raised as a male.

megaly and infertility. An accelerated linear growth velocity, a short final height and an advanced bone age may be other features of this condition.

In cases with genital ambiguity or virilisation, a karyotype and pelvic ultrasound scan to identify the internal organs are mandatory. A raised plasma 17-hydroxyprogesterone level (17 OHP) indicates a diagnosis of 21-hydroxylase deficiency. A urinary steroid profile may help to define the enzyme block. In cases of simple-virilising CAH, a synacthen test (flat cortisol response, raised 17OHP concentrations) with the collection of appropriate plasma and urine samples will assist in the diagnosis. Urea and electrolyte measurements, plasma renin activity and plasma aldosterone concentrations are essential in the diagnosis of salt-losing CAH. A bone age (usually advanced) may be helpful in the management of simple-virilising CAH. Genetic analysis is useful, particularly if future pregnancies are being considered.

Treatment

Initial treatment is as described for primary adrenal insufficiency (see earlier). Salt supplements should be continued until an infant is switched to normal cow's milk and diet. Hydrocortisone clearance can be rapid in the neonate and adolescent and the hydrocortisone may need to be given more frequently than three times a day. Late-onset, simple-virilising CAH is best treated with hydrocortisone in order to suppress the ACTH drive. Puberty may need to be induced in CYP11A/StAR deficiency, 3β-hydroxysteroid dehydrogenase deficiency and 17-hydroxylase deficiency.

Monitoring of the condition is by regular auxology and biochemical monitoring. Both undertreated and over-treated congenital adrenal hyperplasia can result in an abnormal growth pattern, with an increased or decreased growth velocity respectively. Skeletal age is advanced in under-treated congenital adrenal hyperplasia. Measurement of plasma renin activity and 17OHP is useful in monitoring salt-losing CAH.

Prognosis

In well-controlled CAH where compliance with medication is satisfactory, the prognosis for final height and pubertal development is good in males, while that for fertility is more guarded. Females with CAH often develop polycystic ovarian disease and the prognosis for fertility may be affected by this complication. With late diagnosis and/or poor compliance, the children grow extremely rapidly with a considerable advance in bone age and early fusion of the epiphyses leading to a compromised final height.

GLUCOSE METABOLISM

HYPERINSULINISM

Incidence/Genetics

Congenital Hyperinsulinism (CHI) has an incidence of approximately 1 in 40,000 births and is the most common cause of persistent and recurrent hypoglycaemia. To date, mutations have been described in several genes which lead to dysregulated insulin secretion from pancreatic β-cells and account for approximately 50% of cases. CHI is also associated with Beckwith-Weidemann Syndrome. Transient hyperinsulinism is most commonly seen in infants of diabetic mothers and infants with evidence of intrauterine growth restriction.

Pathogenesis/Aetiology

Mutations in the ß-cell membrane KATP channel (*ABCC8* and *KCJN11*) can lead to focal or diffuse areas of hyperinsulinism in the pancreas. Other genes implicated in the disorder include *GLUD1*, *GCK*, *HADH*, *HNF4A*, *HNF1A*, *PMM2* and *FOXA2*. This in turn leads to severe hypoglycaemia with suppression of ketones and fatty acids and failure of counter-regulatory hormone responses.

Diagnosis

The majority present in the first few days after birth with symptoms of neonatal hypoglycaemia. These include tremor, jitteriness, apnoea, hypotonia, feeding difficulties, convulsions and coma. Examination may reveal macrosomia, plethora, hepatomegaly and generalised adiposity. In Beckwith–Wiedemann syndrome, characteristic abnormal somatic features may exist including exomphalos, macroglossia (Figure 13.35), visceromegaly, polycythaemia, hemi-hypertrophy and gigantism. Abnormalities of the ears are also present, and include transverse creases in the ear lobes.

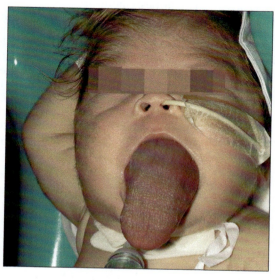

Figure 13.35 Massive macroglossia in a child with Beckwith–Weidemann syndrome. Note the tracheostomy and nasogastric tube.

Detection of insulin and C-peptide concentrations at the time of hypoglycaemia is diagnostic. Concentrations of free fatty acids, ketone bodies, glycerol and branched chain amino acids are low. Serum growth hormone and cortisol concentrations are often raised, although if the concentrations are low, they do not necessarily indicate GH and cortisol deficiency. An increased glucose requirement is also helpful in the diagnosis.

Other investigations including a urine organic acid screen taken at the time of hypoglycaemia and exclusion of metabolic conditions such as hyperinsulinism/hyperammonaemia (HIHA) syndrome are also helpful.

Treatment

The aim of treatment is to establish glucose concentrations > 3.5 mmol/L. Initially glucose infusion rates between 6–20 mg/kg/min may be required. Diazoxide is first line medical treatment and should be given in combination with chlorothiazide, to minimise fluid retention. An echocardiogram is advised to rule out pulmonary hypertension which can be exacerbated by diazoxide. Intravenous fluids should be restricted to 120 mls/kg/day and families counselled that diazoxide can lead to hypertrichosis lanuginosa (Figure 13.36). Octreotide and glucagon may also be helpful to control hypoglycaemia. Longer acting analogues of octreotide and glucagon are potential newer therapies. Where possible, it is important that affected infants maintain some oral intake to minimise later feeding difficulties, although some infants will require gastrostomy feeds to maintain overnight glucose and for emergency glucose delivery.

Genetic testing should be performed early and can help to predict whether disease is focal or diffuse. Positron Emission Tomography (PET) with fluoro-dopa may be useful to further establish focal or diffuse disease. Surgical treatment of focal lesions is potentially curative. A 95% pancreatectomy may be required in diffuse cases that fail medical therapy.

Prognosis

Impaired neurological outcome secondary to hypoglycaemic brain injury is reported in 10–40% of cases and increases with delay in diagnosis. Following a pancreatectomy, the patient is likely to later develop diabetes mellitus, characterised by an excessive sensitivity to insulin. Ketotic hyperglycaemia is very rare. Malabsorption may develop and requires treatment with exocrine pancreatic supplementation.

TYPE 1 DIABETES MELLITUS

Pathogenesis/Aetiology

Absolute insulin deficiency results from autoimmune destruction of the beta cells in the pancreas. HLA-DR and -DQ alleles are associated with varying degrees of predisposition to, and protection

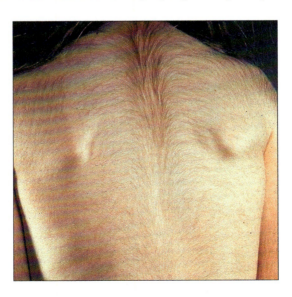

Figure 13.36 Hyperinsulinism: Diazoxide-induced hypertrichosis lanuginosa in a child.

against, the development of type 1 diabetes mellitus. However, 50% concordance rates for Type 1 diabetes in monozygotic twins and a rapid increase in the incidence of Type 1 diabetes over recent decades, suggest that as yet unidentified environmental factors modulate genetic risk.

Epidemiology

Type 1 diabetes is by far the commonest form of diabetes in childhood with an incidence of 24.5 per 100,000 children aged 0 to 15 years in the United Kingdom. The worldwide incidence varies by at least 100-fold, being highest in Finland and lowest in China and it has been increasing worldwide at an annual rate of approximately 3 to 5%.

Presentation

The vast majority of children with Type 1 diabetes will present clinically with the classic triad of polydipsia, polyuria and weight loss. Diabetes may also present with secondary enuresis and recurrent infections. Children may present in diabetic ketoacidosis (DKA) with vomiting, dehydration, abdominal pain, hyperventilation (Kussmaul's breathing), hypovolaemia and altered consciousness.

Necrobiosis lipoidica is a rare skin condition associated with diabetes, but not the level of glycaemic control. It is most commonly found on the shins and is characterised by yellow plaques with a violaceous border, which often scale, crust or ulcerate.

Diagnosis

The diagnosis can be confirmed by a random plasma glucose of > 11.1 mmol/l, HbA1c > 6.5%, a fasting plasma glucose ≥ 7.0 mmol/l, or a two-hour plasma glucose > 11.1 mmol/l during a standard oral glucose tolerance test (OGTT). If these diagnostic criteria are not met, but there is evidence of impaired fasting glycaemia, or impaired glucose tolerance, follow up is essential. In addition to the diagnostic glucose and HbA1c concentrations, blood ketones should be checked to exclude ketoacidosis.

Markers of the process of immune-mediated destruction are present in 85 to 98% of children with newly diagnosed Type 1 diabetes. These include autoantibodies to insulin (IAA), autoantibodies to glutamic acid decarboxylase (GAD65) and autoantibodies to the tyrosine phosphatases IA-2 and IA-2β. Type 2 diabetes or maturity-onset diabetes of the young (MODY) may present with non-ketotic hyperglycaemia and negative antibodies. There is an increased risk of other autoimmune disorders, particularly coeliac disease and hypothyroidism which can be asymptomatic and lead to significant morbidity if left untreated. Addison's disease is a rare but recognised association.

Management

Children in DKA should be treated with intravenous insulin using standardised treatment regimens such as those produced by the British Society of Paediatric Endocrinology and Diabetes (https://www.bsped.org.uk/clinical-resources/bsped-dka-guidelines/). Cerebral oedema is a complication that is associated with high mortality and morbidity.

Treatment requires subcutaneous insulin via multiple daily injections (using insulin injection pens) or continuous infusion (pump therapy). Short acting insulin analogues are given as boluses for meals and correction doses and background insulin is delivered by either long-acting insulin analogue injections or a continuous basal infusion of short acting insulin through the pump. If the pump insulin infusion is disrupted, there is a risk of rapid hyperglycaemia and/or DKA as there is no long-acting insulin present. Therefore, patients using insulin pumps should always have access to injection therapy.

Conversely, immediate access to fast acting glucose is also essential to manage hypoglycaemia. The symptoms and signs of hypoglycaemia relate to autonomic activation (tremor, sweating) and neuroglycopaenia (irritability, headache, confusion, convulsions, coma). Although death is an extremely rare consequence of hypoglycaemia, severe hypoglycaemia may cause long-term neuropsychological impairment.

Insulin doses are based on glucose measurements, carbohydrate intake and activity. Calculations can be automated using smart blood glucose monitors, insulin pumps and diabetes apps. Glucose concentrations may be measured using capillary blood testing or continuous glucose monitoring (CGM) devices which measure interstitial glucose. Automation of insulin delivery through connectivity of CGM and pump devices is now possible with open and closed looping algorithms.

The aim of diabetes management is to achieve optimal time within set glucose targets whilst minimising hypo and hyperglycaemic excursions. Download of CGM data provide percentages for glucose 'Time in Range' (TIR) (standardised as 3.9 mmol/l to 10 mmol/l) and visual data that can aid adjustments to insulin management. A TIR over 75% suggests that glucose targets are being met with minimal glycaemic variation. This is a useful adjunct to three-monthly HbA1c which does not provide information about glucose variability.

Injections and pump cannula insertions should be rotated to avoid lipohypertrophy (Figure 13.37), which results in variable absorption. Lipoatrophy (Figure 13.38) is now rare with the available insulin analogues.

Diabetes care should be provided in a multidisciplinary team setting which includes nursing, medical, dietetic and psychology input by individuals with paediatric diabetes expertise. Access to podiatry and ophthalmology is also essential. Transfer to adult services should be planned with the young person and occur at a time of relative stability.

Prognosis

Glycated haemoglobin (HbA1c) reflects glycaemic control over the past three months and predicts the risk of long-term complications. The relative risk of microvascular complications including retinopathy, nephropathy, neuropathy and microalbuminaemia rise significantly with increasing HbA1c concentrations above 6.5% persisting over the long term. Other rarer clinical manifestations of poor diabetes control include limited finger-joint mobility.

Annual review includes screening for coeliac and thyroid disease, microalbuminuria, lipids and renal function. Retinopathy and foot checks for neuropathy should be performed annually from 12 years of age.

TYPE 2 DIABETES MELLITUS

Aetiology

Type 2 diabetes is the result of beta-cell decompensation which occurs after prolonged hyperglycaemia and insulin insensitivity. The prevalence is rising and it is associated with family history, obesity, ethnicity and socioeconomic deprivation. Risk is increased in those who were born small for gestational age or whose mothers were obese and/or diabetic.

Presentation

Type 2 diabetes should be considered if the child is obese and has a strong family history of diabetes. Ketones at diagnosis are uncommon. Children may have acanthosis nigricans, a velvety thickening of the skin in the neck or axillae (Figure 13.39) and symptoms or signs of polycystic ovarian disease (oligomenorrhoea, hirsutism), both of which are associated with insulin resistance. Investigations include auto-antibodies (islet cell, insulin and GAD), insulin and C-peptide concentrations (fasting and during OGTT) and fasting lipid concentrations.

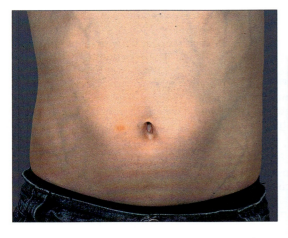

Figure 13.37 Lipohypertrophy in a boy who injected subcutaneously into his abdomen.

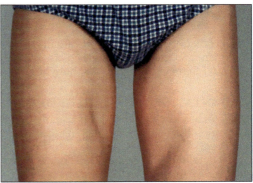

Figure 13.38 Lipoatrophy.

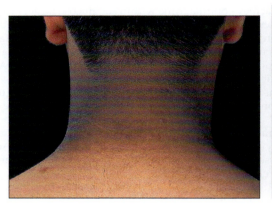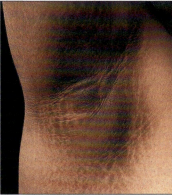

Figure 13.39 Insulin resistance: acanthosis nigricans in (left) the nuchal and (right) axillary folds of a child.

Prognosis

Mortality is two to three times higher among people with Type 2 diabetes than in the general population. In addition, the risk of myocardial infarction is four times greater in those diagnosed with Type 2 diabetes before the age of 45 years.

MONOGENIC DIABETES

Genetics/Incidence

Monogenic diabetes results from the inheritance of a mutation or mutations in a single gene. It may be dominantly or recessively inherited or a *de novo* mutation. It includes MODY, Neonatal diabetes and other genetic syndromes.

MODY affects 1–2% of people with diabetes. It is inherited in an autosomal dominant manner. 87% of the UK MODY is caused by mutations in *HNF1A, HNF4A, GCK, HNF1B, KCNJ11, ABCC8*, and Maternally Inherited Diabetes and Deafness (*MIDD*).

Neonatal diabetes is usually diagnosed in the first six months of life and is classified as transient (TNDM) or permanent (PNDM). The majority of patients with TNDM have an abnormality of imprinting of the *ZAC* and *HYMAI* genes on chromosome 6q while PNDM mutations include those in the *KCNJ11* gene encoding the Kir6.2 subunit of the beta-cell K_{ATP} channel and homozygous or compound heterozygous mutations in glucokinase.

Pathogenesis/Aetiology

Monogenic diabetes results from mutations in genes that regulate beta-cell function. Diabetes resulting from mutations in severe insulin resistance is discussed below. MODY should be considered if the diabetes develops before the age of 25 years and runs in families between generations. Diabetes does not always need insulin treatment and may be treated by diet or sulphonylurea.

Treatment of Mody

Correct diagnosis is important. Patients with mutations in the glucokinase gene rarely require treatment and are not at increased risk of diabetic complications. Those with mutations in *HNF1a* and *HNF4a* may respond to sulphonylurea treatment.

PRESENTATION AND MANAGEMENT OF NEONATAL DIABETES

Diabetes associated with 6q24 is usually diagnosed in the first week of life and resolves in three to six months. The diabetes may recur in later childhood and adolescence. Insulin treatment is required.

Neonatal diabetes due to *Kir6.2* mutations can be managed effectively with sulphonylureas and doses of up to 1 mg/kg/day may be required. Neurological features are seen in 20% of patients and severe defects can lead to developmental delay and epilepsy (Developmental delay, Epilepsy and Neonatal Diabetes (DEND) syndrome).

INSULIN RESISTANCE SYNDROMES

Incidence/Genetics

Syndromes of insulin resistance are rare. They include genetic defects in the insulin receptor (Donohue syndrome; Rabson–Mendenhall syndrome; Type A Insulin Resistance) and downstream insulin signalling defects. Acquired insulin resistance (Type B) may be caused by antibodies against the insulin receptor.

Severe insulin resistance also occurs as a result of adipose tissue abnormalities. These include monogenic obesity syndromes and lipodystrophies. Congenital total lipodystrophies are usually autosomal recessive whilst partial lipodystrophies tend to have an autosomal dominant inheritance.

Pathogenesis/Aetiology

There is a resistance to insulin at the receptor level, although the underlying pathogenetic mechanism is unclear. In the type A syndrome, insulin receptor mutations may cause defects in receptor expression on the cell surface, or in the signalling capacity of the receptor. Similar mutations have been described in patients with Donohue syndrome and lipodystrophy.

Diagnosis

Abnormal glucose homeostasis with raised insulin concentrations develops in all patients although timing and severity is variable, with hypoglycaemia often preceding hyperglycaemia. Acanthosis nigricans (Figure 13.40) is invariably present and is characterised by the presence of hyperkeratotic epidermal papillomatosis with increased melanocytes, leading to hyperpigmented, velvety areas of skin, predominantly in apposed and flexural regions. In girls, the condition is associated with polycystic ovarian disease, where it is associated with hyperandrogenism leading to hirsutism.

Children with Donohue syndrome and Rabson–Mendenhall syndrome also have characteristic features including intrauterine growth retardation, dysmorphic facies, lipoatrophy, acanthosis nigricans, overgrowth of genitalia, and viscera (Figure 13.41).

Disorders of adipose tissue development or function (lipodystrophies) may lead to unusual fat distribution with areas of excessive fat distribution and areas of adipose deficiency. Hypertriglyceridaemia and hepatic steatosis are associated with these conditions. Insulin resistance leads to diabetes mellitus. Causes may be genetic, autoimmune or secondary to drugs, particularly antiretroviral therapies

Treatment

At present, the main form of treatment is dietary restriction with reduced fat intake. Insulin sensitisers such as metformin and anti-androgens may have a role to play. Severe insulin receptor defects may respond to recombinant IGF1 therapy. It is thought to act as an insulin mimetic with similar post-receptor signalling effects.

Prognosis

Donohue syndrome and Rabson–Mendenhall syndrome have limited life expectancy. Other insulin resistant states lead to an increased incidence of diabetes mellitus, hypertension and coronary heart disease.

OTHER FORMS OF DIABETES

Diabetes may also be caused by diseases of the exocrine pancreas (cystic fibrosis), endocrinopathies (Cushing syndrome), drugs or chemicals (glucocorticoids, calcineurin inhibitors) and infections (congenital rubella), and may also be associated with other genetic syndromes (Wolfram syndrome).

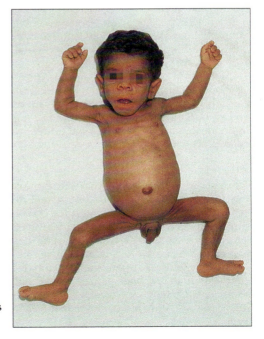

Figure 13.40 Donohue syndrome in a child presenting with hyperinsulinism.

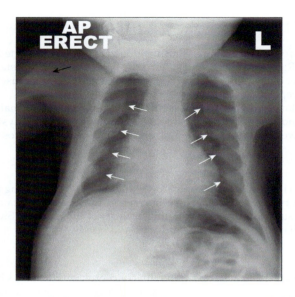

Figure 13.41 Radiograph of left hand and wrist (same patient as in 40). There is marked fraying, cupping, and splaying of the distal radial and ulnar metaphyses, with pseudowidening of the distal radial growth plate.

CALCIUM DISORDERS

RICKETS

Incidence/Genetics

In the United Kingdom, vitamin D deficiency is the most common cause of rickets. It is generally commoner in children in Asian communities, possibly due to a combination of genetic and dietary factors, and a lack of sunlight. Vitamin-D-dependent rickets, which can be due to 1-hydroxylase deficiency (Type 1) or an end-organ receptor resistance to vitamin D (Type 2), is inherited as an autosomal recessive condition. Familial hypophosphataemic rickets is inherited as an X-linked, autosomal dominant or autosomal recessive condition, with a frequency of 1 in 25,000.

Pathogenesis/Aetiology

Calciopenic causes include dietary calcium and vitamin D deficiency, malabsorption, lack of sunlight, hepatic disease, anti-convulsant treatment, renal disease, 1-α hydroxylase deficiency and end-organ resistance to vitamin D. Phosphopenic causes include Fanconi syndrome, X-linked hypophosphataemic rickets, renal tubular acidosis and oculo-cerebro-renal syndrome (Lowe syndrome).

Diagnosis

This condition usually presents with bone deformity exhibiting different patterns, depending on the child's age at the onset of disease and the relative growth rate of different bones. In the first year of life, the most rapidly growing bones are the skull, the upper limbs and ribs. Rickets at this time presents with craniotabes, widening of the cranial sutures, frontal bossing, enlarged swollen epiphyses, particularly of the wrists (Figure 13.42), bulging of the costochondral joints (rachitic rosary) and a Harrison's sulcus (Figure 13.43).

After the first year of life, genu varum (Figure 13.44), genu valgum, abnormal dentition with enamel hypoplasia, bone pain and proximal myopathy are the dominant clinical features. In severe cases, tetany, laryngeal stridor, paraesthesiae and convulsions result from the hypocalcaemia. Growth failure is a common feature. Alopecia is a feature of Vitamin-D-dependent rickets Type 2.

X-linked hypophosphataemic rickets usually presents in the male during late infancy with hypophosphataemia. Subsequently, untreated patients present with slow growth, bowing of the legs and a waddling gait. The clinical presentation is extremely variable, ranging from biochemical

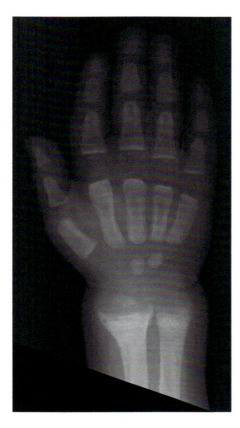

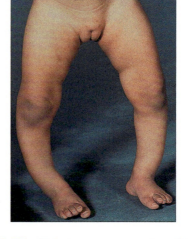

Figure 13.43 Rickets: genu varum in a child.

Figure 13.42 Chest radiograph in a 16-month-old male with severe nutritional rickets. The anterior rib ends are markedly expanded, forming an almost continuous sheet of bone around the anterior chest (white arrows), the radiological correlate of the rachitic rosary.

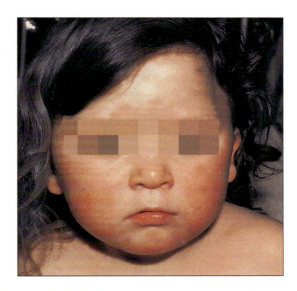

Figure 13.44 Pseudohypoparathyroidism: characteristic facial appearance of a child.

abnormalities to severe bony disease. Other features include poor dental development and abscesses of the teeth.

Biochemically, hypocalcaemia and hypophosphataemia may be present. The alkaline phosphatase concentration is high with low 1,25-dihydroxy vitamin D concentration. The serum parathyroid hormone concentration may be high. Radiologically, widening of the growth plate and fraying, cupping and widening of the metaphyses occur. Pseudofractures and signs of secondary hyperparathyroidism may also be seen (e.g. sub-periosteal erosions). Other investigations may be abnormal, depending on the underlying cause (e.g. acidosis, aminoaciduria, chronic kidney disease, anaemia).

Treatment

Combinations of calcium, phosphate and vitamin D are used in an attempt to correct the clinical, radiological and biochemical abnormalities. In vitamin D deficient states, replacement should be with preparations of cholecalciferol or ergocalciferol. Underlying abnormalities (e.g. coeliac disease) need appropriate treatment. Growth needs to be carefully monitored. In hypophosphataemic rickets, large doses of vitamin D are required. In patients with 1α-hydroxylase deficiency or end-organ resistance to vitamin D, 1,25-dihydroxy-cholecalciferol is usually required in significant doses. Regular renal ultrasound scanning is important to exclude nephrocalcinosis.

Prognosis

The prognosis for growth and cure of radiological and biochemical abnormalities is excellent in most children with rickets, provided that the condition is adequately treated. However, in hypophosphataemic rickets, the prognosis is less certain, and severe deformities of the limbs may result, particularly if compliance is poor.

HYPOPARATHYROIDISM/PSEUDOHYPOPARATHYROIDISM

Incidence/Genetics

When due to polyglandular autoimmune syndrome type I, hypoparathyroidism is inherited as an autosomal recessive condition. DiGeorge syndrome may be due to monosomy 22q11. In pseudohypoparathyroidism, inheritance is autosomal dominant, and the condition is rare. Rarely, hypoparathyroidism may be associated with activating mutations in the gene encoding the calcium sensing receptor

Diagnosis

Usual presentation for both conditions is with symptomatic hypocalcaemia. Children with hypoparathyroidism may present with symptoms and signs of hypocalcaemia *per se*. These include jitteriness, neonatal apnoea, convulsions, tetany, muscle cramps, laryngospasm, carpopedal spasm, positive Chvostek and Trousseau signs, neurodevelopmental delay, basal ganglia calcification and lenticular cataracts.

In DiGeorge syndrome, hypoparathyroidism is associated with thymic aplasia and consequent T-cell defects, congenital heart disease (especially truncus arteriosus) facial anomalies such as micrognathia, cleft lip and palate and ear malformations. (See also the chapter 'Immunology'.)

In pseudohypoparathyroidism, many of the children have neurodevelopmental delay and show unique somatic features, termed Albright's hereditary osteodystrophy. These include short stature, round facies (Figure 13.45), a short neck, obesity and subcutaneous calcification, especially near joints. A pathognomic feature of this condition is shortening of the fourth and fifth metacarpals and metatarsals (Figure 13.46). Symptoms of chronic hypocalcaemia may predominate, and include convulsions, cataracts and ectodermal changes such as dry, scaling skin and enamel hypoplasia.

Hypoparathyroidism is characterised biochemically by hypocalcaemia, hyperphosphataemia and reduced parathyroid hormone concentrations.

In pseudohypoparathyroidism, parathyroid hormone concentrations are elevated, and the diagnosis may be confirmed genetically or clinically by an inability to increase urinary cyclic AMP levels and phosphate excretion in response to an infusion of parathormone. In Albright's syndrome, hormonal resistance may be generalised and the clinical picture includes growth hormone deficiency, hypogonadism and hypothyroidism.

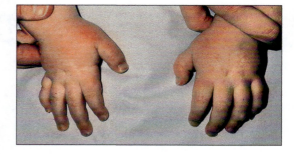

Figure 13.45 Pseudohypoparathyroidism: clinical appearance of the hands, with short fourth and fifth metacarpals.

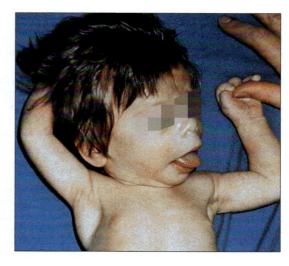

Figure 13.46 Williams syndrome: Typical facies in a child.

A skeletal survey may help in the diagnosis, and reveals short metacarpals and metatarsals with ectopic subcutaneous calcification. Pseudopseudohypoparathyroidism refers to the phenotype associated with pseudohypoparathyroidism but with normal biochemistry.

Pathogenesis/Aetiology

Hypoparathyroidism may be due to mutations in or near the PTH gene on chromosome 11, polyglandular autoimmune syndrome and post-surgery. DiGeorge syndrome is due to developmental defects of the structures which derive from the third and fourth pharyngeal pouches and branchial pouches. Pseudohypoparathyroidism is due to a mutation in the α-subunit of the G-protein coupled to the PTH receptor.

Treatment

Treatment is with calcium supplements and vitamin D, usually in the form of 1α-calcidol, with close biochemical monitoring and regular renal ultrasound scans to detect nephrocalcinosis. An emerging novel therapy is the use of parathyroid hormone given by subcutaneous infusion. In DiGeorge syndrome, recurrent infections need appropriate treatment as do cardiovascular abnormalities.

Prognosis

In DiGeorge syndrome, the prognosis is dictated by the immunological and cardiovascular anomalies. In pseudohypoparathyroidism, mild to moderate neurodevelopmental delay is observed in 50 to 75% of cases. The prognosis in isolated hypoparathyroidism is very good, provided that the condition is not associated with chronic active hepatitis.

HYPERCALCAEMIA

Hypercalcaemia is uncommon in paediatrics and may be attributable to genetic abnormalities of the calcium sensing receptor or mutations that are associated with parathyroid hyperplasia and/or neoplasia such as MEN1. Hypercalcaemia may also be attributable to disorders of bone metabolism or abnormal vitamin D metabolism such as seen in subcutaneous fat necrosis of the newborn.

Presentation

Symptoms may arise once the calcium concentration exceeds 3 mmol/l. Children may present with muscle weakness, vomiting, constipation, abdominal pain and lethargy. Nephrocalcinosis can result from longstanding hypercalcaemia. Investigations for calcium, magnesium, phosphate, alkaline phosphatase, parathyroid hormone and 25-hydroxyvitamin D levels along with a urine calcium: creatinine ratio should be first line. Bone x-rays, renal ultrasound and DNA analysis may also be indicated

WILLIAMS SYNDROME

See also the chapter 'Genetics'.

Incidence/Genetics

The condition is due to a deletion or mutations in the elastin gene on chromosome 7q11.

Pathogenesis/Aetiology

A genetic defect in the elastin gene is responsible for the diverse features of the condition.

Diagnosis

Infantile hypercalcaemia is associated with neurodevelopmental delay, 'cocktail party chatter', facial and cardiovascular features. The facial features include a broad prominent forehead, a short and turned up nose with a flat nasal bridge, full cheeks and lips with a prominent overhanging upper lip, low-set ears, stellate iris, epicanthic folds and strabismus (Figures 13.47 and 13.48). Dental anomalies

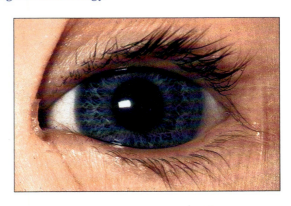

Figure 13.47 Williams syndrome: stellate iris in a child.

393

are characteristic. Cardiovascular anomalies are present in 75% and include supravalvular aortic stenosis and peripheral pulmonary artery stenosis. Low birth weight, short stature, microcephaly, hoarse voice, hyperacusis and kyphoscoliosis are other features. Infantile hypercalcaemia usually resolves spontaneously.

Investigations reveal an elevated serum calcium level, a high normal phosphate level, low normal alkaline phosphatase and PTH concentration, and hypercalciuria. Radiographic features include increased density at the metaphyseal ends of the long bones, osteosclerosis of the base of the skull, nephrocalcinosis and soft tissue calcification. The pathogenesis of the hypercalcaemia remains unclear.

Treatment

The hypercalcaemia usually resolves spontaneously. A low calcium diet is indicated until the calcium level falls. If the calcium concentration is persistently elevated and leads to symptoms, treatment with bisphosphonates or prednisolone may be indicated. The cardiovascular abnormalities will also require treatment.

Prognosis

The prognosis is determined by the cardiovascular anomalies and the neurodevelopmental delay. The outlook for the hypercalcaemia is good.

FURTHER READING

- **Growth hormone deficiency/insufficiency**
- Hage C, Gan HW, Ibba A, et al. Advances in differential diagnosis and management of growth hormone deficiency in children. *Nature Reviews Endocrinology*. 2021;17(10):608–624.
- Gregory LC, Dattani MT. The molecular basis of congenital hypopituitarism and related disorders. *The Journal of Clinical Endocrinology and Metabolism*. 2020;105(6):dgz184.
- **Laron-type dwarfism**
- David A, Hwa V, Metherell LA, et al. Evidence for a continuum of genetic, phenotypic, and biochemical abnormalities in children with growth hormone insensitivity. *Endocrine Reviews*. 2011;32(4):472–497.
- Wit JM, Oostdijk W, Losekoot M, van Duyvenvoorde HA, Ruivenkamp CA, Kant SG. Mechanisms in endocrinology: Novel genetic causes of short stature. *European Journal of Endocrinology*. 2016;174(4):R145–R173.
- **Achondroplasia**
- Savarirayan R, Tofts L, Irving M, et al. Safe and persistent growth-promoting effects of vosoritide in children with achondroplasia: 2-year results from an open-label, phase 3 extension study. *Genetics in Medicine: Official Journal of the American College of Medical Genetics*. 2021:1–5.
- **Russell–Silver syndrome**
- Wakeling EL, Brioude F, Lokulo-Sodipe O, et al. Diagnosis and management of Silver-Russell syndrome: First international consensus statement. *Nature Reviews Endocrinology*. 2017;13(2):105–124.
- **Turner syndrome**
- Gravholt CH, Viuff MH, Brun S, Stochholm K, Andersen NH. Turner syndrome: Mechanisms and management. *Nature Reviews Endocrinology*. 2019;15(10):601–614.
- **Prader–Willi syndrome**
- Butler MG, Miller JL, Forster JL. Prader-Willi Syndrome – Clinical genetics, diagnosis and treatment approaches: An update. *Current Pediatric Reviews*. 2019;15(4):207–244.
- **Pituitary gigantism**
- Keil MF, Stratakis CA. Pituitary tumors in childhood: Update of diagnosis, treatment and molecular genetics. *Expert Review of Neurotherapeutics*. 2008;8(4):563–574.
- Trivellin G, Daly AF, Faucz FR, et al. Gigantism and acromegaly due to Xq26 microduplications and GPR101 mutation. *The New England Journal of Medicine*. 2014;371(25):2363–2674.
- **Late puberty**
- Howard SR, Dunkel L. Delayed puberty-phenotypic diversity, molecular genetic mechanisms, and recent discoveries. *Endocrine Reviews*. 2019;40(5):1285–1317.
- **Early puberty**
- Latronico AC, Brito VN, Carel JC. Causes, diagnosis, and treatment of central precocious puberty. *The Lancet Diabetes & Endocrinology*. 2016;4(3):265–274.

- **Congenital hypothyroidism**
- van Trotsenburg P, Stoupa A, Léger J, et al. Congenital hypothyroidism: A 2020–2021 consensus guidelines update-an ENDO-European reference network initiative endorsed by the European Society for Pediatric Endocrinology and the European Society for Endocrinology. *Thyroid: Official Journal of the American Thyroid Association.* 2021;31(3):387–419.
- **Graves disease**
- Léger J, Carel JC. Diagnosis and management of hyperthyroidism from prenatal life to adolescence. *Best Practice & Research Clinical Endocrinology & Metabolism.* 2018;32(4):373–386.
- **Ambiguous genitalia**
- Ahmed SF, Achermann JC, Arlt W, Balen A, Conway G, Edwards Z, et al. Society for endocrinology UK guidance on the initial evaluation of an infant or an adolescent with a suspected disorder of sex development (Revised 2015). *Clinical Endocrinology.* 2016;84(5):771–788.
- **Congenital adrenal hyperplasia**
- El-Maouche D, Arlt W, Merke DP. Congenital adrenal hyperplasia. *Lancet (London, England).* 2017;390(10108):2194–2210.
- Claahsen-van der Grinten HL, Speiser PW, Ahmed SF, Arlt W, Auchus RJ, Falhammar H, et al. Congenital adrenal hyperplasia – Current insights in pathophysiology, diagnostics and management. *Endocrine Reviews.* 2022;43(1):91–159.

- **Hyperinsulinism**
- Stanley CA. Perspective on the genetics and diagnosis of congenital hyperinsulinism disorders. *The Journal of Clinical Endocrinology and Metabolism.* 2016;101(3):815–826.
- Güemes M, Rahman SA, Kapoor RR, Flanagan S, Houghton JAL, Misra S, et al. Hyperinsulinemic hypoglycemia in children and adolescents: Recent advances in understanding of pathophysiology and management. *Reviews in Endocrine & Metabolic Disorders.* 2020;21(4):577–597.
- **Insulin resistance syndromes**
- Semple RK, Savage DB, Cochran EK, Gorden P, O'Rahilly S. Genetic syndromes of severe insulin resistance. *Endocrine Reviews.* 2011;32(4):498–514.
- **Diabetes Mellitus**
- Chiang JL, Maahs DM, Garvey KC, Hood KK, Laffel LM, Weinzimer SA, et al. Type 1 diabetes in children and adolescents: A position statement by the American Diabetes Association. *Diabetes Care.* 2018;41(9):2026–2044.
- Nadeau KJ, Anderson BJ, Berg EG, Chiang JL, Chou H, Copeland KC, et al. Youth-onset Type 2 diabetes consensus report: Current status, challenges, and priorities. *Diabetes Care.* 2016;39(9):1635–1642.
- Hattersley AT, Greeley SAW, Polak M, Rubio-Cabezas O, Njølstad PR, Mlynarski W, et al. ISPAD Clinical Practice Consensus Guidelines 2018: The diagnosis and management of monogenic diabetes in children and adolescents. *Pediatric Diabetes.* 2018;19(Suppl 27):47–63.

14 Metabolic Diseases

Stephanie Grünewald, Alex Broomfield and Mildrid Yeo

METABOLIC NEWBORN SCREENING (NBS)

Newborn screening (NBS) in the United Kingdom was designed to detect and alter the natural history of conditions that would otherwise cause significant morbidity or mortality within a population. In the United Kingdom, the UK screening programme is regulated by the Department of Health through the National Screening Committee.

All babies born in the United Kingdom should have NBS. The screening sample is collected between day 5–8 of life via heel prick on a blood spot card (Figure 14.1) and is sent to the regional NBS laboratory. Any positive screens are reported immediately to metabolic specialist services.

Since 2015, the UK NBS programme includes six inborn errors of metabolism (Figure 14.2).

AMINO ACID METABOLISM

Phenylketonuria (PKU)

Incidence

Estimated 1:10,0000.

Clinical Presentation

The classical childhood features of phenylketonuria (PKU) are now rarely seen, as a result of the effective neonatal screening programmes. This is based on the detection of elevated phenylalanine (PHE) concentrations. Untreated, PKU leads to progressive mental retardation. Patients may also develop spasticity, abnormal gait, or less commonly focal neurological signs and seizures. Children with untreated PKU may have blond hair, blue eyes and fair skin due to metabolic defect restricting melanin production.

Metabolic Derangements

The disease is caused by a deficiency in the enzyme phenylalanine hydroxylase (co-factor tetrahydrobiopterine BH4) which converts phenylalanine to tyrosine. A proportion of patients are responsive to pharmacological doses of BH4. High phenylalanine levels can result in reduced levels of tyrosine in the blood leading to impaired synthesis of melanin, dopamine and norepinephrine.

Genetics

Autosomal recessive; *PAH* gene.

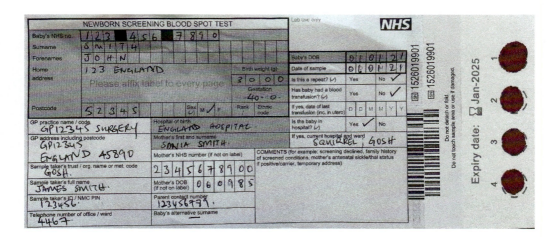

Figure 14.1   Standard NBS card (Guthrie card) used in the United Kingdom.

      DOI: 10.1201/9781003175186-14

Figure 14.2: UK NBS Programme

Newborn screened metabolic conditions since 2015

Inborn errors of metabolism:
- Phenylketonuria (PKU)
- Medium-chain Acyl-CoA Dehydrogenase deficiency (MCADD)
- Glutaric Aciduria Type I (GA1)
- Maple Syrup Urine Disease (MSUD)
- Homocystinuria (HCU)
- Isovaleric aciduria

Diagnosis

In classical severe PKU, PHE levels are above 1200 μmol/l (40–100 μmol/l). Molecular testing is not essential for diagnosis but is increasingly being performed as a means for diagnosis of BH4-responsiveness. Another important differential are pterin defects, which also presents with elevated PHE levels.

Treatment and Prognosis

Treatment for PKU should be commenced as soon as possible with the aim to maintain the phenylalanine concentrations in the range 120–360 μmol/l in the first 12 years, < 600 μmol/l after the 12 years. The immature brain is much more susceptible to hyperphenylalaninaemia and thus good control is essential in early childhood.

The mainstay treatment consists restricting natural protein (phenylalanine) intake and a supplementary phenylalanine-free formula. Compliance is often challenging. The diet can be relaxed in adulthood, except for women contemplating pregnancy. Fetal exposure to high PHE levels can lead to severe complications, therefore, pregnant PKU women need to follow a very strict diet prior to and throughout the pregnancy.

With early treatment, the prognosis is excellent, although there is probably a mild deficit in IQ in some.

Maple Syrup Urine Disease (MSUD)

Incidence

1:120,000 to 1:500,000 (incidence is higher in the Mennonite population).

Clinical Presentation

Clinical phenotypes of MSUD can be classified into five types: classic, intermediate, intermittent, thiamine responsive and E3 deficiency. Classic and E3-deficient MSUD typically present in the neonatal period, while the intermediate, intermittent, and thiamine responsive forms may present at any time of life with metabolic decompensations occurring during periods of illness or stress where a maple syrup odour may be apparent.

In classic MSUD, patients present shortly after birth with irritability, lethargy, poor feeding, apnoea, opisthotonus, 'cycling' movements. If untreated this is leads to coma and early death.

Metabolic Derangements

MSUD is caused by a deficiency of the branched-chain-2-ketoacid dehydrogenase (BCKD) complex. This enzyme catalyses the second common step in the catabolism of three branched-chain amino acids (BCAAs) valine, leucine, isoleucine.

Genetics

Autosomal recessive; *BCKDHA* (E1α subunit of the BCKD complex), *BCKDHB* (E1β), *DBT* (E2) *and DLD* (E3) genes.

Diagnosis

Elevated plasma BCAAs and alloisoleucine and elevated urinary branched-chain ketoacids are observed. An accompanying lactic acidaemia is seen particularly in E3-deficient MSUD. Timely clinical diagnosis remains a challenge in non-classical patients where the biochemical changes may be mild or intermittent. The diagnosis can be confirm by genetic testing.

Treatment and Prognosis

In the acute phase of presentation, haemodialysis/haemofiltration (to remove exogenous toxins) can be considered. This is followed by early introduction of BCAA-free formula. BCAA intake is closely adjusted according to plasma levels.

Long-term management of MSUD comprise of: (1) Life-long strict BCAA restricted diet, and an (2) In an acute decompensation an emergency regimen (ER) consisting of glucose polymer and BCAA-free amino acids. Patients are supplemented with valine and isoleucine supplementation as appropriate.

Liver transplantation in classic MSUD has been a successful treatment in individuals who have poor control despite maintenance treatment. Post-transplant, patients have been able to achieve an unrestricted diet and an apparently abolished risk of metabolic decompensations.

With early treatment, survival is good and patients are generally healthy between episodes of metabolic imbalance. Intellectual outcomes in patients are dependent on the quality of long-term metabolic control as well as the duration of the raised leucine levels at initial presentation prior to treatment. Some patients may present with mental health problems (e.g. inattention, hyperactivity, anxiety and depression) despite good metabolic control.

Isovaleric Aciduria/Methylmalonic Aciduria/Propionic Acidaemia

Clinical Presentation

Isovaleric aciduria (IVA), methylmalonic aciduria (MMA) and propionic acidaemia (PA) are organic acidaemias. These conditions classically present in the neonatal period during episodes of catabolism with unspecific clinical signs, i.e. lethargy, vomiting, irritability and eventually encephalopathy. Milder affected patients may not become clinically unwell until their first significant intercurrent illness, others have subacute presentation with failure to thrive, developmental delay, or late onset cardiomyopathy. Among these disorders, IVA is easily recognised by its unpleasant sweaty feet odour.

Metabolic Derangements

In all three conditions, investigations reveal a severe metabolic acidosis with raised anion gap, ketonuria and often hyperammonaemia. Moderate hypocalcaemia and hyperlactatemia are frequent findings.

IVA is caused by deficiency of isovaleryl-CoA dehydrogenase enzyme which results in the accumulation of derivatives of isovaleryl-CoA, including free isovaleric acid, 3-hydroxyisovaleric acid and N-isovalerylglycine.

PA is caused by deficiency of the mitochondrial enzyme propionyl-CoA carboxylase (PCC; biotin dependent enzyme). This results in increased free propionic acid in blood and urine and propionylcarnitine (C3), 3-hydroxyproprionate and methylcitrate.

MMA is caused by a deficiency of methylmalonyl-CoA mutase enzyme (vitamin B12 dependent enzyme) which results in the accumulation of methylmalonyl-CoA causing increased amounts of methylmalonic acid in plasma and urine. Due to the secondary inhibition of PCC, propionic acid also accumulates and other propionyl-CoA metabolites such those seen in PA can be detected.

Genetics

All conditions are autosomal recessively inherited.

- IVA: *IVD* gene
- PA: *PCCA* or *PCCB* gene
- MMA: *MUT* gene

Diagnosis

The diagnosis is made based on specific urinary organic acid and acylcarnitine profile. On plasma amino acid profiles, hyperglycinaemia, hyperalaninaemia and often normal/low glutamine levels are seen. Confirmation of the diagnosis can be made genetically.

Treatment and Prognosis

Patient with organic acidaemias are on a protein restricted diet and regular L-carnitine supplementation to promote excretion of toxic metabolites.

Aggressive treatment during periods of intercurrent illness with high calories reversing catabolism, either orally or intravenously is essential. In the acute setting patients with severe disease may require haemofiltration until metabolically stable. The long-term prognosis is generally guarded, as these conditions are prone to episodes of recurrent decompensation.

Some patients with MMA may respond to regular vitamin B12 injections. MMA patients frequently suffer chronic renal impairment; cardiomyopathy is more often seen in PA. Liver transplantation, replacing the defective enzyme can be considered for PA and MMA, although some patients have still decompensated post-transplant and long-term neurological complications have still occurred. Renal transplantation might be needed in chronic renal failure in MMA. Various forms of gene therapy offer hope for future treatment.

The prognosis often depends on the severity of decompensation at the first admission. Life expectancy for organic acidaemias have increased over time but patients are often seen with life-long complications.

Glutaric Aciduria Type 1 (GA1)

Incidence

1:100,000 (higher in Amish people, and Irish travellers).

Clinical Presentation

GA1 patients are typically well when they are born. There is often a history of macrocephaly present at or shortly after birth. Prior to the introduction of NBS, patients were often only diagnosed after suffering an acute metabolic encephalopathy, precipitated by an intercurrent illness. This results in severe neurological sequelae secondary to destruction of the striatum leaving children with severe dystonic–dyskinetic movement disorder.

Metabolic Derangements

GA1 is caused by the deficiency of the enzyme glutaryl-CoA dehydrogenase. The enzyme is involved in the catabolism of the amino acid lysine, which is a neurotoxic compound, resulting in a severe permanent neurological insult. Characteristic MRI brain changes observed include changes in the striatum, prominent sylvian fissures and fronto-occipital enlargement of the CSF spaces are observed (Figure 14.3).

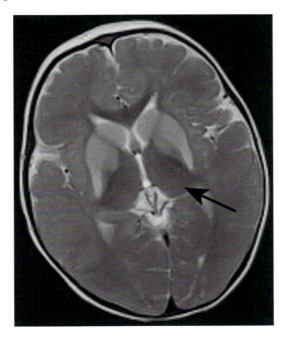

Figure 14.3 Bilateral symmetrical abnormalities of the basal ganglia (arrow) with sparing of the thalamus in a patient with glutaric aciduria Type 1.

Genetics

Autosomal recessive; *GCDH* gene.

Diagnosis

Elevated 3-hydroxyglutarate and glutaric acid (GA) in the urine organic acids characteristic acyl-carnitine profile are diagnostic for GA1.

NBS is very effective in diagnosing the majority of patients. However, low excretors might be missed as they have slight or inconsistent elevation of GA or glutarylcarnitine. In low excretors, diagnosis should be confirmed by enzyme testing in cultured fibroblasts or genetically.

Treatment and Prognosis

The key to treatment is early diagnosis, ideally by NBS and then aggressive treatment of periods of catabolic stress with high carbohydrate intake and supplementation with L-carnitine. When well, a low lysine diet is achieved by the use of a special formulas. This is complemented by oral L-carnitine.

With presymptomatic diagnosis through NBS and aggressive management of catabolic crisis throughout early childhood, the prognosis is excellent and severe neurological sequelae can be prevented. If diagnosis is late and once brain damage has occurred however, the typical severe dystonia and movement disorder is irreversible.

Tyrosinaemia Type I

Incidence

Estimated 1:100,000 (higher in Canada).

Clinical Presentation

Tyrosinaemia is a potentially life-threatening condition that usually presents as 'acute' neonatal liver failure with jaundice, coagulopathy, failure to thrive and often sepsis.

Alternatively, the 'chronic' presentation in later infancy is of failure to thrive, rickets (due to renal tubular dysfunction) (Figure 14.4) and liver dysfunction. Other problems include neurological crises with porphyria-like pain and paraesthesia, renal failure and hepatocarcinoma (Figure 14.5).

Metabolic Derangements

The defect is in the enzyme fumarylacetoacetase, the last enzyme in the breakdown of the

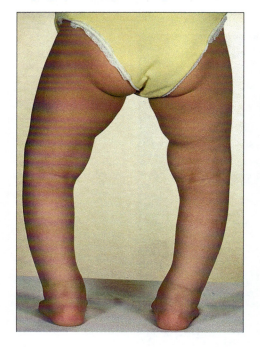

Figure 14.4 Tyrosinaemia: Involvement of the bones (rickets) is seen in untreated tyrosinaemia.

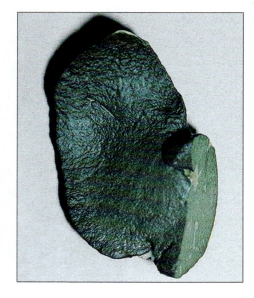

Figure 14.5 Severe liver cirrhosis in tyrosinaemia.

amino acids phenylalanine and tyrosine. The 'upstream' metabolites are alkylating agents and are thought to be responsible for the hepatorenal damage.

Genetics

Autosomal recessive; *FAH* gene.

Diagnosis

The presence of elevated levels of succinylacetone in the urine or in dried blood spot is diagnostic. Raised levels of tyrosine, phenylalanine and methionine are observed.

Decreased activity of fumarylacetoacetase in fibroblasts or lymphocytes, in the presence of the classical biochemical and clinical features, confirms the diagnosis although the diagnosis is usually confirmed genetically.

Treatment and Prognosis

Normal feeds should be stopped and the hepatorenal dysfunction and rickets treated as indicated. Prior to 1991, the only successful long-term treatment of tyrosinaemia was liver transplantation but, with the advent of NTBC (2-(2-nitro-4-trifluoromethylbenzoyl)-1,3-cyclohexanedione) – a potent inhibitor of an upstream enzyme 4-hydroxyphenylpyruvate dioxygenase – effective treatment is now available. NTBC prevents the toxic metabolites forming. Because the children still have a 'metabolic block', they require a low PHE and tyrosine diet with a supplementary PHE-/ tyrosine-free amino acid formula.

Provided there is no substantial liver damage or malignant transformation, the long-term prognosis is likely to be excellent.

Classical Homocystinuria (HCU)

Incidence

1:1800–1:900,000 (highest incidence in Qatar).

Clinical Presentation

There is a wide spectrum of severity (asymptomatic to multisystem involvement). Approximately one-half of individuals with HCU are pyridoxine (Vitamin B6) responsive. Prior to NBS patients with HCU typically presented with mental retardation, ectopia lentis (usually between the ages 6–10 years) and/or thromboembolic episodes. As patients get older, there is increasing skeletal involvement with many patients developing a marfanoid body habitus though with restriction rather than joint laxity.

Metabolic Derangements

HCU is due to cystathionine b-synthase (CBS) deficiency, an enzyme that utilises pyridoxine as a co-factor. This results in increase in homocysteine and methionine (to a lesser extent) in plasma.

Genetics

Autosomal recessive; *CBS* gene.

Diagnosis

A raised plasma total homocysteine and/or methionine with low cysteine is observed. In addition, CBS deficiency should be confirmed by enzyme measurement and/or by mutation analysis.

Treatment and Prognosis

Pyridoxine responsiveness should be assessed. In those patients that do not or only partial respond, a diet low in methionine and homocysteine is recommended. Further adjunctive treatment with betaine, vitamin B12 and folate should be considered.

Good metabolic control reduces the risk of ectopia lentis, osteoporosis and thromboembolic events.

UREA CYCLE DISORDERS (UCDS)

Incidence

Estimated 1:1800–1:44,000.

Clinical Presentation

Ammonia is detoxified by the liver-based urea cycle and converted to non-toxic urea by several enzymatic steps (six enzymes and two transporter proteins). Toxic effects of hyperammonaemia in the neonatal period result in lethargy, poor feeding, apnoea and encephalopathy. These symptoms are often mistaken for signs of sepsis. Over 50% of patients are diagnosed after the age of 2 years presenting with recurrent unexplained encephalopathy, notable gastrointestinal concerns, protein avoidance or unusual psychiatric presentation. Ammonia, the key diagnostic metabolite in the acute setting, is a respiratory stimulant and a respiratory alkalosis may be found early in the illness.

The most common UCD is ornithine transcarbamylase deficiency (OTC). This is the only X-linked inherited UCD. Affected males often die with overwhelming hyperammonaemia in the newborn period. Female carriers, although usually much less severely affected, can also present with hyperammonaemic episodes.

Metabolic Derangements

An ammonia concentration greater than 200 µmol/l in neonates and 100 µmol/l in older children is highly suspicious of a metabolic condition. Depending where the defect is in the urea cycle, the concentration of the amino acids immediately proximal to the enzyme defect will increase and those beyond will decrease. Plasma alanine and glutamine accumulate in all disorders. Urinary orotic acid is raised in defects distal to the formation of carbamoylphosphate (OTC, ASS, ASL and arginase deficiency).

Genetics

All urea cycle disorders other than OTC (X-linked) are inherited in an autosomal recessive manner.

Genes affected:

N-acetyl glutamate dehydrogenase deficiency (NAGS): *NAGS*

Carbamoyl phosphate synthetase deficiency (CPS1): *CPS1*

Ornithine transcarbamoylase deficency (OTC): *OTC*

Argininosuccinate synthetase deficiency (ASS; Citrullinaemia Type 1): *ASS*

Arginosuccinate lyase deficiency (ASL; Argininosuccinic aciduria): *ASL*

Arginase deficiency: *ARG1*

Aspartate-glutamate carrier deficiency (Citrullinaemia Type 2): *SLC25A13*

Ornithine transporter deficiency: *SLC25A15*

Diagnosis

The key investigation of the hyperammonaemic patient are plasma amino acids and urine organic acids differentiating the UCD subtype to be confirmed on genetic testing.

Treatment and Prognosis

Any new hyperammonaemic patient should be transferred to a metabolic centre for acute removal of ammonia. In general, stopping normal feeds and commencing intravenous 10% dextrose at high infusion rates is recommended. The sick neonate will frequently require haemofiltration. Sodium benzoate and sodium phenylbutyrate lower the ammonia by conjugating with amino acids and reducing the nitrogen load.

Depending on the UCD defect, supplementation with arginine or citrulline becomes essential. Once the situation has stabilised, protein is gradually reintroduced. The long-term management includes a protein restricted diet, the use of ammonia scavenger drugs/N-carbamoyl-L-glutamic acid and the use of an ER whenever the child is unwell.

The outcome depends on the diagnosis, severity and duration of the initial hyperammonaemic crisis. Children who present in the neonatal period with severe encephalopathy frequently die and those that survive will invariably have some degree of neurodevelopmental delay. Once treated, children often have further episodes of metabolic decompensation, especially during periods of intercurrent illness. Children with milder disease who present later may do remarkably well, with the outcome dependent on the severity of hyperammonaemic events prior to diagnosis and initiation of treatment. Liver transplantation is increasingly considered for a wide array of urea cycle disorders to enable greater stability and a better quality of life.

CARBOHYDRATE METABOLISM

Classical Galactosaemia

Incidence

1:50,000.

Clinical Presentation

Classically, patients present in the early neonatal period with jaundice, vomiting and lethargy when exposed to milk. Once the lactose (galactose)-containing feeds are stopped, the children improve. The frequent finding of an *Escherichia coli*-positive blood culture may confuse the diagnosis. Less commonly, children may also present in infancy with failure to thrive and vomiting. Hepatomegaly and jaundice are often present on examination and there is usually biochemical evidence of liver dysfunction. Cataracts are characteristically present. In many countries, galactosaemia is part of the NBS.

Metabolic Derangements

The disease is caused by a deficiency in the enzyme Galactose-1-phosphate uridyltransferase (GALT). Lactose, the disaccharide in breast, formula and cow's milk, consists of galactose and glucose. The metabolites of galactose are toxic to the liver and eyes. The cause of dyspraxia, intellectual disability, ataxia and early ovarian failure seen in females in later life is largely unknown with a variety of mechanisms suggested.

Genetics

Autosomal recessive; *GALT* gene.

Diagnosis

Positive urine reducing substances can suggest the diagnosis, but the sensitivity of the test is limited and would be negative in a galactosaemia child that has not yet been exposed to galactose. Direct measurement of the enzyme GALT in red blood cells is diagnostic. The parents of affected children will have GALT levels in the heterozygotes range and this is useful in diagnosing the infant who has received a recent blood transfusion. Affected children should have their eyes and liver function assessed.

Treatment and Prognosis

Galactose (i.e. lactose) should be eliminated from the diet as death from liver failure is seen if patients remains on a lactose diet. Essentially this means switching to a soya based formula and later a dairy products-free and 'minimal galactose containing foods' diet. In later life, the diet can be relaxed as adults appear to be able to tolerate moderate amounts of galactose without apparent clinical problems. Bone health should be monitored and calcium and vitamin D supplements are usually recommended. The cataracts are reversible if treatment is started early.

With treatment, the immediate prognosis is generally good, although early feeding problems and speech delay due to an oral motor dyspraxia are common. Older children and adults might have problems with verbal planning and 'concepts' in mathematics and science. Motor function, co-ordination and balance may also be affected. The majority of women develop hypergonadotrophic hypogonadism and there is a high risk for early ovarian failure. Individually, females need to be assessed and started on hormone replacement therapy as indicated.

Fructuse 1,6-Bisphosphatase Deficiency

Incidence

FBP is very rare; an incidence of 1:350,000 has been reported in The Netherlands.

Clinical Presentation

Around 50% of patients present in the first days of life with metabolic acidosis, marked hypoglycaemia, raised lactate and often a degree of hepatomegaly. Decompensation is triggered by catabolism, e.g. by (febrile) illness and/or refusal to eat. Episodes may also be triggered by large fructose loads (> 1 g/kg/dose). Between attacks, patients are usually well though mild, intermittent or chronic acidosis can persist. The frequency of attacks decreases with age.

Metabolic Derangements

Fructose 1,6-bisphosphatase is a key enzyme in the gluconeogenic pathway, with deficiency impairing the production of glucose from all gluconeogenic precursors including fructose. Children with FBP deficiency have a greater tolerance to fructose than those with hereditary fructose intolerance as they can still metabolise fructose 1-P to lactate.

Genetics

Autosomal recessive; *FBP1* gene.

Diagnosis

Hypoglycaemia, high lactate and a variable degree of ketosis are seen during periods of decompensation. Increased levels of glycerol and lactate excretion may be found on urinary organic acids analysis. The diagnosis can be confirmed by measurement of fructose 1,6-bisphosphatase activity in blood or by mutation analysis.

Treatment and Prognosis

Emergency management is the provision of adequate glucose during decompensations. Additional supplementation of bicarbonate is only occasionally necessary. The cornerstone of therapy is the avoidance of fasting and the restriction of fructose, sucrose and sorbitol, particularly during unwell episodes.

The prognosis is favourable and fasting tolerance improves with age.

Glycogen Storage Disorder (GSD) Type I (Von Gierke) and II (Pompe)

GSD IA and GSD1B

There are two genetically distinct forms of GSD I, called GSD Ia and GSD Ib.

Incidence

1:100,000 with GSD Ia accounting for accounting 80% of the diagnosis.

Clinical Presentation

Children with GSD I usually present in infancy with failure to thrive, abdominal distension secondary to hepatomegaly and/or symptoms of hypoglycaemia. The latter can occur after a short fast, yet the child, especially in early infancy, may surprisingly be asymptomatic. On examination there is often massive hepatomegaly, truncal obesity, short stature, mild hypotonia and a 'doll-like' face.

Metabolic Derangements

GSD Ia is caused by a deficiency of glucose-6-phosphatase. A transport protein, responsible for the transport of glucose-6-phosphate, is defective in GSD Ib. The latter is additionally associated with neutropenia and immune deficiency.

Genetics

Both conditions are autosomal recessively inherited. GSD Ia patients carry mutations in the *G6PC* gene, GSD Ib patients in SLC37A4.

Diagnosis

There is often a significant lactic acidosis that decreases with feeding. Hypertriglyceridaemia and hyperuricaemia are also characteristically present. These findings, along with the typical clinical appearance, are highly suggestive of GSD I and subsequent diagnostic investigations should be based on molecular testing.

Treatment and Prognosis

Maintaining normal glucose homeostasis is the key and is likely to reduce the long-term complications greatly. This is achieved by frequent daytime feeds and a continuous overnight feed via a nasogastric tube or gastrostomy. Specialist dietary input is essential. After the age of 2 years, uncooked cornstarch may be used to improve fasting tolerance. Individual fasting tolerance needs to be assessed. Allopurinol lowers uric acid levels while granulocyte colony stimulating factor (G-CSF) can improve the neutropenia seen in GSD Ib. Long-term management also includes regular monitoring of the biochemistry (lactate, triglycerides and glucose profiles), growth, renal function, liver (ultrasound for adenomas) and bone mineralisation status. Liver transplantation may be an option in some patients.

Adults who have had relatively poorly controlled disease frequently have the complications of short stature, renal disease, osteoporosis and liver adenomas. The latter may become malignant. Good metabolic control is essential for favourable long-term outcome.

GSD II (Pompe Disease)
Incidence
1:40,000.

Clinical Presentation
The classical infantile form presents in early childhood with severe cardiomyopathy, hypotonia, respiratory failure and failure to thrive. The course is fatal in the first year if untreated. Patients with the juvenile/adult form show slowly progressive muscular weakness.

Metabolic Derangements
Pompe patients have a low activity of alpha-glucosidase (acid maltase).

Genetics
Mutations in the *GAA* gene cause Pompe disease which is autosomal recessively inherited.

Diagnosis
There are typical ECG (massive QRS waves and shortened PR interval) changes. The diagnosis is based on abnormal urinary tetrasaccharides, the presence of vacuolated lymphocytes and the diagnosis can be confirmed on enzyme studies in leucocytes and dry blood spots and genetic testing.

Treatment and Prognosis
Early intravenous enzyme replacement therapy should be initiated alongside regular physiotherapy. Long-term prognosis is still guarded, especially as there seems to be an emerging leukodystrophy in the infantile onset cohort.

Glucose Transporter Deficiency 1 (GLUT 1)
Incidence
1:90,000.

Clinical Presentation
Children with GLUT 1 transport deficiency (GLUT 1) typically present with developmental delay and/or epileptic encephalopathy (70%). There may be a history of developmental regression or more commonly failure of developmental progression in the others. There is often a degree of microcephaly. Milder variants might present with (exercise induced) fluctuating movement disorder. Especially in the more mildly affected cases, there is often a history of symptoms being better after eating and worsening after a short fast. Paradoxically there may be a history of the children being more alert or having fewer seizures during a period of significant sickness, reflecting the positive effect of a ketogenic state at the time.

Metabolic Derangements
Mutation in the glucose transporter facilitating transport of glucose across the blood–brain barrier. This results in inadequate glucose being delivered to the brain despite normal blood sugar level.

Genetics
GLUT 1 is caused by an autosomal dominant, usually *de novo*, molecular defect of the glucose transporter (*SLCA1*) gene.

Diagnosis

The critical and relatively easy investigation is the plasma/CSF glucose ratio. This is normally greater than 0.6. If it is less than 0.45, and if there is no other cause of hypoglycorrachia (low CSF glucose), for instance infection, then the diagnosis is highly likely, especially if the result is repeatable. If the ratio is between 0.4 and 0.6, then the diagnosis should still be considered. A repeat sample should be obtained on a fasted sample, e.g. in the morning. An elevated plasma glucose due to stress can lead to a falsely reduced ratio. Of note, lactate levels are usually normal. Erythrocyte glucose uptake can be measured, but usually the diagnosis is confirmed molecularly.

Treatment and Prognosis

The mainstay of treatment is ketogenic diet. This often results in a dramatic decrease of seizures and increase in cognitive function. The diet is burdensome. The ratio of calories deriving from fat to other sources needed is individually different and ranges from 4:1 to a 3 or even a 2.5:1 ratio. In mild cases maintaining high blood glucose levels with regular high carbohydrate meals, including cornstarch supplements, can result in improved neurological function without needing to implement a ketogenic diet.

The earlier the diagnosis and thus the earlier treatment is commenced, the better the prognosis. Early treatment reduces the severity of intellectual disability.

FATTY ACID OXIDATION DISORDER (FAOD) AND KETONE BODY METABOLISM DISORDER

During fasting, ketone bodies are the important fuel for many tissues including cardiac and skeletal muscle and brain, as the latter cannot oxidise fatty acids. Ketone bodies are formed in the liver mitochondria predominantly from fatty acids but also from certain amino acids such as leucine.

FAODs

FAODs are genetic disorders that result in the inability to produce or utilise fat as an energy source in the liver or muscles.

Incidence

The most commonly diagnosed FAOD is medium-chain acyl-CoA dehydrogenase deficiency (MCAD) with a prevalence of 1:20,000. MCAD is usually included in NBS programmes.

Clinical Presentation

Prior to expanded NBS, children with FAODs frequently presented with encephalopathy due to severe hypoketotic hypoglycaemia and hepatic dysfunction. Usually there was a history of a preceding viral-like illness and a period of catabolic stress such as missed meals. There was often little to find on examination apart from some hepatomegaly. 'Found dead in bed' during an intercurrent illness was unfortunately also a relatively common presentation. Thus while MCAD should be suspected in the above clinical scenario, the most common presentation nowadays is with a positive screening test. Babies can, however, become unwell prior to screening and older children born prior to the commencement of expanded NBS might present symptomatically in later life.

Muscle preferentially oxidises fat as an energy source, so alternative presentations for FAODs, especially the so-called long-chain disorders, are cardiomyopathy, especially in infancy, and/or rhabdomyolysis, potentially occurring after significant exercise.

Metabolic Derangements

The fatty oxidation process involves several different enzymes that break down long fats to ketone bodies and acetyl-CoA.

Genetics

The FAODs are inherited in an autosomal recessive manner.

Diagnosis

The finding of hypoglycaemia with inappropriately low ketones (urine or blood) is suggestive of a FAOD. There may be acidosis, hepatic dysfunction, an elevated creatine kinase and/or hyperammonaemia. The specific disorder can usually be diagnosed on the acylcarnitine profile. Cardiological assessment is essential in any suspected cases. Confirmation of the diagnosis is by fatty acid oxidation flux studies of fibroblasts (skin biopsy and culture) and/or on molecular genetic testing.

Treatment and Prognosis

Catabolism should be avoided. The child must not be subjected to significant catabolic stress such as fasting, especially during periods of intercurrent illness. If the child is unwell, they should be commenced on their ER (high calorie carbohydrate drink) until well. If they are not tolerating this, or if there are any other concerns, then they should be admitted to their local hospital.

Regular feeds, in some FAOD even overnight feeds and the avoidance of dietary long-chain fats are recommended, particularly necessary in long-chain disorders (long-chain L-3-hydroxyacyl-CoA dehydrogenase deficiency (LCHAD) and very long-chain L-3-hydroxyacyl-CoA dehydrogenase deficiency (VLCAD).

Once diagnosed and treated, the prognosis for MCAD is generally favourable. The long-term outcome for some of the long-chain disorders are less favourable even on treatment, as the children may develop peripheral neuropathy, recurrent rhabdomyolysis, retinopathy and cardiomyopathy/conduction defects.

Ketone Body Metabolism Disorder

Ketogenesis Disorders

Clinical Presentation

The initial presentation is that of profound hypoglycaemia, metabolic acidosis, inappropriate low ketones. Clinical symptoms are encephalopathy and possible seizures, triggered by catabolic stressors such as infection or decreased oral intake.

Metabolic Derangements

Ketone bodies (acetoacetate and 3-hydroxybutyrate) are metabolites derived from fatty acids and ketogenic amino acids, such as leucine. They are mainly produced in the liver, via reactions catalysed by the ketogenic enzymes 3-hydroxy-3-methylglutaryl-(HMG) CoA synthase and HMG CoA lyase.

Genetics

These conditions are autosomal recessively inherited.

Diagnosis

Any patient with hypoglycaemia should be tested for ketones. There is an abnormal ratio of fatty acids/total ketone bodies > 2.5. Urine organic acids may show a non-specific dicarboxylic aciduria (HMG CoA synthase deficiency) or the presence of diagnostic leucine metabolites (HMG CoA lyase deficiency). Functional enzymatic and genetic testing can be performed.

Treatment and Prognosis

The avoidance of fasting and the use of a high energy carbohydrate ER at times of catabolic stress, e.g. infections, are the cornerstone of management. A low leucine diet has been recommended in HMG CoA lyase patients but the need for this has been questioned. Patients may be given carnitine to avoid secondary deficiencies.

The prognosis is determined by the severity of the first presentation. Overall the prognosis tends to be excellent although individual HMG CoA lyase patients have developed white matter lesions and cardiomyopathies.

Ketolysis Disorders

Clinical Presentation

The initial presentation is that of profound hypoglycaemia and severe ketoacidosis, acute nausea and vomiting triggered by fasting/infection in infancy.

Metabolic Derangements

Failure to utilise ketone bodies synthesised in the liver causes severe ketoacidosis and hyperketotic hypoglycaemia. The rate-limiting enzyme of ketone body utilisation (ketolysis) is succinyl-coenzyme A: 3-oxoacid coenzyme A transferase. The subsequent step of ketolysis is catalysed by

2-methylactoacetyl-coenzyme A thiolase (beta-ketothiolase), which is also involved in isoleucine catabolism.

Genetics

Patients carry either mutations in the *OXCT1* or *AXAT1* gene. These conditions are of autosomal recessive inheritance.

Diagnosis

Any patient with hypoglycaemia should be tested for ketones. Excessive ketones and/or very high unexplained anion gap is suspicious of a ketone disorder, although an exaggerated normal physiological response is a much more common explanation. A clue to the presence of the ketone body utilisation defects can be the persistence of ketones after a meal or its presence in a morning sample after usual overnight fasting in an otherwise well child. Definitive functional enzymatic and genetic testing can be performed.

Treatment and Prognosis

The avoidance of fasting and the use of a high energy carbohydrate ER at times of catabolic stress, e.g. infections, is the cornerstone of management. Most patients make a full recovery following episodes of acidosis particularly when treated quickly.

MITOCHONDRIAOPATHIES-LEIGHS SYNDROME (LS)

Clinical Presentation

LS also called subacute, necrotising encephalopathy, is a devastating neurodegenerative disorder, characterised by defined changes on CNS imaging, i.e. focal, bilaterally symmetric lesions, particularly in the basal ganglia, thalamus and brainstem (Figure 14.6). Patients can exhibit considerable clinical and genetic heterogeneity. The course of the illness is unpredictable, although the onset is frequently in infancy often triggered by an intercurrent illness. The child may present acutely with encephalopathy, respiratory abnormalities or a stroke-like event. Alternatively, there are non-specific symptoms such as failure to thrive, generalised myopathy or polyneuropathy and occasionally developmental delay. The children may have evidence of basal ganglia dysfunction, with variable combinations of abnormal eye movements, dysarthria, dystonia, ataxia and autonomic dysfunction.

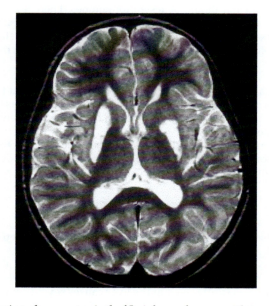

Figure 14.6 MRI showing changes typical of Leigh syndrome, with involvement of the lentiform nuclei bilaterally.

Metabolic Derangements

While LS remains a neuropathological/neuro-imaging-based diagnosis, there are characteristic clinical features and often elevated blood and/or CSF lactate. Low CSF methyltetrahydrofolate can be found. In addition, muscle biopsies can reflect defects in histology, histochemistry, respiratory chain enzymology and coenzyme Q levels.

Diagnosis

Diagnosis confirmed on neuropathological/neuro-imaging and typical clinical features. Overall more than 75 different genes are currently associated with a Leigh like phenotype. While many of the defects are likely to be inherited in an autosomal recessive manner, some forms of LS are caused by mutations in the mitochondrial genome.

Treatment and Prognosis

Treatment is supportive. A variety of vitamins and other medications have been tried with anecdotal reports of their benefit. These include thiamine, riboflavin, coenzyme Q, carnitine, biotin and folinic acid. Ketogenic diet should be considered in pyruvate dehydrogenase defect.

The long-term prognosis is generally poor although there may be long periods of stability. Children with early onset of disease tend to have poorer outcomes.

STEROL METABOLISM

Smith–Lemli–Opitz Syndrome (SLO)

Incidence

1:15,000–1:60,000 in Caucasians. Higher incidences found in some East European countries.

Clinical Presentation

SLO patients usually display characteristic dysmorphic features (Figures 14.7 and 14.8) including syndactyly of the second and third toe, hypospadia and structural visceral and neurological abnormalities. There is usually global developmental delay with very slow progression of development. Challenging behaviour and sleeping difficulties are usually present. Patients need to be carefully clinically assessed as manifestation of SLO can be on any organ system. Structural abnormalities of brain, heart and gastrointestinal systems have been reported. Patients can have life-threatening adrenal crisis.

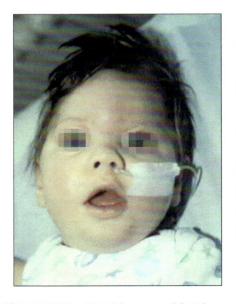

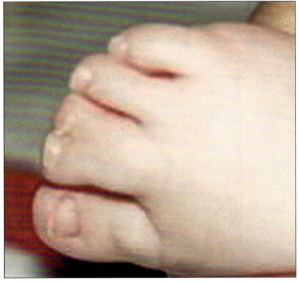

Figure 14.7 Facial features of Smith–Lemli–Opitz syndrome.

Figure 14.8 Smith–Lemli–Opitz syndrome: An example of the 2–3 syndactyly seen.

Metabolic Derangements

SLO is caused by deficiency of 7-dehydrocholesterol reductase which catalyses the reduction of 7-dehydrocholesterol to cholesterol.

Genetics

Autosomal recessive; *DHCR7* gene.

Diagnosis

Low cholesterol levels might be seen on baseline testing. A falsely normal total cholesterol level may be reported if the SLO specific 7- and 8-dehydrocholesterol are measured together. The diagnosis is usually confirmed on genetic testing.

Treatment and Prognosis

There is no curative treatment. Supplementation of cholesterol has been reported to improve growth and behavioural challenges of some patients. Melatonin can be useful in some patients to improve sleep quality. Occasionally statins have been used with few proven benefits.

General health of the patient is usually satisfactory.

LYSOSOMAL METABOLISM

Mucopolysaccharidosis Type 1 (MPS I; Hurler Disease)

Clinical Presentation

Classical MPS I (Hurler disease) presents in infancy with delayed developmental milestones, respiratory concerns, hepatomegaly, thickened skin, 'claw-like' hands (Figure 14.9), corneal clouding (Figure 14.10), macrocephaly and the classical 'coarse' facial features. Radiologically confirmed dysostosis multiplex is evident early, and later results clinically in short stature and lumbar gibbus.

Deafness, cardiac valvular disease, carpal tunnel disease and joint contractures are typically seen later. The milder end of the phenotypic spectrum, historically called Scheie disease, presents in late childhood with mainly bone and joint disease but without cognitive impairment. The intermediate phenotype Hurler–Scheie can display all the visceral problems of those with Hurler diseases but with no or mild cognitive impairment.

Metabolic Derangements

Raised dermatan sulphate and heparan sulphate are seen on urine glycosaminoglycan (GAG) electrophoresis. Alpha-L-iduronidase activity is low.

Genetics

Autosomal recessive; *IDUA* gene.

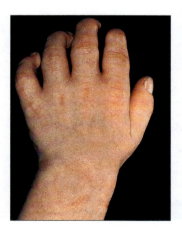

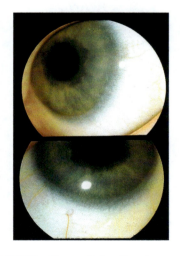

Figure 14.9 Typical 'claw' hand of mucopolysaccharidosis disease.

Figure 14.10 Corneal clouding in a patient with Hurler disease.

Diagnosis

Enzyme assay and/or genetics.

Treatment and Prognosis

Early (< 18 months) haematopoietic stem cell transplant (HSCT) significantly slows the progression of the disease but does not reverse bone or pre-existing neurological disease. Enzyme replacement therapy (ERT) can improve some visceral manifestations of the disease but does not penetrate the blood–brain barrier. The use of ERT prior to induction of HSCT has improved transplant outcome.

The prognosis for untreated classic Hurler is poor, with progressive and severe neurodevelopmental regression. Death usually occurs before the age of 10 years from cardiac, respiratory or neurological causes.

Mucopolysaccharidosis Type II (MPS II; Hunter Syndrome)

Clinical Presentation

MPS II patients' symptoms emerge between the ages of 18 months and 4 years (depending on the disease severity). The first symptoms may include abdominal hernias, recurrent otitis media or respiratory infections. Physical appearances develop overtime including short statures, macrocephaly, coarse facial features, prominent forehead, flattened nasal bridge and macroglossia. In severe cases developmental decline are evident around 18 months. Valvular heart disease, obstructive airway disease, hepatomegaly and joint stiffness also develop.

Metabolic Derangements

Raised dermatan sulphate and heparan sulphate are seen on urine GAG electrophoresis. Iduronate-2-sulphatase (I2S) activity is low.

Genetics

X-linked recessive; *IDS* gene.

Diagnosis

Enzyme assay and/or genetics.

Treatment and Prognosis

ERT reduces somatic symptoms. Cognitive manifestations are not expected to improve due to inability of the enzyme to cross the blood–brain barrier.

HSCT is not recommended for MPS II because there is no evidence of neurocognitive stabilisation in these patients that are usually diagnosed late.

Life expectancy varies according to disease severity.

Mucopolysaccharidosis Type 3 (MPS III; Sanfilippo Syndrome)

Clinical Presentation

MPS III is the most common of the MPSs. There are four types of MPS III (A–D) which are caused by one of the four enzymes required in the break down of heparan sulphate. Unlike the other MPSs, the predominant manifestations are neurological rather than visceral. Patients typically present with mild speech delay and increasing behavioural problems that usually start around the age of 3–5 years and consist of restlessness, destructive, chaotic and aggressive behaviour and sleep difficulties. The behavioural problems decline with age and eventually disappear with progressive mental retardation which ultimately results in patient becoming fully bedridden.

Metabolic Derangements

Raised heparan sulphate is seen on urine GAG electrophoresis. Low enzyme activity of heparan-N-sulphatase is measured in MPS IIIA, N-acetylglucosaminidase in MPS IIIB, acetyl-CoA glucosaminide N-acetyltransferase in MPS IIIC and N-acetylglucosamine 6-sulphatase in MPS IIID.

Genetics

All MPS III types are autosomal recessively inherited.
MPS IIIA: *SGSH*
MPS IIIB: *NAGLU*

MPS IIIC: *HGSNAT*
MPS IIID: *GNS*

Diagnosis

Enzyme assay and/or genetics.

Treatment and Prognosis

Treatment is mainly supportive. Intrathecal ERT and gene therapies are in development.

Mucopolysaccharidosis Type IV (MPS IV; Morquio Syndrome)
Clinical Presentation

Patients with MPS IV usually present around the age of 3 years, with unusual skeletal features including short trunk, pectus carinatum, kyphosis, scoliosis, genu valgum and abnormal gait. Odontoid hypoplasia is the most critical skeletal feature, which in combination with the ligamentous laxity can result in atlantoaxial subluxation, cervical myelopathy or even death (Figure 14.11). Patients usually require cervical spinal fixation. Pulmonary compromise, valvular heart disease, hearing loss, hepatomegaly, corneal clouding, coarse facial features and abnormal dentition are common. Patients with MPS IV have normal intelligence.

Metabolic Derangements

Raised keratin sulphate is seen on urine GAG electrophoresis. Low enzyme activity of N-acetylgalactosamine-6-sulphatase is seen in MPS IVA, beta-galactosidase in MPS IVB.

Genetics

Autosomal recessive:
  MPS IVA: *GALNS*
  MPS IVB: *GLB1*

Diagnosis

Enzyme assay and/or genetics.

Treatment and Prognosis

ERT for MPS IVA is available however the mainstay of treatment remains supportive. Orthopaedic and spinal interventions are commonly required.

Mucopolysaccharidosis Type VI (MPS VI)
Clinical Presentation

MPS VI patients share many physical symptoms found in MPS I. However, they usually have normal intelligence. Patients gradually develop multisystemic clinical manifestations. Other features are skeletal dysplasia including short stature, dysostosis multiplex, degenerative joint disease, coarse facial features, obstructive/restrictive respiratory disease, cardiac valvular disease, corneal clouding, hearing loss and hepatosplenomegaly. Symptoms are usually apparent before the age of 2 years.

Metabolic Derangements

Raised dermatan sulphate is seen on urine GAG electrophoresis. N-acetylgalactosamine-4-sulphatase activity is low.

Genetics

Autosomal recessive; *ARSB* gene.

Diagnosis

Enzyme assay and/or genetics.

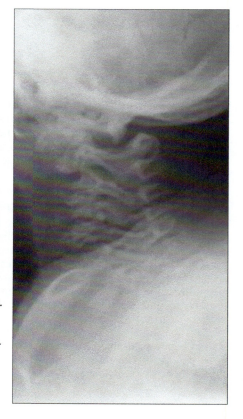

Figure 14.11 Cervical x-ray showing atlantoaxial subluxation in a patient with Morquio syndrome.

Treatment and Prognosis

The primary treatment for MPS VI is ERT with Galsulfase. Very early and continuous ERT has been shown to slow the rate of disease progression (except for skeletal or eye disease).

The risk-benefit profile of HSCT in patients with MPS VI is less clear than in other types of MPS.

The life expectancy of individuals with MPS VI varies depending on the severity of symptoms. Without treatment, some individuals may survive through late childhood or early adolescence. Patients with milder forms of the disorder usually live into adulthood. Heart disease and airway obstruction are major causes of death in MPS VI.

PEROXISOMAL METABOLISM

Adrenoleukodystrophy (ALD)

Clinical Presentation

ALD is a peroxisomal X-linked inherited disorder with a variable phenotype. The most severe form is childhood onset cerebral ALD (COCALD) occurring in up to 35% of patients. This typically presents between the ages of 4 and 10 years with progressive neurological impairment. This may manifest as behavioural problems, deterioration in school performance, focal neurological symptoms and/or hearing/visual impairment. Alternatively, they may present with an adrenal crisis. About 8–10% may have only Addison disease; the patient is abnormally tanned and have adrenal insufficiency. Approximately 30% of patients present in early adult life with evidence of spinal cord and peripheral nerve involvement; this form is known as adrenomyeloneuropathy (AMN). These patients can develop cerebral involvement and dementia. A number of ALD patients may remain entirely asymptomatic. Up to 50% of women who are heterozygous for ALD develop an AMN-like syndrome in adulthood.

Metabolic Derangements

Elevated very long-chain fatty acids (VLCFAs). Abnormal C26:22 and C24:22 ratios.

Genetics

X-linked disorder caused by a defect in a peroxisomal transmembrane transporter protein (*ABCD1* gene).

Diagnosis

Elevated VLCFAs in the presence of suggestive clinical features are diagnostic. Specific MRI brain findings are illustrated in Figure 14.12.

Treatment and Prognosis

Cortisol and very occasionally fludrocortisone are used to manage the adrenal insufficiency. Lorenzo's oil, a mixture of monounsaturated fatty acids, inhibits the elongation of docosanoic acid (22:0) to 26:0 and improves/normalises the VLCFA level in many patients. However, normalising VLCFAs have not consistently shown positive neurological outcomes. HSCT if performed in the early stages of COCALD does prevent the progression of the neurological disease but needs to be performed before there is significant neurological impairment and carries significant risks. Thus, asymptomatic patients are monitored with regular cerebral imaging.

The prognosis of COCALD without HSCT is very poor. Once neurological regression has commenced there is rapid progression. The prognosis for AMN is variable; the role of gene therapy, Lorenzo's oil and HSCT is unclear.

CONGENITAL DISORDERS OF GLYCOSYLATION (CDG)

Many enzymes, transport and membrane proteins, hormones etc. require post-translational modification by attaching polysaccharide chains. CDG comprise a large, continuous growing number of monogenic diseases affecting the attachment of polysaccharide chains to proteins or lipids as well as the biosynthesis of proteoglycans.

Clinical Presentation

Congenital disorders of glycosylation (CDG) are a group of inherited conditions, usually presenting as multi-organ disease, and often affecting the CNS.

The most frequently diagnosed deficiency of phosphomannomutase (PMM), PMM-CDG, presents with the diagnostic triad of cerebellar hypoplasia, abnormal fat pads and inverted nipples

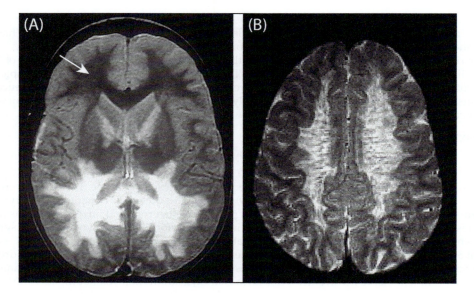

Figure 14.12 Adrenoleukodystrophy (ALD). (A) MRI scan showing moderately advanced leukodystrophy in a boy with COCALD. This pattern of severe temporal and parieto-occipital involvement is typical for ALD; (B) in contrast, more diffuse white matter involvement is seen in metachromatic leukodystrophy.

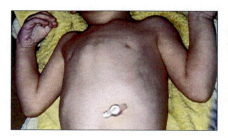

Figure 14.13 Features suggestive of congenital disorders of glycosylation 1a: inverted nipples.

(Figures 14.13 to 14.15). Very few CDG disorders (over 100 genetic disorders are known) present with normal neurological development. In PMI-CDG, due to phosphoisomerase deficiency, patients primarily present with gastrointestinal symptoms (failure to thrive, protein-losing enteropathy and liver fibrosis). Other CDG diseases, belonging to the group of muscular dystroglycanopathies, affect primarily the muscle, brain and eye.

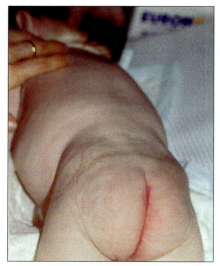

Figure 14.14 Features suggestive of congenital disorders of glycosylation 1a: abnormal fat pads.

Metabolic Derangements

CDGs affect the glycosylation of glycoproteins and glycolipids. Defects can be localised to the cytoplasma, endoplasmatic reticulum or Golgi network. Depending on the defects, disorders are grouped as N- or O-glycosylation defects, combined defects or others.

Genetics

CDGs are usually inherited in an autosomal recessive matter, but X-linked and autosomal dominant CDG subtypes are known.

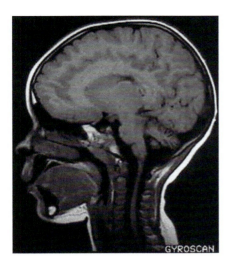

Figure 14.15 Features suggestive of congenital disorders of glycosylation 1a: cerebellar hypoplasia.

Diagnosis

The most commonly used screening test for N-glycosylation defects is transferrin isoelectric focusing; the majority of O-glycosylation defect can be detected by IEF of ApoCIII. However, only specific enzyme and/or molecular genetic testing can identify the precise CDG subtype of the patient.

Treatment and Prognosis

There is no curative treatment available for any CDG disorder. Supplementation of several different carbohydrates, such as mannose in PMI-CDG or galactose in galactose transporter deficiency SLC35A2-CDG, has been reported to be of some benefit.

The prognosis of CDG patients depends on the subtype of the disease. Around 30% of PMM-CDG patients die in early infancy secondary to complications such as liver failure, cardiomyopathy and severe seizures. Regression of skills is rarely seen in patients with CDG.

METABOLISM OF VITAMINS AND TRACE METALS
Biotin Disorders
Clinical Presentation

There are two main forms of biotin disorders: holocarboxylase synthetase (HCS) and biotinidase deficiency, the latter presenting in infancy whereas HCS patients presents earlier. The presentation is variable and patients might have neurological symptoms such as ataxia, hypotonia and seizures. Patients are usually diagnosed in an acute metabolic decompensation. There may be a characteristic erythematous rash, which may be generalised or confined to the perioral regions (Figures

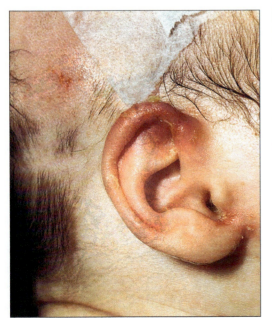

14.16 and 14.17). There may be blepharoconjunctivitis and glossitis. Both conditions can be diagnosed by NBS, so ideally patients will be treated prior to symptoms and they will remain asymptomatic.

Metabolic Derangements

Acutely unwell children have lactic acidaemia with a diagnostic urine organic acid profile (elevated 3-methylcrotonylglycine and 3-hydroxy-isovaleric acid).

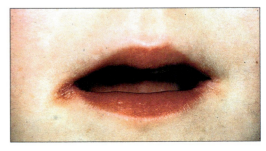

Figure 14.16 Typical skin manifestations of biotinidase deficiency.

Figure 14.17 Typical skin manifestations of biotinidase deficiency.

Genetics

Autosomal recessive.
   HSC deficiency: *HLCS*
   Biotinidase deficiency: *BTD*

Diagnosis

Enzymology +/– genetics.

Treatment and Prognosis

Patients respond rapidly to biotin supplementation (5–20 mg/day). Seizures tend to improve but significant neurological impairments to hearing, vision and cognition may remain.

Menkes Disease

Incidence

1:250,000.

Clinical Presentation

Menkes disease is a disorder of copper transport which causes severe neurological disease. Apart from neonatal jaundice, children are usually relatively normal during early infancy but develop symptoms of poor feeding, vomiting and failure to thrive at 2–4 months (Figure 14.18). Seizures and developmental delay are often the presenting features. Neurological regression is rapid, and seizures are often difficult to control.

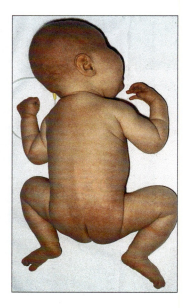

Figure 14.18   Infant with Menke disease who presented with failure to thrive and seizures.

The facial appearance is highly characteristic, with a pale complexion, sagging jowls, wide nasal bridge and abnormal hair. The hair is lustreless, brittle and has an unkempt appearance (Figures 14.19 and 14.20). Microscopically it shows pili torti. Menke patients, because of the role of copper in elastin and collagen synthesis, can also have problems with joint laxity, bladder diverticulum and rupture, arterial bleeds and bony abnormalities. These features are also seen in the milder forms of the disease such as the occipital horn syndrome.

Metabolic Derangements

Menkes disease is caused by a defect in copper transmembrane transporter (ATP7A protein) resulting in enhanced uptake but decreased efflux in intestinal and renal tubular cells. Low copper and caeruloplasmin levels are characteristic. Cellular copper deficiency affects copper-containing enzymes such as cytochrome oxidase and lysyl oxidase, essential in cellular energy production and collagen/elastin synthesis, respectively.

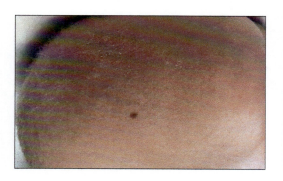

Figure 14.19   The short, brittle hair of Menke disease.

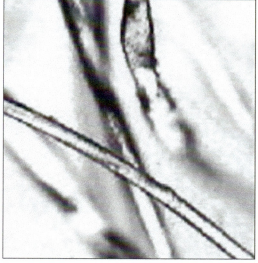

Figure 14.20   Pili torti and trichorrhexis nodosa seen in Menke disease.

Genetics

X-linked recessive; *ATP7A* gene.

Diagnosis

The clinical features and low serum copper and caeruloplasmin establish the diagnosis. Copper levels can be (very) low in the normal neonate and thus biochemical diagnosis at this age can be difficult. Copper uptake and release studies in fibroblasts and/or genetics are the gold standard confirmatory test.

Treatment and Prognosis

Treatment is symptomatic. Intravenous or subcutaneous copper histidine therapy may be partially successful if started very early (< 1 month old) although these children still have a significant morbidity, with a severe connective tissue disorder and developmental delay.

REFERENCES

- Newborn blood spot screening: Programme overview [Internet]. 2013 Jan 1 [updated 2018 Nov 1]. Available from: https://www.gov.uk/guidance/newborn-blood-spot-screening-programme-overview.
- van Wegberg AMJ, MacDonald A, Ahring K, et al. The complete European guidelines on phenylketonuria: Diagnosis and treatment. *Orphanet J Rare Dis.* 2017 Oct 12;12(1):162. doi:10.1186/s13023-017-0685-2.
- Blackburn PR, Gass JM, Vairo FPE, et al. Maple syrup urine disease: Mechanisms and management. *Appl Clin Genet.* 2017 Sep 6;10:57–66.
- Forny P, Hörster F, Ballhausen D, et al. Guidelines for the diagnosis and management of methylmalonic acidaemia and propionic acidaemia: First revision. *J Inherit Metab Dis.* 2021 May;44(3):566–592. doi:10.1002/jimd.12370. Epub 2021 Mar 9.
- Boy N, Mühlhausen C, Maier EM, et al. Proposed recommendations for diagnosing and managing individuals with glutaric aciduria type I: Second revision. *J Inherit Metab Dis.* 2017 Jan;40(1):75–101. doi:10.1007/s10545-016-9999-9. Epub 2016 Nov 16. PMID: 27853989.
- Chinsky JM, Singh R, Ficicioglu C, et al. Diagnosis and treatment of tyrosinemia type I: A US and Canadian consensus group review and recommendations. *Genet Med.* 2017 Dec;19(12). doi:10.1038/gim.2017.101. Epub 2017 Aug 3.
- Morris AA, Kožich V, Santra S, et al. Guidelines for the diagnosis and management of cystathionine beta-synthase deficiency. *J Inherit Metab Dis.* 2017 Jan;40(1):49–74. doi:10.1007/s10545-016-9979-0. Epub 2016 Oct 24.
- Häberle J, Boddaert N, Burlina A, et al. Suggested guidelines for the diagnosis and management of urea cycle disorders. First Revision. *J Inherit Metab Dis.* 2019 Nov;42(6):1192–1230.
- Welling L, Bernstein LE, Berry GT, et al.; Galactosemia Network (GalNet). International clinical guideline for the management of classical galactosemia: Diagnosis, treatment, and follow-up. *J Inherit Metab Dis.* 2017 Mar;40(2):171–176. doi:10.1007/s10545-016-9990-5. Epub 2016 Nov 17.
- Kishnani PS, Austin SL, Abdenur JE, et al.; American College of Medical Genetics and Genomics. Diagnosis and management of glycogen storage disease type I: A practice guideline of the American College of Medical Genetics and Genomics. *Genet Med.* 2014 Nov;16(11):e1.
- Klepper J, Akman C, Armeno M, et al. Glut1 Deficiency Syndrome (Glut1DS): State of the art in 2020 and recommendations of the international Glut1DS study group. *Epilepsia Open.* 2020 Aug 13;5(3):354–365. doi:10.1002/epi4.12414.
- Lake NJ, Compton AG, Rahman S, Thorburn DR. Leigh syndrome: One disorder, more than 75 monogenic causes. *Ann Neurol.* 2016 Feb;79(2):190–203.
- Nowaczyk MJM, Wassif CA. Smith-Lemli-Opitz Syndrome. 1998 Nov 13 [Updated 2020 Jan 30]. In: Adam MP, Ardinger HH, Pagon RA, et al., editors. GeneReviews® [Internet]. Seattle (WA): University of Washington; 1993–2021. Available from: https://www.ncbi.nlm.nih.gov/books/NBK1143/.
- Clarke LA. Mucopolysaccharidosis Type I. 2002 Oct 31 [Updated 2021 Feb 25]. In: Adam MP, Ardinger HH, Pagon RA, et al., editors. GeneReviews® [Internet]. Seattle (WA): University of Washington; 1993–2021. Available from: https://www.ncbi.nlm.nih.gov/books/NBK1162/.
- Scarpa M. Mucopolysaccharidosis Type II. 2007 Nov 6 [Updated 2018 Oct 4]. In: Adam MP, Ardinger HH, Pagon RA, et al., editors. GeneReviews® [Internet]. Seattle (WA): University of Washington; 1993–2021. Available from: https://www.ncbi.nlm.nih.gov/books/NBK1274/.

- Wagner VF, Northrup H. Mucopolysaccharidosis Type III. 2019 Sep 19. In: Adam MP, Ardinger HH, Pagon RA, et al., editors. GeneReviews® [Internet]. Seattle (WA): University of Washington; 1993–2021. Available from: https://www.ncbi.nlm.nih.gov/books/NBK546574/.
- Regier DS, Oetgen M, Tanpaiboon P. Mucopolysaccharidosis Type IVA. 2013 Jul 11 [Updated 2021 Jun 17]. In: Adam MP, Ardinger HH, Pagon RA, et al., editors. GeneReviews® [Internet]. Seattle (WA): University of Washington; 1993–2021. Available from: https://www.ncbi.nlm.nih.gov/books/NBK148668/.
- Akyol MU, Alden TD, Amartino H, et al.; MPS Consensus Programme Steering Committee; MPS Consensus Programme Co-Chairs. Recommendations for the management of MPS VI: Systematic evidence- and consensus-based guidance. *Orphanet J Rare Dis.* 2019 May 29;14(1):118.
- Engelen M, Kemp S, de Visser M, van Geel BM, Wanders RJ, Aubourg P, Poll-The BT. X-linked adrenoleukodystrophy (X-ALD): Clinical presentation and guidelines for diagnosis, follow-up and management. *Orphanet J Rare Dis.* 2012 Aug 13;7:51.
- Ondruskova N, Cechova A, Hansikova H, et al. Congenital disorders of glycosylation: Still "hot" in 2020. *Biochim Biophys Acta Gen Subj.* 2021 Jan;1865(1):129751. doi:10.1016/j.bbagen.2020.129751. Epub 2020 Sep 28.
- Vairo FPE, Chwal BC, Perini S, Ferreira MAP, de Freitas Lopes AC, Saute JAM. A systematic review and evidence-based guideline for diagnosis and treatment of Menkes disease. *Mol Genet Metab.* 2019 Jan;126(1):6–13.

15 Genetics

Richard H. Scott, Angela Barnicoat, Emma Wakeling and Philip J. Ostrowski

INTRODUCTION

The management of genetic disorders is a major part of the role of a paediatrician in high income countries. Approximately 50–60% of admissions and deaths in paediatric hospitals are due to malformations or genetic disorders, including many of the conditions discussed elsewhere in this book.

The correct diagnosis of genetic disorders, and their differentiation from sporadic or environmentally caused malformations is important in the proper care of children and their families. It allows the institution of optimal management and surveillance programmes for the affected individuals, and guides advice regarding natural history and prognosis, as well as the risk of recurrence of the disorder in further pregnancies.

COMMON CONGENITAL MALFORMATIONS

About 2–3% of newborns have a major congenital anomaly (Table 15.1). This rate doubles with follow-up throughout childhood. Monozygous twins have double the rate of malformations. Infants of diabetic mothers and mothers on some anti-epileptic medications have about double the risk of congenital malformation. Alcohol and other drugs also increase the risk.

Genetic Aetiology/Pathogenesis

Most isolated malformations are described as having a multifactorial aetiology caused by a combination of environmental and genetic effects. It is important to assess if the malformation is an isolated anomaly or part of a syndrome where the prognosis and inheritance pattern are specific to that syndrome.

Natural History

Dependent on the specific condition.

Differential Diagnosis

See Table 15.1. If the malformation is not isolated, consider syndromes where the specific malformation is a frequently found feature.

Treatment/Management/Surveillance

Good control of diabetes mellitus in mothers in a subsequent pregnancy and high dose folic acid to prevent recurrence of neural tube defects. Prenatal diagnosis may be possible in future pregnancies by ultrasound scan.

Table 15.1: Incidence of Congenital Malformations

Malformation	Livebirth incidence	Syndromes to consider
Congenital heart disease	7 in 1000	Chromosomal trisomy, del 22q11, Noonan syndrome, CHARGE syndrome
Hypospadias	1 in 156 males	*WT1*-associated syndromes, Smith–Lemli–Opitz syndrome
Neural tube defects	1 in 500	Occipital encephalocoele: Meckel syndrome, muscle–eye–brain disease
Talipes equinovarus (club foot)	1 in 625	Congenital myotonic dystrophy
Cleft lip and palate	1 in 700 to 1000	Van der Woude syndrome
Cleft palate	1 in 2500	Stickler syndrome
Diaphragmatic hernia	3 in 10,000	30% have chromosomal abnormality

DOI: 10.1201/9781003175186-15

Table 15.2: Incidence of Structural Chromosome Abnormalities

Deletion	8% of abnormal results based on G-banded analysis
Duplication	2% of abnormal results based on G-banded analysis
Inversion	Many are normal variants; 1 in 100 population
Balanced reciprocal translocation	1 in 500 population

GENETIC TESTING

The range of genetic tests available in clinical practice has expanded considerably in recent years. There is no single 'best' genetic test, and understanding their strengths and weaknesses is crucial in selecting the correct test for each patient. It is important to remember which types of abnormality each test can identify – and, conversely, which diagnoses they can miss.

Most genetic tests fall into two broad categories – **sequencing tests** and **cytogenetic tests**:

- On a fine scale, DNA is a strand of nucleotides which form a genetic code. **Sequencing tests** read the code at this level and compare it to a known reference sequence.

- On a larger scale, the DNA strand is assembled into chromosomes. **Cytogenetic tests** look for structural abnormalities at this level (e.g. regions which are deleted, duplicated or rearranged) – without reading the detailed sequence.

Clinical geneticists and genetic counsellors often use the analogy of a library – a sequencing test is like opening a book and looking for spelling mistakes, while a cytogenetic test is like looking around a library to check if any books are missing, duplicated, or on the wrong shelf.

Sequencing Tests

The traditional method, Sanger sequencing, works by sequencing DNA one nucleotide at a time. For many applications, it has been supplanted by next-generation sequencing (NGS), which allows for a large number of genes to be sequenced in parallel.

While there are situations where either Sanger sequencing or NGS is technically preferable, the most clinically relevant question is often not the choice of sequencing method, but the breadth of the test – *i.e.*, how many genes are being sequenced. The most common options are:

- **Single-gene testing:** Sequencing a single gene associated with a specific phenotype (e.g. the *NF1* gene in neurofibromatosis type 1), or testing for a known genetic change which has been identified in a patient's relative. This can be a relatively quick and cost-effective approach, but analysis is limited to a single gene.

- **Gene panel:** Sequencing a predetermined selection of genes associated with a similar phenotype (*e.g.*, genes associated with skeletal dysplasias)

- **Exome sequencing:** Sequencing the coding regions (exons) of a wide range of genes. Based on the patient's phenotype, a specific 'virtual panel' of genes is usually selected for initial analysis – however, unlike a gene panel, the analysis can be extended to include additional genes if required. Exome sequencing can be further subclassified as:

  - **Clinical exome sequencing:** Sequencing the exons of genes known to be associated with disease

  - **Whole-exome sequencing (WES):** Sequencing the exons of all known genes. Analysis can include genes which have not previously been associated with a clinical phenotype, which can allow for novel genetic conditions to be identified.

- **Whole-genome sequencing (WGS):** Sequencing the entire genome, including non-coding regions (*e.g.*, introns and intergenic regions). As with exome sequencing, analysis can be performed with a 'virtual panel' of genes of interest, but can also be broadened to look for changes in other genes – including genes which have not previously been associated with a clinical phenotype.

The main limitation of sequencing tests is that they are not designed to identify structural changes at the chromosomal level. Some bioinformatic tools for NGS analysis are able to identify copy-number changes (deletions/duplications) or the breakpoints of structural changes (inversions/translocations), but if a chromosomal abnormality is suspected, a cytogenetic test would be more appropriate.

Cytogenetic Tests

The two main types of cytogenetic tests are **chromosomal microarrays** and **karyotyping**. Other, less commonly used cytogenetic tests (*e.g.*, FISH) are applied in specific scenarios.

- **Chromosomal microarrays** (including **array CGH** and **SNP array**) use a series of probes spread across the chromosomes to determine how many copies of DNA are present at each locus. This can be used to identify changes in copy number, affecting an entire chromosome (e.g. Turner syndrome, Down syndrome) or part of a chromosome (*e.g.*, 22q11 deletion syndrome). Microarrays are often used as an initial test in children with multiple congenital abnormalities and/or developmental delay.

- **Karyotyping** uses staining to directly examine the chromosomes under a microscope and look for changes in their number or structure.

- **qfPCR** (quantitative fluorescence polymerase chain reaction) is a rapid method of detecting chromosome copy number, using a series of microsatellite markers. qfPCR is primarily used in the prenatal setting, to test for trisomy 13/18/21 and/or sex chromosome aneuploidies. An abnormal qfPCR result will indicate a specific chromosomal imbalance (e.g. trisomy 21), but does not provide information on chromosome structure (*e.g.*, it will not distinguish between an extra chromosome and a translocation) – therefore, abnormal results are often followed up by karyotype to inform the recurrence risk.

Due to its limited resolution and time-consuming nature, karyotyping has largely been replaced by microarrays or qfPCR for most applications, but it remains the only method for directly visualising the chromosomes, which is required in some scenarios. In particular, microarrays and qfPCR may *not* identify the following abnormalities, which require a karyotype if suspected:

- Structural rearrangements (*e.g.*, translocations, inversions): Microarrays and qfPCR are quantitative tests which provide information on DNA copy number, but do not directly visualise the chromosomes, and therefore are not able to identify structural changes such as balanced translocations.

- Mosaicism: Chromosomal mosaicism can sometimes be detected on microarray or qfPCR, but karyotyping may be more appropriate, as it allows for direct examination of the chromosomes of individual cells (sometimes from tissues other than blood) – particularly if low-level mosaicism is suspected.

Other Tests

Some genetic conditions are caused by more complex mechanisms which may not be identified by standard sequencing or cytogenetic tests. Common examples include:

- **Methylation disorders** (*e.g.*, Beckwith–Wiedemann, Silver–Russell, Prader–Willi and Angelman syndromes): These conditions can be caused by epigenetic changes which affect DNA methylation, rather than the DNA sequence itself. Methylation analysis is used for diagnosis.

- **Repeat disorders** (*e.g.*, fragile X syndrome, myotonic dystrophy, Huntington disease): These conditions are caused by expansion of a repeated sequence of nucleotides. Repetitive sequences are technically difficult to quantify using standard sequencing techniques, and other methods (*e.g.*, Southern blot or triplet-primed PCR) must be used.

- **Somatic or mosaic disorders** (*e.g.*, McCune–Albright, Pallister–Killian and segmental overgrowth syndromes): These conditions are caused by changes which are present in some, but not all cells of the body. Standard genetic testing is usually performed using peripheral blood samples, which may not be representative of the affected tissues. Biopsy of an affected region may be required to obtain tissue for testing.

It is important to remember these exceptions, because they may require targeted testing. For example, a normal microarray and whole-genome sequencing would not rule out Prader–Willi syndrome – methylation studies are required to confirm or exclude this diagnosis.

Variant Interpretation

There is an enormous amount of natural variation in the human genome. Genetic testing compares a patient's DNA to a standard reference sequence, but each individual person has millions of variants compared to this sequence, the vast majority of which are harmless. Genetic laboratories apply specific criteria for variant interpretation, which attempt to distinguish between normal variation and damaging changes which significantly affect a gene. If there is strong evidence either way, a variant is termed (likely) benign or (likely) pathogenic, but if the evidence is inconclusive, it is considered a 'variant of uncertain significance'. When interpreting the results of a test, it is important to remember that simply identifying a 'variant' in a particular gene does not constitute a diagnosis, unless there is enough evidence to suggest that it is significantly affecting gene function.

When discussing genetic test results with patients or in the literature, it is generally preferable to use the term 'variant' rather than 'mutation' – both because it avoids a negative connotation, and because it does not imply pathogenicity ('variant' is a neutral term, while 'mutation' suggests a disease-causing change). The term 'mutation' is used in this chapter for clarity, as shorthand for 'pathogenic or likely pathogenic variant'.

See Richards et al. (2015) in references.

Diagnostic Versus Predictive Testing

The application of genetic testing in clinical practice is broadly divided into diagnostic and predictive testing:

- **Diagnostic testing** attempts to identify a diagnosis in a patient who has symptoms suggestive of a genetic condition.

- **Predictive testing** is testing a patient who is *not* clinically symptomatic, but is at risk of developing a particular condition in future (*e.g.*, due to a family history).

This distinction is particularly important in paediatrics, as predictive testing in children is only indicated if it would change management or screening in childhood. For example, if a child is at risk of an adult-onset condition like Huntington disease, it would be inappropriate to offer a predictive test in childhood – there would be no clinical benefit (since there is no specific treatment or screening), and this would remove the patient's autonomy to make an informed decision about testing.

CHROMOSOME DISORDERS

Chromosomes – Structural Abnormalities and Imbalance

Genetic Aetiology/Pathogenesis

Loss or gain of the DNA content of the chromosome is known as an unbalanced rearrangement. The chromosome structure can be altered by:

- Deletion of part of a chromosome

- Duplication of part of a chromosome

- Inversion of part of a chromosome – two breaks form on a single chromosome and the middle section rotates through 180° (Figure 15.1)

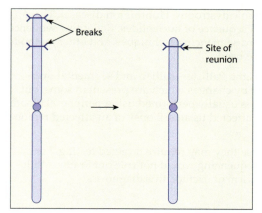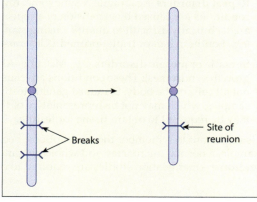

Figure 15.1   Chromosome deletion. (With permission from Oxford University Press, Firth, Hurst and Hall, *Oxford Desk Reference – Clinical Genetics*, 2005.)

■ Translocation of part of a chromosome to another chromosome. This can either result in a *balanced translocation* if there is no overall gain or loss of chromosome material (Figure 15.2), or an *unbalanced translocation* if there is a net loss or gain of chromosomal material. Translocations are also classified as either *reciprocal*, where there is an exchange between two chromosomes, or *Robertsonian* (Figures 15.4 and 15.5) where two acrocentric chromosomes are joined. Carriers of balanced translocations are at increased risk of unbalanced offspring and miscarriage or infertility. The size of this risk will depend on a number of factors – for Robertsonian translocations the sex of the carrier parent (higher risk for females) and the involved chromosomes are relevant; for reciprocal translocations the size of the fragments and potentially specific genes involved can be important.

Clinical Presentation

A child with congenital malformations and/or developmental delay.

Diagnosis

Cytogenetic analysis – in most cases, microarray to detect copy-number imbalance (Figure 15.3), unless the family history suggests a structural abnormality without gain/loss of material (*e.g.*, translocation or inversion), where karyotype is needed.

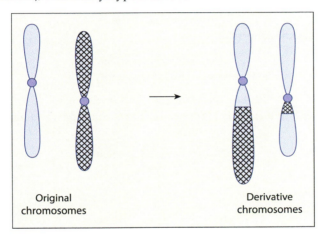

Original chromosomes

Derivative chromosomes

Figure 15.2   Balanced reciprocal chromosome translocation.

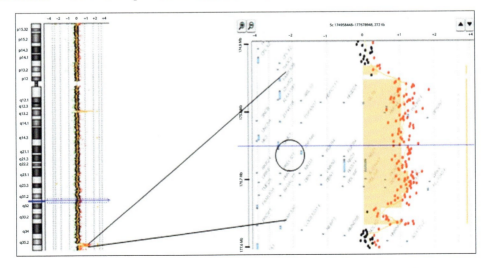

Figure 15.3   Ideogram of chromosome 5 and array CGH data, showing a 1.91 Mb deletion at 5q35.2, including *NSD1*, identified using an Oxford custom 4 × 180 K array; deletion of *NSD1* causes Sotos syndrome.

Inheritance

Deletions and duplications usually follow a dominant pattern of inheritance. The inheritance of inversions and translocations is more complex and requires referral to clinical genetics. They may be associated with a high miscarriage rate or risk of a child with severe developmental delay and malformation caused by chromosome imbalance.

Natural History

Although the natural history of the common deletion syndromes is well delineated, the majority of chromosome abnormalities are unique to a family. Databases such as DECIPHER can give guidance about the phenotype and prognosis.

Differential Diagnosis

Single gene and environmental causes of syndromes and malformations.

Treatment/Management/Surveillance

Refer to clinical genetics; family follow-up and chromosome testing are necessary. Prenatal testing can be offered.

Natural History

As for specific chromosome abnormality.

Differential Diagnosis

Other chromosomal mechanisms can cause the same phenotype.

Treatment/Management/Surveillance

Carrier testing of parents and extended family; prenatal chromosome and uniparental disomy testing as appropriate.

Chromosome Mosaicism
Incidence

- 1 in 50 chorionic villus samples
- 1 in 200 amniocentesis samples

Genetic Aetiology/Pathogenesis

Chromosome mosaicism is the presence of two or more cell lines with different chromosomal complements. Mosaicism can also occur for point mutations in single-gene disorders (e.g. neurofibromatosis type 1).

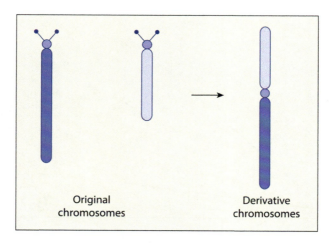

Original chromosomes

Derivative chromosomes

Figure 15.4 Balanced Robertsonian translocation. (With permission from Oxford University Press, Firth, Hurst and Hall, Oxford Desk Reference – Clinical Genetics, 2005.)

Clinical Presentation

- Hypomelanosis of Ito
- Mosaic trisomy 8
- Mosaic tetrasomy 12p (Pallister–Killian syndrome)
- Mosaic uniparental disomy 11p15 (Beckwith–Wiedemann syndrome)

Diagnosis

Extended karyotype, microarray, or testing of another tissue (buccal swab or skin biopsy) is required.

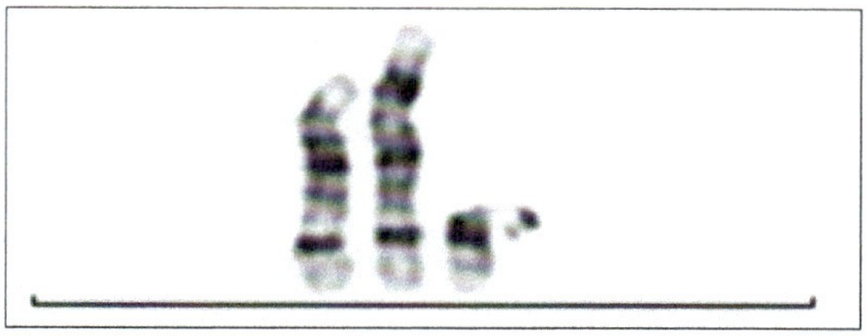

Trisomy 13 (Patau Syndrome)
Incidence

1 in 50,000 livebirths (increases with maternal age).

Genetic Aetiology/Pathogenesis

- Trisomy 13: 90% of cases, associated with increased maternal age. Low recurrence risk in future pregnancies, although risk is dependent on maternal age and if prenatal diagnosis is offered.
- Translocation: 5 to 10% of cases: Robertsonian translocation.
- Mosaic trisomy 13: up to 5% of cases. The phenotype is milder and babies live longer but the developmental outcome is poor.

Clinical Presentation

Children present with low birth weight, major facial malformations (holoprosencephaly sequence, clefts, microphthalmia) (Figure 15.6), postaxial polydactyly, cardiac defects and exomphalos.

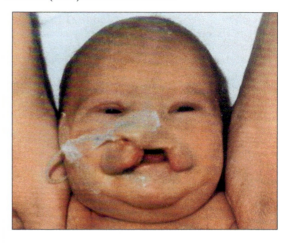

Figure 15.5 A Robertsonian translocation rob (14:21), the cause of 2% of Down syndrome. A normal chromosome 14 is pictured on the left, a normal chromosome 21 on the right, and a derivative rob (14:21) between the two.

Figure 15.6 A child with trisomy 13 (Patau syndrome).

Diagnosis

A rapid result is obtained by qfPCR; confirmation by karyotype can be sought to exclude Robertsonian translocation.

Inheritance

- Trisomy 13 (including mosaicism): Sporadic, maternal age-related
- Robertsonian translocation: Refer to clinical genetics for advice regarding risks in future pregnancies

Natural History

Median survival 7–10 days, 5–10% survive after their first birthday.

Differential Diagnosis

Autosomal recessive disorders such as ciliopathies and severe Smith–Lemli–Opitz syndrome; other unbalanced chromosome abnormalities.

Treatment/Management/Surveillance

After confirmation of the diagnosis, supportive treatment only is indicated unless mosaic.

Trisomy 18 (Edwards Syndrome)

Incidence

1 in 12,500 livebirths (increases with maternal age).

Genetic Aetiology/Pathogenesis

Trisomy 18. Most are due to an error during meiosis and 85% are of maternal origin. The aetiology is associated with increased maternal age.

Clinical Presentation

Prematurity is common and many trisomy 18 foetuses are lost spontaneously during pregnancy. The birth weight is low and the head shape is abnormal with a prominent occiput. Limb abnormalities are found with contractures of the fingers, short hallux, prominent heels and sometimes a radial deficiency of the forearms; 90% have congenital heart disease and the sternum is short. Cleft lip and palate, exomphalos and diaphragmatic hernia are common additional malformations (Figure 15.7).

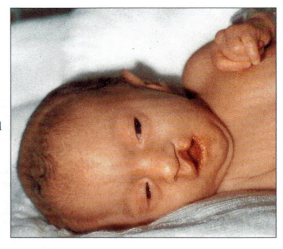

Figure 15.7   A child with trisomy 18 (Edwards syndrome).

Diagnosis

A rapid result is obtained by qfPCR, with confirmation by karyotype. The phenotype is not as distinctive as trisomy 21 or 13 so it is wise to wait for the rapid qfPCR result before discussing the diagnosis with the parents.

Inheritance

There is a low recurrence risk in future pregnancies, though risk is dependent on maternal age.

Natural History

Mean survival after birth is four days with failure to establish respiration probably secondary to CNS malformation with contribution from chest and heart malformations.

Differential Diagnosis

Other chromosome abnormalities; syndromic causes of distal arthrogryposis

Treatment/Management/Surveillance

Given the guarded prognosis, treatment options are mainly supportive.

Trisomy 21 (Down Syndrome)

Incidence

The incidence is 1 in 600, but the livebirth rate is influenced by the uptake and availability of prenatal screening and is about 1 in 1100 in the United Kingdom. There is an increase with maternal age from 1 in 1500 at 17 years to 1 in 100 at 40 years.

Genetic Aetiology/Pathogenesis

- Trisomy 21: 95% of cases (Figure 15.8). There is a low recurrence risk in future pregnancies, although risk is dependent on maternal age.

- Translocation – 2% of cases: Robertsonian translocation.

- Mosaic Down syndrome – 2% of cases: phenotype may be milder but the ratio of normal to Down syndrome cells in blood or prenatal testing is not a reliable indicator of the ratio in other tissues. The level of mosaicism cannot therefore be used to predict prognosis.

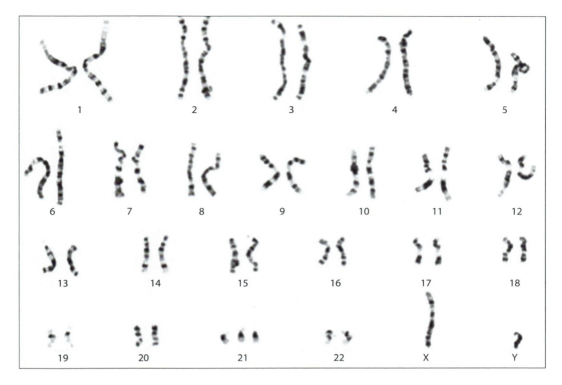

Figure 15.8 G-banded karyotype showing trisomy 21.

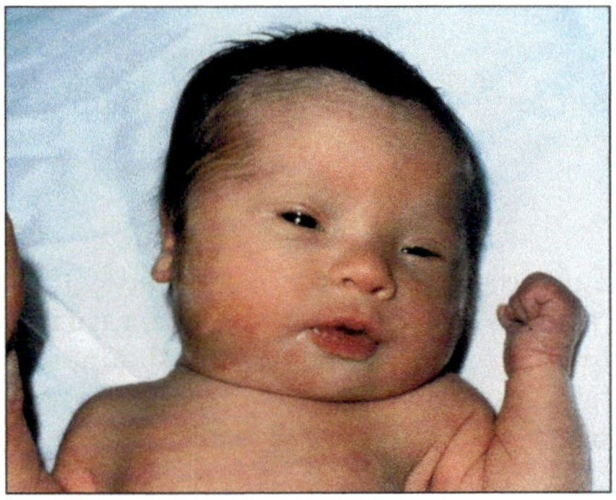

Clinical Presentation

Paediatricians are familiar with the clinical features (Figure 15.9). Enquire about screening in pregnancy. The child typically presents as a floppy neonate with upslanting palpebral fissures, flat facial profile, large fontanelle(s), poor suck and cardiac murmur; 50% have congenital heart disease and there is a two-fold increase for all congenital anomalies.

Diagnosis

A rapid result is obtained by qfPCR, with confirmation by karyotype to exclude Robertsonian translocation.

Figure 15.9 Down syndrome.

Inheritance

- Trisomy 21: Sporadic, maternal age-related

- Robertsonian translocation: Refer to clinical genetics

- Mosaic: Refer to clinical genetics. An individual with mosaic Down syndrome may have a child with complete trisomy 21.

Natural History

Median survival is close to 50 years unless there is a significant cardiac or other malformation. Mean IQ for young adults is 45–50 but this declines later due to early-onset dementia.

Differential Diagnosis

Usually no diagnostic difficulty but:

- Mosaic trisomy 21: May not be detected with basic genetic testing

- Deletion of chromosome 9q34.3 (Kleefstra syndrome): Has a similar facial profile
- Zellweger syndrome: Extremely floppy with large fontanelle

Treatment/Management/Surveillance

Echocardiogram for cardiac disease. Referral to a community paediatrician for surveillance of medical (thyroid function, visual and hearing checks, increased risk for coeliac disease, increased risk of leukaemia) and developmental issues is necessary.

Turner Syndrome, 45, X and Variants
Incidence

1 in 2500 female livebirths.

Genetic Aetiology/Pathogenesis

The clinical features are due to monosomy (one copy) of all or part of the X chromosome in females. About 50% of females with Turner have 'pure' monosomy X, whereas the other 50% shows mosaicism for a second cell line (Table 15.3). There is a high rate of loss during pregnancy of about 65% between 12 and 40 weeks.

Clinical Presentation

- Neonate: A history of increased nuchal measurement, cystic hygroma or hydrops in pregnancy is almost always found and prenatal karyotype may have been performed. Peripheral oedema, excess skin around the neck. coarctation of the aorta and renal anomalies may be present.
- Childhood: Short stature, neck webbing, ptosis (Figure 15.10)
- Adolescent: Primary ovarian failure with scant or no pubertal development and amenorrhoea

Diagnosis
Karyotype with 30-cell count to investigate possible mosaicism.

Inheritance
Turner syndrome occurs sporadically. The majority of women with Turner are infertile. *In vitro* fertilisation (IVF) with donor oocytes has resulted in successful pregnancy for some women with Turner syndrome.

Natural History
Although there are some well documented behavioural and specific developmental difficulties, the majority of girls attend mainstream school and have a normal independent adult life.

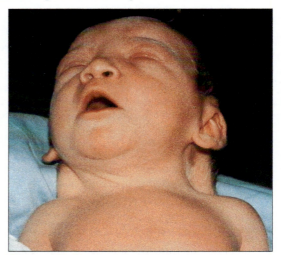

Figure 15.10   A child with Turner syndrome with neck webbing.

Table 15.3: X Chromosome Abnormalities Found in Turner Syndrome

X chromosome abnormality	Frequency
45,X	50%
45,X/structural abnormality of other X	20%
45,X/46,XX	20%
46,XX with structural abnormality of second X	10%

Differential Diagnosis

- Other causes of primary ovarian failure

- Syndromes with overlapping features (e.g. Noonan syndrome)

Treatment/Management/Surveillance

- Neonate: Echocardiogram, renal ultrasound, audiogram

- Childhood: Paediatric endocrinology review. Short stature can be partially corrected by administration of growth hormone in childhood.

- Adolescents/adults: In addition to primary ovarian failure, adults with Turner syndrome are also susceptible to a range of disorders, including osteoporosis, hypothyroidism and renal and gastrointestinal disease. They have a particularly high cardiovascular risk and it is imperative that patients are assessed by a cardiologist and advised of the potential risks before attempting to become pregnant by *in vitro* fertilisation as there is a 2% risk of rupture or dissection of the aorta.

Williams Syndrome
Incidence

1 in 20,000.

Genetic Aetiology/Pathogenesis

Williams syndrome is due to a monoallelic deletion of chromosome 7q11.23 encompassing the elastin (*ELN*) gene. This microdeletion is not detectable by karyotype but identified by microarray.

Clinical Presentation

The typical cardiac defects are supravalvular aortic stenosis and supravalvular pulmonary stenosis. There is a history of poor feeding and developmental delay. Facial features include periorbital oedema, small nose with upturned nasal tip, wide mouth with full lips and sagging cheeks due to elastin deficiency (Figures 15.11 and 15.12). The facial features coarsen with age.

There is a typical behavioural phenotype that has been well delineated. There are visual-spatial deficits but strengths in communication. Hyperacusis is a problem to some. Adults are not usually able to live an independent life.

Diagnosis

Microarray or FISH

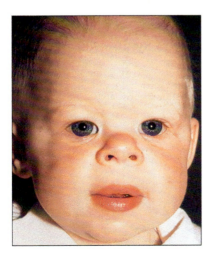

Figure 15.11   A baby with Williams syndrome.

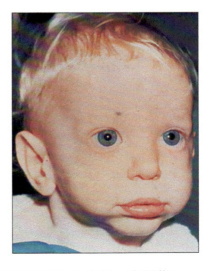

Figure 15.12   A child with Williams syndrome.

Inheritance

The vast majority arise *de novo*, the remainder have a parent with the deletion. Inheritance is autosomal dominant with full penetrance. Parents are offered the availability of prenatal diagnosis in a subsequent pregnancy but the risk is low when parents do not have Williams syndrome.

Differential Diagnosis

- Elastin mutation
- Noonan syndrome

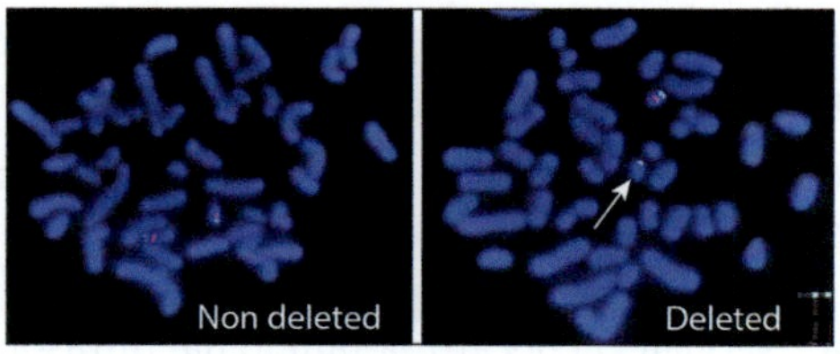

Figure 15.13 FISH using specific 22q11 probe (red) and control chromosome 22 probe (green) showing 22q11 deletion (absent red signal on the deleted chromosome).

Treatment/Management/Surveillance

- Screening for hypercalcaemia and nephrocalcinosis (see the chapter 'Endocrinolgy')
- Surveillance for later onset arterial hypertension and renal artery stenosis
- Referral to clinical genetics to discuss parental testing and prenatal diagnosis

22q11 Deletion Syndrome (DiGeorge/Velocardiofacial Syndrome)

Incidence

1 in 2000 to 4000.

Genetic Aetiology/Pathogenesis

DiGeorge syndrome is due to a monoallelic deletion of chromosome 22q11 (del22q11.2) (Figure 15.13). These microdeletions are typically ~3 Mb of genomic DNA and are not detectable by G-banded karyotype. The *TBX1* gene within the area of deletion is of particular importance in the phenotype.

Clinical Presentation

In the neonate, cardiac defects and cleft palate lead to identification of the deletion. In older children speech delay, velopharyngeal insufficiency and the facial features are more common reasons for testing. The facial features are not distinctive but there are subtle changes to the shape of the nose and ears. The ear abnormalities include overfolded or squared off helices. A prominent nasal root and bulbous nasal tip is sometimes observed in older children. (See other features in Table 15.4.)

Diagnosis

Microarray or FISH.

Table 15.4: Features of 22q11 Deletion (DiGeorge Syndrome)

Age	Feature	Frequency
Infant	Congenital heart disease (all types but particularly associated are tetralogy of Fallot, pulmonary atresia – ventricular septal defect, interrupted aortic arch, truncus arteriosus)	75%
	Cleft palate, including submucous cleft	15%
	Hypocalcaemia	Up to 60%
	Defects in cell-mediated immunity (hypoplasia of the thymus) and recurrent infections	1% have a major immune defect
	Renal anomalies	30–40%
Child	Speech delay and velopharyngeal insufficiency	30%
	Hypocalcaemia/hypoparathyroidism	30%
Older child	Schooling and learning difficulties Hypocalcaemic seizures	60–70%
Adult	Psychiatric problems	15–20%

Inheritance

Approximately 90% arise as new mutations, the remainder have a parent with the deletion. Inheritance is autosomal dominant with full penetrance but huge variability of expression. Parents are offered prenatal diagnosis in a subsequent pregnancy. If parents do not have the deletion, risk to a subsequent pregnancy is about 1–2% due to gonadal mosaicism.

Differential Diagnosis

- CHARGE syndrome
- VATER/VACTERL association
- Goldenhar/oculo-auricular-vertebral syndrome

Treatment/Management/Surveillance

Immune function should be checked prior to vaccination with live vaccines and whole blood transfusion; referral to clinical genetics should be offered to discuss family testing and prenatal diagnosis.

Common Neurosusceptibility Loci

Incidence

Variable but of order of magnitude 1 in 5000 to 10,000 births depending on locus.

Genetic Aetiology/Pathogenesis

The disorders are likely to arise from mismatched crossing over at meiosis due to low copy-number repeat segments of DNA.

Clinical Features

Microarray technology has led to the identification of a significant number of common sub-microscopic copy-number changes of the chromosomes.

A proportion of these are linked to (usually) mild developmental delay and learning problems and behavioural features such as autistic spectrum disorders and attention deficit hyperactivity disorder.

Neurosuceptibility loci

The link to congenital abnormalities is much weaker than with typical larger chromosomal changes and in most cases the phenotype is confined to the developmental disorder.

These copy-number changes are considered risk factors for these phenotypes rather than being directly causal and may depend on other genetic or environmental factors for the development of the associated phenotype. Penetrance data is available for some of the more common microdeletions and microduplications.

Diagnosis

Microarray.

Inheritance

Autosomal dominant with variable penetrance (i.e. not all relatives who inherit the neurosusceptibility locus will be similarly affected).

Treatment/Surveillance

The disorders are quite variable within families because of the variable penetrance and it is not infrequent to find an unaffected parent harbouring the change identified in a child.

An offer of cascade screening to close relatives may be appropriate in some cases. Prenatal diagnosis would not usually be considered because of the inability to predict the phenotype.

MODES OF INHERITANCE

Single-Gene Disorders

The human genome contains approximately 20,000 genes and many disorders are caused by mutations affecting just one gene. Often referred to as single-gene disorders, they can follow a number of different patterns of inheritance depending on whether the affected gene resides on an autosome or sex chromosome and whether disease is caused by mutations affecting one or two alleles (copies) of the gene.

Mutations in single-gene disorders can be single nucleotide alterations, for example inserting a premature 'stop' codon. They can also be larger scale, for example deletions affecting a several exons of the gene or even the whole gene. Testing for single-gene disorders can be performed by DNA sequencing (searching for single nucleotide and other small-scale sequence alterations) and copy-number testing (looking for deletions or duplications).

Clinical Pedigrees

Drawing and interpretation of clinical pedigrees are important skills and aid the recognition of the likely underlying pattern of inheritance (Figure 15.14). A pedigree is usually started from the presenting individual (the consultand), who is marked with an arrow. The person through whom the family was first brought to medical attention is referred to as the proband. A three-generation pedigree is usual but can be more extensive if appropriate. Enquiries should specifically but tactfully be made about consanguinity, miscarriages and stillbirths.

Autosomal Dominant Inheritance

Autosomal dominant (AD) disorders are caused by mutations in genes on the autosomes (chromosomes 1–22) (Table 15.5).

Children (and adults) with AD conditions have a mutation on one of the two alleles of the gene ('monoallelic' or heterozygous mutation). Aspects of inheritance in AD disorders include:

- Differences in expression with inter- and intrafamilial variability

- Penetrance: the percentage of individuals who have any features of the disorder. This may be age-dependent penetrance or incomplete penetrance (not all mutation carriers will develop the condition).

- Somatic mosaicism: A new mutation arising at an early stage in embryogenesis may result in a partial or modified phenotype.

- Germline/gonadal mosaicism: A new mutation arising during gametogenesis may cause no phenotype in the parent but can be transmitted to the offspring.

- Paternal age effect: For some AD disorders the chance of a new mutation from the father increases with his age.

- Anticipation: Worsening of disease severity in successive generations

Some AD conditions are more commonly encountered in adults (due to age-dependent penetrance). Others are more frequently considered in children (see Table 15.5), particularly those severe dominantly inherited conditions that have arisen as the result of a new mutation or where anticipation is a feature of the condition.

Carrier and predictive testing should be considered for the wider family. However, there are ethical considerations in the testing of children with adult-onset conditions and this is usually only performed when the diagnosis will lead to better treatment and/

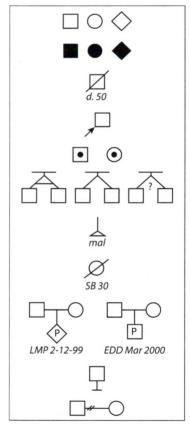

Figure 15.14 Standard symbols for pedigree drawing. (See further Bennett RL et al. 1995. Recommendations for standardised human pedigree nomenclature. Pedigree Standardization) Task Force of the National Society of Genetic Counselors. *Am J Hum Genet* 1995; 56: 745–752.)

Table 15.5: **Common Autosomal Dominant Conditions**

Disease	Incidence	Gene	Particular features
Osteogenesis imperfecta	1 in 500 incidence 1 in 1000 prevalence	COL1A1/A2 and others	Severe types lethal Gonadal and somatic mosaicism
Neurofibromatosis type 1	1 in 5000	NF1	Variable expression, age-dependent expression, somatic mosaicism
Myotonic dystrophy	1 in 8000	DMPK	Anticipation
Tuberous sclerosis	1 in 10,000	TSC1/2	Variable expression, age-dependent expression, somatic and gonadal mosaicism
Craniosynostosis (Apert/ Crouzon/Pfeiffer)	Apert: 1 in 100,000 Crouzon: 1 in 50,000	FGFR2	Paternal age effect
Achondroplasia	1 in 27,000	FGFR3	Paternal age effect

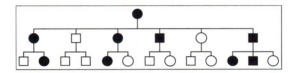

Figure 15.15 A typical family tree showing AD inheritance. An affected parent has a 50% risk of transmitting the condition to each child whether they are male or female. (With permission from Oxford University Press, Firth, Hurst and Hall, *Oxford Desk Reference – Clinical Genetics*, 2005.)

Table 15.6: **Common Autosomal Recessive Conditions**

Disease	Carrier frequency in general population	Gene
α1-antitrypsin deficiency	1 in 25 for Z allele and 1 in 17 for S allele in north European populations	SERPINA1
Congenital adrenal hyperplasia	1 in 50 for CYP21	CYP21
Cystic fibrosis	1 in 23 in north European populations	CFTR
Gaucher disease	1 in 25 in Ashkenazi Jewish population	GBA
Haemochromatosis	1 in 10 in north European populations	HFE
Phenylketonuria	1 in 50	PAH
Sickle cell disease	> 1 in 10 in equatorial Africa	HBB
Spinal muscular atrophy	1 in 50	SMN1
Tay Sachs disease	1 in 30 in Ashkenazi Jewish population	HEXA
Beta-thalassaemia	1 in 30 in Greek/Italian population	HBB

or surveillance. Surveillance for age-dependent features that require treatment (e.g. aortic dilatation in Marfan syndrome) should be carried out. Prenatal diagnosis is often possible in future pregnancies.

Autosomal Recessive Inheritance

Autosomal recessive (AR) disorders are caused by mutations affecting both alleles of genes on the autosomes (chromosomes 1–22). Table 15.6 presents common AR conditions.

Affected children have mutations in both of the two alleles of the gene ('biallelic' mutation). They are either homozygotes (two identical mutations) or compound heterozygotes (two different mutations). Individuals with a mutation in one allele are known as carriers. They either do not have features of the condition (e.g. cystic fibrosis), or if they do this is very mild in comparison with the disease state (e.g. sickle cell trait vs. sickle cell disease). Many of the more common AR conditions have higher frequencies in certain populations (Table 15.6). Rare AR conditions are more common in the children of consanguineous parents.

Autosomal recessive inheritance is depicted in Figure 15.16. There is a 25% risk of an affected child in any pregnancy, independent of sex. The diagram on the right illustrates a consanguineous

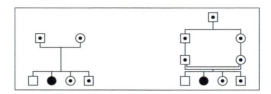

Figure 15.16 Family trees to illustrate autosomal recessive inheritance. (With permission from Oxford University Press, Firth, Hurst and hall, *Oxford Desk Reference – Clinical Genetics*, 2005.)

Table 15.7: **Common X-linked Conditions**

Disease	Frequency in males	Gene	Particular features
Duchenne muscular dystrophy	1 in 3000 to 4000	*DMD*	High new mutation and gonadal mosaic risk
Haemophilia A	1 in 5000	*F8*	Most mothers of affected boys are carriers
Fragile X syndrome	1 in 5500	*FMR1*	Anticipation, normal transmitting males, premutations, premature ovarian failure in carrier females

relationship between first cousins. A common ancestor is a carrier for a recessive mutation that may occur in homozygous form in a descendent as a consequence of consanguinity.

Carrier testing for the wider family may be appropriate. Prenatal diagnosis is often possible in future pregnancies.

X-Linked Inheritance

X-linked (XL) disorders are due to mutation in genes on the X chromosome. There can be a spectrum from dominant to recessive

■ X-linked recessive (XLR) – males are hemizygous and affected; females are heterozygous carriers and usually show no or mild symptoms.

■ X-linked dominant (XLD) conditions are often lethal to males and the affected individuals are heterozygous females (e.g. Rett syndrome).

Some common X-linked conditions are shown in Table 15.7.

In some disorders females have symptoms due to non-random X-inactivation and age-dependent penetrance.

In Duchenne or Becker muscular dystrophy, there is a significantly high gonadal mosaic risk.

XL conditions should be considered where a genetic condition affects males more severely and there is no male-to-male transmission of the condition.

Inheritance of X-linked conditions is shown in Figure 15.17.

It is appropriate to refer families to clinical genetics to evaluate the family history and so females at risk of being carriers can be offered testing. Prenatal diagnosis is often possible in future pregnancies.

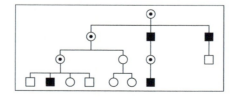

Figure 15.17 A typical family tree showing X-linked recessive inheritance. The condition is expressed in males, but not in females. For a carrier female, on average, 50% of her sons will be affected and 50% of her daughters will be carriers. All daughters of an affected male are obligate carriers and none of his sons inherit the condition. (With permission from Oxford University Press, Firth, Hurst and Hall, *Oxford Desk Reference – Clinical Genetics*, 2005.)

Mitochondrial Conditions and Inheritance

These conditions often present insidiously and diagnosis can be delayed. Key clinical features are myoclonus, external ophthalmoplegia, ptosis, sensorineural deafness, cardiac conduction defects and diabetes mellitus.

Diagnosis is based on a combination of biochemical abnormalities (raised lactate in blood/CSF), characteristic muscle biopsy 'ragged red fibres', brain MRI and genetic testing.

Mitochondrial DNA (mtDNA) is exclusively maternally inherited (Figure 15.18) and for the purposes of genetic counselling the risk of paternal inheritance of a mitochondrial mutation is zero. The severity in children is difficult to predict.

It is important to distinguish between conditions caused by mutations in mtDNA, as opposed to conditions caused by mutations in nuclear genes encoding mitochondrial proteins (which can cause a 'mitochondrial' phenotype, but follow standard autosomal or X-linked inheritance patterns).

Imprinting Disorders

The majority of genes are expressed from both parental copies. However, a small number of genes are only expressed from either the maternally or paternally inherited copy, with the opposite allele remaining silent. These genes are known as 'imprinted genes'. Imprinted genes have a wide range of roles in growth, development, metabolism and behaviour, as well as tumour suppression.

Imprinting disorders result from changes in the expression of imprinted genes. A number of different mechanisms can result in altered expression:

a) uniparental disomy (inheritance of two copies of the same chromosome from one parent)

b) copy-number variants (CNVs)

c) epigenetic changes (usually loss or gain of parental-specific methylation)

d) variants within imprinted genes

Variants will result in a phenotype depending on their parent of origin. For example, only *maternally* derived variants in the maternally expressed *UBE3A* gene will result in Angelman syndrome.

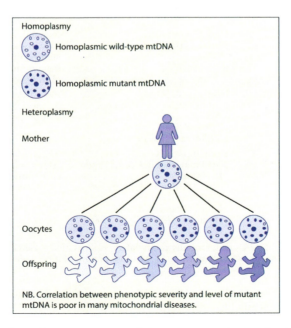

NB. Correlation between phenotypic severity and level of mutant mtDNA is poor in many mitochondrial diseases.

Figure 15.18 Illustration of maternal transmission of a mitochondrial mutation. (With permission from Oxford University Press, Firth, Hurst and Hall, *Oxford Desk Reference – Clinical Genetics*, 2005.)

Table 15.8: Common Mitochondrial Conditions

Disease	Features	Mechanism	Inheritance
Kearns Sayre	Chronic progressive external ophthalmoplegia (CPEO), ataxia, cardiac conduction defect	mtDNA deletion	Sporadic or rarely maternally inherited
Leber's hereditary optic neuropathy	Loss of vision	mtDNA mutation	Maternal
Leigh syndrome	Developmental delay/regression, seizures, raised lactate, abnormal brain MRI	Both mtDNA mutations (*NARP* mutations) and nuclear encoded gene mutation	Maternal and autosomal recessive
Aminoglycoside deafness	Progressive sensorineural deafness	mtDNA mutation, usually m.A1555G	Maternal
Pearson syndrome	Transfusion dependent anaemia, exocrine pancreatic failure	mtDNA deletion	Usually sporadic

Table 15.9: Common Imprinting Disorders

Imprinting disorder	Chromo-some	Genetic aetiology/pathogenesis	Clinical presentation
Silver–Russell syndrome (Figure 15.19) – see Wakeling et al. (2017) in references	7 11p15.5	Upd(7)mat: 5–10% 11p15 LOM: 30–60% 11p15 CNVs: (< 1%) Upd(11p15)mat (rare) *CDKN1C, IGF2, HGMA2, PLAG1* variants (~4%)	IUGR, short stature, relative macrocephaly at birth, body asymmetry, prominent forehead, feeding difficulties in early childhood
Beckwith–Wiedemann syndrome (Figure 15.20) – see Brioude et al. (2018) in references	11p15.5	Segmental upd(11)pat: 20% Paternal duplications: (2–4%) Deletions: 1–5% IC2 LOM: 50% IC1 GOM: 5% *CDKN1C* variants 5% (40% in familial cases)	Macroglossia, exomphalos/umbilical hernia, hemihypertrophy, hyperinsulinaemic hypoglycaemia, predisposition to embryonal tumours, especially Wilms tumour, increased birth weight, facial naevus flammeus, ear pits and/or creases Note: risk of Wilms tumour is dependent on genetic aetiology. There is no evidence of increased Wilms risk in cases with IC2 LOM
Prader–Willi syndrome	15q11.2	Upd(15)mat: 42% 15q11q13 paternal deletion: 55% IC defect: 2%	Neonatal hypotonia, feeding difficulties in infancy, hypogonadism, short stature, intellectual disability, behavioural problems, hyperphagia, obesity, small hands and feet
Angelman syndrome	15q11.2	Upd(15)pat: 5% 15q11q13 maternal deletion: 70% IC defect: 5% *UBE3A* variants: 10%	Severe intellectual disability, ataxia, seizures, EEG abnormalities, bouts of inappropriate laughter
Pseudohypo-parathyroidism	20q13	Upd(20)pat: (Type 1b – rare) 20q13 maternal deletion (Type 1a – rare) *GNAS* DMRs LOM: (Type 1b –~100%) Maternally derived *GNAS* variants: 62–82% (Type 1a & 1c)	PTH resistance, TSH resistance, Albright hereditary osteodystrophy, early-onset obesity, subcutaneous ossifications

CNV – copy-number variant; DMR – differentially methylated region; GOM – gain of methylation; IC – imprinting centre; IUGR – intrauterine growth retardation; LOM – loss of methylation; Upd – uniparental disomy

Imprinting centres (ICs) are regions of DNA which control the expression of surrounding imprinted genes. They typically have differentially methylated regions (DMRs) in which methylation depends on the parental origin of the allele. Testing for imprinting disorders relies on detection of aberrant methylation patterns within the DMRs. The most common method of testing is methylation sensitive MLPA (MS-MLPA). This will detect uniparental disomy, CNVs and epigenetic changes. Single-gene variants will not be detected by MS-MLPA.

It is important to determine the underlying mechanism as this will determine the recurrence risk for parents. Epigenetic changes and uniparental disomy are associated with a very low recurrence risk. Copy-number and single-gene variants can be associated with a 50% recurrence risk, depending on parental inheritance.

SELECTED SINGLE-GENE DISORDERS

Fragile X Syndrome

Incidence

Approximately 1 in 5000 males.

Genetic Aetiology/Pathogenesis

Most cases of fragile X syndrome are caused by a triplet repeat expansion within the *FMR1* gene. Repeat lengths of > 200 are referred to as 'full mutations' and cause fragile X syndrome. Alleles with 55 to 200 repeats are referred to as 'premutations' and are associated with an increased risk of expansion to > 200 repeats when transmitted.

Clinical Presentation

Males with fragile X typically have moderate learning difficulties. Behavioural difficulties, often leading to a diagnosis of autism, are common. Physical features present in some include relative macrocephaly, a long face, prominent ears, squint, joint laxity, mitral valve prolapse and (post-pubertally) large testes (Figure 15.21). Affected females typically have mild learning difficulties.

Additional adult phenotypes are associated with some premutation changes including premature ovarian insufficiency and a progressive neurological phenotype with ataxia.

Diagnosis

Southern blotting and/or PCR analysis to identify the expansion in the *FMR1* gene.

Inheritance

X-linked incompletely dominant, with risk of anticipation as the expansion size can increase in female meiosis.

Natural History

The features of the fragile X syndrome are largely static.

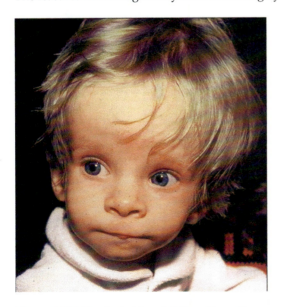

Figure 15.19   A child with Silver-Russell syndrome.

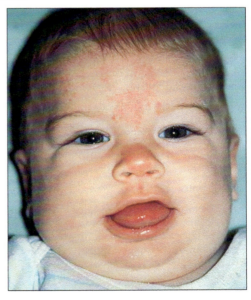

Figure 15.20   A child with Beckwith-Wiedemann syndrome.

437

Differential Diagnosis

- Chromosome abnormalities

- Sotos syndrome

- Non-syndromic autism of unknown cause

Treatment/Management/Surveillance

Developmental evaluation and support should be provided as appropriate, including speech therapy and behavioural management. Children should receive routine medical management of concomitant problems such as strabismus or mitral valve prolapse.

Carrier testing should be offered for the wider family; prenatal diagnosis can be offered in future pregnancies.

Neurofibromatosis Type 1
Incidence

One of the most common genetic disorders – approximately 1 in 3000.

Genetic Aetiology/Pathogenesis

Neurofibromatosis type 1 (NF1) is caused by pathogenic sequence or copy-number variants in the neurofibromin 1 gene (*NF1*). The phenotype can be more severe in patients with deletions of the entire *NF1* gene, and milder or localised in patients with mosaic NF1.

Clinical Presentation

NF1 is a neurocutaneous disorder which can usually be diagnosed clinically, but features are variable; some are common in the general population (*e.g.,* up to a few *café-au-lait* macules), while others evolve with age (*e.g.,* neurofibromas usually appear in adolescence or adulthood). The cardinal signs of NF1 are incorporated into the diagnostic criteria (see below), but other suggestive features include malignant peripheral nerve sheath tumours, hypertension, seizures, relative macrocephaly, scoliosis, and learning difficulties and/or behavioural problems (in 50–70% of patients). Careful assessment of patients with suspected NF1 is essential to ensure that affected patients have appropriate screening.

Diagnosis

Diagnosis of NF1 is based on the presence of *two or more* of the following criteria:

- Six or more *café-au-lait* macules (over 5 mm in greatest diameter in prepubertal individuals and over 15 mm in greatest diameter in post-pubertal individuals) *(a)* (Figure 15.22)

- Freckling in the axillary or inguinal region *(a)* (Figure 15.23)

- Two or more neurofibromas of any type (Figure 15.24) or one plexiform neurofibroma (Figure 15.25)

- Optic pathway glioma

- Two or more iris Lisch nodules identified by slit lamp examination or two or more choroidal abnormalities (defined as bright, patchy nodules imaged by optical coherence tomography [OCT]/near-infrared reflectance [NIR] imaging)

- A distinctive osseous lesion such as sphenoid dysplasia *(b)*, anterolateral bowing of the tibia, or pseudarthrosis of a long bone

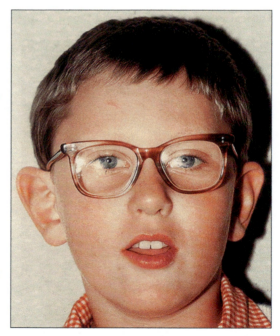

Figure 15.21 A child with Fragile X syndrome.

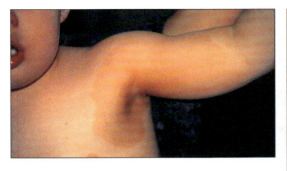

Figure 15.22 Cafe-au-lait macules.

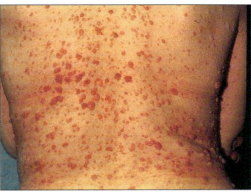

Figure 15.24 Neurofibromas.

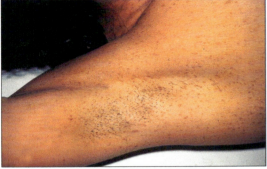

Figure 15.23 Axillary freckling.

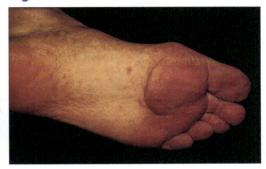

Figure 15.25 Plexiform neurofibroma.

- A heterozygous pathogenic *NF1* variant with a variant allele fraction of 50% in apparently normal tissue such as white blood cells

A child of a parent with NF1 (where the parent meets the diagnostic criteria above) merits a diagnosis of NF1 if *one or more* of the criteria are present:

Notes:

(a) If only *café-au-lait* macules and freckling are present, the diagnosis is most likely NF1 but exceptionally the person might have another diagnosis such as Legius syndrome (*SPRED1*). At least one of the two pigmentary findings (*café-au-lait* macules or freckling) should be bilateral.

(b) Sphenoid wing dysplasia is not a separate criterion in case of an ipsilateral orbital plexiform neurofibroma.

See Legius et al. (2021) in the references.

Inheritance

Autosomal dominant. Approximately 50% of patients have inherited NF1 from an affected parent (who may or may not have been previously diagnosed). The remaining half of cases are due to a *de novo* variant in *NF1*.

Differential Diagnosis

- Legius syndrome (*SPRED1*)
- Neurofibromatosis type 2 (NF2)
- Schwannomatosis
- Constitutional mismatch repair deficiency syndrome
- Noonan syndrome, Noonan syndrome with multiple lentigines (formerly LEOPARD syndrome), and other RASopathies

- McCune–Albright syndrome

Treatment/Management/Surveillance

- Cardiovascular: Regular monitoring of blood pressure (risk of renal artery stenosis and phaeochromoctyoma)

- Ophthalmological: Regular surveillance in childhood (risk of optic glioma)

- Neurological: Developmental assessment in childhood, monitoring for neurological symptoms (risk of developmental delay and cranial glioma)

- Dermatological: Monitoring of skin lesions (risk of malignant transformation)

- Musculoskeletal: Assessment of pseudarthrosis and/or scoliosis if present

- Other: Enhanced breast cancer screening in adult females (moderately increased risk)

See Ferner et al. (2007) in references.

Stickler Syndrome
Incidence
Approximately 1 in 7500. Stickler syndrome is particularly common in patients with Pierre–Robin sequence (present in up to one in three cases).

Genetic Aetiology/Pathogenesis
Stickler syndrome is caused by pathogenic sequence or copy-number variants in one of the following collagen genes: *COL2A1, COL11A1, COL11A2, COL9A1, COL9A2, COL9A3.*

Clinical Presentation
Stickler syndrome is a multisystem disorder with can include the following features:

- Craniofacial:
  - Pierre–Robin sequence, micrognathia, cleft palate, bifid uvula
  - Midface hypoplasia
- Ophthalmological:
  - Myopia (congenital, non-progressive)
  - Vitreous anomaly
  - Retinal detachment
  - Cataracts
- Auditory:
  - Sensorineural hearing impairment
  - Conductive hearing impairment
  - Recurrent otitis media
- Musculoskeletal:
  - Short stature (usually mild)
  - Early-onset arthritis
  - Spondyloepiphyseal dysplasia
  - Joint hypermobility
  - Scoliosis
- Cardiac:
  - Mitral valve prolapse

Diagnosis

The diagnosis can be made clinically (particularly in the presence of characteristic abnormalities on ophthalmological examination), but can be confirmed by genetic testing. Some forms of Stickler syndrome present with an isolated ocular phenotype – the absence of other systemic features should therefore not rule out the diagnosis.

Inheritance

- Autosomal dominant (most cases): *COL2A1* (~80%), *COL11A1* (~20%), *COL11A2*
- Autosomal recessive (rare): *COL9A1, COL9A2, COL9A3*

Differential Diagnosis

- Loeys–Dietz syndrome (cleft palate, hypermobility)
- Isolated Pierre–Robin sequence
- 22q11.2 deletion syndrome (Pierre–Robin/cleft palate, hearing impairment)
- Marfan syndrome (myopia, retinal detachment, hypermobility, mitral valve prolapse)
- Kniest syndrome and spondyloepiphyseal dysplasia congenita (hearing loss, cleft palate, short stature)

Treatment/Management/Surveillance

- Airway management for micrognathia/Pierre–Robin (can require tracheostomy in severe cases)
- Assessment for cleft palate
- Regular ophthalmological monitoring (retinal detachment can cause permanent loss of vision if untreated)
- Regular audiological monitoring (hearing loss can be progressive)
- Speech/language therapy
- Management of musculoskeletal symptoms

See Snead et al. (2020) in the references.

Marfan Syndrome
Incidence

1 in 5000 to 10,000.

Genetic Aetiology/Pathogenesis

Marfan syndrome is caused by pathogenic sequence or copy-number variants in the fibrillin 1 gene (*FBN1*).

Clinical Presentation

Marfan syndrome is a connective tissue disorder of variable severity which can be diagnosed at any age. The cardinal features are aortic root dilatation and displacement of the ocular lens (ectopia lentis). Many patients have a characteristic habitus, but tall stature alone is not a uniquely 'Marfanoid' feature – more specific abnormalities include long limbs (dolichostenomelia) and fingers (arachnodactyly). Other musculoskeletal signs include pectus carinatum or excavatum, scoliosis, and hindfoot deformity and/or pes planus. The diagnostic criteria incorporate a 'systemic score' (see below), which facilitates objective assessment of a patient's phenotype.

Diagnosis

Diagnosis of Marfan syndrome is based on the Ghent criteria (see Loeys et al. [2010] in references):

- In the **absence** of family history:
  - **Aortic root dilatation** (Z score $\geq$ 2) *and* **Ectopia lentis**
  - **Aortic root dilatation** (Z score $\geq$ 2) *and* **FBN1** pathogenic variant

- **Aortic root dilatation** (Z score ≥ 2) *and* **Systemic score** ≥ 7 points (see below)
- **Ectopia lentis** *and* *FBN1* pathogenic variant (variant must have been previously associated with aortic dilatation)

- In the **presence** of family history:
  - **Ectopia lentis** *and* **Family history** of Marfan syndrome (meeting the criteria above)
  - **Systemic score** ≥ 7 points *and* **Family history** of Marfan syndrome (meeting the criteria above)
  - **Aortic root dilatation** (Z score ≥ 2 above 20 years old or ≥ 3 below 20 years) *and* **Family history** of Marfan syndrome (meeting the criteria above)

The systemic score is calculated based on the following features:

Feature	Score
Wrist *and* thumb sign	3
Wrist *or* thumb sign	1
Pectus carinatum deformity	2
Pectus excavatum or chest asymmetry	1
Hindfoot deformity	2
Plain flat foot (pes planus)	1
Pneumothorax	2
Dural ectasia	2
Protrusio acetabulae	2
Reduced upper segment/lower segment (< 0.85 [white]/0.78 [black]) and increased arm span/height ratio (> 1.05)	1
Scoliosis or thoracolumbar kyphosis	1
Reduced elbow extension	1
Three of five facial features: Dolichocephaly Downward slanting palpebral fissures Enophthalmos Retrognathia Malar hypoplasia	1
Skin striae	1
Myopia	1
Mitral valve prolapse	1

Inheritance

Autosomal dominant. The majority of patients (~75%) have inherited Marfan syndrome from an affected parent (who may or may not have been previously diagnosed). The remaining ~25% of cases are due to a *de novo* variant in *FBN1*.

Differential Diagnosis

- Loeys–Dietz syndrome
- Congenital contractural arachnodactyly (Beals syndrome)
- Specific monogenic forms of Ehlers–Danlos syndrome (e.g. vascular EDS)
- Homocystinuria
- Non-syndromic thoracic aortic dilatation syndromes

Treatment/Management/Surveillance

- Cardiovascular: Regular surveillance including echocardiogram and cross-sectional imaging (CT/MRI) by a cardiologist with experience of Marfan syndrome, pharmacotherapy to reduce risk of aortic dilatation (beta-blockers and/or angiotensin receptor blockers), prophylactic aortic root surgery if indicated

- Ophthalmological: Regular surveillance by an ophthalmologist with experience of Marfan syndrome, correction of refractive errors, surgery for ectopia lentis (rarely required)

- Musculoskeletal: Physiotherapy, surgery for severe scoliosis or pectus excavatum (rarely required), cardiothoracic management of recurrent pneumothorax

- Lifestyle: Avoid contact sports, rapid acceleration/deceleration, and significant pressure changes

Noonan Syndrome and Other Rasopathy Syndromes

Incidence

Estimated up to 1 in 1000.

Genetic Aetiology/Pathogenesis

Noonan syndrome is genetically heterogeneous. The most common causes are gain-of-function variants in the *PTPN11* gene, accounting for ~50% of cases. The remaining cases are due to variants in genes including *SOS1, RAF1, RIT1, KRAS, NRAS, BRAF, MAP2K1* and *LZTR1*. These genes are part of the Ras-MAPK signalling pathway, which regulates cell growth, differentiation, and proliferation. Other genetic disorders affecting this pathway can present with overlapping phenotypic features, and are collectively termed 'RASopathies' (see below) – see Rauen (2013) in the references.

Clinical Presentation

The main features of Noonan syndrome are:

- Facial features: Hypertelorism with down-slanted palpebral fissures, low-set and posteriorly rotated ears (Figure 15.26)

- Cardiovascular: Pulmonary stenosis, hypertrophic cardiomyopathy, atrial septal defect

- Growth: Short stature, poor feeding in infancy (usually normal birthweight)

- Pectus carinatum or excavatum, broad chest, broad/webbed neck

- Cryptorchidism

- Lymphatic malformations

- Coagulopathy

- Hearing loss (usually conductive rather than sensorineural)

- Renal defects

- Developmental delay (variable, usually mild-to-normal)

- Leukaemia and myeloproliferative disorders (e.g. juvenile myelomonocytic leukaemia)

Similar combinations of features can be observed in other RASopathies, which include:

- Noonan syndrome with multiple lentigines (formerly known as LEOPARD syndrome) (*PTPN11, RAF1*)

- Cardiofaciocutaneous (CFC) syndrome (*BRAF, MAP2K1, MAP2K2, KRAS*)

- Costello syndrome (*HRAS*)

- Neurofibromatosis type 1 (*NF1*)

- Legius syndrome (*SPRED1*)

RASopathies can also present in the prenatal setting, with features including increased nuchal translucency, cardiac defects, fetal hydrops, renal defects, and polyhydramnios.

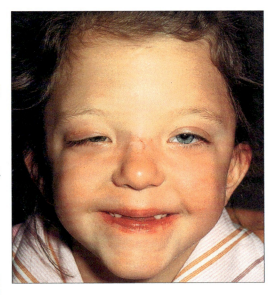

Figure 15.26 Child with Noonan syndrome.

Diagnosis

Noonan syndrome and other RASopathies are diagnosed based on the presence of characteristic clinical features and/or a pathogenic variant in a relevant Ras-MAPK pathway gene.

Inheritance

Most RASopathies follow autosomal dominant inheritance, with the exception of a rare autosomal recessive form of Noonan syndrome associated with the *LZTR1* gene. Up to 70% of cases of Noonan syndrome are due to *de novo* variants, with the remainder inherited from an affected parent. Since some patients are mildly affected, it is not uncommon for a parent to be diagnosed with Noonan syndrome after having a more severely affected child.

Differential Diagnosis

- Other RASopathies (see above)
- Turner syndrome
- Chromosomal abnormalities (*e.g.,* Williams syndrome)
- Aarskog syndrome

Treatment/Management/Surveillance

- Cardiovascular: Echocardiogram at diagnosis and in adolescence/adulthood, routine treatment for any abnormalities
- Growth: Regular monitoring with use of Noonan-specific growth charts, may consider growth hormone if significant short stature (rarely required)
- Cryptorchidism: Routine treatment
- Development: Regular assessment throughout childhood
- Hearing: Regular assessment
- Coagulopathy: Clotting studies, particularly before surgical procedures
- Renal: Ultrasound at diagnosis, routine treatment for structural abnormalities

Kabuki Syndrome
Incidence

Approximately 1 in 30,000.

Genetic Aetiology/Pathogenesis

Loss-of-function mutations in *KMT2D* (approx. 75% of cases) or *KDM6A* (approx. 5%). The cause in the remainder is unknown.

Clinical Presentation

The facial appearance is characteristic but may be difficult to recognise in early infancy. Features include arched eyebrows with lateral sparseness, long palpebral fissures with eversion of the lateral portion of the lower lid and prominent cupped ears (Figures 15.27 and 15.28). Growth retardation including microcephaly occurs, often with other congenital anomalies including congenital heart disease, cleft palate and structural renal abnormalities. Immune dysfunction is often present. Hypotonia is common in infancy and development is delayed. Learning difficulties are typically moderate.

Diagnosis

Diagnosis is clinical, with recognition of the characteristic facial appearance in the context of other supportive features. Mutation analysis is particularly useful in cases where the diagnosis is uncertain.

Inheritance

KMT2D: Autosomal dominant. However, the large majority of cases arise as a result of *de novo* mutations, meaning that the parents of an affected child are usually at low risk of having a further affected child.

   KDM6: Both males and females are affected, though females tend to have milder features.

Treatment/Management/Surveillance

Initial work-up should include echocardiogram, renal ultrasound scan, hearing assessment, T-cell subsets and immunoglobulins, and formal palatal assessment. Subsequently management focuses on monitoring and support of development, growth and specific abnormalities identified in initial work-up.

Rubinstein–Taybi Syndrome

Incidence

1 in 125,000 to 300,000.

Genetic Aetiology/Pathogenesis

This syndrome is caused by heterozygous deletions or loss-of-function mutations affecting the *CREBBP* gene in 50 to 70% of cases. Heterozygous loss-of-function mutations in the *EP300* gene have been found in a small number of cases (approximately 3%). The cause in the remainder is unknown.

Clinical Presentation

Children present with microcephaly with short stature and developmental delay. Learning difficulties are moderate to severe. The facial appearance is often recognisable with downslanting palpebral fissures, prominent columella and a grimacing smile (Figure 15.29). Thumbs and great toes are often broad and medially deviated (Figure 15.30). Structural cardiac and renal tract abnormalities are common and cryptorchidism is almost invariably present in males. The phenotype may be more subtle in individuals with *EP300* mutations.

Diagnosis

Diagnosis is by recognition of the characteristic facial and other physical features in the context of other supportive features. *CREBBP* copy-number and mutation analysis and *EP300* mutation analysis can provide molecular confirmation.

Inheritance

Rubinstein–Taybi syndrome is autosomal dominant; the large majority of cases arise as a result of *de novo* mutations, meaning that the parents of an affected child are usually at low risk of having a further affected child.

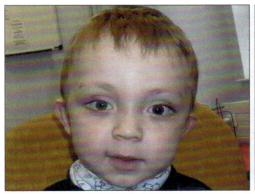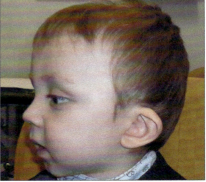

Figures 15.27, 15.28   Facial features of Kabuki syndrome.

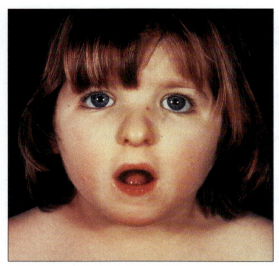

Figure 15.29 Facial features in Rubinstein–Taybi syndrome.

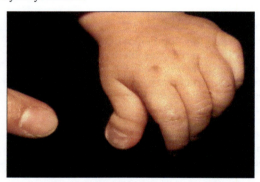

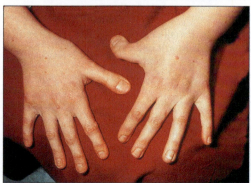

Figure 15.30 Appearance of digits in Rubinstein–Taybi syndrome.

Differential Diagnosis

Floating–Harbor syndrome (*SRCAP* gene – in the same pathway as *CREBBP*)

Treatment/Management/Surveillance

Initial evaluation should include echocardiogram and renal ultrasound scan. Subsequent management focuses on monitoring and support of development, growth and other specific abnormalities.

Cornelia De Lange Syndrome
Incidence

1 in 10,000 to 30,000.

Genetic Aetiology/Pathogenesis

Heterozygous deletions and loss-of-function mutations of the *NIBPL* gene cause typical Cornelia de Lange syndrome (CdLS). Mutations in other genes occur in a small percentage of cases (usually with atypical features). Around 20% of individuals with CdLS are mosaic for the gene mutation.

Clinical Presentation

The facial appearance is characteristic including synophrys, long thick eyelashes, upturned nasal tip, long smooth philtrum and thin upper lip (Figures 15.31 and 15.32). Additional features are pre- and postnatal growth retardation with microcephaly, limb abnormalities (Figure 15.33), hirsutism and learning difficulties. Limb defects range from phocomelia or ectrodactyly to more subtle hand abnormalities such as proximally placed thumbs or fifth finger clinodactyly. Most children with typical CdLS have severe learning difficulties.

Diagnosis

The diagnosis of CdLS can be made clinically based on the characteristic facial and physical features. Genetic testing can provide molecular confirmation.

Inheritance

NIBPL mutations are autosomal dominant. However, the large majority of cases arise as a result of *de novo* mutations, meaning that the parents of an affected child are usually at low risk of having a further affected child. *SMC1A* and *HDAC8* mutations are X-linked .

Treatment/Management/Surveillance

Children are monitored and given support for development, growth and other specific abnormalities including limb defects. Management of gastro-oesophageal reflux is often required.

Sotos Syndrome
Incidence

1 in 10,000 to 20,000.

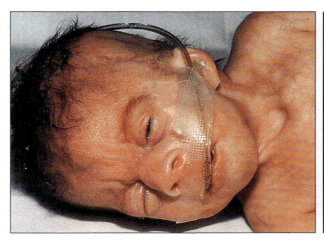
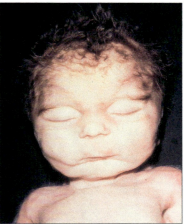

Figures 15.31, 15.32 Facial features of Cornelia de Lange syndrome.

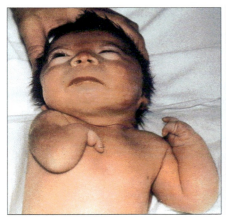
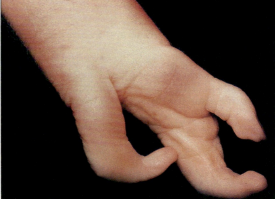

Figures 15.33, 15.34 Limb defects in Cornelia de Lange syndrome.

Genetic Aetiology/Pathogenesis

Heterozygous loss-of-function mutations and deletions in the *NSD1* gene occur in 90% of cases.

Clinical Presentation

Sotos syndrome is an overgrowth disorder, which often initially presents with pre- and postnatal macrosomia including macrocephaly. Bone age is advanced in the majority of cases. The facial appearance is characteristic with a tall forehead, high frontal hairline, downslanting palpebral fissures and a prominent chin (Figure 15.35). Developmental delay is very common and learning difficulties are usually present, but to a variable degree.

Diagnosis

Diagnosis is on characteristic facial appearance in the context of overgrowth and developmental delay/learning difficulties. *NSD1* mutation and copy-number analysis provides molecular confirmation.

Inheritance

Inheritance is autosomal dominant; more than 95% of *NSD1* mutations arise as *de novo* mutations meaning that the parents of an affected child are usually at low risk of having a further affected child.

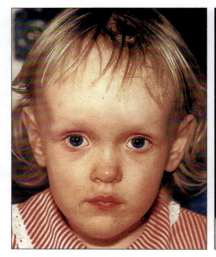 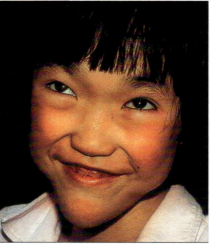

Figures 15.35, 15.36 Facial features of Sotos syndrome.

Differential Diagnosis
Other overgrowth syndromes and fragile X syndrome.

Treatment/Management/Surveillance
Children are monitored and given support for development, growth and other specific abnormalities. Annual surveillance should include assessment for scoliosis and blood pressure measurement. Unlike some overgrowth syndromes, additional cancer screening is not recommended.

Bardet–Biedl Syndrome
Incidence
1 in 150,000.

Genetic Aetiology/Pathogenesis
Bardet–Biedl syndrome (BBS) is caused by biallelic loss-of-function mutations in one of more than 22 currently known genes associated with the function of cilia. BBS is part of a group of conditions with overlapping features known as 'ciliopathies'.

Clinical Presentation
BBS causes truncal obesity (in 70%) and mild to moderate learning difficulties. Postaxial polydactyly (that may affect all four limbs) is often also present. Other features include progressive rod–cone dystrophy and renal disease with cystic kidneys and chronic kidney disease. Additional features include male hypogonadotropic hypogonadism and complex female genital abnormalities (e.g. hydrometrocolpos).

Diagnosis
Gene panel testing for known BBS genes. Renal ultrasound, renal function testing and ophthalmological assessment including electrodiagnostic testing are useful in detecting occult renal and ophthalmological disease.

Inheritance
Autosomal recessive.

Natural History
Initial presentation is with pre- or early postnatal detection of structural physical abnormalities such as postaxial polydactyly (Figure 15.37) or cystic kidney disease. Truncal obesity is present in approximately 70% and usually develops during the first year (Figure 15.38). Progressive rod–cone

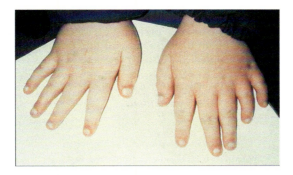

Figure 15.37   Postaxial polydactyly in Bardet–Biedl syndrome.

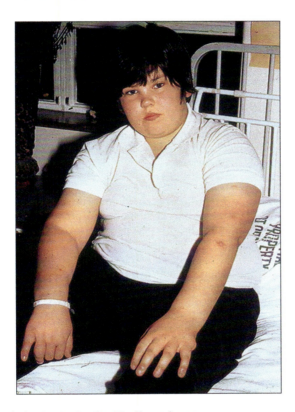

Figure 15.38   Truncal obesity in Bardet–Biedl syndrome.

dystrophy causes night blindness by eight years. The mean age of registered visual loss is 15 to 16 years. Renal disease is also progressive and end-stage kidney disease is present in 10% of patients. Diabetes mellitus and abnormal lipid profiles are also features.

Differential Diagnosis

- Other causes of childhood obesity/macrosomia
- Other disorders caused by mutations in ciliary genes (e.g. AR polycystic kidney disease, Joubert syndrome)
- Alstrøm syndrome (retinal dystrophy, obesity, sensorineural deafness, cardiomyopathy)
- Autosomal dominant HNF1β mutations (renal cysts, diabetes)

449

Treatment/Management/Surveillance

Regular ophthalmologic evaluation should be performed with monitoring of renal function, blood pressure, blood lipids and screening for diabetes mellitus and annual blood pressure measurement. Prenatal diagnosis may be available in future pregnancies.

CHARGE Syndrome

Incidence

Approximately 1:10,000 to 15,000.

Genetic Aetiology/Pathogenesis

Heterozygous pathogenic variants in *CHD7* on chromosome 8q12 are found in 80–90% of patients with clinical and radiological findings suggestive of CHARGE syndrome.

Clinical Presentation

The acronym CHARGE stands for Coloboma, *H*eart defect, *A*tresia choanae, *R*etarded growth and development, *G*enital hypoplasia, *E*ar anomalies and/or deafness. The most characteristic features are coloboma, choanal atresia and characteristic ears (external ear anomalies and small or absent semicircular canals). Cranial nerve abnormalities, including anosmia and facial palsy are common. Some patients have additional structural abnormalities including renal and tracheoesophageal anomalies. Affected individuals commonly have variable developmental delay and intellectual disability. Normal intelligence is seen in 30–50%.

Diagnosis

A molecular diagnosis can be confirmed by testing for gene variants in *CHD7*, either by single-gene sequencing or gene panel testing. A small proportion of patients (around 2%) have intragenic copy-number variants.

Inheritance

The condition is usually sporadic. Inheritance is autosomal dominant. The recurrence risk for unaffected parents is 1–2%. An affected individual has a 50% offspring risk, though the condition is commonly associated with hypogonadotropic hypogonadism and infertility.

Natural History

Most patients with CHARGE syndrome have difficulty with hearing, balance and vision, resulting in delayed motor development and communication difficulties. Intelligence can be underestimated as a result. Around 30% of patients with *CHD7* variants develop seizures. Overall life expectancy is reduced, especially in the first two years of life. However, those patients with relatively few medical complications can have normal lifespan.

Differential Diagnosis

- Mandibulofacial dysostosis with microcephaly (*EFTUD2*)
- Treacher Collins syndrome (*TCOF1, POLR1C, POLR1D*)
- Cat-eye syndrome (marker chromosome 22 with 22pter-22q11 inverted duplication)
- Syndromic microphthalmia (including *SOX2, OTX2*)

Treatment/Management/Surveillance

Management needs a multidisciplinary approach, taking into account problems with hearing, balance and vision. A checklist for health surveillance has been published by Trider et al. (2017) – see the references.

Goldenhar Syndrome (Hemifacial Microsomia)

Incidence

1 in 5000.

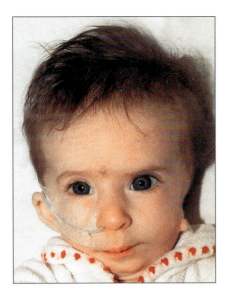

Figure 15.39 Facial features in Goldenhar syndrome.

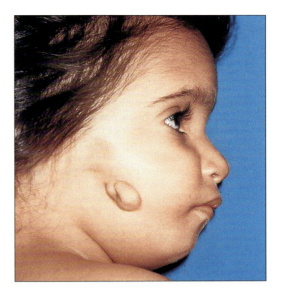

Figure 15.40 Facial features in Goldenhar syndrome.

Genetic Aetiology/Pathogenesis

Goldenhar syndrome is considered to be a non-genetic disorder that results from a vascular insult early in development.

Clinical Presentation

This is a disorder principally affecting the derivatives of the first and second branchial arches. Its features include facial asymmetry, macrostomia with lateral oral clefting, cleft palate and microtia (Figure 15.39). Preauricular ear tags and epibulbar dermoids of the eye are key features (Figure 15.41). Microphthalmia and coloboma also occur. Common extracranial features include hemivertrebrae, fused vertebrae and structural cardiac and renal abnormalities. Hearing is often affected.

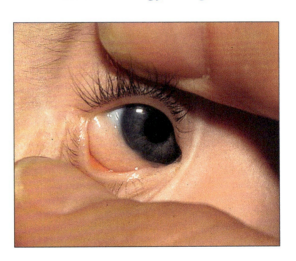

Figure 15.41 An epibulbar dermoid in a child with Goldenhar syndrome.

Diagnosis

Based on clinical findings and eliminating other diagnoses.

Inheritance

Sporadic.

Differential Diagnosis

Chromosome 22 abnormalities, particularly duplication and additional marker 22.

Treatment/Management/Surveillance

Management is best co-ordinated by a multidisciplinary craniofacial team including craniofacial surgeons, speech therapists, audiologists and ophthalmologists.

451

FURTHER READING

- **General Genetics Texts**
- Firth HV, Hurst JA. *Oxford Desk Reference – Clinical Genetics*, 2nd edn. Oxford: Oxford University Press, 2017. ISBN 9780199557509.

Web Resources

- Health Education England Genomics Education Programme (includes fact sheets on common genetic conditions): https://www.genomicseducation.hee.nhs.uk/.
- GeneReviews (this includes reviews of the majority of the single gene and epigenetic disorders covered in this text): https://www.ncbi.nlm.nih.gov/books/NBK1116/.
- OMIM – Online Mendelian Inheritance in Man: www.ncbi.nlm.nih.gov/omim/.
- Orphanet (supported by the European Commission, provides high-quality information on rare diseases, through a consortium of 40 countries): https://www.orpha.net/.
- DECIPHER database of chromosomal imbalance and phenotype: https://www.deciphergeno mics.org/.
- UNIQUE (Support group for rare chromosome and gene disorders providing free Information Guides to specific chromosome and gene disorders): https://rarechromo.org/.

Dysmorphology Texts

- Jones KL, Jones MC, Del Campo Casanelles M, eds. *Smith's Recognisable Patterns of Human Malformations*, 8th edn. Elsevier, 2021.
- Hennekam RCM, Krantz ID, Allanson JE, eds. *Gorlin's Syndromes of the Head and Neck*, 5th edn. Oxford: Oxford University Press, 2010.

Other Key References

- British Society for Human Genetics report on Genetic testing in children (2010).
- Joint Committee on Genomics in Medicine report on Consent and confidentiality in genomic medicine (2019).
- Brioude F, Kalish JM, Mussa A, et al. Expert consensus document: Clinical and molecular diagnosis, screening and management of Beckwith-Wiedemann syndrome: An international consensus statement. *Nat Rev Endocrinol*. 2018;14(4):229–249. doi:10.1038/nrendo.2017.166.
- Ferner RE, Huson SM, Thomas N, et al. Guidelines for the diagnosis and management of individuals with neurofibromatosis 1. *J Med Genet*. 2007;44(2):81–88. doi:10.1136/jmg.2006.045906.
- Legius E, Messiaen L, Wolkenstein P, et al. Revised diagnostic criteria for neurofibromatosis type 1 and Legius syndrome: An international consensus recommendation. *Genet Med*. 2021;23(8):1506–1513. doi:10.1038/s41436-021-01170-5.
- Loeys BL, Dietz HC, Braverman AC, et al. The revised Ghent nosology for the Marfan syndrome. *J Med Genet*. 2010;47(7):476–485. doi:10.1136/jmg.2009.072785.
- Rauen KA. The RASopathies. *Annu Rev Genomics Hum Genet*. 2013;14:355–369. doi:10.1146/annurev-genom-091212-153523.
- Richards S, Aziz N, Bale S, et al. Standards and guidelines for the interpretation of sequence variants: A joint consensus recommendation of the American College of Medical Genetics and Genomics and the Association for Molecular Pathology. *Genet Med*. 2015;17(5):405–424. doi:10.1038/gim.2015.30.
- Snead M, Martin H, Bale P, Shenker N, Baguley D, Alexander P, McNinch A, Poulson A. Therapeutic and diagnostic advances in Stickler syndrome. *Ther Adv Rare Dis*. 2020;1:263300402097866. doi:10.1177/2633004020978661.
- Trider CL, Arra-Robar A, van Ravenswaaij-Arts C, Blake K. Developing a CHARGE syndrome checklist: Health supervision across the lifespan (from head to toe). *Am J Med Genet A*. 2017;173:684–691.
- Wakeling EL, Brioude F, Lokulo-Sodipe O, et al. Diagnosis and management of Silver-Russell syndrome: First international consensus statement. *Nat Rev Endocrinol*. 2017;13(2):105–124. doi:10.1038/nrendo.2016.138.

16 Immunology

Austen Worth, Winnie Ip and Liam Reilly

BACKGROUND

Primary Immunodeficiency, more recently known as Inborn Errors of Immunity (IEI), are rare disorders affecting the development and function of the innate and/or adaptive immunity. The collective incidence varies depending on the population and epidemiological methodology. Reported rates of IEI vary from around 1 in 1200 people in the United States to 1 in 22,000 in France. There are 485 single gene defects described so far, according to the 2022 Update of International Union of Immunological Societies (IUIS) Phenotypical Classification for Human Inborn Errors of Immunity.

Secondary immunodeficiencies are more common. They are due to factors extrinsic to the immune system that impair its function, such as immunosuppressive medication, malignancy, and infections such as HIV/AIDS. Secondary immunodeficiency will not be discussed further in this chapter.

PRESENTING FEATURES OF IEI

Infection is the traditional hallmark of IEI, although only 10% of those referred with recurrent infection have IEI. Screening tools for PID include the 'Ten Warning Signs' (Table 16.1) and 'SPUR' (Box 16.1). Other signs include opportunistic infection, complication of live immunisations, chronic diarrhoea, poor wound healing, and granulomatous inflammation. Increasingly immunodysregulatory features of IEI are being recognised, including allergy, autoimmunity, organ-specific inflammation (e.g. inflammatory bowel disease, arthritis), predisposition to malignancy, and haemophagocytic lymphohistiocytosis (HLH).

BOX 16.1   SPUR

S – Severe
P – Persistent
U – Unusual
R – Recurrent

Children are less likely to have IEI if they have normal growth and development, respond quickly to appropriate treatment, recover completely, and are healthy between infections. Alternative causes for recurrent infection should be sought, such increased pathogen exposure (e.g. starting at nursery), poor housing, unimmunised, anatomical abnormalities, predisposing illnesses (e.g. IDDM).

NEWBORN SCREENING (NBS)

Treatment of IEI prior to the development of infections or other complications leads to improved outcomes. NBS for Severe Combined Immunodeficiency (SCID), has been introduced in several countries, including the United States, Germany, Israel, Taiwan and New Zealand, and data suggest improved survival and neurodevelopmental outcomes. Modelling suggests prevention of complications will make screening cost effective. A pilot study of NBS for SCID in the United Kingdom started in 2021 and is ongoing.

NBS for SCID detects T-cell receptor excision circles (TRECs) by PCR from dried bloodspots taken from infants in the first few days of life. TRECS are fragments of non-replicating DNA discarded during T-cell receptor formation. They are a marker of newly produced T-cells – recent thymic emigrant T-cells/naive T-cells (RTEs). Low TRECs detect severe T-cell disorders including.

CLASSIFICATION OF IEI

The IUIS have developed an internationally accepted classification of IEI summarised in Table 16.3. Antibody deficiencies are the most common, whilst isolated T-cell defects, including SCID are rare.

DOI: 10.1201/9781003175186-16

Table 16.1: The Ten Warning Signs of Primary Immunodeficiency (Adapted from Jeffery Modell Foundation)

Four or more new ear infections within one year

Two or more serious sinus infections within one year

Two or more months on antibiotics with little effect

Two or more episodes of pneumonia within one year

Failure to thrive in an infant

Recurrent deep skin, or internal organ abscesses

Persistent oral candidiasis or fungal skin infections (see Figure 16.1)

Need for intravenous antibiotics to clear infections

Two or more deep seated infections, including septicaemia

A family history of IEI

Table 16.2: Classification of IEI (Adapted from Bousfiha et al.)

Category	Subcategory
I. Immunodeficiencies affecting cellular and humoral immunity {Combined Immunodeficiencies (CID)}	(a) SCID
	(b) Combined Immunodeficiencies less severe than SCID
II. CID with associated or syndromic features	
III. Predominantly antibody deficiencies	Hypogammaglobulinaemia
	Other antibody deficiencies
IV. Diseases of Immune Dysregulation	HLH and susceptibility to Epstein–Barr Virus (EBV)
	Syndromes with autoimmunity
V. Congenital phagocyte defects	Neutropenia
	Functional
VI. Defects in Innate and Intrinsic immunity	Predisposition to invasive bacterial infection
	Predisposition to parasitic and fungal infection
	Predisposition to mycobacterial infection
	Predisposition to viral infection
VII. Autoinflammatory disorders	
VIII. Complement deficiencies	
IX. Bone marrow failure	
X. Phenocopies of IEI	

Table 16.3: Histiocyte Society Diagnostic Criteria (HLH2004)(5)

Criterion A	Genetic mutation consistent with Primary HLH
Criterion B	Five or more of the following:

- Fever
- Splenomegaly
- Cytopenia in 2 lineages (Hb <90g/L, Platelets < 100 x 10^3/ml, Neutrophils < 1 x 10^3/ml)
- Raised triglycerides or low fibrinogen
- Raised ferritin
- sCD25 > 2400 U/ml
- Haemophagocytosis in blood or bone marrow
- Low or absent NK-cell killing

OVERVIEW OF IEI MANAGEMENT

Stabilisation

Initial management must focus on aggressive treatment of infectious and inflammatory/autoimmune complications, in parallel with IEI investigations. Prolonged courses of intravenous antibiotics, and investigation of covert sites of infection should be considered.

Supportive Care

Appropriate anti-infective prophylaxis (against bacteria, fungi, viruses and *Pneumocystis jiroveci* (PCP)) and immunoglobulin replacement therapy (IgRT) should be started. IgRT is usually continued lifelong and may be given intravenously (IVIG) or subcutaneously (SCIG). Patients and families are routinely taught to give SCIG themselves at home whereas IVIG is usually administered as a day case. In specific conditions targeted therapies may be available.

Preventative measures such as protective isolation in hospital or the community is advised for the most severe disorders (SCID), however for most children with IEI, normal activities should continue, and it is essential not to restrict the child inappropriately.

Minimisation of cryptosporidium exposure by only drinking pre-boiled tap or bottled water, minimising contact with farm animals and avoiding swimming until avoidance of swallowing water can be guaranteed, is important for specific conditions.

Children on IgRT do not require vaccination, and specialist advice should be sought for live vaccinations (e.g. BCG, MMR, rotavirus), which are contraindicated in some IEIs. Other patients with IEIs should follow national vaccination programmes. Extra immunisations are advised in conditions such as hyposplenism.

Curative Treatment

Haematopoietic Stem Cell Transplantation (HSCT) is appropriate in severe conditions. HSCT may be lifesaving but carries significant mortality and morbidity, and risks must be considered carefully. Gene therapy, is available for ADA-SCID as a licenced therapy, and for highly selected other patients in the context of clinical trials (X-SCID, WAS, CGD, LAD1). Thymus transplant is the treatment of choice for congenital athymia (absence of thymus), such as in complete DiGeorge syndrome.

SPECIFIC DISORDERS

SEVERE COMBINED IMMUNODEFICIENCY (SCID)

Gene/inheritance	XL or AR
Gene defect	Various
IUIS Class	Ia
Treatment	HSCT standard

SCID is a clinical syndrome caused by absent T-cell development. It is defined by absent or very low RTEs. Over 25 genetic causes of SCID are described. Neutrophil, B and NK-cell development

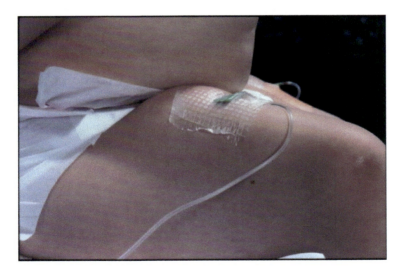

Figure 16.1 A 3-year-old girl with subcutaneous immunoglobulin infusion (markedly swollen thigh during infusion: normal finding).

may also be impaired. B-cells will not be able to function effectively due to the lack of T-cell co-stimulation. It is usually fatal in the first years of life without treatment. SCID can be caused by disorders of;

- Cytokine or T-cell receptor signalling
- DNA recombination (inhibitor T or B-cell receptor development)
- Metabolic defects leading to lymphocyte toxicity
- Congenital athymia

Presentation
Recurrent or opportunistic infections (particularly severe respiratory/gastrointestinal viral infections). Failure to thrive and persistent diarrhoea. There may be a family history of SCID.

Investigations
Very low RTEs (CD4+ve RTEs < 10%). Severe T-cell lymphopenia if no Omenn syndrome. Absent T-cell proliferative responses.

OMENN SYNDROME
Omenn syndrome is caused by oligoclonal dysregulated T-cells in a child with SCID, causing inflammatory immunopathology. This manifests as erythrodermic dermatitis, lymphadenopathy, hepatosplenomegaly, eosinophilia, and raised IgE levels. There is a normal or high lymphocyte count, but T-cells are highly activated, have abnormal T-cell proliferations, and oligoclonal expansions on V-beta repertoire analysis. Immunoglobulin levels are decreased. General management is the same as other forms of SCID, but they may also require immunosuppression with systemic steroids and cyclosporin, and intensive topical skin care, to manage inflammation.

RADIOSENSITIVE SCID
Radiosensitive SCID disorders are associated with a global disorder including short stature, microcephaly, facial dysmorphism and intellectual impairment. These disorders are caused by defects in DNA repair mechanisms. Some patients develop hypomorphic (mild or partial) SCID which can present with autoimmunity, granulomatous inflammation and infections.

ADENOSINE DEAMINASE (ADA) DEFICIENCY
ADA deficiency results in impaired purine metabolism, leading to build up of toxic metabolites which kills lymphocytes. ADA is also expressed in non-haematopoietic cells, resulting in neurodevelopmental delay, deafness, and skeletal abnormalities, although the severity of these complications is highly varied. Reduced ADA enzyme levels are found in haematopoietic cells, with increased toxic metabolite concentrations in plasma and urine. Treatment with pegylated Adenosine Deaminase (Peg-ADA) can be given intramuscularly as a bridge to either gene therapy or HSCT; however the non-haematopoietic manifestations can't be corrected.

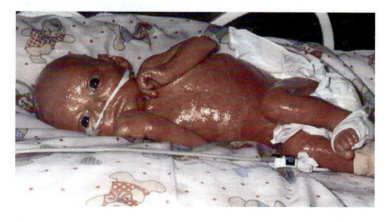

Figure 16.2   Omenn syndrome: showing erythrosquamous exanthema and hair loss.

Treatment

Patients should be transferred urgently to a specialist centre. They should be nursed in protective isolation and investigated for intercurrent infection, including the complications of live immunisations such as BCG infection. Patients require prophylaxis against bacteria, PCP, and fungal infections, as well as IgRT. They may be malnourished at presentation, which requires careful multidisciplinary management with enteral and parenteral feeding alongside monitoring for refeeding syndrome.

HSCT is the definitive treatment in most cases except thymic transplant for congenital athymia All blood products should be CMV negative (unless already CMV infected) and irradiated to prevent transmission of CMV infection and the possibility of transfusion associated graft versus host disease (TA-GvHD).

Prognosis

SCID is fatal without treatment, but survival rates with HSCT are around 70–95% depending on the genetic defect, stem cell donor source and tissue typing, and clinical condition when starting treatment.

CD40 LIGAND DEFICIENCY (X-LINKED HYPER IGM SYNDROME)

Gene/inheritance	XL
Gene defect	CD40LG
IUIS Class	Ib
Treatment	HSCT most

CD40 ligand (CD154) is a T-cell co-stimulatory receptor which interacts with CD40 on B-cells to induce class switching from IgM to affinity matured IgG or other immunoglobulin classes. Without this stimulation, B-cells are only able to produce low affinity IgM. CD40 ligand deficiency is the most common cause of Hyper IgM syndrome. Rarer autosomal recessive Hyper IgM disorders include CD40, AID, and UNG deficiencies, which also impair class switching. Hyper IgM syndrome may also be triggered by congenital rubella syndrome, medications (e.g. phenytoin), and malignancy.

CD40 ligand deficiency is a T-cell disorder which causes B-cell dysfunction, and therefore has clinical features of T- and B-cell deficiencies.

Presentation

Affected infants usually present with either PCP or recurrent bacterial infections after maternal IgG has waned (6 months old). They are particularly susceptible to cryptosporidium infection and

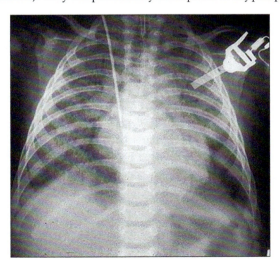

Figure 16.3 Chest x-ray of a boy with ADA-SCID and *P. jirovecii* pneumonitis. Note the interstitial infiltration predominantly in the left upper lobe and absence of a thymic shadow.

457

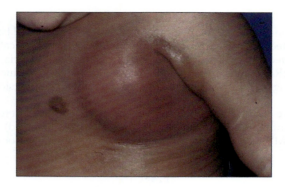

Figure 16.4 BCG abscess in a child with severe combined immunodeficiency (SCID).

may develop sclerosing cholangitis. Neutropenia and oral ulcers are common. They also have an increased risk of autoimmunity and malignancy.

Investigations
Normal or high IgM with very low IgG and IgA. Lymphocyte subsets usually normal. Absence of CD40 ligand expression following T-cell activation.

Treatment
IgRT should be started. Prophylaxis against PJP and cryptosporidium avoidance advice. Patients must be monitored for the development of liver and autoimmune disease.

Prognosis
HSCT is curative with excellent outcomes if performed prior to complications. Survival to adulthood with conservative treatment is typical, but bronchiectasis and liver sclerosis are life limiting (median survival 25–30 years).

WISKOTT–ALDRICH SYNDROME (WAS)

Gene/inheritance	XL
Gene defect	WASP
IUIS Class	IIa
Treatment	HSCT standard

WAS is a triad of eczema, thrombocytopenia and infections with a high risk of both autoimmunity and malignancy.

Presentation
Patients present with easy bruising or bleeding, severe eczema, cows' milk protein allergy, early onset inflammatory bowel disease, and recurrent infections of the upper and lower respiratory tracts. Only one-third of cases have a positive family history. X-linked thrombocytopenia (XLT) is a milder phenotype without significant immunodeficiency also caused by mutations in WASP. Patients frequently develop autoimmune haemolytic anaemia and/or thrombocytopenia, vasculitis, and lymphoma.

Investigations
Thrombocytopenia with a low mean platelet volume is characteristic. Lymphocyte subsets are normal initially. Immunoglobulins show a low IgM, normal IgG, and raised IgA. WASP protein expression is absent or reduced in peripheral blood mononuclear cells (PBMCs).

Treatment
Antibiotic prophylaxis, IgRT, and eczema treatment should be started. Autoimmune complications may require immunosuppressive treatment.

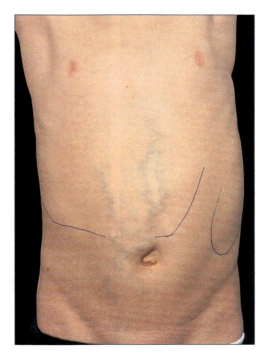

Figure 16.5 Caput medusae and hepatosplenomegaly (outlined) in a boy with CD40 ligand deficiency complicated by sclerosing cholangitis.

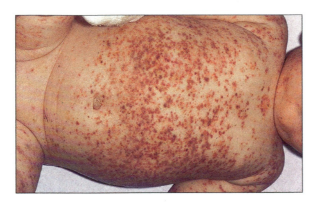

Figure 16.6 Wiskott–Aldrich syndrome: Extensive eczema and purpuric skin rash.

Prognosis

Prognosis is generally poor without definitive treatment. Although some boys will survive into adulthood they usually have significant complications. HSCT is curative and outcomes are excellent.

CARTILAGE HAIR HYPOPLASIA (CHH)

Gene/inheritance	AR
Gene defect	RMRP
IUIS Class	IIa
Treatment	HSCT standard

459

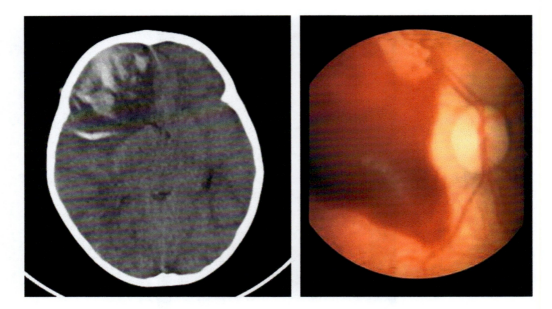

Figure 16.7 Intracranial haemorrhage and retinal haemorrhage after mild trauma in a patient with Wiskott–Aldrich syndrome.

RNase Mitochondrial RNA processing (RMRP) deficiency causes a syndrome of immunodeficiency and disproportionate (McKusick type) short stature. Clinical severity is highly variable and immunodeficiency is not always present but may be progressive. CHH is a rare cause of SCID, which is not always accompanied by skeletal dysplasia. Although rare, CHH is common in Finnish and Amish populations.

Presentation
Skeletal dysplasia may be evident antenatally with shortening and bowing of the femur. Other features include skin hypopigmentation, fine, sparse hair (hypotrichosis), nail dysplasia, and microdontia. Average adult height is reduced, typically 110–140 cm. Congenital gastrointestinal malformations may also be present. Recurrent or opportunistic infections may occur, including severe varicella zoster infection. Incidence of malignancy is increased.

Investigations
Lymphopenia may be seen, with reduced T-cells and reduced RTEs but normal B- and NK-cells.

Treatment
Prophylactic antibiotics and IgRT may be required. Live immunisations should be withheld until initial investigations are completed. HSCT will cure the associated immunodeficiency but will not affect skeletal manifestations. CHH patients are at increased risk of gastrointestinal obstruction, and malignancy such as leukaemia and lymphoma.

Prognosis
The prognosis is variable and depends on the degree of immunodeficiency, as well as autoimmunity and malignancy.

ATAXIA TELANGIECTASIA (AT)
See also the chapter 'Neurology'.

Gene/inheritance	AR
Gene defect	ATM
IUIS Class	IIa
Treatment	Conservative

The ATM protein is responsible for cell cycle regulation and DNA repair. Deficiency causes cerebellar ataxia, oculocutaneous telangiectasia, and immunodeficiency. Patients are radiation sensitive and predisposed to malignancy.

Presentation

Around 70% of AT patients have variable immunodeficiency. Recurrent respiratory infections, exacerbated by recurrent aspiration, may result in the development of bronchiectasis. Neurological features include cerebellar and extrapyramidal signs, and muscle weakness. Ocular telangiectasias may develop over time. Gonadal atrophy, poor pubertal developmental, growth failure, and insulin resistant diabetes may develop.

Investigations

Common immunological abnormalities include T-cell lymphopenia, IgA deficiency, IgG subclass deficiency and impaired T-cell proliferations. Serum alpha fetoprotein is usually raised. Assays of DNA double strand break repair are available in specialist laboratories.

Treatment

Antibiotic prophylaxis and IgRT may be required. HSCT can cure the immunological defect but will not change the alter the progression of neurological disease, and therefore is not routinely recommended.

Prognosis

The neurological features of AT are progressive with most patients being wheelchair users in the second decade of life. The median age of death is 25 years old.

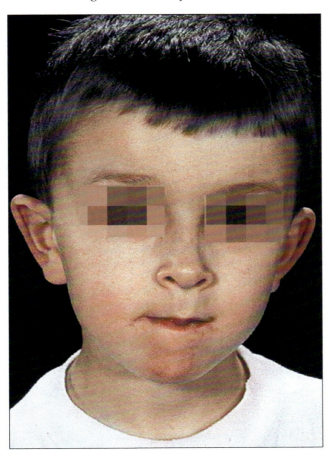

Figure 16.8 Ataxia telangiectasia: typical facial appearance.

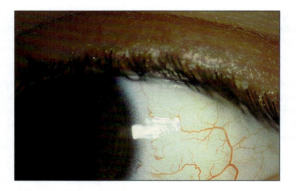

Figure 16.9 Ataxia telangiectasia: appearance of the eye.

DIGEORGE SYNDROME (22Q11.2 DELETION SYNDROME, VELOCARDIOFACIAL (VCF) SYNDROME)

Gene/inheritance	Usually spontaneous (may be AD)
Gene defect	*22q11* microdeletion, rarely *10p* del, *TBX1* (AR), *CHD7* (AD)
IUIS Class	IIa
Treatment	Conservative

Immunodeficiency varies from the rare complete DiGeorge syndrome with an absence of T-cells, to the more common phenotype of mild lymphopenia. Similar thymic defects may be part of other conditions such as CHARGE association.

Presentation
The clinical phenotype is a spectrum involving multiple organ systems (see section X). Patients with DiGeorge syndrome generally have more respiratory tract and sino-pulmonary infections, which are a consequence of both their underlying immunodeficiency and their anatomy and other complications.

Investigations
Lymphocyte subsets may show low T-cells with reduced RTEs. T-cell numbers may increase in the first years of life. B-cell and NK-cell numbers are normal, with normal antibody levels, however, vaccine responses may be poor. Patients with complete DiGeorge syndrome have extremely low RTEs with no functional immunity.

Treatment
Management depends on the level of immunodeficiency, ranging from thymus transplant in complete DiGeorge, to antibiotic prophylaxis, IgRT, and active monitoring. Irradiated blood products and avoidance of live immunisations until immunology investigations are concluded and complete Di George syndrome is excluded.

All patients will require multidisciplinary follow up with a general or neurodevelopmental paediatrics, psychology and psychiatry, Speech and Language, and other teams depending on the patient's other co-morbidities.

Prognosis
The outcome depends on the degree of immunodeficiency and non-immune manifestations.

AUTOSOMAL DOMINANT HYPER IGE SYNDROME (JOB SYNDROME, ADHIES)

Gene/inheritance	AD
Gene defect	STAT3
IUIS Class	IIb
Treatment	HSCT selected

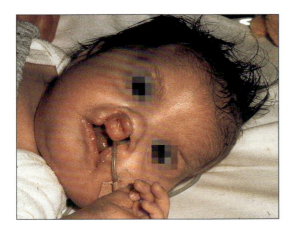

Figure 16.10 DiGeorge syndrome: characteristic facies.

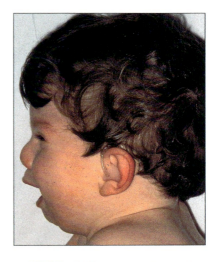

Figure 16.11 DiGeorge syndrome: lateral view of face showing small jaws and low ears.

Dominant negative mutations in *STAT3* lead to loss of function, resulting in impaired Th17 T-cell differentiation and T-cell subset imbalance.

Presentation

Typically, patients will have severe atopic eczema with recurrent staphylococcal skin and chest infections. They may develop coarse facial features, delayed loss of primary dentition, scoliosis, hypermobility and an increased fracture risk. Pneumatoceles develop following lower respiratory tract infections, and are at risk of superinfection with *Aspergillus* spp. Almost 50% have allergies. There is increased risk of vascular complications (strokes, early coronary artery disease) in adults.

Investigations

All patients develop high IgE levels, typically > 2000 IU/ml, although IgE may be normal at presentation. Other immunoglobulins are normal. There may be eosinophilia, reduced memory T- and B-cells, and impaired vaccine responses. Th17 T-cells will be low or absent.

Treatment

Anti-staphylococcal and antifungal prophylaxis is required. IgRT may be appropriate in some patients.

Prognosis

Death in childhood is uncommon. Quality of life for children and adults is variable, with many patients functionally limited by their disease. HSCT cures the immunodeficiency but not the non-haematological complications.

DOCK8 DEFICIENCY (AUTOSOMAL RECESSIVE HYPER IGE SYNDROME)

Gene/inheritance	AR
Gene defect	DOCK8
IUIS Class	Ib
Treatment	HSCT standard

Presentation

Similar to ADHIES, there are lower respiratory tract infections, severe eczema and recurrent staphylococcal skin infections. Additionally, there is an excess of cutaneous viral infections, allergies, and autoimmunity. Gastrointestinal manifestations such as enteropathy lead to chronic diarrhoea, failure to thrive, and impaired growth. Unlike ADHIES there are no skeletal or pneumatocele complications.

Investigations

T-cell lymphopenia with reduced RTEs and poor T-cell proliferation to anti-CD3. Immunoglobulin G, A and M are low, with high IgE. Th17 numbers are usually reduced.

Treatment

Antibiotic prophylaxis, IgRT and cryptosporidium avoidance measures should be started, before moving to HSCT.

Prognosis

Median survival without transplant is currently estimated to be between 20 and 30 years of age.

X-LINKED AGAMMAGLOBULINAEMIA (XLA)

Gene/inheritance	XL
Gene defect	BTK
IUIS Class	IIIa
Treatment	Conservative

XLA is caused by a block in B-cell development leading to an absence of B-cells and abrogated antibody production. Around one-third have a positive family history.

Clinical Presentation

Maternal IgG is transferred to the foetus across the placenta and provides initial protection for the newborn. Affected boys usually present following maternal IgG decline (6 months of age) with recurrent bacterial infections. Neutropenia can complicate infections. There is an increased risk of enterovirus meningoencephalitis.

Investigations

There is extremely low or absent immunoglobulins, B-cells and antibody response to immunisations. The BTK protein is absent on PBMCs.

Treatment

IgRT is the mainstay of treatment. IgG trough levels should be maintained > 8 g/L. Antibiotic prophylaxis may be required in some cases. Bronchiectasis is the most frequent complication, so interval chest imaging required.

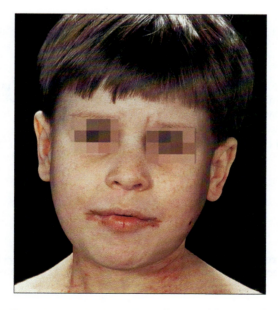

Figure 16.12   Hyper IgE syndrome: the face of an affected child showing coarse, pitted skin.

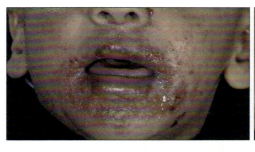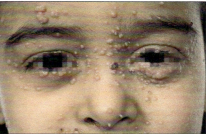

Figures 16.13, 16.14 DOCK-8 deficiency. Extensive perioral herpes simplex (16.13) and facial viral warts (16.14) in a 5-year-old boy.

Prognosis

Long term survival is excellent but development of bronchiectasis in adulthood is common.

COMMON VARIABLE IMMUNODEFICIENCY (CVID)

Gene/inheritance	Variable or spontaneous
Gene defect	Approximately 10% gave monogenic cause identified. Others genetically undefined
IUIS Class	IIIa
Treatment	HSCT selected

CVID is a heterogeneous group of IEIs with impaired antibody production and a variable degree of functional T-cell defect. It is likely to be polygenic with environmental triggers in most cases. There is an increased familial incidence but no clear inheritance pattern.

Presentation

CVID develops in late childhood or adulthood, typically with recurrent sinopulmonary infections, or unusually severe manifestations of common infections. Non-infectious presenting features include chronic diarrhoea, autoimmune cytopenia, inflammatory bowel disease and bronchiectasis.

Investigations

Diagnostic criteria are increased vulnerability to infection, autoimmune manifestations, poor antibody titres (IgG low + IgA or IgM), impaired vaccine responses, and exclusion of other causes of antibody deficiency.

Treatment

IgRT is required, plus antibiotic prophylaxis in selected cases. Monitoring is required to detect the development of bronchiectasis. There is an increased risk of malignancy, as well as autoimmune and inflammatory complications. These complications may be managed with immunosuppressive therapy.

Prognosis

Prevention of organ damage correlates with a good outcome for CVID patients. Inflammatory and lymphoproliferative complications have a poor outcome. In selected cases, HSCT may be offered.

ACTIVATED PHOSPHOINOSITIDE 3-KINASE Δ SYNDROME (APDS)

Gene/inheritance	AD
Gene defect	PIK3CD GOF (APDS1), PIK3R1 (APDS2)
IUIS Class	III
Treatment	HSCT most

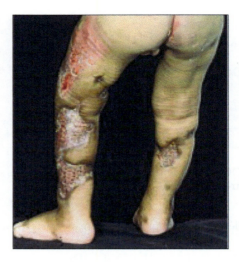

Figure 16.15   Severe pseudomonas fasciitis in XLA requiring skin grafting.

These disorders are caused by uncontrolled activity of PI3 kinase, a pathway involved in lymphocyte proliferation, survival and differentaition. This results in T-cell senescence and subsequent immunodeficiency and immune dysregulation.

Presentation
Patients usually present within the first five years of life, but diagnosis is difficult to make and therefore frequently delayed. Almost all patients develop recurrent respiraotry tract infections and are at high risk of developong bronchiectasis. Lymphoproliferation and autoimmunity is common. Patients are at high risk of developing EBV-driven lymphoma.

Investigations
T-cell lymphopenia with reduced RTEs is common, but not always present. Immunoglobulin G and A are usually reduced with impaired vaccine responses. Abnormalities of B-cell differentiation are common.

Treatment
IgRT is required, plus antibiotic prophylaxis is usually recommended. Close monitoring of lymphoproliferation and EBV to detect malignancy early is recommended. HSCTis recommended in most cases.

Prognosis
Early bronciectasis and lymphoma are both common, with median survival of 30–40 years of age. HSCT is curative, but challenging with high rejection rates.

TRANSIENT HYPOGAMMAGLOBULINAEMIA OF INFANCY (THI)

Gene/inheritance	Unknown
Gene defect	Unknown
IUIS Class	IIIb
Treatment	Conservative

THI is an exaggeration of the physiological fall in immunoglobulin levels after birth. It is a diagnosis of exclusion. Most children will have normal immunoglobulin levels by the age of 4 years old, but some do not reach normal levels until older. No specific treatment is required, although prophylactic antibiotics may be helpful if the patient has recurrent infections. Very occasionally, IgRT is required.

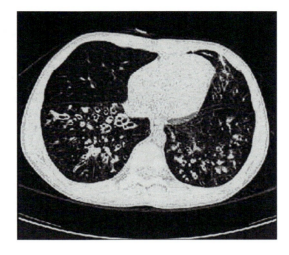

Figure 16.16   Bronchiectasis in common variable immunodeficiency.

SELECTIVE IGA (SIGA) DEFICIENCY

Gene/inheritance	Unknown
Gene defect	Unknown
IUIS Class	IIIb
Treatment	Conservative

This is the most common primary immunodeficiency, with an incidence of 1 in 600, however about 85% of people with sIgA deficiency are asymptomatic. It should be differentiated from other causes of low IgA, including THI. Children should be followed up annually to monitor for the development of associated conditions, including autoimmune cytopenias, coeliac disease, and recurrent infections. Progression to CVID is possible, so immunoglobulins should be measured annually.

HAEMOPHAGOCYTIC LYMPHOHISTIOCYTOSIS (HLH)

Primary HLH is HLH which develops in association with an IEI. This may be familial HLH (fHLH), where HLH is the predominant complication or as part of a wider immune disorder. There is uncontrolled hyperinflammation leading to persistent fevers, cytopenias, and organ damage such as coagulopathy, hepatitis, and CNS involvement. The untreated mortality rate is high. Currently accepted best practice is to follow the HLH2004 treatment guidelines with progression to early HSCT.

X-LINKED LYMPHOPROLIFERATIVE DISEASE (XLP-1)

Gene/inheritance	XL
Gene defect	SH2D1A
IUIS Class	IVa
Treatment	HSCT most

Presentation

XLP-1 may present as fulminant EBV disease with HLH, lymphoproliferation, aplastic anaemia, or progressive hypogammaglobulinemia.

Investigations

Bloods may demonstrate a reversed CD4:CD8 ratio, absence of NKT-cells and panhypogamma-globulinaemia. SAP expression in PBMCs is absent. There is a family history in 30%.

Treatment

Rituximab may be helpful in managing EBV infection. HLH2004 guidance should be followed for HLH, with progression to early HSCT. Milder phenotypes may be managed with immunoglobulin replacement.

Prognosis

Median survival into adulthood with conservative management is approximately 50%. Mortality is high after the development of HLH.

X-LINKED INHIBITOR OF APOPTOSIS (XIAP) DEFICIENCY (XLP2)

Gene/inheritance	XL
Gene defect	XIAP/BIRC4
IUIS Class	IVa
Treatment	HSCT selected

Presentation

XIAP deficiency has great variability in clinical severity and age of presentation. It may present with HLH, inflammatory bowel disease, antibody deficiency or autoimmune complications.

Investigations

XIAP expression in PBMCs is absent.

Treatment

Treatment is individualised targeted toward clinical and immunological complications. Early research into treatment of inflammation with biologic agents is encouraging.

Prognosis

Over 90% of patients survive long term into adulthood although quality of life is variable. HSCT is associated with high mortality particularly if GVHD develops.

CHEDIAK–HIGASHI SYNDROME (CHS)

Gene/inheritance	AR
Gene defect	LYST
IUIS Class	IVa
Treatment	HSCT most

Lyst deficiency causes impaired lysosomal trafficking and failure of granule release by cytotoxic cells.

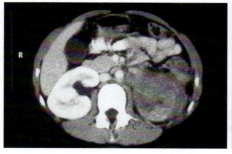 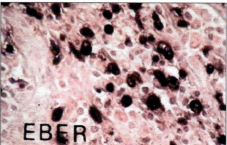

Figures 16.17, 16.18 Patient with APDS developed EBV-driven lymphoproliferation as a renal mass (16.17). Histology (16.18) showed xanthogranulomatous pyelonephritis, with positive Epstein–Barr encoding region (EBER) *in-situ* hybridisation which demonstrates active EBV replication.

Presentation

Partial oculocutaneous albinism and grey hair may be noted. Recurrent infections (viral and bacterial), antibody deficiency and neutropenia are common. In the stable phase there is a varying degree of immunodeficiency, but there is a risk of progression to an accelerated phase with HLH.

Investigations

Diagnosis is suggested by the typical clinical features. Large inclusions in neutrophils seen on blood film and abnormal pigment banding on hair microscopy have a pathognomonic appearance.

Treatment

HLH is managed as per HLH2004 protocols. The stable phase may be managed with antibiotic prophylaxis and elective HSCT to prevent the development of the accelerated phase.

Prognosis

Those who remain in the stable phase do well without HSCT, but the outcome is poor for those who develop HLH. Neurological sequelae can develop in adulthood, which HSCT does not prevent.

AUTOIMMUNE LYMPHOPROLIFERATIVE SYNDROME (ALPS)

Gene/inheritance	AD (FAS, Caspase10), AR (FASLigand)
Gene defect	TNFRSF6, TNFSF6, CASP10
IUIS Class	IVb
Treatment	Conservative

ALPS is characterised by failure of lymphocyte apoptosis. It is most commonly caused by FAS deficiency, although other extremely rare causes are described.

Presentation

ALPS often presents in childhood with widespread lymphadenopathy and hepatosplenomegaly. There is a risk of progression to haematological malignancy. Autoimmune cytopenia are common.

Investigations

This is an increased CD3+ CD4– CD8– (double negative T-cell) cells. Serum vitamin B12 and soluble FAS ligand are elevated. Functional testing of FAS mediated apoptosis is impaired.

Treatment

Monitoring for development of lymphoma is required. Parents should be counselled about the risks of trauma with splenomegaly. Autoimmunity is treated with immunosuppression, such as sirolimus.

Table 16.4: Genetic Diagnoses of Primary HLH (After Ishii (5))

Condition	Gene	Gene product/function
fHLH 1	Unknown	Unknown
fHLH 2	PRF 1	Perforin – apoptosis
fHLH 3	UNC13D	Munc 13 – granule release
fHLH 4	STX11	Granule trafficking
fHLH 5	STXBP2	Syntaxin binding protein 2
XLP-1	SH2D1A	SAP
XLP-2	XIAP	XIAP
Griscelli Syndrome Type 2	RAB27A	Granule trafficking
Chediak–Higashi	LYST	Granule release
Hermansky Pudlak type 2	AP3B1	Granule trafficking

REGULATORY T-CELL (T-REG) DISORDERS

Condition	Gene	Inheritance	Targeted treatment	Definitive treatment
IPEX syndrome	FOXP3	XL	Sirolimus	HSCT most
CTLA4 deficiency	CTLA4	AD	Abatacept	HSCT selected
LRBA deficiency	LRBA	AR	Abatacept,	HSCT selected
STAT3 gain of function	STAT3	AD	JAK inhibitor Tocalizumab	HSCT selected

All IUIS group IVb adapted from Cepika et al.

T-regs supress effector T-cell function and regulate B-cell activation, in order to maintain self-tolerance and minimise immune mediate damage. T-reg disorders often present with auto-immunity, enteropathy, lymphoproliferation and recurrent infections. Treatment is with immuno-suppression (steroids, cyclosporin) and targeted therapies (abatacept, sirolimus, JAK inhibitors). HSCT is usually challenging in these disorders but remains appropriate for selected patients.

CHRONIC GRANULOMATOUS DISEASE (CGD)

Gene/inheritance	XL (gp91) or AR (p47, p22, p40, p67)
Gene defect	CYBB (XL), NCF1, CYBA, NCF4, NCF2 (AR)
IUIS Class	Vb
Treatment	HSCT Standard

Neutrophils in CGD may phagocytose bacteria but there is a failure of NADPH oxidase to produce the oxidative burst within the phagolysosome, leading to defective pathogen killing. X-CGD accounts for two-thirds of cases.

Presentation

CGD may present at any age. Invasive infection with *Staphylococcus aureus*, *Salmonella* spp., *Aspergillus* spp. is common. Skin inflammation, poor wound healing, tiredness, and lethargy may also be seen. Inflammatory bowel disease is common. Granulomatous inflammation may cause strictures in hollow viscera, such as bladder or gastric outlet obstruction. X-linked carriers may have inflammatory complications but are not immunodeficient.

Investigations

Nitroblue tetrazolium (NBT) and Dihydrorhodamine (DHR) testing are functional tests of phagolysosome oxidative burst. Western blotting for CGD proteins can confirm the type of CGD.

Treatment

Co-trimoxazole is given for antibacterial prophylaxis due to its high intracellular concentration. Antifungal prophylaxis against *Aspergillus*, such as itraconazole, is required. Immunosuppression is frequently required for inflammatory complications.

Prognosis

Survival into adulthood without HSCT is possible but with increasing co-morbidities and ongoing risk of invasive infection. Outcomes from successful childhood HSCT are excellent.

LEUKOCYTE ADHESION DISORDER 1 (LAD1)

Gene/inheritance	AR
Gene defect	ITGB2
IUIS Class	Vb
Treatment	HSCT Standard

LAD1 is caused by mutations in the integrin *CD18* gene, resulting in impaired neutrophil adherence to the endovascular epithelium, and preventing neutrophils from leaving the blood stream to invade inflamed tissues. Two other extremely rare forms of LAD exist.

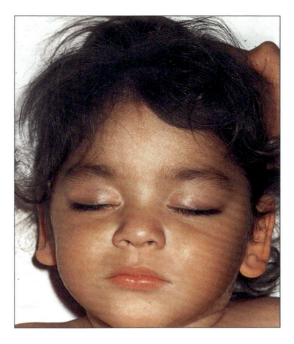

Figure 16.19 Chediak–Higashi syndrome in a boy, with greyish appearance of the hair.

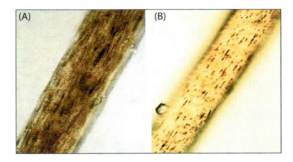

Figure 16.20 Chediak–Higashi syndrome. (A) Appearance of normal hair under the microscope; (B) patient with Chediak–Higashi syndrome.

Presentation

Neonates commonly present with delayed umbilical cord separation (> 21 days), omphalitis, and neonatal sepsis. LAD patients cannot form abscesses or pus and have impaired wound healing. They have high baseline neutrophil counts since their neutrophils cannot leave the bloodstream. Gingivitis and periodontitis are seen in older children.

Investigations

Baseline neutrophilia is seen in almost all cases. CD18 is absent from neutrophils in LAD1.

Treatment

Antibiotic prophylaxis and good dental hygiene are useful preventative measures.

Prognosis

HSCT outcomes are excellent. Some patients with late presentation and milder disease survive with conservative management, however usually prognosis is poor without HSCT.

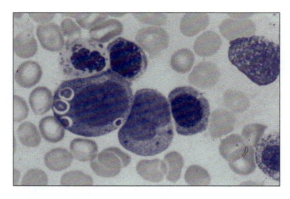

Figure 16.21 Blood film with giant inclusions in Chediak–Higashi syndrome.

CHRONIC MUCOCUTANEOUS CANDIDIASIS (CMC)

This is a group of illnesses characterised by recurrent and chronic fungal infections of the skin and mucosae. Invasive fungal infection is unusual. It is caused by a wide range of IEIs all impacting on IL17 function (IL17/IL17R defects, antibodies against IL17, or defective Th17 signalling (Hyper IgE syndromes).

AUTOIMMUNE POLYENDOCRINE CANDIDIASIS ECTODERMAL DYSTROPHY (APECED, APS1)

Gene/inheritance	AR/AD
Gene defect	AIRE
IUIS Class	IVb
Treatment	Conservative

APECED is a thymic defect causing impaired central tolerance, It is characterised by multiple auto-antibodies associated with endocrinopathies (Addison's disease, IDDM, Hypoparathyroidism). Autoantibodies to IL17 and other cytokines are associated with CMC. Treatment is supportive with immunosuppression for autoimmune complications, and specialist endocrinology input.

STAT1 GAIN OF FUNCTION (STAT1GOF)

Gene/inheritance	AD
Gene defect	STAT1
IUIS Class	VIa
Treatment	HSCT Selected

STATGOF1 may present with recurrent infections (viral, bacterial), autoimmunity or CMC. IL17 receptor signalling is impaired. Treatment is supportive, and targeted treatment with JAK inhibitors maybe helpful in severe cases. Anti-fungal prophylaxis is not recommended as this promotes resistance, but clinically evident infections should be treated. Published HSCT outcomes are currently poor.

MENDELIAN SUSCEPTIBILITY TO MYCOBACTERIAL DISEASE (MSMD)

Interferon gamma (IFNg) and IL12 pathway defects increase the risk of infection with environmental and weakly pathogenic mycobacteria, such as BCG. Over 35 monogenic disorders associated with increased risk of mycobacterial infection have been identified, with all modes of inheritance and variable penetrance.

Presentation

Mycobacterial infection is the hallmark of MSMD. There is also increased risk of non-typhoid salmonella infection.

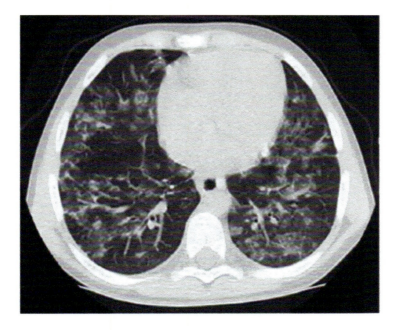

Figure 16.22   Granulomatous lymphocytic interstitial lung disease (GLILD), as a lymphoproliferative complication in a patient with a T-regulatory cell disorder.

Investigations
Cytokine stimulation assays can demonstrate a block in IFNg–IL12 signalling.

Treatment
BCG vaccination should be avoided. IFNg infusion may be given alongside anti-mycobacterial
chemotherapy for active infections. HSCT has been successful in severe disorders, but is extremely
challenging with established mycobacterial infection or active inflammation.

Prognosis
The outcomes vary with the underlying genetic Investigations.

ANHIDROTIC ECTODERMAL DYSPLASIA WITH IMMUNODEFICIENCY (AED-ID, NEMO)

Gene/inheritance	XL
Gene defect	IKBKG
IUIS Class	IIb
Treatment	HSCT Selected

AED-ID is caused by mutations in the NFkB essential modulator (NEMO) gene. It is one of over
20 disorders which disrupt signalling through the NFkB pathway. These disorders have variable
clinical phenotypes with features of CID/CVID, ectodermal dysplasia, mycobacterial susceptibility
disorders and T-reg defects.

Presentation
Typical facial features include frontal bossing, depressed nasal bridge, hypodontia with peg
shaped teeth. These children have sparse hair and eczema as well as absent sweat glands. They
often present with failure to thrive and diarrhoea. Recurrent bacterial, mycobacterial, and herpes-
virus infections are common. AED-ID is associated with autoimmunity.

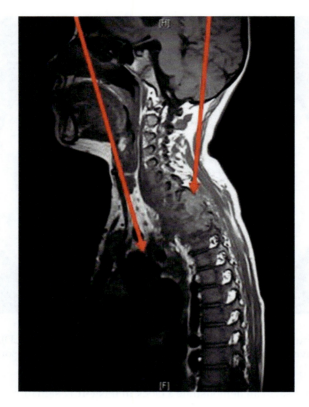

Figure 16.23 Invasive *Aspergillus* infection in a patient with CGD. Typical lung mass (left arrow) has spread and causes destruction of the spinal column (right arrow).

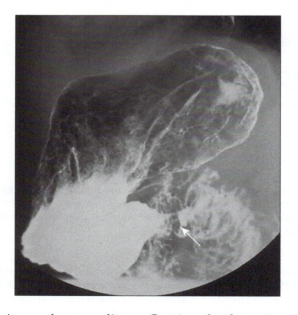

Figure 16.24 Chronic granulomatous disease: Gastric outlet obstruction.

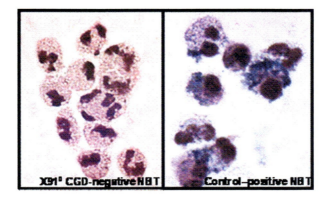

Figure 16.25   Chronic granulomatous disease: Nitro-blue tetrazolium test shows impaired oxi-dative burst activity in a patient with X-CGD (left, pink granules) compared to control (right, blue granules).

Investigations
Immune testing is highly variable. T- and NK-cell numbers and function can be reduced. Immunoglobulins may be low with suboptimal vaccine responses.

Treatment
Prophylaxis against infection should be started and HSCT considered.

Prognosis
Highly variable according to clinical phenotype and underlying genetic disorder. HSCT will cure immunodeficiency but does not cure all features of these disorders.

MYD88 AND IRAK4

Gene/inheritance	AR
Gene defect	IRAK4, MYD88
IUIS Class	VIa
Treatment	Conservative

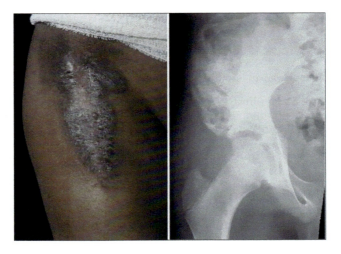

Figure 16.26   *Aspergillus* osteomyelitis and skin infection in a 6-year-old boy with X-linked chronic granulomatous disease before subsequent successful gene therapy.

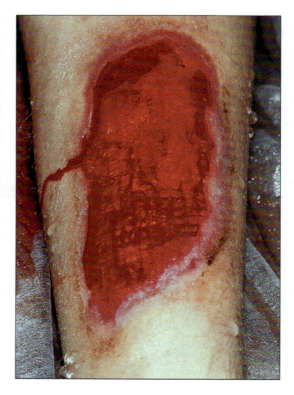

Figure 16.27 Large clean ulcer in leukocyte adhesion defects.

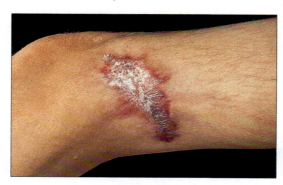

Figure 16.28 Dysplastic scar in leukocyte adhesion defects.

IRAK4 and MyD88 form a signalling complex downstream from several Toll like receptors (TLRs), which are important innate immune system pathogen receptors. This complex leads to activation of NFkB pathway and ultimately transcription of genes responsible for proinflammatory cytokines.

Presentation

IRAK4 deficiency leads to increased susceptibility to bacterial infection, including *Staphylococcus aureus*, *Pseudomonas aeruginosa* and *Streptococcus pneumoniae*. Importantly, infection in IRAK4 and MyD88 deficient patients may not cause a fever or a CRP rise. Delayed umbilical cord separation occurs in 20%.

Investigations

CD62 ligand shedding after TLR stimulation of granulocytes is impaired. Serum IL6 is inappropriately low.

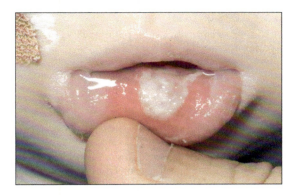

Figure 16.29 Persistent *Candida* infection in the mouth despite recurrent courses of topical therapy in Chronic Mucocutaneous Candidiasis (CMC).

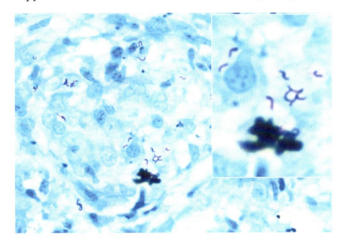

Figure 16.30 Atypical mycobacterial infection in a lymph node from a boy with NEMO, one of the Mendelian Susceptibility to Mycobacterial Disease (MSMD) disorders.

Treatment

Life-long antibiotic prophylaxis is recommended. Children may benefit from IgRT. Suspected infection should be managed aggressively.

Prognosis

Without prophylaxis there is a high mortality rate for children, but the incidence of infection appears to normalise by the end of the second decade of life.

FREQUENTLY USED ABBREVIATIONS

AD: Autosomal dominant inheritance
AR: Autosomal recessive inheritance
HSCT: Haematopoietic Stem Cell Transplantation
HLH: Haemophagocytic lymphohistiocytosis
IgRT: Immunoglobulin replacement therapy
IEI: Inborn Errors of Immunity
NBS: Newborn Screening
RTEs: Recent thymic emigrant T-cells/naive T-cells
SCID: Severe Combined Immunodeficiency
TRECs: T-cell receptor excision circles
XL: X-linked inheritance

111111111111111111

DEFINITIVE TREATMENT ABBREVIATIONS

HSCT standard: HSCT standard of care, almost all patients HSCT treated
HSCT most: Majority of patients treated by HSCT
HSCT selected: HSCT offered in selected cases
Conservative: Conservative therapy standard of care (exceptional patients may be treated by HSCT)

REFERENCES AND FURTHER READING

- Arlabosse T, Booth C, Candotti F. Gene therapy for inborn errors of immunity. *J Allergy Clin Immunol Pract*. 2023.
- Bousfiha A, Moundir A, Tangye SG, Picard C, Jeddane L, Al-Herz W, et al. The 2022 update of IUIS phenotypical classification for human inborn errors of immunity. *J Clin Immunol*. 2022 Oct 1;42(7):1508–1520.
- Castagnoli R, Delmonte OM, Calzoni E, Notarangelo LD. Hematopoietic stem cell transplantation in primary immunodeficiency diseases: Current status and future perspectives. *Front Pediatr*. 2019 Aug 8;7:295–295.
- Cepika AM, Sato Y, Liu JMH, Uyeda MJ, Bacchetta R, Roncarolo MG. Tregopathies: Monogenic diseases resulting in regulatory T-cell deficiency. *J Allergy Clin Immunol*. 2018 Dec 1;142(6):1679–1695.
- Delafontaine S, Meyts I. Infection and autoinflammation in inborn errors of immunity: Brothers in arms. *Curr Opin Immunol*. 2021;72:331–339.
- La Rosee, P Horne, AC Hines, M et al. Recommendations for the management of hemophagocytic lymphohistiocytosis in adults. *Blood*. 2019;133(23):2465–2477.
- Slatter MA, Gennery AR. Advances in the treatment of severe combined immunodeficiency. *Clin Immunol*. 2022 Sep 1;242:109084.

17 Rheumatology

Samantha Cooray, Clarissa Pilkington and Paul Brogan

INTRODUCTION

There have been many recent advances in paediatric rheumatology. New genetic diagnostics and more targeted therapies have improved the treatment of the inflammatory disorders resulting in better disease control and less organ injury.

JUVENILE IDIOPATHIC ARTHRITIS

Juvenile idiopathic arthritis (JIA) is the most common rheumatic disease of childhood and represents a heterogenous group of clinically and genetically distinct forms of chronic arthritis (persistent inflammation for six or more weeks with onset prior to age of 16 years). The UK incidence is 1 in 10,000; and prevalence is 1 in 1000 in children under 16 years.

SYSTEMIC (S)JIA

- Incidence: 0.3 to 0.8/100,000 children under 16 years.

- Onset: 1 to 5 years old; sJIA can occur throughout childhood and into adult years.

- Pathogenesis: Poorly defined, and complex; dysfunction of the innate immune system, in particular elevation of interleukin (IL)1β and IL6, is important.

- Genetic association: *HLA-DRB1*11* confers the strongest risk in sJIA.

Diagnosis

- Arthritis ≥ 1 joint.

- Rash: Salmon pink, macular and evanescent (not fixed), but can be erythematous, urticarial, or pruritic (Figure 17.1).

- Spiking fevers (Figure 17.2) lasting for two weeks with a quotidian (once a day) pattern for at least three days.

- Generalised lymphadenopathy with or without hepato-splenomegaly.

- Pericarditis, peritonitis (mimicking acute abdomen) and pleuritis can occur.

- Growth failure is common, secondary to disease or high-dose corticosteroids.

Treatment

High dose NSAIDs are used to control fever, pain and stiffness. Oral or intravenous corticosteroids are required by most patients. Methotrexate is used as a second-line agent when arthritis is the predominant clinical feature, although efficacy in clinical trials in not proven for sJIA. IL1 and IL6R-blockade (canakinumab and tocilizumab, respectivley) have proven efficacy in large

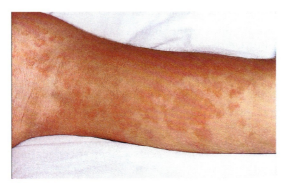

Figure 17.1 Typical 'salmon-pink' rash in the axilla and upper arm of a child with systemic onset juvenile idiopathic arthritis.

DOI: 10.1201/9781003175186-17

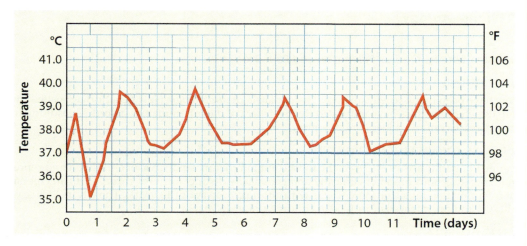

Figure 17.2 Swinging high fever chart in a child with systemic onset juvenile idiopathic arthritis.

randomised controlled trials for sJIA.' Anakinra (IL1 receptor antagonist) is used for macrophage activation syndrome (MAS), and/or if systemic features (fever and rash) persist. Rehabilitation, including physiotherapy and occupational therapy, are essential.

Prognosis

Biologics targeting IL1 and IL6 have improved outcomes significantly, with up to 75% in remission and off treatment after five years (Nienke M Ter Haar et al., 2019; Klein et al., 2020).

POLYARTICULAR ONSET: Rheumatoid Factor (RF-)Negative JIA
Incidence and Prevalence

RF-negative poly-JIA incidence is 0.3 to 6.5 per 100,000 children; prevalence is 1.64 to 33.4 per 100,000 children. The commonest onset is under 6 years of age, but it is seen throughout childhood.

Diagnosis

■ Five or more joints are involved within six months of onset.

■ Affects both large and small joints.

■ Early predilection for cervical spine and temperomandibular joint (TMJ) involvement with resultant micrognathia is common (Figures 17.3 and 17.4).

■ Knee, ankle, wrist, hip and elbow joints are frequently involved.

■ Contractures of joints or fusion of cervical vertebrae can occur if untreated.

■ Up to 50% of patients are antinuclear antibody (ANA) positive, with increased risk of chronic anterior uveitis in one-third of patients (Figure 17.5).

Treatment

■ NSAIDs.

■ Corticosteroids (either as intra-articular injection or systemically).

■ Methotrexate.

■ Anti-tumour necrosis factor (TNF)-alpha agents (etanercept or adalimumab) and tocilizumab are second-line treatments for resistant disease.

■ Physiotherapy, occupational therapy and podiatry.

■ Regular eye screening for anterior uveitis.

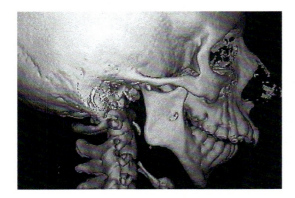

Figure 17.3 3D CT scan reconstruction, showing severe micrognathia in a 12-year-old boy with juvenile idiopathic arthritis.

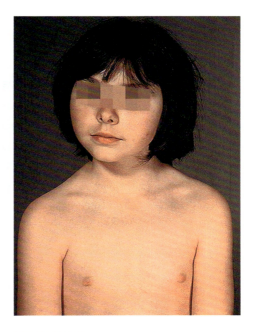

Figure 17.4 Torticollis due to cervical spine involvement in an 8-year-old girl with juvenile. idiopathic arthritis.

Prognosis

50% remit two to ten years after onset. The remainder continue with disease activity into adult years.

POLYARTICULAR RF-POSITIVE JIA

The incidence of RF-positive JIA is 0.3 to 0.7 per 100,000 children under 16 years.

Diagnosis

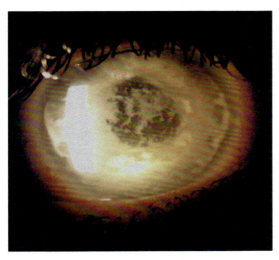

Figure 17.5 Uveitis: end-stage chronic anterior uveitis with visible calcium deposits of band keratopathy.

The disease is the equivalent to RF-positive rheumatoid arthritis. Onset is usually over 8 years, most commonly in females. Children present with symmetrical polyarthritis, involving proximal interphalangeal joints (PIP), metacarpophalangeal joints (MCP), wrists, knees, and feet. There is a high risk of erosion if not treated promptly.

Treatment/Prognosis

Treatment is as for RF-negative polyarthritis, with rapid escalation of therapy, in patients who fail to respond adequately to methotrexate, to biologics including anti-TNF agents (usually etanercept or adalimumab), tocilizumab or the anti-T-cell agent, abatacept. Physiotherapy is mandatory. Intra-articular joint injection with corticosteroid can be used concurrently with systemic treatments. Surgery may be required.

The disease is destructive unless treated early and has a worse long-term remission rate compared with RF-negative polyarthritis.

OLIGOARTICULAR ARTHRITIS

Incidence

Oligoarticular arthritis is the most common type of JIA (50–80% of cases); incidence 7 per 100,000 children under 16 years. It is commonest in females, with onset between 1 and 5 years of age; peak onset 1 to 3 years of age.

Diagnosis

- Fewer than five joints involved.
- ANA positive (> 75%).
- Risk of anterior uveitis (approximately 25%):
  - Clinically silent, diagnosed on slit-lamp examination.
  - Usually occurs in the first five years after onset of arthritis.
  - Slit-lamp examinations are recommended every three months.
  - Untreated uveitis can lead to visual impairment or blindness.
- Arthritis is usually asymmetric, involving knees and ankles in particular.
- Extends to multiple (5 or more) joints in up to 25% of cases after the first six months: extended oligoarticular JIA, identical to polyarticular JIA.

Treatment

- NSAIDs.
- Intermittent intra-articular corticosteroid injections.
  - Uveitis: topical corticosteroids and mydriatics.
  - Methotrexate is used for ongoing eye or joint disease.
  - Anti-TNF agents may be considered for resistant and/or extended cases.

Prognosis

Significant bony overgrowth may occur in affected joints, which leads to leg-length discrepancies and angular deformity (Figure 17.6). The extended form affects 10 to 20%, with greater risk for joint destruction and loss of function; 75% or more of patients tend to go into remission in late childhood, but the disease can persist especially in extended disease.

ENTHESITIS-RELATED ARTHRITIS

Formerly known as juvenile onset spondyloarthropathy or juvenile ankylosing spondylitis.

Incidence

1 in 100,000 children per year, typically in males > 8 years of age.

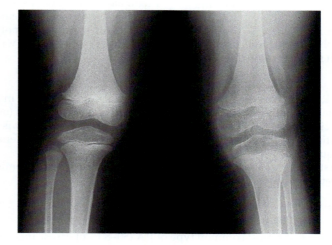

Figure 17.6　X-ray of a 6-year-old boy with oligoarticular arthritis of the left knee, showing medial overgrowth of the femoral and tibial condyles, osteoporosis, and early valgus deformity.

Pathogenesis

Th17 cells have been implicated as playing a role. Presence of HLA-B27 antigen or a family history of HLA-B27 associated disorders is common.

Diagnosis

The pattern is of a lower limb, large joint, asymmetric arthritis (Figure 17.7). Acute, painful, anterior uveitis occurs, but rarely causes permanent visual loss if treated. Enthesitis (inflammation of ligament and tendon insertions) is typical. It affects the insertions of the Achilles tendon and plantar fascia into the calcaneum; inflammation of patella tendon (quadriceps) insertion also occurs.

Spinal and sacroiliac involvement (ankylosing spondylitis) is uncommon in childhood but may occur in later life (Figure 17.8). Arthritis may progress to involve hip joints in adolescence and be very destructive.

Treatment

- NSAIDs.

- Corticosteroid intra-articular joint injections.

- Disease-modifying agents: sulphasalazine, methotrexate.

- Anti-TNF therapy for refractory or axial disease.

- Physiotherapy and occupational therapy.

Prognosis

Enthesitis-related arthritis persists or recurs intermittently into adult years. In some, remission occurs in late childhood. Ankle and hip arthritis are associated with a worse prognosis.

PSORIATIC ARTHRITIS

- Incidence: < 1 in 100,000 children.

- Diagnosis:

  - Arthritis associated with psoriasis (Figure 17.9).

  - May have oligo- or polyarticular course.

  - Characteristic dactylitis or swelling of toes/fingers (sausage-shaped).

  - Nail pitting and a psoriatic rash (or a first degree relative with psoriasis) are part of the diagnostic criteria.

  - Psoriasis may occur many years after the onset of arthritis.

  - ANA positive in 50% of patients, with increased risk of chronic anterior uveitis.

- Treatment: as for oligo/polyarticular JIA; skin disease may respond to corticosteroids, methotrexate, or sulfasalazine. Anti-TNF agents are also helpful.

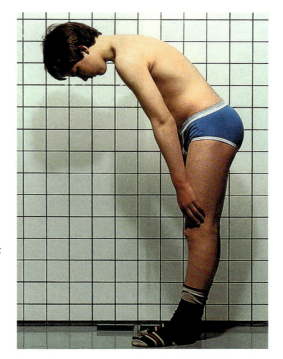

Figure 17.7 A 12-year-old boy with juvenile ankylosing spondylitis showing limited flexion of the lumbar spine and loss of lumbar lordosis.

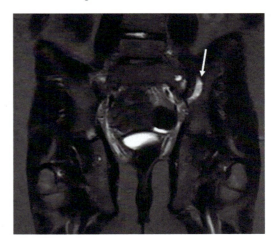

Figure 17.8 Sacroiliitis: short T1 inversion recovery MRI left sacroiliac joint showing bone marrow oedema (arrow).

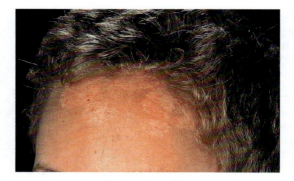

Figure 17.9 Psoriasis on the forehead of a child with psoriatic arthritis.

■ Prognosis: remission may occur in late childhood but can persist into adulthood.

ARTHRITIS ASSOCIATED WITH OTHER CHRONIC DISEASES
Inflammatory Bowel Disease

■ Arthritis occurs in 10–20% of inflammatory bowel disease patients with ulcerative colitis or Crohn disease.

■ Treatment of underlying bowel disease typically improves peripheral arthritis, but axial skeletal involvement may require more aggressive treatment despite good control of IBD.

■ Sulphasalazine may be useful. Methotrexate and anti-TNF (infliximab or adalimumab) may improve both gut and joint symptoms.

■ Arthritis and growth failure may precede symptomatic bowel disease.

Cystic Fibrosis (CF)

■ Between 2 and 8.5% of CF patients may develop an inflammatory arthropathy.

■ It is commonest in teenagers and young adults and is episodic.

■ Arthritis usually responds to NSAIDs, rarely destructive.

■ Hypertrophic osteoarthropathy in 5%: associated with severe lung disease: periosteal reactions of long bones.

■ Ongoing arthritis may require methotrexate.

Immunodeficiency

■ Humoral and cellular deficiency syndromes may be associated with inflammatory arthritis.

■ Rarely destructive or deforming. Treat with NSAIDs, physiotherapy and in some cases methotrexate.

Associated Syndromes

Patients with trisomy 21, Turner syndrome or DiGeorge (22q11.2 deletion) syndrome may all develop inflammatory arthritis requiring treatment.

SCLERODERMA

Scleroderma is characterised by thickened fibrotic skin and subcutaneous tissue. It is considered to be a vasculopathy with secondary changes in collagen and connective tissue.

SYSTEMIC SCLEROSIS

Incidence

The systemic form of scleroderma, systemic sclerosis (SS), affects internal organs; 0.27 to 1 per million children per year; and is much less common than the localised form.

Diagnosis

The progressive form has widespread skin and internal organ involvement. Skin changes are typically on the face and limbs, with loss of subcutaneous tissues, hardening and tightening of the skin with telangiectasia and calcinosis. Joint contractures are common, especially of the hands (Figure 17.10).

In the limited form there is oesophageal involvement and skin changes in the distal extremities. Raynaud's and nail-bed capillary changes are almost universal. Involvement of kidneys, lungs or heart can be life threatening.

Treatment

■ Avoid excess sun exposure. Topical skin-softening treatments. Dynamic splints.

■ Corticosteroids; methotrexate; mycophenolate mofetil; intravenous cyclophosphamide, although disease may be unresponsive in some patients.

■ Raynaud's: Nifedipine, glyceryl trinitrate patches, iloprost if severe.

■ Bosentan and ACE inhibitors, for cardiopulmonary and renal disease respectively.

Prognosis

Mortality is 5–10% during childhood but is improved with early treatment of complications such as pulmonary hypertension and renal disease.

LOCALISED SCLERODERMA (MORPHOEA)

Incidence

Morphoea affects 0.34 to 2.7 in 100,000 children per year.

Diagnosis

Children may present with morphoea (round or oval patches of indurated, hyper- or hypopigmented skin), which may become widespread (diffuse form). Linear scleroderma usually affects limbs (upper and / or lower) or face (*en coup de sabre*) or trunk. The *en coup de sabre* lesion is associated with uveitis and cerebral involvement (seizures) (Figure 17.11).

Disease may be severe, with thickening of superficial skin, loss of subcutaneous tissue, deformity of long bones, and failure of limb growth (Figure 17.12). Contractures of joints are common.

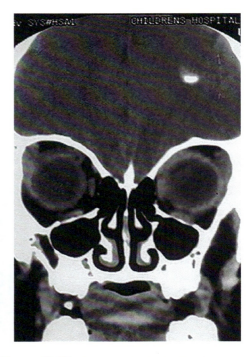

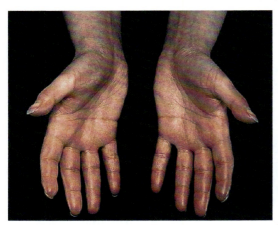

Figure 17.10 Severe sclerodactyly in a 15-year-old girl with systemic sclerosis.

Figure 17.11 Intracerebral calcification shown on CT scan in a 5-year-old child with localised scleroderma of the face on the same side.

Treatment/Prognosis

Methotrexate with or without corticosteroids may halt progress of the disease. Mycophenolate mofetil can be used if methotrexate is not tolerated. Physical therapies are essential to improve function.

Active disease occurs in many for five to six years; disease may progress despite treatment.

JUVENILE DERMATOMYOSITIS

A rare autoimmune vasculopathy that mainly affects the skin but also affects joints and other organs.

Incidence

Juvenile dermatomyositis (JDM) affects 1.9 to 4.1 cases in 1 million children per year. The mean age of onset is 7 years; 25% of cases occur before the age of 4 years; more common in girls. There is no association with malignancy (unlike adult cases).

Diagnosis

- Typical heliotrope rash (bluish-purple colour) over the eyelids with periorbital oedema (Figure 17.13).

- Gottron's papules: thickened erythematous, scaly rash over extensor surfaces (Figure 17.14).

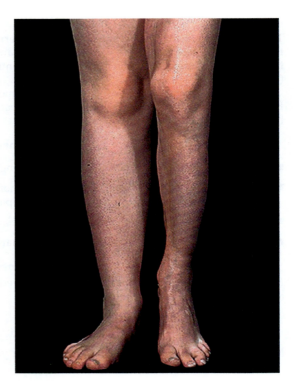

Figure 17.12 Severe localised scleroderma of the left leg in a 6-year-old girl showing tissue atrophy and local growth failure.

- Progressive proximal muscle weakness of hip, shoulder, trunk, and neck muscles.

Other features:

- Systemic symptoms (fever, malaise, anorexia, weight loss, irritability).
- Arthritis, myalgia, contractures.
- Dysphagia, dyspnoea, dysphonia: oesophageal muscle involvement.
- Lipoatrophy, calcinosis, skin ulceration, oedema.
- Respiratory failure – respiratory muscle involvement.
- Interstitial lung disease (ILD) in 5–10%.

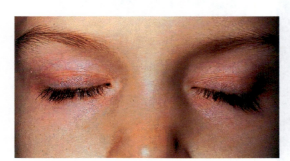

Figure 17.13 Typical heliotrope rash on the eyelids of a 7-year-old girl with juvenile dermatomyositis.

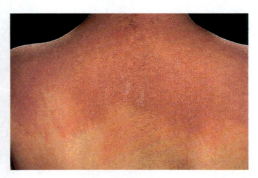

Figure 17.14 A photosensitive 'shawl' distribution rash in a 10-year-old girl with juvenile dermatomyositis.

There is elevation of muscle enzymes early on in the disease, including creatinine kinase, lactate dehydrogenase, aspartate aminotransferase and alanine aminotransferase. Muscle involvement on MRI findings; characteristic muscle biopsy appearance. Enzymes may not be elevated in chronic JDM, particularly if muscle-wasting is present.

Treatment

High-dose long-term corticosteroids (often intravenous followed by oral) are used with disease-modifying anti-rheumatic drugs or DMARDS (e.g. methotrexate, intravenous immunoglobulin [IVIg] or mycophenolate mofetil) together with vitamin D supplementation and photoprotective measures. Hydroxychloroquine may be useful for persistent severe rash. Intravenous cyclophosphamide, tacrolimus, or anti-TNF agents are used in resistant or severe disease. Physical therapies are essential to prevent contractures and improve function. Disease activity is monitored clinically with muscle strength, skin involvement, nail-bed capillary involvement, as well as, muscle enzymes. MRI (Figure 17.15) can be useful to monitor myositis.

Prognosis

The mortality rate is 1–2%. Mortality is associated with severe disease (ulceration, ILD, gastrointestinal involvement). Poorer outcome occurs with delayed diagnosis and late treatment, with loss of muscle, contractures, and calcinosis. Skin disease is often difficult to control.

VASCULITIDES

IgA VASCULITIS (IgAV)

See also the chapter 'Kidney Diseases'.

Incidence/Pathogenesis

IgAV is the commonest vasculitis in childhood, with an incidence of 3 to 26.7 per 100,000 children. The pathogenesis is unknown, but there is a probable polygenic contribution. It presents as a vasculitis with deposition of IgA1 in small vessels of the skin, gut, and glomeruli. IgAV nephritis (IgAVN) arises from deposition of immune complexes comprised of galactose-deficient IgA1 and anti-glycan antibodies resulting in mesangial deposition, and renal injury. Disease is more common in winter and may be triggered by a bacterial or viral infection.

Clinical Presentation

Classification criteria are palpable purpura (Figure 17.16) in a predominantly lower limb distribution with at least one of:

- Diffuse abdominal pain.

- Any biopsy showing IgA deposition.

- Arthritis and/or arthralgia.

- Haematuria or proteinuria.

Presentation is variable:

- 60% have arthritis and/or arthralgia: usually knees and ankles.

- 25 to 60% have renal involvement.

- 68% have gastrointestinal involvement: intermittent colicky abdominal pain, vomiting, with or without haematemesis or melaena. Intussusception, appendicitis, cholecystitis, pancreatitis, orchitis, gastrointestinal haemorrhage, ulceration, infarction or perforation can occur.

- 43% of patients: abdominal pain precedes rash by 1 to 14 days.

- Of those who develop renal involvement, 76% do so within four weeks of disease onset; and 97% will develop IgAVN within three months.

Diagnosis

Skin histology can be helpful in atypical cases, and shows a leucocytoclastic cutaneous vasculitis with predominant IgA deposition. Renal involvement demonstrates focal and segmental proliferative glomerulonephritis, sometimes crescentic glomerulonephritis (Figure 17.17). Serum IgA

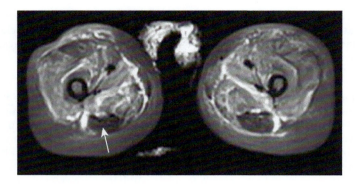

Figure 17.15   MRI of the thighs of a 3-year-old boy with juvenile dermatomyositis showing widespread muscle oedema due to inflammation.

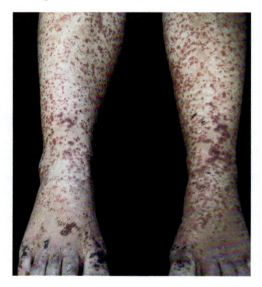

Figure 17.16   Typical (severe) palpable purpura of IgA Vasculitis in a 13-year-old female without renal involvement.

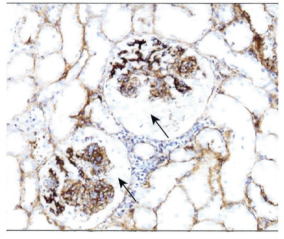

Figure 17.17   Immunohistochemistry of renal histology from a 16-year-old male with IgAV and heavy proteinuria, showing: Diffuse mesangial matrix expansion and thickening of capillary walls; strong diffuse granular mesangial and capillary wall IgA deposition; fibrocellular crescentic change is also present in both the glomeruli (arrowed).

may be elevated. It is essential to measure BP, monitor urine dipstick for haematuria and proteinuria and check renal function.

Differential Diagnosis

- Sepsis.
- Other systemic vasculitides.
- Monogenetic autoinflammatory vasculitides (e.g. mevalonate kinase deficiency; several others).

Treatment

Treatment is symptomatic, including rest and analgesia. Corticosteroids do not prevent renal or gastrointestinal involvement, but may be therapeutically useful should these develop. Indications for corticosteroids include renal, gastrointestinal, severe facial and/or scrotal involvement. Severe renal involvement may require additional immunosuppressive agents, antiproteinuric and antihypertensive agents (see the chapter 'Kidney Diseases').

Prognosis

The severity of IgAVN is the main prognostic determinant, causing 1.6–3% of all childhood end-stage kidney disease in the United Kingdom. Some patients show a relapsing course: one-third have symptoms for up to a fortnight, one-third for up to one month and one-third with recurrence of symptoms within four months.

KAWASAKI DISEASE

Incidence

Kawasaki disease (KD) is the second commonest vasculitis and the leading cause of acquired heart disease in children in developed countries. It has a worldwide distribution, with a male preponderance. UK incidence is 4.9 in 100,000 children under 5 years old; in Japan the incidence is 308 in 100,000 children under 5 years old.

Pathogenesis

KD has a pronounced seasonality, with occasional epidemics and clustering of cases. No single infectious agent has been found. The exact aetiology of KD remains unknown; it may result from an infection evoking an abnormal immunological response in genetically susceptible individuals. Children with features in common with KD have been observed three to four weeks after infection with SARS-CoV-2 as part of a spectrum of disease referred to as paediatric multisystem inflammatory syndrome temporally associated with COVID-19 (PIMS-TS); however it is now generally accepted that PIMS-TS is a separate entity from KD.

Diagnosis

Diagnosis requires five of six criteria of:

■ Fever persisting for five days or more.

■ Reddening of the palms and soles, indurative oedema, and subsequent desquamation.

■ A polymorphous exanthem (Figure 17.18).

■ Bilateral conjunctival injection or congestion.

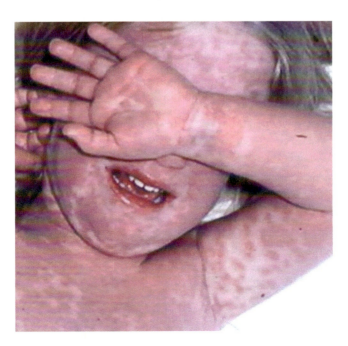

Figure 17.18 Characteristic polymorphous exanthema and reddening of the lips in a 4-year-old with Kawasaki disease. (Courtesy of Prof. N. Klein.)

- Lips and oral cavity changes (reddening or cracking of lips, strawberry tongue, oral and pharyngeal injection).

- Acute non-purulent cervical lymphadenopathy.

- Can be diagnosed less than five days if coronary artery aneurysm (CAA) or dilatation are present.

Symptoms and signs may present sequentially. Patients can develop coronary artery aneurysms (CAA): 15–40% in untreated cases, usually falling to 4% with treatment. More recently, CAA outcomes have been described as poorer, despite IVIg treatment, leading to exploration of other treatments in clinical trials. Other clinical features include arthritis, aseptic meningitis, pneumonitis, uveitis, gastroenteritis, meatitis and dysuria and otitis.

Differential Diagnosis

- Scarlet fever.

- Rheumatic fever.

- Streptococcal or staphylococcal toxic shock syndrome.

- Staphylococcal scalded skin syndrome.

- PIMS-TS.

- sJIA.

- Infantile polyarteritis nodosa.

- SLE.

- Adenovirus, enterovirus, EBV, CMV, parvovirus, influenza virus.

- *Mycoplasma pneumoniae* infection.

- Measles.

- Lymphoma – particularly for IVIg resistant cases.

Treatment

IVIg 2 g/kg is given as a single infusion over 12 hours. IVIg should be given even after ten days if there are signs of persisting inflammation such as elevated C-reactive protein. IVIg resistance occurs in up to 20 to 30% of cases. A second dose of IVIg and/or corticosteroids should be considered. Severe cases including those deemed at high risk of IVIg resistance should have corticosteroids plus IVIg as primary therapy. A major international trial of adjunctive corticosteroids is ongoing for KD, across the United Kingdom and Europe.

For fever, aspirin 30 to 50 mg/kg/day can be given in four divided doses; the dose of aspirin is reduced to 2 to 5 mg/kg/day when the fever settles, continued for a minimum of six weeks.

Refractory cases, consider:

- Infliximab (anti-TNF agent).

- Anakinra (IL1 receptor antagonist).

- Patients with giant aneurysms require life-long anticoagulation, in addition to aspirin.

Prognosis

Treatment with IVIg and aspirin reduces CAA from 25% for untreated cases to 4%. Clinical trials now suggest the addition of corticosteroids to IVIg as primary therapy for severe cases.

IVIg resistance is associated with a higher risk of CAA. The acute mortality rate due to myocardial infarction is < 1% but the disease may contribute to the burden of adult cardiovascular disease.

POLYARTERITIS NODOSA

Incidence/Pathogenesis

PAN is a necrotising vasculitis associated with aneurysmal nodules along the walls of medium-sized muscular arteries. It affects approximately two to nine per million individuals annually. Peak age of onset in childhood is 7 to 11 years, with slight male preponderance.

Pathogenesis is unknown. Deficiency of adenosine deaminase Type 2 (DADA2) is a monogenic disease with features of PAN.

Clinical Presentation

Malaise, fever, weight loss, skin rash, myalgia, abdominal pain and arthropathy. Vasculitic skin lesions include livedo reticularis (Figure 17.19), skin nodules, superficial skin infarctions, deep skin infarctions and peripheral tissue (nose and ear tips) necrosis/gangrene.

Haematuria, proteinuria, hypertension, abdominal pain, gastrointestinal haemorrhage, perforation, and pancreatitis can present. Neurological features such as focal defects, hemiplegia, visual loss, mononeuritis multiplex and organic psychosis may also be present.

Classification criteria for PAN in children are histopathology or angiographic abnormalities (mandatory) plus one of:

- Skin involvement.
- Myalgia/muscle tenderness.
- Hypertension.
- Peripheral neuropathy.
- Renal involvement.

Diagnosis

Selective visceral digital subtraction catheter angiography (Figure 17.20) shows abnormalities in medium-vessel walls (e.g. aneurysms). Tissue biopsy (Figure 17.21) demonstrates medium-vessel vasculitis.

Differential Diagnosis

- Other vasculitides.
- Monogenetic autoinflammatory diseases: MVK deficiency; interferonopathies; DADA2; others.
- Other autoimmune connective tissue diseases.
- Infections:
    - Bacterial, particularly streptococcal infections, and subacute bacterial endocarditis.
    - Viral, particularly hepatitis B/C, CMV, EBV, parvovirus B19 and consider HIV.
- Malignancy: lymphoma, leukaemia and other malignancies can mimic PAN.

Treatment

Induce and maintain remission.

Induction therapy: High-dose corticosteroid with an additional cytotoxic agent such as intravenous cyclophosphamide monthly for three to six months. A recent clinical trial has suggested that

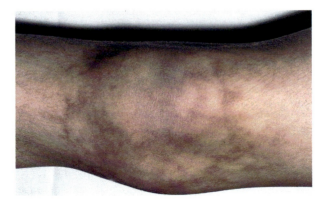

Figure 17.19   Livedo reticularis.

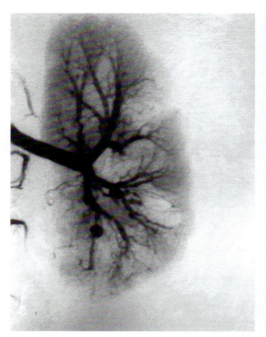
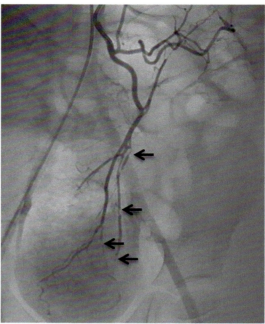

Figure 17.20 (A) Selective renal digital subtraction arteriography in an 8-year-old girl with polyarteritis nodosa. Large aneurysms, small aneurysms, renal, parenchymal perfusion defects, and calibre variation of intrarenal arteries are demonstrated. Perfusion defects in the renal cortex are also present; (B) selective mesenteric digital subtraction arteriography in a 6-year-old boy with partially treated polyarteritis nodosa. More subtle changes, including calibre variation and beading of medium-sized mesenteric arteries are demonstrated (arrowed) and these are unlikely to have been detected using non-invasive angiography such as CT angiography or MR angiography.

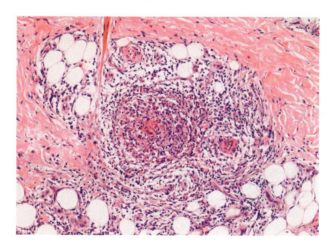

Figure 17.21 High-power view of a skin biopsy from a 4-year-old boy with polyarteritis nodosa. Biopsy shows a neutrophilic vasculitis affecting medium and small arteries in the deep dermis and subcutis. There is also an associated lobular panniculitis.

mycophenolate mofetil (600 mg/m^2 twice daily) is probably as effective as cyclophosphamide for induction of remission in cPAN. Aspirin 1–5 mg/kg/day can be considered as an antiplatelet agent.

Once remission is achieved, **maintenance therapy:** Daily low-dose prednisolone and azathioprine for up to 18 to 24 months. Other maintenance agents include methotrexate, or mycophenolate mofetil. Use of anti-TNF agents (infliximab, adalimumab), rituximab, or anti-IL6R (tocilizumab) may be considered in those who do not respond to initial therapy.

For mild, predominantly cutaneous disease, corticosteroid alone may be appropriate, with careful monitoring of clinical and laboratory parameters as this is weaned.

Prognosis

Remission was achieved in up to 80% within six months in a recent clinical trial (the MYPAN trial), with no relapses over 18 months. However, relapses can occur outside of clinical trials. If treatment is delayed or inadequate, life-threatening complications can occur. The mortality rate of almost 100% prior to corticosteroid use is now reduced to close to 0%. The relapse rate is approximately 0–35%, although many relapsing cases may historically have had the genetic form of PAN (DADA2).

ANTI-NEUTROPHIL CYTOPLASMIC ANTIBODY-ASSOCIATED VASCULITIDES

Incidence/Aetiology

The ANCA-associated vasculitides (AAV) are:

- Granulomatosis with polyangiitis (GPA).

- Microscopic polyangiitis (MPA).

- Eosinophilic granulomatosis with polyangiitis (EGPA).

AAV is rare in children, with an incidence of < 1 in 100,000. GPA is the commonest AAV seen in childhood.

Pathogenesis

It is not known why patients develop ANCA. There are two main types, anti-proteinase 3 (PR3) and anti-myeloperoxidase (MPO) ANCA:

- PR3 ANCA is mainly associated with GPA.

- MPO-ANCA is mainly associated with MPA.

ANCA activate cytokine-primed neutrophils, leading to bystander damage of endothelial cells and an escalation of inflammation with recruitment of mononuclear cells. Other factors such as HLA type may influence genetic susceptibility.

Clinical Presentation

- **GPA:** Granulomatous inflammation involving the respiratory tract and necrotising vasculitis affecting predominantly small vessels.

- **MPA:** Necrotising vasculitis, with few or no immune deposits, affecting predominatly small vessels; necrotising arteritis involving small and medium-sized arteries may be present; pulmonary capillaritis often occurs. Clinically, it often presents with rapidly progressive pauci-immune glomerulonephritis, in association with perinuclear ANCA, (MPO-ANCA) positivity.

- **EGPA:** Eosinophil-rich and granulomatous inflammation involving respiratory tract; necrotising vasculitis affecting small to medium-sized vessels; association with asthma and eosinophilia.

- **Renal limited vasculitis:** Rapidly progressive glomerulonephritis, often with ANCA positivity (usually MPO-ANCA) but without other organ involvement.

Clinical Features of GPA

- Upper respiratory tract:
  - Epistaxis.
  - Otalgia, and hearing loss (conductive and/or sensorineural); chronic otitis media; mastoiditis.
  - Nasal septal involvement with cartilaginous collapse results in the characteristic saddle nose deformity (Figure 17.22).

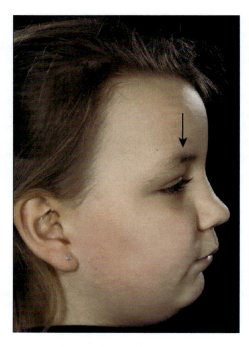

Figure 17.22 10-year-old girl with granulomatosis with polyangiitis. Note the typical saddle nose deformity, and orbital mass lesion from granulomatous inflammation (arrowed).

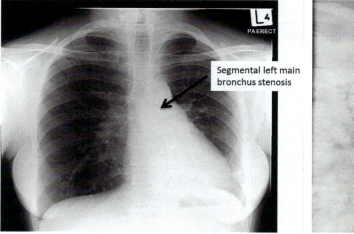 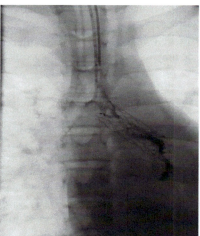

Figure 17.23 (A) Chest x-ray from a 14-year-old girl with granulomatosis with polyangiitis, demonstrating left main bronchus narrowing; (B) bronchogram performed in the same patient following insertion of a left main bronchial stent.

- Chronic sinusitis.
- Glottic and subglottic polyps and/or large and medium-sized airway stenosis (Figure 17.23).
- Lower respiratory tract manifestations include (singly or in combination):
  - Granulomatous pulmonary nodules (Figure 17.24) with or without central cavitation.
  - Pulmonary haemorrhage with respiratory distress (Figure 17.25), frank haemoptysis and/or evanescent pulmonary shadows (on chest x-ray).

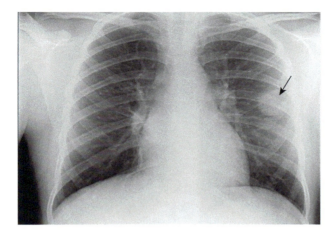

Figure 17.24 Chest x-ray from a 12-year-old girl with granulomatosis with polyangiitis, revealing pulmonary nodule (arrowed).

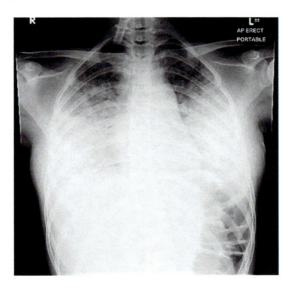

Figure 17.25 Diffuse alveolar haemorrhage in granulomatosis with polyangiitis (GPA). Chest x-ray from a 14-year-old girl with diffuse alveolar haemorrhage due to GPA with high titre PR3 antineutrophil cytoplasmic antibody (ANCA).

- Interstitial pneumonitis.

■ Renal involvement: Typically, a focal segmental necrotising glomerulonephritis, with pauci-immune crescentic glomerular changes (Figure 17.26). The clinical manifestations associated with this lesion are:

- Hypertension.
- Significant proteinuria.
- Nephritic and/or nephrotic syndrome.
- Other manifestations of acute kidney injury and chronic kidney disease.

■ Ophthalmological disease: retinal vasculitis, conjunctivitis, episcleritis, uveitis, optic neuritis. Unilateral or bilateral proptosis may be caused by granulomatous inflammation affecting the orbit (pseudotumour) (Figure 17.23).

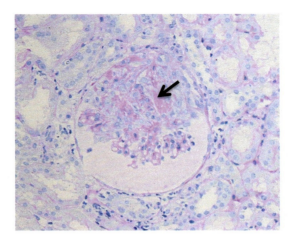

Figure 17.26 Renal biopsy from a 12-year-old girl with granulomatosis with polyangiitis, renal impairment, heavy proteinuria and microscopic haematuria. Fibrocellular crescentic nephritis associated with glomerular necrotising tuft lesions (arrowed). Immunohistochemical staining with IgG, IgM, IgA, C1q and C3 was negative (pauci-immune focal segmental necrotising glomerulonephritis).

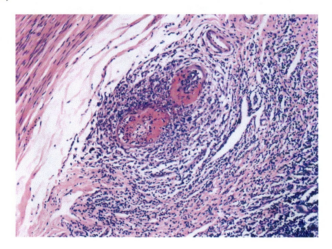

Figure 17.27 Fibrinoid necrosis of small vessels within the appendix of a 15-year-old girl who presented with acute appendicitis as a feature of granulomatosis with polyangiitis (PR3 ANCA positive).

- Malaise, fever, weight loss or growth failure, arthralgia, and arthritis.
- Other manifestations include peripheral gangrene with tissue loss, and vasculitis of the skin, gut (including appendicitis, Figure 17.27), heart, CNS and/or peripheral nerves (mononeuritis multiplex), salivary glands, gonads, and breast.

Diagnosis

- GPA: cytoplasmic staining pattern of ANCA by indirect immunofluorescence (IIF), and enzyme linked immunosorbent assay (ELISA) reveals specificity against PR3 (PR3 ANCA).
- MPA and renal limited AAV are typically associated with pANCA by IIF and with MPO-ANCA specificity on ELISA.
- ANCA-negative forms of GPA, MPA, renal limited vasculitis, and EGPA are well described in children.

- ANCA is probably unreliable for monitoring of disease activity in many GPA patients.

- Tissue diagnosis: renal (also skin, nasal septum, or other tissue) biopsy can be important.

Differential Diagnosis

- Other primary systemic vasculitides.

- Chronic infections, including *Mycobacterium tuberculosis*, and atypical mycobacterial infections; other granulomatous infections.

- Immunodeficiencies including chronic granulomatous disease; transporter associated with antigen processing (TAP) deficiency; COPA syndrome; and many others.

- Sarcoidosis.

- Idiopathic orbital pseudotumour of the young.

- Orbital foreign body and other trauma including non-accidental injury.

- Cocaine abuse (associated with cartilaginous nasal destruction, sometimes hypertension).

- Malignancy.

Treatment

The initial aim of treatment is to induce remission using corticosteroids plus rituximab, mycophenolate mofetil, or cyclophosphamide; plasma exchange is no longer routinely recommended since a major clinical trial (PEXIVAS) failed to demonstrate efficacy. To maintain remission (typically after three to six months), low-dose corticosteroids and azathioprine; or six-monthly rituximab are used. Co-trimoxazole is used as prophylaxis against opportunistic infection and as a possible disease-modifying agent in GPA, particularly with upper respiratory tract involvement. Clinical trials involving children with AAV now support the use of mycophenolate mofetil or rituximab as remission induction agents, combined with corticosteroids.

Prognosis

Mortality for GPA from one historic paediatric series was 12% over a 17-year period of study inclusion. The largest paediatric series of patients with GPA reported 40% of cases with chronic kidney disease at 33 months of follow-up despite therapy. Mortality for MPA has been reported as 0–14%, while for EGPA in children, the most recent GOSH series (the largest single centre study to date) reported a mortality of 15%.

TAKAYASU ARTERITIS

Incidence/Pathogenesis

Takayasu arteritis (TA) is a rare large-vessel vasculitis, affecting the aorta and its main branches, with incidence less than 1 in 100,000 children. The pathogenesis is unknown.

Clinical Presentation

Classification criteria for childhood TA are angiographic abnormalities of the aorta or its main branches (also pulmonary arteries) showing aneurysm/dilatation (mandatory criterion), plus one out of the following criteria:

- Pulse deficit or claudication.

- Four limb blood pressure discrepancy.

- Bruits.

- Hypertension.

- Acute phase response.

Clinical features are usually non-specific: fever and acute phase response, initial florid inflammatory vasculitic phase followed by a later fibrotic phase of the illness. A proportion of children present in this late fibrotic/stenotic phase of the disease, usually with hypertension. Common presentations include headache, abdominal pain, claudication of extremities, fever, weight loss, hypertension (89%), absent pulses and arterial bruits. Aortic and mitral valve involvement is recognised, as is myocardial involvement and formation of ventricular aneurysms, sometimes with calcification.

Diagnosis

Clinical features plus findings on MRA (Figure 17.28) are important diagnostically, and for monitoring disease progression catheter arteriography and CT angiography are sometimes required. Doppler USS is useful for assessing carotid and renal arteries. Positron emission tomography (PET) co-registered with MR or CT angiography (PET-MR or CT) can be helpful to detect large-vessel vasculitis.

Differential Diagnosis

- Other vasculitides
- Infections:
  - Bacterial endocarditis.
  - Septicaemia without true endocarditis.
  - Tuberculosis.
  - Syphilis.
  - HIV.
  - Borreliosis (Lyme disease).
  - Brucellosis (very rare).
- Other autoimmune diseases: SLE; rheumatic fever; sarcoidosis.
- Non-inflammatory large-vessel vasculopathy of congenital cause:
  - Fibromuscular dysplasia.
  - Williams syndrome.
  - Coarctation of the aorta.

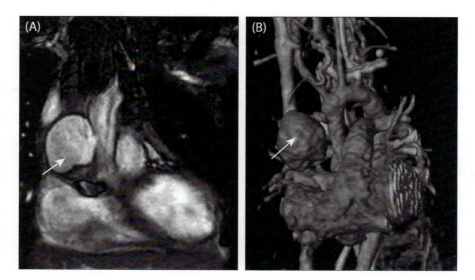

Figure 17.28   (A) MRA performed in a 13-year-old boy with Takayasu arteritis. Massive saccular aneurysm with narrow peduncle arising from the ascending aorta (arrowed); (B) three-dimensional construct of the same study. In addition, he had a left ventricular aneurysm (repaired twice) and aortic root dilatation with increased uptake in the wall demonstrated on FDG PET scanning (not shown). There was also a giant aneurysm of the right coronary artery (not shown).

- Midaortic syndrome.

- Ehlers–Danlos Type IV; Marfan syndrome; Neurofibromatosis Type 1; tuberous sclerosis; and many other genetic aortopathies.

■ Other: post radiation therapy.

Treatment/Prognosis

Treatment is with corticosteroids, usually in combination with methotrexate +/– anti-TNF (adalimumab or infliximab) anti-IL6 (tocilizumab); or rituximab. Cyclophosphamide may also be used for induction of remission. Maintenance agents include methotrexate, azathioprine, and increasingly anti-TNF or anti-IL6 agents. Surgical revascularisation procedures may be required.

TA is a relapsing and remitting disorder. The five-year mortality rate in children has been reported as high as 35%. Poor prognostic factors include diagnostic delay, severe aortic regurgitation, severe hypertension, cardiac failure, and aneurysms.

Other Vasculitides

Behçet's disease, vasculitis secondary to infection (particularly TB), malignancy, drugs, vasculitis associated with other connective tissue diseases and primary angiitis of the CNS are also seen in children but are beyond the scope of this chapter.

SYSTEMIC LUPUS ERYTHEMATOSUS

Incidence

The incidence of paediatric SLE is 0.4–2.5 per 100,000 children (Africans > Asians > Caucasians). Onset is commonest in girls over 12 years (rare under 8 years).

Aetiology/Pathogenesis

Abnormal regulation of Type I interferons and defective clearance of apoptotic cells which leads to polyclonal B-cell activation with generation of autoantibodies and immune complex deposition and T cell dysregulation.

Diagnosis

Onset is commonly insidious, with fever, fatigue, weight loss, rash, and polyarthritis. Acute onset demonstrates serositis; CNS or renal involvement; an erythematous photosensitive malar or butterfly rash with nasolabial fold sparing. Rashes may occur in other sun-exposed sites. Discoid lesions can occur and become thicker causing scarring (e.g. discoid lupus, Figure 17.29). Vasculitic rashes occur, especially on fingertips. Raynaud's may be present.

Arthritis is polyarticular and painful but is usually not destructive. Renal involvement presents with proteinuria, albuminuria, and casts in urine; renal involvement with glomerulonephritis requires percutaneous renal biopsy to confirm and grade severity. If there is severe renal involvement, renal dysfunction (elevated plasma creatinine with reduced glomerular filtration rate [GFR]) is seen.

CNS features include seizures, chorea, depression, or cognitive changes. CSF findings are non-specific, MRI findings may be supportive. ANA are found in virtually all patients (95%) and antibodies to double stranded DNA are found in > 60%, especially with nephritis; anti-Sm antibodies, present in 20%, are very

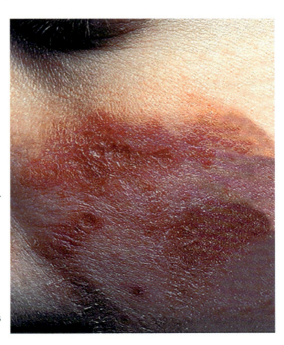

Figure 17.29 Typical malar rash in a 15-year-old showing some discoid lesions.

specific and anticardiolipin (antiphospholipid) antibodies are present in $\geq 25\%$ and are associated with risk of thrombosis.

Risk of thrombosis is greatest in patients with lupus anticoagulant; autoantibodies that target domain 1 of the beta 2 glycoprotein are also particularly thought to be associated with thrombotic risk. Patients with only anticardiolipin antibodies and thromboses or recurrent miscarriages have primary antiphospholipid syndrome.

Treatment

- Sun avoidance and use of sunblock.

- Mild disease: hydroxychloroquine, low-dose steroids and NSAID.

- Moderate disease: oral corticosteroids and immunosuppressive treatment such as azathioprine, methotrexate, or mycophenolate mofetil.

- Severe disease (includes renal and CNS) requires high-dose corticosteroids with mycophenolate mofetil, rituximab (an anti-CD20 monoclonal antibody) and/or cyclophosphamide.

- Antiplatelet treatment with low-dose aspirin in antiphospholipid antibody positive patients.

- Thrombosis: Requires warfarin, cover initial warfarinisation with heparin until therapeutic INR is achieved.

Prognosis

The five-year survival for SLE has improved ($\geq 90\%$), although renal involvement and glucocorticoid toxicity contribute significant morbidity. Deaths occur due to overwhelming disease or infection (especially fungal). There is increased risk of atherosclerosis and cardiovascular disease longer term.

OVERLAP CONNECTIVE TISSUE DISEASE

- Incidence: uncommon: 1 in 50,000 to 100,000, mostly females.

- Diagnosis: Patients develop clinical features of two different connective tissue diseases (CTD):

- Overlapping features of SLE, JDM, JIA and scleroderma.

  - Often ANA positive.

  - Undifferentiated CTD: Moderate features of several disorders, but insufficient to fulfil one diagnosis.

- Mixed CTD (MCTD): May be a subgroup of SLE.

  - MCTD: Ribonucleoprotein positive, Raynaud's, sclerodactyly, arthritis and lung involvement possible, renal and CNS involvement absent or late.

Treatment and Prognosis

As for the underlying CTD.

CHRONIC RECURRENT MULTIFOCAL OSTEOMYELITIS

Incidence

Chronic recurrent multifocal osteomyelitis (CRMO) is rare, incidence of 2–80 in 100,000 children. The aetiology is unknown; CRMO is increasingly classified as an autoinflammatory bone disease.

Diagnosis

- Multifocal bone pain swelling and fever.

- Joints usually normal.

- X-rays: Osteolytic metaphyseal lesions, osteitis, new bone formation (Figure 17.30).

- Bone scan: Often helpful, with increased uptake at sites of osteitis.

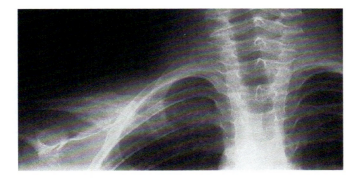

Figure 17.30   Clavicular osteitis in a 9-year-old boy with chronic recurrent multifocal osteomyelitis.

- Bone biopsy: Chronic inflammation consistent with osteomyelitis but with negative cultures, and exclusion malignancy.
- Pustular rash: Synovitis, acne, pustulosis, hyperostosis and osteitis (SAPHO) syndrome.

Treatment

- NSAIDs may improve symptoms.
- Pamidronate (or other bisphosphonate).
- Corticosteroids may help resolve persistent lesions.
- MTX may improve any associated arthritis and anti-TNFα therapy has been used in severe cases unresponsive to pamidronate.

Prognosis

Remissions and painful relapses can continue into late adolescence. Bony overgrowth or loss of growth may cause leg-length discrepancy or joint deformity.

PERIODIC FEVER SYNDROMES/AUTOINFLAMMATORY DISEASES

INTRODUCTION

The periodic fever syndromes are disorders of innate immunity, now usually referred to as autoinflammatory diseases. They are characterised by the following:

- Recurring episodes of fever and constitutional upset.
- Systemic inflammatory symptoms affecting:
  - Serosal surfaces.
  - Joints.
  - Skin.
  - Eyes.
- Biochemical markers of inflammation: raised ESR, CRP and leucocytosis.
- Near normal life expectancy, except for risk of developing AA amyloidosis in later life.
- There are now almost 30 recognised inherited fever syndromes. Many are extremely rare; the most well described are (Table 17.1):
  - Familial Mediterranean fever (FMF).
  - TNF receptor-associated period syndrome (TRAPS).

Table 17.1: Hereditary Autoinflammatory Diseases

Periodic fever syndrome	Gene	Mode of inheritance	Predominant ethnic groups	Usual age at onset	Potential precipitants of attacks	Distinctive clinical features	Typical duration of attacks	Typical frequency of attacks	Characteristic laboratory abnormalities	Treatment
FMF	MEFV Chromosome 16	Autosomal recessive (dominant in rare families)	Eastern Mediterranean	Childhood/early adult	Usually none Occasionally menstruation, fasting, stress, trauma	Short severe attacks Colchicine responsive Erysipelas-like erythema	one to three days	Variable	Marked acute phase response during attacks	Colchicine
TRAPS	TNFRSF1A Chromosome 12	Autosomal dominant, can be de novo	Northern European but reported in many ethnic groups	Childhood/early adult	Usually none	Prolonged symptoms	More than one week, may be very prolonged	Variable, may be continuous	Marked acute phase response during attacks Low levels of soluble TNFR1 when well	Etanercept High-dose corticosteroids
HIDS	MVK Chromosome 12	Autosomal recessive	Northern European	Infancy	Immunisations	Diarrhoea and lymphadenopathy	three to seven days	one to two monthly	Elevated IgD & IgA, acute phase response, and mevalonate aciduria during attacks.	Anti-TNF and anti-IL1 therapies
CAPS	NLRP3 Chromosome 1	Autosomal dominant or sporadic	Northern European	Neonatal/infancy	Marked diurnal variation Cold environment but less marked than in FCAS	Severity spectrum including: urticarial rash conjunctivitis sensorineural deafness aseptic chronic meningitis deforming arthropathy	Continuous, often worse in the evenings	Often daily	Varying but marked acute phase response most of the time	Anti-IL1 therapies (mainly anakinra; canakinumab)
PAPA	PSTPIP1 (CD2BP1) Chromosome 15	Autosomal dominant	Northern European (only three families reported)	Childhood	None	pyogenic arthritis, pyoderma gangrenosum Cystic acne	Intermittent attacks with migratory arthritis	Variable, may be continuous	acute phase response during attacks	anti-tNF therapy or anti-IL1 therapies
DIRA	IL1RN Chromosome 2	Autosomal recessive	hispanic and European (few families reported)	Neonatal	None	Sterile multifocal osteomyelitis, periostitis and pustulosis	Continuous	Continuous	Marked acute phase response	IL1ra
Blau syndrome	NOD2 (CARD15) Chromosome 16	Autosomal dominant	None	Childhood	None	Granulomatous polyarthritis, iritis and dermatitis	Continuous	Continuous	Sustained modest acute phase response	Corticosteroids, anti-tNF, anti-IL1

- Mevalonate kinase deficiency (MKD) (also known as hyperimmunoglobulin D and periodic fever syndrome [HIDS]).

- Cryopyrin-associated periodic syndrome (CAPS) (subdivided into familial cold autoinflammatory syndrome [FCAS], Muckle Wells syndrome [MWS] and chronic infantile, neurological, cutaneous, and articular syndrome/neonatal onset multisystem inflammatory disease [CINCA/NOMID]).

- Pyogenic arthritis, pyoderma gangrenosum and acne (PAPA) syndrome.

- Deficiency of IL1 receptor antagonist (DIRA).

- Blau syndrome/early onset sarcoidosis (EOS).

- Deficiency of IL36 antagonist (DITRA).

- Chronic atypical neutrophilic dermatosis with lipodystrophy and elevated temperature (CANDLE).

- Deficiency of adenosine deaminase 2 (DADA2).

- STING-associated vasculopathy with onset in infancy (SAVI).

- Majeed syndrome.

Treatment is effective for most patients with FMF, CAPS and DIRA; good treatments are available for most of the other syndromes.

Disorders of unknown aetiology that share some features with the inherited syndromes include:

- Periodic fever, aphthous stomatitis, pharyngitis, and cervical adenitis (PFAPA) syndrome.

- Behcet's disease.

- CRMO.

- sJIA.

FAMILIAL MEDITERRANEAN FEVER

Incidence/Aetiology

FMF is commonest in Middle Eastern populations; prevalence is 1 in 250 to 1000 but occurs worldwide. It has a recessive inheritance, with mutations in the *MEFV* gene on chromosome 16, but has been observed in heterozygotes and there is a rarer autosomal dominant form.

Clinical Presentation

- Attacks last 12 to 72 hours but occur irregularly, precipitated by minor physical or emotional stress, menstrual cycle, or diet with clinical features including:

  - Fever.

  - Aseptic peritonitis in 85%.

  - Pleuritic chest pain in 40%.

  - Erysipelas-like rash in 20%.

  - Meningitic headache occurs rarely.

  - Orchitis occurs rarely.

  - Joint involvement is rare and generally mild affecting the lower limbs.

  - Neutrophil leucocytosis and a dramatic acute phase response occur with attacks.

  - Protracted febrile myalgia (rare): Severe muscle pain, may have vasculitic rash, usually responds to high-dose corticosteroids.

Diagnosis

Recurrent self-limiting attacks of fever and serositis, prevented by colchicine; mutation in *MEFV* is confirmatory. Differential diagnosis is other periodic fever syndromes (Table 17.1).

Treatment

Colchicine is the prophylactic treatment of FMF, and is required life-long:

- Continuous use reduces/prevents symptoms of FMF in at least 95%.

- Almost completely eliminates the risk of developing AA amyloidosis.

- Mechanism of action is pleiotropic; children respond to 0.25–2 mg/day.

Prognosis

The long-term outlook is excellent with life-long treatment. Prior to colchicine treatment 60% of Turkish patients developed AA amyloidosis.

TUMOUR NECROSIS FACTOR RECEPTOR-ASSOCIATED PERIODIC SYNDROME

Incidence/Aetiology

Tumour necrosis factor receptor-associated periodic syndrome (TRAPS) is rare, with an estimated prevalence of about 1 per million in Europe. TRAPS is caused by autosomal dominant, gene mutations in *TNFRSF1A* on chromosome 12; 64% have a family history

Clinical Presentation

Prolonged attacks occur, lasting one to three weeks (symptoms are near continuous in 30%). Features include:

- Fever in ~90%.

- Arthralgia and myalgia in 85%, often with centripetal migration.

- Abdominal pain in 74%.

- Rash in 64%: erythematous, oedematous plaques, discrete reticulate or serpiginous lesions (Figure 17.31).

- Headache, pleuritic pain, lymphadenopathy, conjunctivitis, and periorbital oedema.

- Symptoms are accompanied by a marked acute phase response.

Diagnosis

Diagnosis requires confirmatory genetic testing. However, the difficulty is in interpretation of the significance of two common polymorphisms, *R92Q* (Caucasian) and *P46L* (African/Arab origin); found in around 4–10% of the normal population, and usually not associated with an inflammatory syndrome. Differential diagnosis is other periodic fever syndromes (Table 17.1).

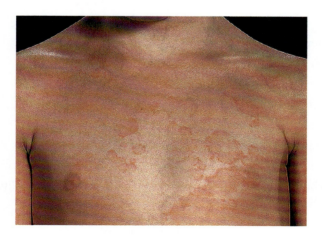

Figure 17.31 Erythema multiforme rash in a 7-year-old girl with tumour necrosis factor receptor-associated periodic syndrome.

Treatment

Acute attacks are treated with high-dose corticosteroids, but these do not reduce the frequency of attacks. IL1 blockade seems to be the most effective treatment, as confirmed in a major clincal trial of canakinumab (the CLUSTER trial). Recombinant IL1 receptor antagonist (anakinra) is also effective; the longer-acting IL1 blocking agent canakinumab is now more commonly used in the United Kingdom than anakinra.

Prognosis

Without treatment > 25% develop AA amyloidosis. Patients have poor growth, interrupted schooling, and poor fertility. Life-long treatment is needed, but there is a good long-term outlook as long as inflammatory attacks are prevented/minimised throughout life.

MEVALONATE KINASE DEFICIENCY

Incidence/Aetiology

MKD is extremely rare. Most patients are North European, many in the Netherlands, but can occur in other ethnicities. The disease is caused by an autosomal recessive mutation in the gene for mevalonate kinase (*MVK*), the enzyme downstream of HMG CoA reductase.

Clinical Presentation

Onset of MKD is below 1 year of age. Children experience irregular attacks lasting four to seven days, that may be precipitated by vaccination, minor trauma, surgery, or stress. Fever, unilateral or bilateral cervical lymphadenopathy, abdominal pain with vomiting and diarrhoea, headache, arthralgia, large joint arthritis, erythematous macules, and papules and aphthous ulcers are common. A history of high fevers or a full attack with vaccination is often evident.

Diagnosis

- High serum IgD, IgE and IgA (none of these are sensitive or specific, however).

- Presence of mevalonic acid in the urine during attacks is notoriously impractical to document, and rarely used in clinical practice in the United Kingdom.

- Genetic confirmation is required for a secure diagnosis +/– intracellular leucocyte MVK enzyme activity.

Treatment/Prognosis

IL1 blockade is the most effective treatment, as confirmed in a major clinical trial of canakinumab. Recombinant IL1 receptor antagonist (anakinra) can either be used continuously or to abort attacks. Long-term IL1beta inhibition with canakinumab is usually required. Curative allogeneic haematopoietic stem cell transplantation has been described in patients who have failed biologic therapy. Symptoms may partially improve with age. AA amyloidosis is seen, but less commonly than in FMF, TRAPS or CAPS. Gene therapies may be curative in the future but are still at preclinical stages of research.

CRYOPYRIN-ASSOCIATED PERIODIC SYNDROME

CAPS includes a spectrum of conditions ranging from mild to severe, and includes three syndromes:

- FCAS.

- MWS.

- CINCA/NOMID.

Incidence/Aetiology

CAPS is extremely rare, with an incidence of probably < 1 in 500,000. CAPS is due to mutations in *NLRP3* on chromosome 1q44, that encodes the key component of the IL1 activation complex: the inflammasome. A dominant inheritance occurs in about 75% of patients with FCAS and MWS, whereas CINCA is usually due to *de novo* mutations.

Clinical Presentation

Onset is in early infancy, often from birth; there is no sex bias. Children present with a characteristic appearance of flattened nasal bridge and bossing of the skull (Figure 17.32).

- FCAS: Attacks of fever, urticarial rash, arthralgia, and conjunctivitis precipitated by cold or damp exposure.

- MWS: Daily attacks (afternoon/evenings); may be exacerbated by the cold. Acute symptoms include fever, urticarial rash, arthralgia and myalgia, conjunctivitis, headache, and fatigue. Rash can be persistent (Figure 17.33). Deafness occurs later and is often missed in the early stages.

- CINCA/NOMID: Continuous inflammation with additional severe chronic aseptic meningitis, raised intracranial pressure, uveitis, deafness and arthropathy.

Diagnosis

- FCAS and MWS usually have mutations in *NLRP3*, although *NLRP3* mutation negative cases are recognised in some.

- Clinical diagnosis for CINCA/NOMID: Mutations are found in only 50%. Differential diagnosis (see Table 17.1).

Treatment

Treatment is IL1 blockade with anakinra or (more commonly in the United Kingdom) canakinumab.

Prognosis

If untreated:

- ~25% develop AA amyloidosis.

- Complications of chronic CNS inflammation: Severe in CINCA, less in MWS.

- 40% sensorineural deafness; blindness due to optic atrophy or uveitis; developmental delay.

- CINCA arthropathy: Cartilage and bony overgrowth (patella), joint destruction can occur.

- MWS and CINCA: 17% clubbing of the fingernails.

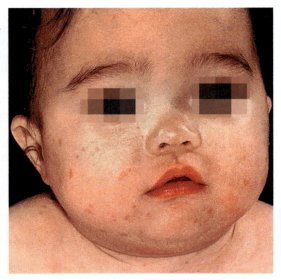

Figure 17.32 Typical facial features of chronic infantile, neurological, cutaneous, and articular syndrome (CINCA) in a child at 11 months, showing flattened nasal bridge and hydrocephalus.

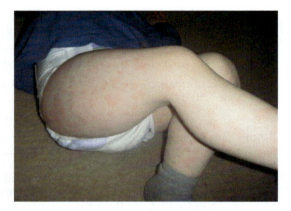

Figure 17.33 Typical rash of Muckle Wells syndrome in a 2-year-old boy. The rash completely resolved within 24 hours of receiving the first dose of canakinumab.

PERIODIC FEVER, APHTHOUS STOMATITIS, PHARYNGITIS AND ADENITIS

PFAPA was first described in 1987 (as Marshall syndrome). It has an unknown aetiology, and the epidemiology is poorly described. PFAPA is the commonest periodic fever syndrome in childhood and is not caused by monogenetic mutation.

- **Diagnosis** is clinical, in the absence of evidence of recurrent upper respiratory tract infections or cyclic neutropenia:

- Regular recurrent fever of early onset.
- Oral aphthous ulcers.
- Cervical lymphadenopathy.
- Pharyngitis.

■ **Treatment**:

■ Single dose of corticosteroid (1–2 mg/kg) given at the start of an attack.

- Tonsillectomy: approximately 50% success reported.
- Long-term colchicine prophylaxis may ameliorate symptoms.

■ **Prognosis** is good; most outgrow their symptoms by adolescence.

Other Diseases

There are many other emerging and recently described genetic autoinflammatory diseases (see Table 17.1), beyond the scope of this chapter.

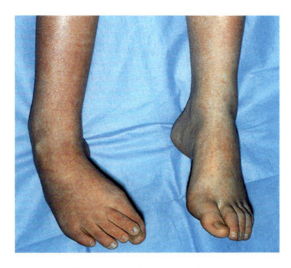

Figure 17.34   Long-standing reflex sympathetic dystrophy in a 13 year old, showing skin colour changes and flexion posture of the right foot.

CHRONIC PAIN SYNDROME

■ Can be localised or diffuse, pain needs to have lasted at least three months.

■ Includes forms similar to adult fibromyalgia.

■ Overlaps with chronic fatigue syndrome and post viral fatigue syndrome.

■ All of these conditions have major psychological components, which are either aetiological or result from the inciting illness.

■ Psychological intervention and, usually, physiotherapy are mandatory in these conditions.

COMPLEX REGIONAL PAIN SYNDROME

Incidence

This was previously called reflex sympathetic dystrophy or algodystrophy. It is uncommon, < 1 in 50,000, predominantly in females over 8 years of age.

Diagnosis

Diagnosis is clinical, possibly an exaggerated response to minor trauma or minor pathology. It has psychosocial features. Early on there is soft tissue swelling, sweating and oedema; later on, children develop cold skin, increased hair growth, allodynia (severe skin hypersensitivity to light stimuli) and pseudoparalysis.

Untreated there is atrophy of skin and undergrowth of bone (Figure 17.34). Bone scans may show increased uptake in the early phases and reduced uptake later on with disuse of the limb. X-rays may show osteoporosis with long-standing disease.

Treatment/Prognosis

Intensive physiotherapy and psychological input are essential. Skin massage and desensitisation can be helpful. Medical therapies are limited but, in addition to regular analgesics, gabapentin and pregabalin may help neuropathic pain. Amitriptyline may have a specific role to help the burning sensation. There is little evidence for nerve blocks or skin patches.

Patients improve significantly with treatment, but recurrences do occur. Any delay in diagnosis causes prolonged morbidity and disability and many patients persist with various symptoms into their adult years. Psychosocial issues may predispose patients to chronicity and poor treatment response.

JOINT HYPERMOBILITY SYNDROME

Incidence

This is common: children have a greater range of normal joint mobility than adults and 25–50% of normal children have either localised or generalised hypermobility (up to 10% of which becomes symptomatic). Genetic syndromes include Marfan syndrome and Ehlers–Danlos syndrome.

Diagnosis

The joints commonly affected include the knees, ankles, elbows, wrists and feet. Recurrent minor 'sprains', subluxation/dislocation lead to recurrent arthralgias and occasional joint effusions. 'Growing pains' are commonly related to hypermobility. Adolescents may present with back pain.

Treatment/Prognosis

Treatment is with physiotherapy, with specific muscle strengthening and joint protection measures, such as supportive shoes and insoles. Anti-inflammatories and analgesics are unhelpful.
  Prognosis is generally good; many improve with age and function is usually maintained.

FURTHER READING

- Petty R, Laxer R, Lindsley C, et al. *Textbook of Pediatric Rheumatology*, 8th edn. Elsevier, 2020.
- Cobb JE, Hinks A, Thomson W. The genetics of juvenile idiopathic arthritis: Current understanding and future prospects. *Rheumatology* (Oxford) 2014;*53(4)*:592–599.
- De Benedetti F, Brunner HI, Ruperto N, et al. Randomized trial of tocilizumab in systemic juvenile idiopathic arthritis. *N Engl J Med* 2012;*367(25)*:2385–2395.
- Foster H, Brogan PA. *The Oxford Handbook of Paediatric Rheumatology*. Oxford: Oxford University Press, 2012.
- Hinks A, Cobb J, Marion MC, et al. Dense genotyping of immune-related disease regions identifies 14 new susceptibility loci for juvenile idiopathic arthritis. *Nat Genet* 2013;*45(6)*:664–669.
- Lovell DJ, Giannini EH, Reiff A, et al.; Pediatric Rheumatology Collaborative Study Group. Etanercept in children with polyarticular juvenile rheumatoid arthritis. *N Engl J Med* 2000;*342(11)*:763–769.
- Magni-Manzoni S, Malattia C, Lanni S, Ravelli A. Advances and challenges in imaging in juvenile idiopathic arthritis. *Nat Rev Rheumatol* 2012;*8(6)*:329–336.
- Prakken B, Albani S, Martini A. Juvenile idiopathic arthritis. *Lancet* 2011;*377(9783)*:2138–2149.
- Ringold S, Weiss PF, Beukelman T, et al. 2013 update of the 2011 American College of Rheumatology recommendations for the treatment of juvenile idiopathic arthritis: Recommendations for the medical therapy of children with systemic juvenile idiopathic arthritis and tuberculosis screening among children receiving biologic medications. *Arthritis Care Res* (Hoboken) 2013;*65(10)*:1551–1563.
- Ruperto N, Brunner HI, Quartier P, et al. Two randomized trials of canakinumab in systemic juvenile idiopathic arthritis. *N Engl J Med* 2012;*367(25)*:2396–2406.
- Schulert GS, Grom AA. Macrophage activation syndrome and cytokine-directed therapies. *Best Pract Res Clin Rheumatol* 2014;*28(2)*:277–292.
- van Dijkhuizen EH, Wulffraat NM. Early predictors of prognosis in juvenile idiopathic arthritis: a systematic literature review. *Ann Rheum Dis* 2014;*74(11)*:1996–2005.
- Watts R, Conaghan P, Denton C, Foster H, Isaacs J, Muller-Ladner U, eds. *Oxford Textbook of Rheumatology*, 4th edn. Oxford: Oxford University Press, 2018.

18 Neonatal and General Paediatric Surgery

Dhanya Mullassery and Simon Blackburn

GENERAL PAEDIATRIC SURGERY CONDITIONS
Inguinoscrotal Swellings

Inguinoscrotal swellings are one of the most common presentations to a paediatric surgery clinic. The most common pathologies and their management are outlined below.

Inguinal Hernia
Incidence

Inguinal hernia occurs in 1–2 per 100 live births, but may be present is as many as 20–30% of premature infants. Male infants are four times more frequently affected than females and the right side twice as often as the left.

Clinical Presentation

An inguinal hernia in a child is typically an indirect hernia caused by protrusion of intra-abdominal contents (commonly bowel or bladder) into the patent processus vaginalis. They present as intermittent swelling in the groin and/or scrotum (Figures 18.1 and 18.2). In girls, the hernia may present as a bulge in the groin that may extend into the labium and can contain an ovary (Figure 18.3). In infancy, the risk of incarceration is as high as 30% and the first presentation may well be with an incarcerated hernia.

Diagnosis

The presence of a reducible inguinal or inguinoscrotal swelling or a good history of such a swelling provided by the parents is diagnostic.

Treatment

In infancy there is a high risk of irreducibility and urgent surgery is generally recommended in the form of open or laparoscopic inguinal herniotomy. Irreducible hernias will usually reduce spontaneously following the administration of the analgesia or with manual reduction. A strangulated hernia requires urgent resuscitation followed by surgical reduction of viable contents, resection of any necrotic intestine and herniotomy.

Hydrocoele

Failure of the processus vaginalis to undergo obliteration leads to the development of an inguinal hernia. When the communication to the peritoneal cavity is very narrow, the passage of peritoneal fluid only is possible and this results in the formation of a hydrocoele, which may occupy the tunica vaginalis and surround the testis (scrotal hydrocele) or may occur as a localised swelling anywhere along the cord (hydrocoele of the cord).

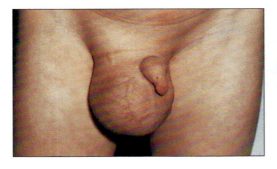

Figure 18.1 Uncomplicated right inguinal hernia.

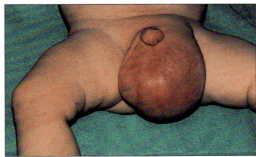

Figure 18.2 Incarcerated left inguinal hernia.

DOI: 10.1201/9781003175186-18

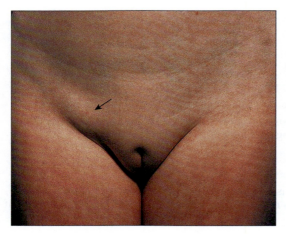

Figure 18.3 Right inguinal hernia in a girl (arrow).

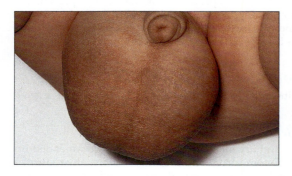

Figure 18.4 Hydrocoele: Bilateral scrotal swellings.

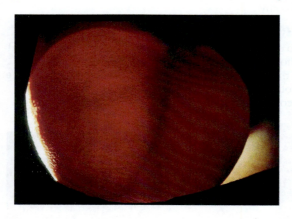

Figure 18.5 Hydrocoele: Transillumination depicting fluid in the scrotal sac.

Clinical Presentation

A scrotal hydrocoele appears as a soft, non-tender, fluid-filled sac that is transilluminable. This sign should be interpreted with caution in neonates, in whom the bowel within a hernia may transilluminate. The swelling may fluctuate somewhat in size and it is usually possible to palpate a normal cord above the swelling. A hydrocoele of the cord presents as a well-circumscribed, fluid-filled mass in the inguinal region (Figures 18.4 and 18.5).

Treatment

Operative correction is reserved for scrotal hydrocoeles which fail to spontaneously regress in the first 2–3 years of life. The procedure is a PPV ligation, an operation almost indistinguishable from an inguinal herniotomy, with ligation and division of the patent processus vaginalis and evacuation of fluid from the scrotum.

Please see the chapter 'Urology' for undescended testis and acute scrotum.

Phimosis

Phimosis is the inability to retract the foreskin over the glans. It is physiological in the early years of life (Figure 18.6).

Clinical Presentation

Pathological phimosis is usually secondary to balanitis xerotica obliterans (BXO) and rarely occurs before the age of 6 years. The foreskin is scarred and whitish in appearance and the opening is severely narrowed resulting in non-retractability (Figure 18.7). Pathologically this is a form of lichen sclerosis.

Treatment

Pathological phimosis secondary to BXO is an absolute indication for circumcision. Preputial adhesions are common in the first few years of life and normally resolve spontaneously – they do not constitute an indication for circumcision. A non-retractile foreskin following puberty is another indication for intervention, which may take the form of circumcision or preputioplasty.

Other swellings of the foreskin which may concern parents include ballooning during micturition and the presence of aggregations of smegma under the skin of the prepuce (so called 'smegmal cysts' or 'preputial pearls'). These are both physiological phenomena and do not constitute an indication for circumcision.

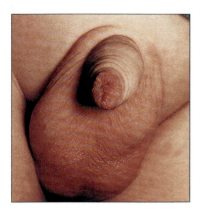

Figure 18.6 Non-retractile foreskin – a normal phenomenon.

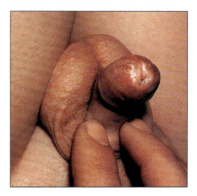

Figure 18.7 Phimosis showing evidence of scarring of the foreskin resulting in nonretractability – a pathological condition.

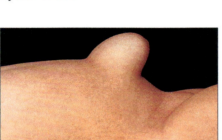

Figure 18.8 Umbilical hernia of moderate size.

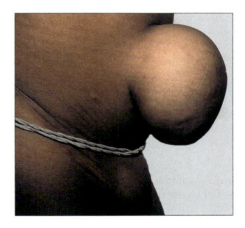

Figure 18.9 Umbilical hernia: Large, truncated.

Umbilical Hernia
Clinical Presentation

The hernia occurs through a defect in the umbilical cicatrix and usually contains omentum only (Figure 18.8). These hernias tend to resolve spontaneously by the time children reach the age of 3 years. Incarceration is extremely unlikely except in the large truncated variety (Figure 18.9).

Treatment

Elective surgery is undertaken following failure to close spontaneously after the age of 3 years. The operative procedure consists of closure of the fascial defect at the base of the hernia with sutures.

Umbilical Anomalies
Types

- **Umbilical granuloma**: due to failure of the umbilical cord to separate completely. Application of silver nitrate to the granulation tissue will result in its resolution (Figure 18.10).

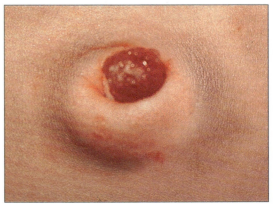

Figure 18.10 Umbilical granuloma: an infected remnant of the umbilical cord that has failed to separate completely.

511

- **Umbilical polyp:** Due to persistence of a remnant of the umbilical end of a vitello-intestinal duct at the umbilicus. It is covered by mucosa that requires formal excision (Figure 18.11).

- **Patent vitello-intestinal duct:** Due to persistence of an open vitello-intestinal duct at the umbilicus through which intestinal content passes out onto the umbilicus. Urgent surgery is required to excise the fistula from the umbilicus to the ileum and restore intestinal continuity by end-to-end anastomosis (Figure 18.12).

- **Patent urachus:** Due to persistence of communication between the bladder dome and the umbilicus and may produce a persistent urinary leak. It is important to exclude a bladder outlet obstruction (e.g. posterior urethral valves) before attempting closure of the urachal remnant (Figure 18.13).

Appendicitis
Incidence
Appendicitis is one of the most common causes of acute abdominal pain in children.

Clinical Presentation
The classical presentation is with acute onset of vague periumbilical pain that rapidly radiates and localises in the right iliac fossa, where it becomes continuous in nature. The pain is accompanied by anorexia, nausea and vomiting. Diarrhoea may be present when there is pelvic appendicitis. Most children have a low-grade pyrexia. Physical examination reveals localised tenderness in the right lower quadrant of the abdomen. Infants under the age of 2 years generally present with perforated appendicitis and peritonitis.

Diagnosis
Investigation results typical of appendicitis include:

- Leukocytosis of $10–15 \times 10^9/\mathrm{l}$.

- An elevated C reactive protein (CRP).

- Ultrasound scan – thickening of the appendix (if it can be be identified) (diameter > 6 mm) with free fluid in the right iliac fossa.

- CT scan in selected patients where there is diagnostic dilemma and high risk of general anaesthesia.

- Diagnostic laparoscopy.

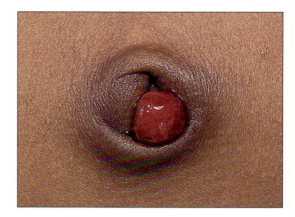

Figure 18.11   Umbilical polyp: Mucosal remnant of the vitello-intestinal duct at the umbilicus.

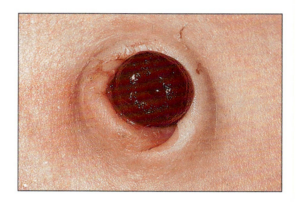

Figure 18.12   Patent vitello-intestinal duct due to persistence of the duct, which allows discharge of faeces.

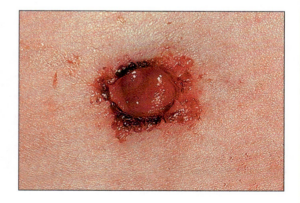

Figure 18.13   Patent urachus causing a urinary discharge from the orifice of the duct.

Treatment

Standard treatment is by an open or laparoscopic appendicectomy (Figure 18.14). Conservative management using antibiotics has, however, recently been shown to be effective in simple appendicitis. Where the diagnosis is in doubt, a period of active observation in hospital should be undertaken for 24–48 hours.

In patients with perforated appendicitis and peritonitis, a period of active resuscitation with intravenous fluids and intravenous antibiotics is essential prior to appendicectomy. In the presence of an established mass conservative treatment with antibiotics alone and delayed appendicectomy should be undertaken.

Pyloric Stenosis

Incidence

Pyloric stenosis occurs in 1 in 400 infants. The muscle of the pylorus undergoes hypertrophy causing gastric outlet obstruction. A family history is common. Male to female ratio is 4:1.

Clinical Presentation

Non bilious vomiting (typically projectile) usually commences at 2–4 weeks of age. This may lead to weight loss, dehydration and electrolyte disturbance characterised by hypokalaemic hypochloraemic metabolic alkalosis. Visible gastric peristalsis may be seen on the abdomen with the palpation of the typical olive-shaped pyloric 'tumour' in the right upper. Ultrasound assessment of the pylorus shows thickened pyloric musculature measuring > 16 mm in length and > 4 mm thickness (Figures 18.15).

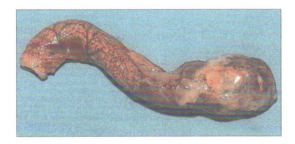

Figure 18.14   Appendicitis: Operative specimen of an acute appendicitis.

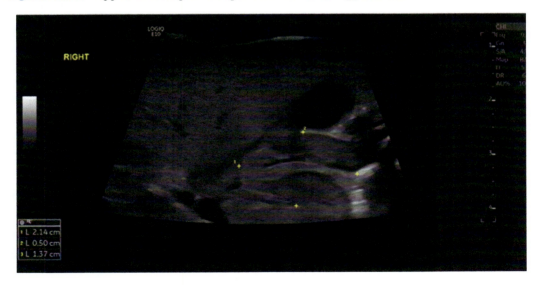

Figure 18.15   Ultrasound scan showing thickened pyloric musculature – canal length (1) measures 21 mm, and muscle thickness (2) measures 5 mm.

513

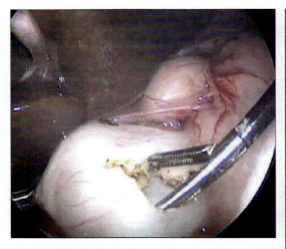

Figure 18.16 Operative view of pyloromyotomy at laparoscopic surgery, showing split thickened pyloric muscle down to, but not including mucosa.

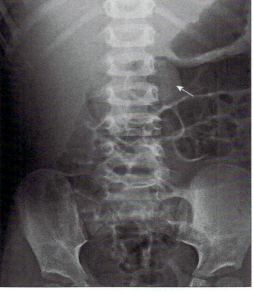

Figure 18.17 Intussusception: plain abdominal x-ray showing obstructed small intestinal loops and an 'empty' right iliac fossa and flank. The arrow shows a soft tissue mass of the apex of the intussusception.

Treatment

Electrolyte disturbance is corrected followed by pyloromyotomy (open or laparoscopic) preserving the mucosal layer (Figure 18.16).

Intussusception
Incidence

Intussusception occurs in 1 in 250 infants. An intussusception consists of invagination of one part of the intestine into the adjacent bowel. This causes an incomplete obstruction which, if unrelieved, leads to complete obstruction together with impairment of the vascularity to the invaginated (intussusceptum) bowel, initially venous congestion but ultimately ischaemic necrosis. The ileocaecal region is the most common site but any portion of the intestinal tract may be involved.

Peak incidence is 6–9 months of age, with a seasonal variation of increased incidence in spring and early summer and again in mid-winter.

Pathophysiology

Over 95% of cases of intussusception in children aged 3–24 months do not have a recognisable pathological lead point and are assumed to occur as a result of an enlarged Peyer's patch (musosa associated lymphoid tissue), secondary to an enteral infection. Pathological lead points occur in 5% of cases and may comprise polyps, a Meckel's diverticulum, duplications or a tumour.

Clinical Presentation

The cardinal signs of intussusception include colicky abdominal pain, during which the infant draws up his/her legs, vomiting (initially of food only but, as the obstructive element develops, becoming bilious and eventually faeculent) and the passage of 'redcurrant jelly'-like stools *per rectum*. It may be possible to palpate a 'sausage-shaped' mass in the right upper quadrant of the abdomen. The concurrence of all of these signs is rare, meaning a high index of suspicion is required. The diagnosis should form part of the differential in a collapsed child of typical age where the cause is unclear.

Diagnosis

Diagnosis is by history, clinical examination and with investigations. Plain abdominal x-ray may show an absence of gas in the right iliac fossa (Figure 18.17).

Ultrasonography: shows the intussusception with a 'doughnut' appearance (Figures 18.18).

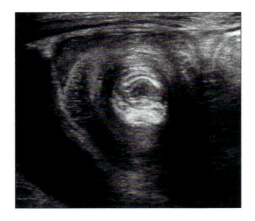

Figure 18.18 Ultrasound scan of an intussusception showing 'doughnut' appearance.

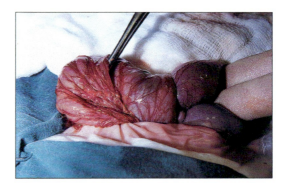

Figure 18.19 Intussusception: Operative appearance of an ileocolic intussusception.

Treatment

Following adequate resuscitation non-operative reduction using air or contrast (hydrostatic) under fluoroscopic or ultrasound control is recommended. Contraindications for non-operative reduction are the presence of shock/toxicity, evidence of necrotic intestine or perforation. Operative treatment consists of reduction of a viable intussusceptum (Figure 18.19) or resection and primary anastomosis for necrotic intestine or to resect a pathological lead point (Figure 18.20).

CONGENITAL MALFORMATIONS NEEDING SPECIALIST PAEDIATRIC SURGERY

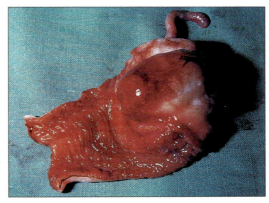

Figure 18.20 Intussusception with a duplication cyst as the lead point.

Oesophageal Atresia

Incidence and Types

Oesophageal atresia occurs in 1 in 4500 live births.

- Proximal atresia with distal tracheo-oesophageal fistula – 85% (Figure 18.21)

- Isolated oesophageal atresia – 7% (Figure 18.22)

- H-type tracheo-oesophageal fistula without atresia – 4%

- Atresia with proximal tracheo-oesophageal fistula – 1%

- Atresia with proximal and distal fistulae – 3%

Classification

The Spitz classification gives prognostic information:

Group I infants with birthweight > 1500 g and no major congenital cardiac defect (98.5% survival).

Group II birthweight < 1500 g or a major cardiac defect (82% survival).

Group III birthweight < 1500 g and major cardiac defect (50% survival).

Associated Anomalies

Congenital cardiac malformations and VACTERL (V – vertebral; A – anorectal; C – cardiac; TE – tracheo-oesophageal; R – radial and/or renal anomalies; L – limb) associations are the most common.

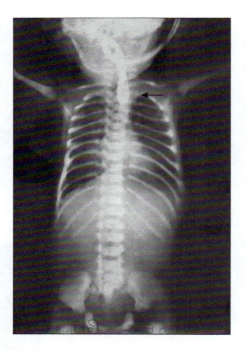

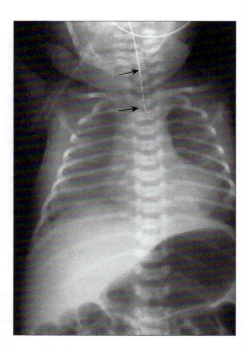

Figure 18.22 Oesophageal atresia without tracheo-oesophageal fistula. X-ray of chest and abdomen showing a radio-opaque catheter in the upper oesophagus and the complete absence of gas in the bowel.

Figure 18.21 Oesophageal atresia with distal tracheo-oesophageal fistula. X-ray of chest and abdomen showing a radio-opaque catheter in the upper, blind, oesophageal pouch and gas in the gastrointestinal tract.

Prenatal Diagnosis

Polyhydramnios with absence of a detectable stomach 'bubble' on prenatal ultrasound scan provides evidence for the presence of an isolated atresia without tracheo-oesophageal fistula. In addition, the upper oesophageal pouch may be seen to be dilated and obstructed on the ultrasound scan.

Postnatal Diagnosis

An oesophageal atresia should be suspected when the infant is 'excessively mucousy' at birth. Coughing and cyanosis coinciding with the first feed is a consequence of delayed diagnosis.

Inability to advance a No. 8–10F nasogastric tube by mouth beyond 10 cm from the lower gum margin and an x-ray showing the tip of the tube in the upper thorax provides confirmation of the diagnosis. The presence of gas within the gastrointestinal (GI) tract is indicative of a distal tracheo-oesophageal fistula.

Treatment

Optimal treatment is ligation of the tracheooesophageal fistula and primary oesophageal anastomosis. Occasionally, primary anastomosis is not possible and delayed repair is required. In rare circumstances, oesophageal replacement is necessary.

Congenital Diaphragmatic Hernia (CDH)

Incidence

CDH occurs in 1 in 3500 live births. The herniation of abdominal contents occurs through a defect in the pleuroperitoneal canal (foramen of Bochdalek), which fails to close during intrauterine development.

Pathophysiology

Herniation occurs more frequently on the left side (4:1) and causes compression of the ipsilateral developing lung and shift of the mediastinal structures to the opposite side. This is associated with lung hypoplasia and pulmonary hypertension which are the main causes of mortality and morbidity in this condition.

Diagnosis

The majority of CDH are detected on prenatal ultrasound scan at around 20 weeks of gestation. Early assessment for lethal chromosomal defects and congenital cardiac anomalies is vital.

Clinical Presentation

Respiratory distress is usually present at birth with decreased breath sounds on the ipsilateral side, and a flat or even scaphoid abdomen.

Diagnosis

Plain chest and abdominal x-ray will reveal loops of intestine in the chest, shift of the mediastinal structures to the contralateral side and an absence of bowel gas shadows in the abdomen (Figures 18.23 and 18.24). In late presenting cases or when the diagnosis is doubtful, upper GI contrast studies will show contrast-filling intestinal loops within the pleural cavity.

Treatment

Postnatal care includes neonatal resuscitation and stabilisation prior to surgery. This consists of gastric decompression using a nasogastric tube, endotracheal intubation, gentle mechanical ventilation with permissive hypercapnoea and elective sedation and paralysis. In refractory cases high-frequency oscillating ventilation, nitric oxide and extracorporeal membrane oxygenation (ECMO) may be used. Operative repair consists of reduction of the herniated contents into the abdomen and closure of the diaphragmatic defect primarily or using a prosthetic patch.

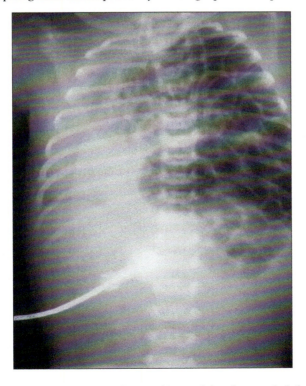

Figure 18.23 Congenital diaphragmatic hernia. X-ray of the chest and abdomen showing intestinal gas shadows in the left chest, a shift of the mediastinum to the right and absence of bowel in the abdomen.

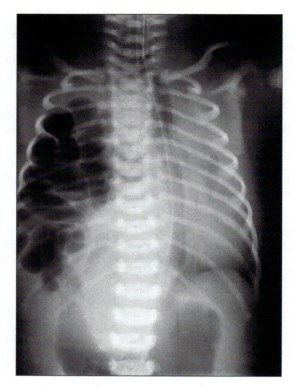

Figure 18.24 Congenital diaphragmatic hernia. X-ray of the chest and abdomen showing a right-sided diaphragmatic hernia, which is less common than left-sided hernia.

Prognosis

Although postoperative survival has improved in recent decades to over 90%, population level survival rates remain around 50% following antenatal diagnosis, with most deaths occurring prenatally or prior to surgery, due to failure of stabilisation of cardiorespiratory function.

NEONATAL INTESTINAL OBSTRUCTION

See Table 18.1 for an overview.

Table 18.1: Intestinal Obstruction in the Neonate

Mechanical

Intraluminal	Meconium ileus – Meconium obstruction of the newborn
Intramural	Atresia: duodenal, intestinal – Anorectal anomalies – Hirschsprung's disease
Extraluminal	Malrotation – Duplication – Hernia – Cysts – Tumours

Paralytic ileus
Septicaemia
Necrotising enterocolitis
Symptomatology
Bile-stained vomiting
Abdominal distension
Failure to pass meconium
Oedema and/or erythema of the anterior abdominal wall
  indicates peritonitis, perforation or gangrenous intestine

Meconium Ileus
Incidence

Meconium ileus occurs in 1 in 2500 live births.

Aetiology/Pathophysiology

Meconium ileus is intraluminal obstruction caused by tenacious meconium in cystic fibrosis. This is caused by a genetic defect involving the long arm of chromosome 7, the commonest mutation being a single amino acid substitution, ΔF508. Cystic fibrosis is inherited as an autosomal recessive characteristic with 25% transmission. Meconium ileus occurs in 10–15% of infants with cystic fibrosis. The risk of meconium ileus varies according the gnetic abnormality underlying the cystic fibrosis.

Due to the pancreatic exocrine deficiency, the meconium becomes tenacious and sticky and cannot be propelled by peristalsis through the GI tract. The resultant obstruction causes proximal dilatation, which may culminate in volvulus with or without atresia, or perforation with meconium peritonitis.

Clinical Presentation

Bilious vomiting occurs soon after birth in these infants, who are usually born with a distended abdomen (Figure 18.25). It may be possible to palpate the distended loops of intestine impacted with meconium through the abdominal wall. No meconium will be passed and a small amount of mucus may follow rectal probing.

Diagnosis

The plain abdominal x-ray shows dilated loops of intestine of varying calibre (Figure 18.26) and, unless there is an atresia or volvulus, an absence of air–fluid levels. Calcification suggests the occurrence of an antenatal intestinal perforation. A 'ground-glass' appearance of impacted meconium may be seen on the plain x-ray. In meconium peritonitis, the abdomen may be opaque due to the presence of ascites.

Chromosomal analysis will reveal the ΔF508 defect in 90% of cases. Sweat test with pilocarpine iontophoresis is diagnostic when the volume of sweat obtained is over 100 g and the sodium and chloride content is in excess of 60 mEq/l.

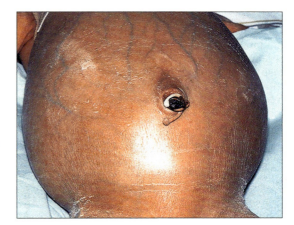

Figure 18.25 Meconium ileus. Infant with abdominal distension present at birth.

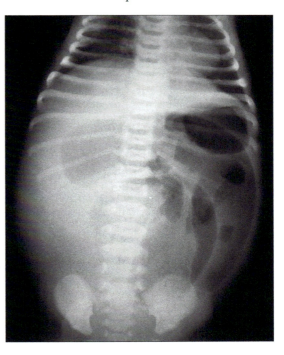

Figure 18.26 Meconium ileus. Abdominal x-ray showing dilated loops of intestine of varying calibre and an absence of air–fluid levels.

Treatment

For uncomplicated meconium ileus, a carefully performed gastrografin enema may relieve the intraluminal obstruction (Figure 18.27). Surgery is required for complicated meconium ileus and when gastrografin enema fails to relieve the obstruction (Figure 18.28). The procedure consists of either enterotomy or stoma formation with washout of the obstructing meconium or resection and primary anastomosis of the intestine.

Prognosis

Although neonatal survival is close to 100%, life-long replacement of pancreatic enzymes is required due to the presence of pancreatic insufficiency, as is physiotherapy to improve the drainage of bronchial secretions and intensive antibiotic management of respiratory infections.

Duodenal Atresia

Incidence and Type

Duodenal atresia occurs in 1 in 7500 live births.

- Duodenal atresia – in continuity, with fibrous connection, or with gap

- Duodenal web – perforated and/or windsock

- Duodenal stenosis

Associated Anomalies

Down's syndrome (30%), cardiac malformations, malrotation and atresias involving other parts of the alimentary canal, especially oesophageal and anorectal anomalies.

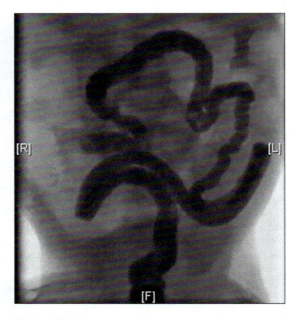

Figure 18.27 A carefully performed gastrografin enema may relieve the intraluminal obstruction.

Clinical Presentation

The presence of polyhydramnios should alert the clinician to the diagnosis of a proximal GI obstruction. Prenatal ultrasound scan will show the typical 'double-bubble' of duodenal atresia.

Postnatally, bilious vomiting is the most prominent symptom when the obstruction is below the level of the ampulla of Vater (two-thirds of cases). In higher obstructions, the vomitus is clear but persistent. There is usually upper abdominal distension and visible gastric peristalsis may be seen.

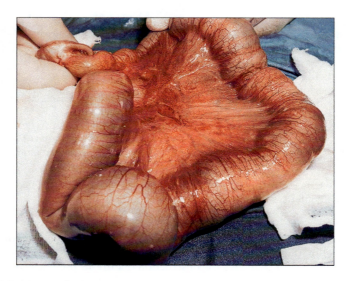

Figure 18.28 Meconium ileus. Operative appearance of the intestine showing dilated small intestine distended with impacted meconium.

Diagnosis

Plain abdominal x-ray will reveal the 'double-bubble' diagnostic of duodenal atresia (Figure 18.29). In incomplete obstructions, a contrast study may be required to reveal the partial duodenal obstruction.

Treatment

Duodenoduodenostomy (open or laparoscopic).

Intestinal Atresia

Incidence and Types

Intestinal atresia occurs in 1 in 6000 live births.

- Type 1 – atresia in continuity
- Type 2 – atresia with fibrous connection
- Type 3 – atresia with gap in mesentery
- Type 4 – multiple atresias

Aetiology

Intrauterine vascular insufficiency to the involved segment of intestine (e.g. strangulation, intussusception, volvulus) results in isolated intestinal atresia, although additional anomalies may be found in up to 10% of cases.

Clinical Presentation

The presence of an intestinal atresia may be suspected on prenatal ultrasound scan by the presence of dilated or echogenic bowel.

Postnatally, neonates present with bilious vomiting associated with abdominal distension proportional to the level of the obstruction (with massive distension sufficient to cause respiratory embarrassment sometimes occurring in low obstructions). A small amount of meconium may be passed but, in general, only mucus may be present in the rectum and air is never passed.

Diagnosis

Plain abdominal x-ray shows dilated loops of proximal intestine with an absence of gas distally (Figure 18.30). It is not possible to differentiate small from large intestine on plain x-ray and occasionally it may be necessary to perform contrast studies to document the level of the obstruction.

Treatment

Surgical management consists of excising the ends of atretic segments followed by anastomosis (Figure 18.31).

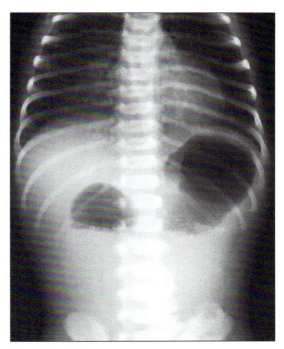

Figure 18.29 Duodenal atresia. Abdominal x-ray showing the typical 'double-bubble'.

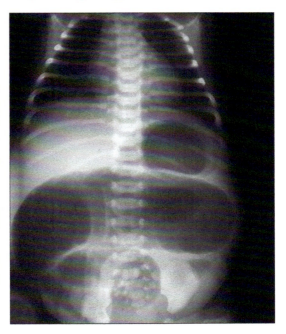

Figure 18.30 Intestinal atresia. Abdominal x-ray showing large dilated loops of obstructed proximal small intestine.

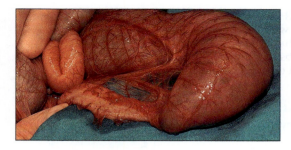

Figure 18.31 Intestinal atresia. Operative appearance, showing dilated proximal and collapsed distal bowel.

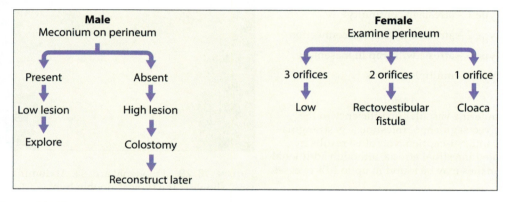

Figure 18.32 Diagnosis of anorectal anomalies.

Table 18.2: Commonest Anatomical Varieties of Anorectal Anomalies

	High (supralevator)	Low (translevator)
MALE	Rectourethral fistula	Covered anus
FEMALE	Cloacal or rectovaginal fistula	Ectopic anus or rectovestibular fistula

Anorectal Anomalies

Incidence

Anorectal anomalies occur in 1 in 3000 live births. Anorectal anomalies arise from a failure of complete development of the hindgut.

Associated Anomalies

Most frequent are anomalies of the urinary system (dysplastic kidney, hydronephrosis, vesicoureteric reflux, neuropathic bladder), sacral defects and VACTERL association.

Diagnosis

See Figure 18.32.

Anatomical Types

The number and variety of abnormalities is vast but a few basic principles in diagnosis and treatment should be adhered to (Table 18.2 and Figures 18.33 and 18.38)

Treatment

- High anomaly – colostomy followed later by posterior sagittal anorectoplasty

- Low anomaly – local perineal procedure either as an anoplasty or limited posterior sagittal repair

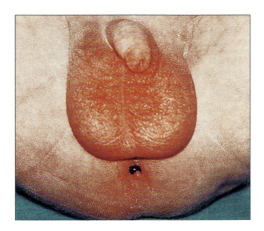

Figure 18.33 Low anorectal anomaly in a male infant, showing a spot of meconium on the perineum.

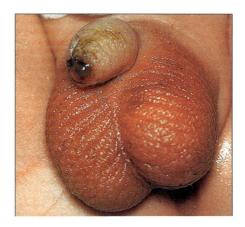

Figure 18.34 A high anorectal anomaly in a male infant, showing a 'flat' perineum and meconium in the urine.

Prognosis

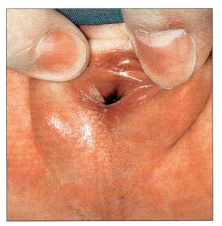

Figure 18.35 High anorectal anomaly in a female infant with a single opening on the perineum (a cloacal anomaly).

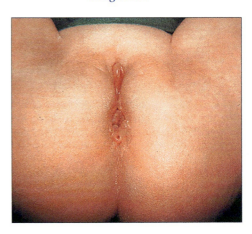

Figure 18.36 Low anterior ectopic anus, located immediately posterior to the fourchette, in a female infant.

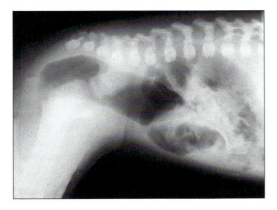

Figure 18.37 A low lesion shown by a cross table lateral radiograph with bowel gas well below the pelvic muscles.

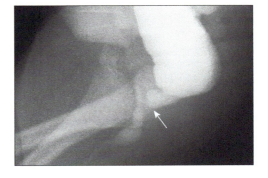

Figure 18.38 Rectourethral fistula. A distal colonogram showing the terminal rectum entering the bladder outlet in the region of the prostatic urethra.

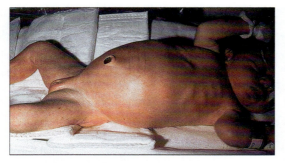

Figure 18.39 Hirschsprung disease: appearance of an infant showing a distended abdomen with dilated loops of bowel visible.

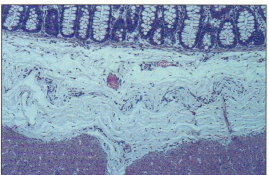

Figure 18.40 Hirschsprung disease: Rectal biopsy (H&E) showing absence of ganglion cells and large nerve trunks in the submucosal layer.

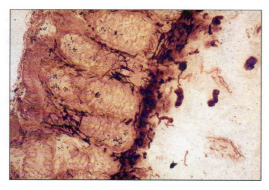

Figure 18.41 Hirschsprung disease: Histochemistry of rectal biopsy showing increased acetylcholinesterase positive nerve fibres in the submucosa and in the lamina propria.

The outlook for normal continence will depend on the anatomy of the lesion and the presence of associated spinal abnormalities. In general the higher the lesion and the more affected is the sacral spine the less likely there is to be normal faecal continence.

Hirschsprung's Disease
Incidence

Hirschsprung's disease characterised by the absence of ganglion cells in the distal intestine, occurs in 1 in 5000 live births. The anorectal region is always affected, with 75% of cases being confined to the rectosigmoid area and 10% including the entire colon (total colonic aganglionosis), extending for a greater or lesser extent into the small bowel.

Genetics

There is a definite familial pattern of inheritance. Males are affected four times as frequently as females. There is a 25% risk of inheritance in total colonic aganglionosis, where the male to female ratio is 1:1. One of the genes responsible for Hirschsprung disease has been isolated on the RET proto oncogene.

Clinical Presentation

Typical presentation is with delayed passage of meconium, in excess of 24 hours after birth, abdominal distension and bilious vomiting, which may be relieved following rectal probing or washout, only for the symptoms to recur shortly afterwards (Figure 18.39). Chronic intractable constipation may only occur in later childhood

Diagnosis

The plain abdominal x-ray may show dilated loops of intestine with an absence of gas in the rectum. A contrast enema may show a contracted rectum with dilated bowel proximally, but in the neonatal period this feature may be absent. Anorectal manometry reveals failure of relaxation of the internal anal sphincter in response to proximal distension. The definitive diagnosis is on histopathological examination of a rectal suction biopsy (Figures 18.40 and 18.41). Typically, this will show an absence of ganglion cells with large nerve trunks present in the submucosa. Histochemistry shows a proliferation of acetylcholinesterase fibres in the submucosa and particularly in the lamina propria.

Treatment

Definitive surgical treatment consists of treatment involving excising the aganglionicn intestine and anastomosing ganglionic bowel to the rectum. A number of surgical techniques are available of which the Duhamel, Swenson and Soave are most commonly employed. All of these operations may be carried out as a single or staged procedure.

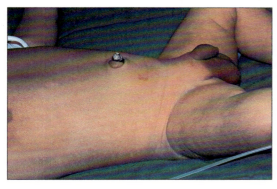

Figure 18.42 Malrotation: Clinical appearance of an infant showing an non-distended abdomen in the presence of bile-stained vomiting.

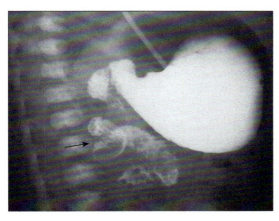

Figure 18.43 Malrotation: Lateral upper gastrointestinal contrast study showing 'corkscrew' appearance of the duodenum signifying a volvulus.

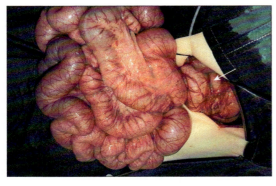

Figure 18.44 Malrotation: Operative appearance of the twist in the mesentery of the midgut. the intestine is viable.

Complications

Enterocolitis can be a life-threatening complication of Hirschsprungs, and is characterised by profuse diarrhoea and toxicity in combination with gross abdominal distension and, if untreated, can culminate in hypovolaemic shock. Enterocolitis may affect children before or after reconstructive surgery.

Malrotation
Aetiology

Failure of the intestine (midgut) to rotate normally in the first 12 weeks of development results in an abnormally mobile midgut with a short narrow based mesentery that has the propensity to twist, causing life-threatening midgut volvulus.

Clinical Presentation

Bile-stained vomiting may be the only symptom. The infant's abdomen is usually flat and non-distended (Figure 18.42). In the presence of volvulus, there may be additional signs such as blood-stained nasogastric aspirate and/or bloody mucusy stools and hypovolaemic shock in cases with advanced intestinal necrosis.

In older children, malrotation may present with gastro-oesophageal reflux (see the chapter 'Gastroenterology') with the occasional bilious vomit, faltering growth, symptoms suggestive of anorexia nervosa or recurrent abdominal pain.

Diagnosis

Plain abdominal x-ray may show absence of intestinal gas especially in the neonatal period. A contrast upper GI study will reveal the abnormally rotated duodenum with a 'corkscrew' pattern in the case of midgut volvulus (Figure 18.43). An ultrasound scan may show abnormal orientation of the superior mesenteric vessels, with the artery anterior or lateral to the vein.

Treatment

Urgent surgical intervention, following rapid and intense fluid resuscitation, is required to prevent or treat volvulus. The procedure consists of straightening the duodenal loop, widening the base of mesentery of the small intestine by dividing fibrous adhesions and placing the intestines in a non-rotated position, with the small bowel on the right side and the caecum and large bowel on the left side of the abdomen (Figure 18.44). Where volvulus has already occurred, the intestines should be de-rotated and inspected for viability. In extreme cases (no viable bowel) it is advisable to resect

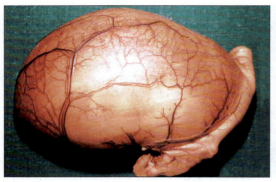

Figure 18.45   Cystic duplication.

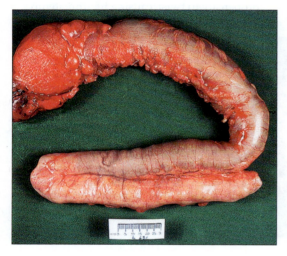

Figure 18.46   Tubular duplication.

frankly gangrenous intestine and to carry out a 'second-look' laparotomy 24 hours later. It may then be possible to salvage sufficient intestine for normal GI function.

Duplications of the Alimentary Tract

Incidence/Aetiology

Duplications can occur anywhere in the alimentary tract, from the mouth to the anus. They most commonly occur in the small bowel mesentery. Duplications comprise a mucosal lining, frequently of an area remote from the site of duplication, and a muscular wall. They may be cystic or tubular in form.

Clinical Presentation

Cystic duplications (Figure 18.45) cause symptoms from pressure on the adjacent intestine and can present with intestinal obstruction in association with a palpable mass. Tubular duplications (Figure 18.46) cause symptoms from peptic ulceration of the intestine due to an acid-secreting mucosal lining.

Diagnosis

An ultrasound scan will reveal the cystic nature and bowel wall signature of the mass. In tubular duplication, a technetium pertechnetate scan may reveal the presence of ectopic gastric mucosa.

Treatment

Excision of the duplication with or without the adjacent intestine and end-to-end anastomosis is the treatment of choice. Where long lengths of intestine are involved or when the site of duplication is in a critical area (duodenum), stripping of the mucosal lining is the best option.

Necrotising Enterocolitis

Incidence

Necrotising enterocolitis (NEC) occurs predominantly in the stressed premature infant and is currently one of the most common neonatal surgical emergency conditions.

Aetiology and Pathogenesis

Although not completely clear, it would appear that certain factors (e.g. prematurity, the presence of intraluminal substrate [breast milk is protective] and micro-organisms [*Klebsiella*, *E coli*, *Clostridia*]) are commonly present. Other contributing factors, such as hypoxia, hypovolaemia, hyperviscosity, hypotension and hypothermia, may be important. The most frequently affected parts of the GI tract are the terminal ileum and caecum and the splenic flexure of the colon. The final common pathway in the pathogenesis of the condition is an ischaemic process.

The mesenteric ischaemia leads progressively from mucosal ulceration through to full-thickness necrosis and perforation with peritonitis.

Clinical Presentation

Typical presentation is intolerance to feed followed rapidly by bilious vomiting or nasogastric aspirate, the passage of blood and mucus in the stool and abdominal distension (Figure 18.47).

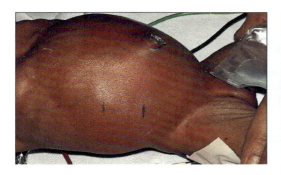

Figure 18.47 Premature infant with necrotising enterocolitis, displaying a distended abdomen, with redness and oedema of the abdominal wall.

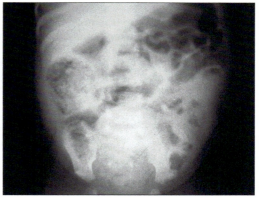

Figure 18.48 Necrotising enterocolitis: Plain x-ray showing pneumatosis intestinalis (gas in the bowel wall).

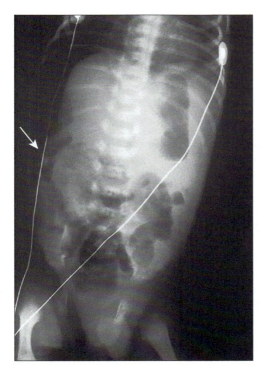

Figure 18.49 Necrotising enterocolitis: Plain x-ray showing pneumoperitoneum indicative of a perforation.

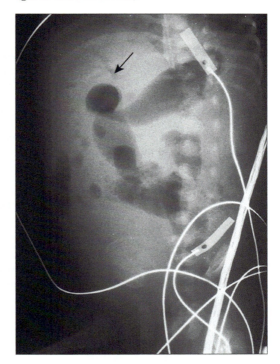

Figure 18.50 Necrotising enterocolitis: Plain x-ray showing portal venous gas.

Erythema and/or oedema of the anterior abdominal wall is indicative of impending intestinal gangrene with perforation. In severe cases, the infant becomes shocked and hypovolaemic.

Diagnosis

The hallmark of the diagnosis is the finding of pneumatosis intestinalis on plain abdominal x-ray. Free air (pneumoperitoneum) is indicative of perforation. Gas in the portal venous system may be a sign of advanced disease (Figures 18.48 to 18.50).

Treatment

Immediate resuscitation is required in all cases. Conservative treatment consists of nasogastric aspiration, broad-spectrum antibiotics and complete GI rest for seven to ten days, during which total parenteral nutrition is administered.

Indications for surgery are intestinal perforation, intestinal obstruction or failure to respond to conservative measures. Late indication for surgery is stricture formation.

Operative procedures comprise resection with primary anastomosis or resection with stoma formation.

Exomphalos

Incidence/Aetiology

Exomphalos occurs in 1 in 5000 live births and is due to failure of the physiological umbilical hernia to reduce fully into the abdominal cavity by the 12th week of gestation.

Clinical Presentation

The anomaly can be detected early in intrauterine life on ultrasound scan as anterior abdominal wall defect covered by a sac comprising of amnion, Wharton's jelly and peritoneum. It can be associated with cardiac and chromosomal anomalies and Beckwith Weidman syndrome (exomphalos, gigantism, macroglossia and hypoglycaemia). Exomphalos is classified as minor or major depending of the size of defect > 5 cm or containing liver (Figures 18.51 and 18.52).

Treatment

Prenatal counselling should be offered, including exclusion of a chromosomal anomaly; cardiac ECHO and detection of associated defects. Exomphalos minor is associated with more chromosomal anomalies whereas both exomphalos major and minor are equally associated with cardiac defects.

Postnatally, the sac must be covered with plastic wrap to prevent excessive fluid and heat loss. Minor lesions are amenable to primary closure of the defect. Major lesions may be treated by surgical application of a silo (preformed or surgically applied), with gradual progressive reduction of the contents into the abdomen or by allowing the sac to epithelialise with a view to delayed closure at a later date.

Prognosis

Poorer prognosis is associated with larger defect size and presence of other major anomalies.

Gastroschisis

Incidence

Gastroschisis occurs in 1 in 3000 live births with increase in incidence in recent decades. The typical abdominal wall defect is to the right of an intact umbilicus with extrusion of part of the intestine.

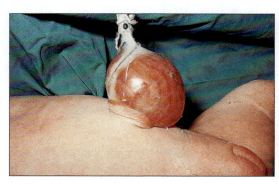

Figure 18.51 Minor exomphalos.

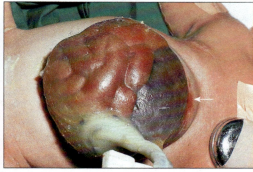

Figure 18.52 Major exomphalos including liver (arrow).

Diagnosis

The lesion is usually recognised on antenatal scan (Figure 18.53). It is not accompanied by any other major congenital anomaly. The diagnosis is self-evident at birth (Figure 18.54) if not detected prenatally.

Treatment

The lesion with the extruded bowel, which may be grossly thickened and oedematous, should be covered with plastic wrap to prevent fluid and heat loss. The bowel can then be reduced surgically, with primary repair of the defect, if the abdominal domain permits this, or placed in a silo to allows staged reduction and secondary closure of the defect.

Prognosis

Prognosis is excellent, except in infants with associated intestinal atresia or short-bowel syndrome.

GASTROINTESTINAL HAEMORRHAGE IN CHILDREN

The presence of blood in the stool needs to be assessed to determine the nature and quantity of blood loss as well as looking for associated hypovolaemic shock, anaemia or bilious vomiting. Swallowed maternal blood may lead to the appearance of blood in the vomitus or in the stool. To differentiate between maternal and fetal blood, the Apt test is used. Mixing the material with sodium hydroxide will colour adult haemoglobin brown while fetal haemoglobin remains pink.

Diagnosis

The age of the patient may be an important determinant of the likely cause of haemorrhage:

- Age < 2 years: volvulus, NEC, intussusception, Meckel's diverticulum, cow's milk protein allergy
- Age > 2 years: oesophageal varices, peptic ulceration, colonic polyps, inflammatory bowel disease

A diagnostic scheme for children presenting with rectal bleeding is shown in Figure 18.55.

Meckel's Diverticulum
Incidence

Meckel's diverticulum represents persistence of the intestinal end of the vitello-intestinal duct. It is present in 2% of the population, is located around 60 cm (2 feet) from the ileocaecal junction and may remain asymptomatic throughout life.

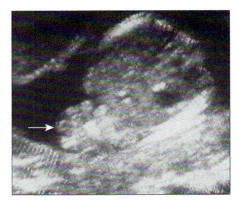

Figure 18.53 Gastroschisis: Prenatal scan showing intestinal loops outside the peritoneal cavity of the fetus (arrow).

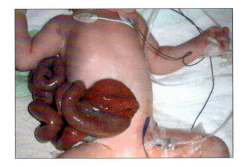

Figure 18.54 Gastroschisis: Appearance of the infant at birth with a large amount of intestine extruding through a defect in the abdominal wall just to the right of the umbilical cord.

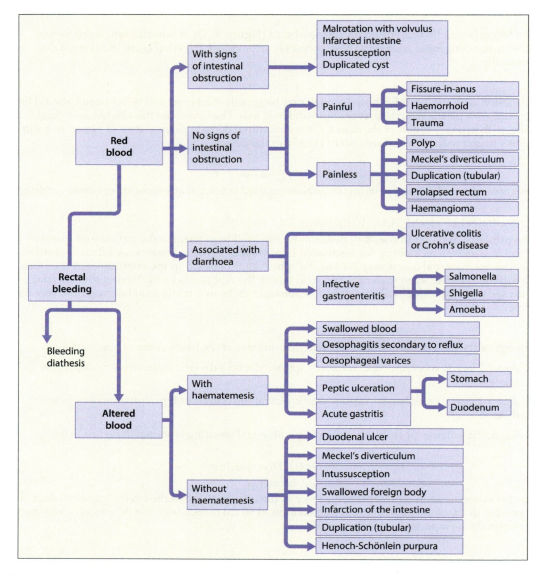

Figure 18.55   Diagnostic approach to rectal bleeding.

Clinical Presentation

Ectopic gastric mucosa causing ulceration in the adjacent ileal mucosa can lead to altered blood in stools. Haemorrhage can be significant. Intestinal obstruction may be due to kinking of the intestine by a fibrous band arising at the mesenteric attachment, or intussusception with the Meckel diverticulum at its apex, or volvulus around a band connecting the Meckel diverticulum to the umbilicus. Meckel's diverticulitis can mimic acute appendicitis.

Diagnosis

In the presence of ectopic gastric mucosa, a Meckel's scan will often detect uptake of technetium within the Meckel's, which localises the gastric mucosa contained within it (Figure 18.56).

Treatment

Operative management consists of wedge-resection of the diverticulum (Figure 18.57) with or without a segment of the adjacent ileum (Figure 18.58) and end-to-end anastomosis.

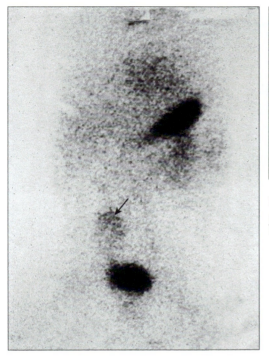

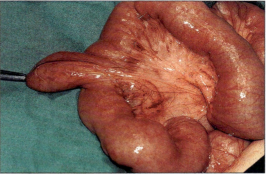

Figure 18.57   Typical appearance of a Meckel diverticulum originating on the antimesenteric border of the distal ileum.

Sacrococcygeal Teratoma

Incidence and Types

Sacrococcygeal teratoma occurs in 1 in 40,000 live births and is classified into the following Altmann Types: I: external sacrococcygeal mass (46%); II: mostly external but with presacral extension (35%); III: mostly presacral but with external element (9%); IV: entire presacral in location (10%). The tumour contains derivatives of all three germ cell elements (ectoderm, endoderm and mesoderm).

Figure 18.56   Technetium (TC99) isotope scan showing simultaneous appearance of isotope in the stomach, Meckel diverticulum and bladder.

Clinical Presentation

Prenatal ultrasound scans now pick up a majority of the lesions. The mode of delivery may be dictated by the size of the lesion, with elective caesarean section recommended for large lesions capable of causing dystocia or bleeding or rupture during delivery.

Postnatally most are visible as sacrococcygeal tumour at birth (Figures 18.59 and 18.60). Rectal examination will determine the extent of presacral extension.

Diagnosis

Clinical examination and imaging (USS/ MRI) will help diagnose and define the extent of the lesion. Alphafetoprotein is measured at diagnosis as it can be secreted by the tumour.

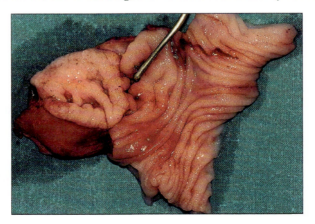

Figure 18.58   Opened Meckel diverticulum showing typical ectopic gastric mucosa leading to ulceration at the junction with the ileum. the ulcer may bleed or perforate.

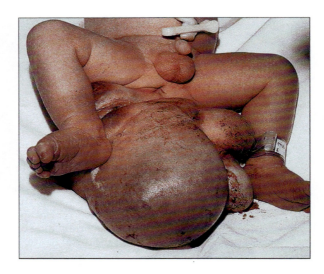

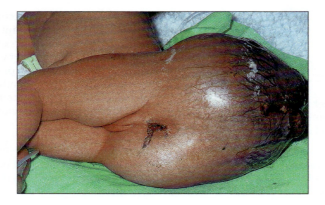

Figures 18.59, 18.60 Clinical appearance of infants with massive sacrococcygeal teratomas.

Treatment

Resection of the tumour *en bloc* with the coccyx is performed soon after birth. Incidence of malignancy increases with age after birth.

Prognosis

Children are followed for recurrence and also for urinary and anorectal dysfunction in the longer term.

Biliary Atresia

Incidence/Aetiology

Biliary atresia occurs in 1 in 12,000 live births. Theories proposed for its aetiology include genetic susceptibility and metabolic, infective and anatomical factors; such as an abnormally long common channel at the junction of the biliary and pancreatic ducts.

Classification (Figure 18.61):

- Type 1: atresia of the common bile duct, which may be associated with a dilatation of the common hepatic duct at the porta hepatis (5%).

- Type 2: atresia of the common hepatic duct with residual patency of the right and left hepatic ducts (3%).

- Type 3: atresia of the whole of the extrahepatic biliary system (92%).

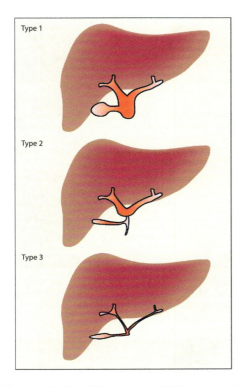

Figure 18.61 Three types of biliary atresia.

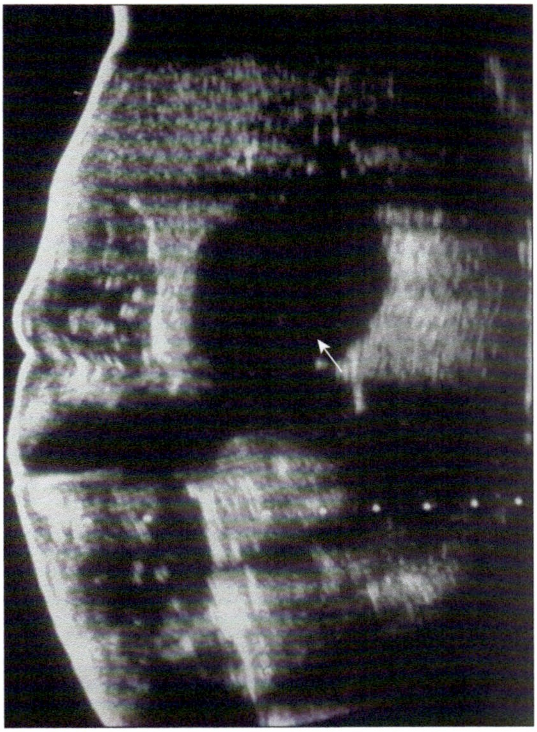

Figure 18.62 Choledochal cyst: Ultrasound scan revealing the cystic lesion inferior to the liver.

Clinical Presentation

Prolonged jaundice occurs in the first few weeks of life and is associated with pale stools.

Investigations

Elevated conjugated serum bilirubin would be assessed using ultrasound scan, percutaneous liver biopsy and operative cholangiography for definitive diagnosis.

Differential Diagnosis

- Neonatal hepatitis, α-1-antitrypsin deficiency.

Treatment

Exploration of the extrahepatic biliary system and hepaticojejunostomy is performed with a Roux-en-Y loop.

Prognosis

Optimal outcomes are reported when drainage of the biliary system is achieved within the first three months of life. Liver transplantation is a viable option for children who fail to respond to portoenterostomy or who develop intractable liver cirrhosis at a later age.

Choledochal Cyst

A choledochal cyst is a dilatation of the biliary system, which may affect the extrahepatic and/or the intrahepatic bile ducts (Figures 18.62 and 18.63).

Classification

- Type I: cystic dilatation of the extrahepatic bile ducts with or without dilatation of the intrahepatic ducts.

- Type II: fusiform dilatation of the extra-hepatic ducts with or without dilatation of the intrahepatic ducts, which are also fusiformly dilated.

- Type III: miscellaneous:

  a. diverticulum of common bile duct

  b. intraduodenal choledochocele

  c. intrahepatic dilatation alone (Caroli)

Aetiology

The aetiology is unknown, but two factors appear to be implicated:

- Weakness of the wall of the bile duct

- Distal obstruction

Clinical Presentation

In infancy, obstructive jaundice occurs with pale stools or a palpable mass in the right hypochondrium. **In older children**, intermittent mild jaundice maybe associated with abdominal pain or a palpable mass. Rarely, ascending cholangitis or pancreatitis are present.

Diagnosis

Diagnosis is based on abdominal ultrasonography and MRCP.

Treatment

The treatment of choice is excision of the cyst and gall bladder and Roux-en-Y hepaticojejunostomy. Postoperatively lifelong follow up is essential due to the risk of malignancy.

NECK LESIONS

During childhood, a variety of lesions occur in the neck. These are remnants of embryonic structures that have failed to resorb completely during development.

Cystic Hygroma

Cystic hygromas are multi-cystic malformations of the lymphatic system and comprise innumerable small cystic spaces or larger single cysts.

Incidence

The majority of lymphatic malformations are located in the neck, but they also occur in the axilla, abdomen and groin.

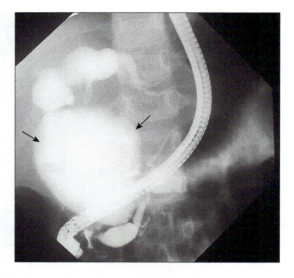

Figure 18.63 Choledochal cyst: Endoscopic retrograde cholangiogram showing the cystic dilatation of the common bile duct.

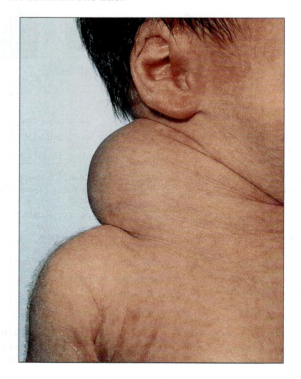

Figure 18.64 Small, posterior, cervical cystic hygroma that is soft and fluctant and transilluminates brilliantly.

They appear as soft, cystic, discrete non-tender masses that are transilluminable. (Figures 18.64 and 18.65). Rapid enlargement can present as a result of inflammation; this can cause acute respiratory distress from compression of the airway, or dysphagia from compression of the oesophagus.

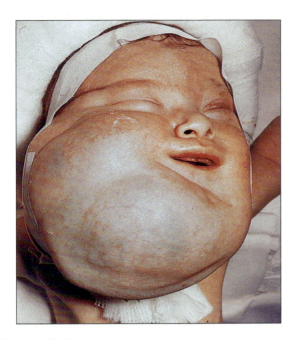

Diagnosis

Diagnosis is on clinical examination followed by ultrasonography to confirm the cystic nature of the lesion and also the extent of involvement. MRI will define the lesion more accurately and is helpful for delineating anatomy and associated strictures especially if planning surgical excision.

Treatment

Spontaneous regression of the lymphatic malformation is rare. Injection sclerotherapy is now the main treatment of choice (e.g. hypertonic saline, bleomycin, doxycycline, OK-432) for macrocystic lesions. Surgical excision is reserved for microcystic or persistent or recurrent lesions and maybe technically challenging due to 'infiltration' of the cysts between vital structures (e.g. carotid artery, internal jugular vein, phrenic nerve, cranial nerves). It is important NOT to sacrifice vital structures but to accept that recurrences will occur, which can then be treated on their merits.

Please also refer to the sections on thyroglossal and branchial remnants in

Figure 18.65 Massive cystic hygroma, extending from the temporal region across the parotid and cheek to cross the midline of the neck. the lesion caused respiratory embarrassment necessitating the tracheostomy.

the chapter 'Otorhinolaryngology' and vascular malformations in the chapters 'Paediatric and Reconstructive Surgery and 'Dermatology'.

CONJOINED TWINS

Incidence

The frequency of conjoined twins is around 1 in 250,000 live births. 60% die during gestation or at birth. Females predominate in the ratio of 3:1.

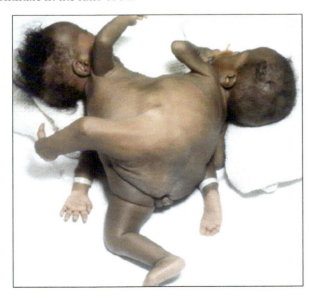

Figure 18.66 Thoracopagus conjoined twins.

Aetiology

Two theories are proposed: 1. secondary fusion between two originally separate monovular embryonic discs at around 13–15 days gestation; or 2. failure of complete separation of the embryonic disc.

Classification

Thoracopagus (**Figure 18.66**)	40%
Omphalopagus	33%
Pygopagus	19%
Ischiopagus (**Figure 18.67**)	6%
Craniopagus	2%

Diagnosis

The abnormality can be detected from 12 weeks on antenatal ultrasound. Detailed scanning at 20 weeks can accurately define the extent of union and indicate the shared organs. Fetal echocardiography is necessary to exclude fused hearts. After birth more detailed CT/MRI scans are valuable in planning the separation.

Treatment

- Non-operative management – for fused hearts of cerebral fusion; all will die.

- Emergency separation – when one twin is dead or dying threatening the survival of its twin; 25–30% survival.

- Planned separation – ideally at 2–4 months of age; 90% survival.

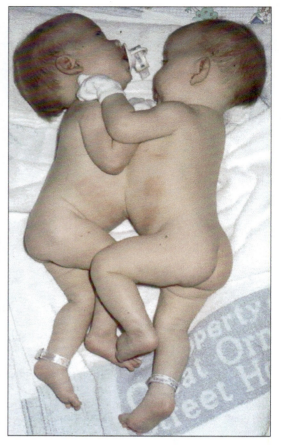

Figure 18.67 Ischiopagus twins.

19 Otorhinolaryngology

Paula Coyle and Chris Jephson

OTITIS MEDIA WITH EFFUSION ('GLUE EAR')

Incidence

High, prevalence: 5–10% unilaterally and 20% bilaterally under 6 years of age. More common in Native Americans, Inuit, Aborigines and Maori. Male:Female = 2:1.

Aetiology

Eustachian tube dysfunction (ETD), viral, bacterial acute otitis media, craniofacial abnormalities and allergy. Associated factors include season of the year, adenoidal hypertrophy, dairy-product diet, bottle feeding, day-care attendance, reflux disease and passive smoking. Local inflammation leads to epithelial metaplasia and collection of liquid in middle ear. The effusion is mucous or sero-mucous in nature.

Classification

Presence of fluid (serous, mucoid or mucopurulent) in an inflamed middle ear cleft without acute signs or symptoms (Figure 19.1).

Genetics

Craniofacial abnormalities, e.g. T21, Turners.

Clinical Presentation

Hearing loss, speech and learning disability with behavioural problems. May be associated with recurrent acute otitis media, or the child may be asymptomatic. Common findings on pneumatic otoscopy include dullness, loss of the light reflex, reduced mobility and retraction of an atrophic tympanic membrane over the ossicles, with a visible air–fluid meniscus. Tympanometry is a sensitive test. Hearing loss can be demonstrated by age-appropriate testing.

Treatment

First, active monitoring for at least three months. Decongestants, antibiotics and antihistamines are of no proven benefit, intranasal steroid therapy may be effective when there is an underlying rhinitis. Grommet (ventilation tube) insertion (Figure 19.2) remains the most efficacious treatment for persistent hearing loss. Adenoidectomy has been shown to have an additive effect in the resolution of OME when combined with grommets. Hearing aids can be offered as an alternative

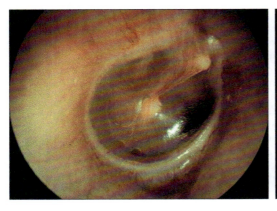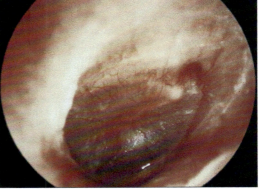

Figure 19.1   (Left): Normal tympanic membrane. (Right): Otitis media with effusion (glue ear).

DOI: 10.1201/9781003175186-19

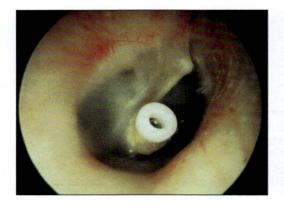

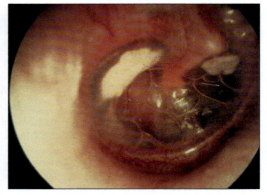

Figure 19.2 Grommet (ventilation tube) *in situ* in right tympanic membrane.

Figure 19.3 Tympanosclerotic plaque and otitis media with effusion.

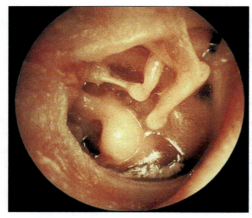

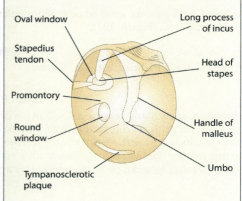

Figure 19.4 (Left): Retraction of the tympanic membrane onto the ossicles. (Right): Line diagram demonstrating features shown in left image.

to surgical intervention. NICE guideline CG60 offers specific advice for treating OME in patients with Down syndrome and in patients with cleft lip and palate.

Prognosis

Half of cases resolve spontaneously within three months and 95% within one year. Local complications of OME include tympanosclerosis, perforation, ossicular erosion, retraction pocket formation and cholesteatoma. Tympanosclerosis (Figure 19.3) is the result of hyaline degeneration and dystrophic calcification and produces characteristic 'chalk patches' in the tympanic membrane; it also occurs with repeated grommet insertion and attacks of acute otitis media. Perforations are most commonly central but can be marginal and these are more likely to be associated with cholesteatoma. Tympanic membrane retraction pockets (Figures 19.4) can be of the pars tensa or flaccida and result from negative middle ear pressures secondary to ETD. Ossicular erosion (most commonly affecting the long process of the incus) may result if the tympanic membrane becomes draped over the ossicles. Cholesteatoma may arise in a retraction pocket.

ACUTE OTITIS MEDIA

Incidence

Half of children under 5 years of age will have at least one episode of AOM. 50% of episodes occur in those under 5 years of age. Males > females, lower socioeconomic groups are more affected. Prevalence is higher in the winter months.

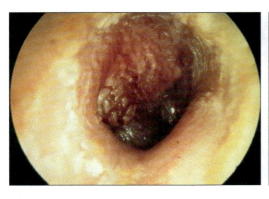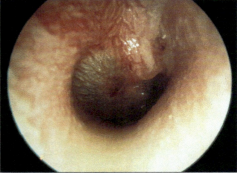

Figure 19.5   (Left): Acute otitis media with bulging of the tympanic membrane. (Right): Early acute otitis media.

Aetiology

Bacterial infection (*Haemophilus influenzae, Streptococcus pneumoniae* and *Moraxella catarrhalis* being the commonest pathogens) or viral infection. Associated factors include adenoidal hypertrophy, ETD, allergy, immunodeficiency, cleft palate and some craniofacial syndromes.

Classification

Acute otitis media (AOM) is defined as an acute infection of the middle ear cleft (Figure 19.5).

Genetics

Human leukocyte antigen (HLA) 2 and *HLA3*.

Clinical Presentation

Otalgia, pyrexia and systemic malaise. If perforation has occurred, otorrhoea may also be present. Tympanic membrane is erythematous and often bulging. Hyperaemia may extend onto the canal wall.

Differential Diagnosis

Otitis media with effusion, Cholestatoma

Pathology

Infection, causing oedema and hyperemia of the subepithelial space, followed by the infiltration of polymorphonuclear (PMN) leukocytes. There is mucosal metaplasia and the formation of granulation tissue.

Treatment

Analgesia and an antibiotic added if symptoms persist beyond 72 hours, or otorrhea or < two years with bilateral ear infection (NICE guideline *NG91*). Amoxicillin is the initial treatment of choice. In cases of incomplete resolution, the immunocompromised or in the presence of a complication, Grommet insertion is necessary, along with a sample for microbiology.

Prognosis

Commonly lasts three days but can persist up to a week. Mastoiditis occurs when the infection involves the mastoid portion of the temporal bone where it may cause osteitis, erosion and suppuration. Features include fever and inflammatory swelling behind the ear with auricular protrusion (Figure 19.6). Treatment is intravenous high-dose broad-spectrum antibiotics with antipseudomonal and staphylococcal activity. Occasionally a cortical mastoidectomy is necessary. Labyrinthitis may occur due to infection extending into the labyrinth via the round or oval window. Vertigo and associated hearing loss can last weeks to months, treat with antibiotics, steroids and labyrinthine sedatives. Sigmoid sinus thrombosis is uncommon and results from thrombophlebitis developing adjacent to the middle ear cleft in the sigmoid sinus. The classical sign is spiking pyrexia in a patient with AOM or mastoiditis (without any evidence of an abscess elsewhere). The thrombus requires prompt evacuation via a cortical mastoidectomy. Meningitis, early

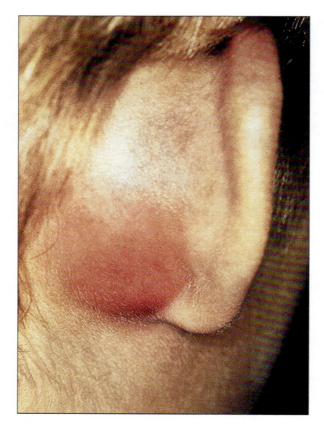

Figure 19.6 Acute mastoiditis showing postauricular swelling, erythema and protrusion for the pinna.

recognition and treatment is mandatory. Brain abscess, abscesses of the temporal lobe are twice as common as cerebellar abscesses. Spread is mainly via venous channels and preformed anatomical pathways. Treatment requires neurosurgical drainage of the abscess together with a mastoidectomy, and antibiotic therapy. Brain abscess formation is estimated to occur in less than 1% of cases of AOM in the paediatric population.

CHOLESTEATOMA

Incidence
Congenital or acquired. Incidence is 0.3–1.6 in 10,000 per year.

Aetiology
Keratinising squamous epithelium within the middle ear or temporal bone. Continuing desquamation causes the cholesteatoma to enlarge, with consequent erosion of bone and the risk of intracranial complications.

Genetics
Likely family genetics but no specifics found yet.

Clinical Presentation
Congenital: Intact tympanic membrane (Figure 19.7) in a patient without a history of otitis media. Asymptomatic, white mass seen on otoscopy behind the tympanic membrane, usually in the anterosuperior quadrant (where a squamous epithelial cell rest may persist at the site of the primitive epidermoid body).

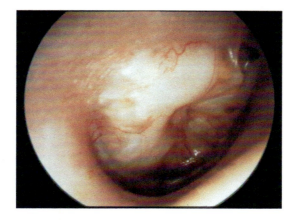

Figure 19.7   Congenital cholesteatoma behind an intact tympanic membrane.

Acquired: Chronic suppurative otitis media (CSOM) with an attic or posterior marginal tympanic membrane perforation. Tympanic membrane perforation or retraction with discharge is the characteristic presentation.

Differential Diagnosis
AOM, Otitis media with effusion.

Pathology
ETD, reduced ventilation in the middle ear, causing keratinising squamous epithelium in be in wrong anatomical place. Multiple theories.

Treatment
Cholesteatoma requires surgical extirpation by means of a mastoidectomy.

Prognosis
In children, cholesteatoma is more aggressive than in adults and so prompt surgery is required to reduce the long-term morbidity. Conductive hearing loss due to perforation, ossicular erosion and recurrent infection is usual; less commonly, vertigo may occur due to erosion of the horizontal semicircular canal and, rarely, facial nerve paralysis can develop due to pressure and inflammation from the cholesteatoma.

CHRONIC SUPPURATIVE OTITIS MEDIA
Incidence
Between 1–6%. Higher in Tanzania, India, Solomon Islands, Guam, Australian Aborigines, Greenland.

Aetiology
CSOM is defined as chronic inflammation of the mucosa of the middle ear in the presence of a tympanic membrane perforation of at least six weeks duration, resulting in otorrhoea and hearing loss.

Genetics
Low *HLA2.*

Clinical Presentation
Otoscopy reveals a perforation with chronic inflammation of the middle ear. There is a conductive hearing loss and intermittent discharge. The perforation can be central (Figure 19.8) or marginal (Figure 19.9). There can also be an associated cholesteatoma (Figure 19.10). Discharge may be precipitated by an upper respiratory tract infection, or by water getting into the ear.

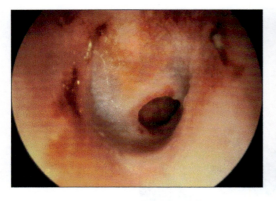

Figure 19.8 Chronic otitis media: central tympanic membrane perforation.

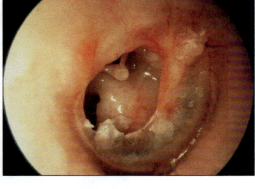

Figure 19.9 Chronic otitis media: posterior marginal tympanic membrane perforation.

Differential Diagnosis

AOM, Otitis media with effusion, cholesteatoma

Pathology

AOM, ETD, Tympanic membrane perforation.

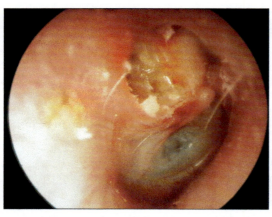

Figure 19.10 Acquired cholesteatoma arising from an attic retraction pocket.

Treatment

Aural toilet, microbiological culture of the discharge and appropriate topical antibiotic ear drops. Audiometry once the discharge has settled. Simple perforations can be repaired by myringoplasty; more advanced disease may require mastoidectomy +/– tympanoplasty to reconstruct the tympanic membrane and ossicular chain.

Prognosis

Good prognosis managing infections; hearing restoration is variable.

OTITIS EXTERNA

Incidence

Lifetime prevalence is 10%.

Aetiology

Inflammation of the skin of the external auditory canal (Figure 19.11), most commonly due to bacterial or fungal infection (Figure 19.12).

Genetics

ELANE gene.

Clinical Presentation

Pain, irritation, discharge and hearing loss. Predisposing factors: Local trauma, irritants, meatal exostoses, a discharging perforation, dermatological conditions and swimming (particularly in tropical waters, spas and hot pools). Skin conditions: dermatitis or psoriasis are less common aetiologies. Common organisms include Pseudomonas aeruginosa, *Staphylococcus aureus*, *Proteus* and *Escherichia coli*. Furunculosis may produce a particularly severe otitis externa secondary to *S. aureus* infection of the hair follicles located in the cartilaginous portion of the ear canal. A short history of severe otalgia with a localised area of swelling, erythema and pus formation is typical. Recurrent episodes are associated with staphylococcal carrier status.

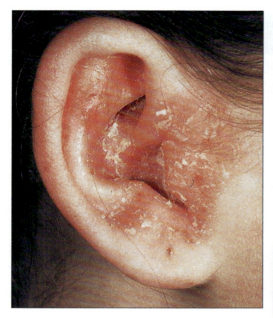

Figure 19.11 Bacterial otitis externa with involvement of the pinna.

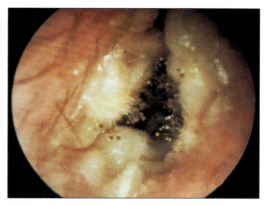

Figure 19.12 Fungal otitis externa.

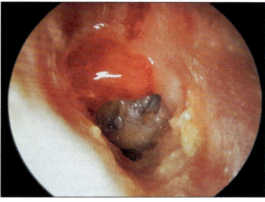

Figure 19.13 Benign aural polyp.

Differential Diagnosis
CSOM, AOM with otorrhea

Pathology
Localised inflammation typically due to bacterial infection. Worse with skin compromise eg. eczema.

Treatment
Meticulous aural toilet, bacteriological swabs and, if necessary, the use of wicks with antibiotic/antifungal/steroid drops. If cellulitis spreads beyond the canal onto the auricle, systemic antibiotics are necessary. It is important to keep the ear dry and continue treatment for several days after the acute episode has settled. Furunculosis may require incision and drainage.

Prognosis
Good prognosis with well managed infections. However, can progress to aural polyps. Most are benign (Figure 19.13) and consist of granulation tissue arising as a result of infection. Occasionally, there may be an underlying cholesteatoma. A differential diagnosis of rhabdomyosarcoma, glomus tumour or facial nerve neuroma should be considered. CT scan may be useful. Treatment includes aural toilet, removal of the polyp and antibiotic ear drops.

AURAL FOREIGN BODIES

Incidence
Foreign bodies in the ear are common in the 2–4 year age group.

Clinical Presentation
Inert foreign bodies may cause local pain due to secondary infection. Foreign bodies such as button batteries, vegetable material and insects produce an intense reaction with ulceration and otitis externa. There may be tympanic membrane perforation and, occasionally, ossicular disruption.

Treatment
Removal under a microscope is required, which frequently occurs under general anaesthesia.

CONGENITAL ANOMALIES OF THE EAR PREAURICULAR SINUS AND ABSCESS

Incidence
1% unilateral; 0.3% bilateral.

Aetiology
Preauricular sinuses (Figure 19.14) arise from the inclusion of ectodermal elements between the six mesenchymal hillocks during embryological development of the pinna. They lie close to the anterior, ascending limb of the helix, running a tortuous branching course that is usually superficial to the temporalis fascia.

Clinical Presentation
Often asymptomatic but can become infected, discharge, occasionally with abscess formation.

Treatment
Recurrently infected sinuses require excision, with meticulous wide dissection including a bit of the Helix cartilage to ensure complete removal. Abscesses require initial incision and drainage, followed by excision once settled.

EXTERNAL EAR ANOMALIES
Range from minor abnormalities such as 'bat ears', as a result of abnormal folding of the cartilage, through varying degrees of microtia (Figure 19.15), to complete absence of the pinna (anotia) with atresia of the external auditory meatus. Anomalies may occur in isolation or in combination with other craniofacial or genetic syndromes. Cosmetic deformities may also have a conductive hearing loss. The facial nerve may follow an abnormal course.

Incidence
1/5–6000 births; 90% unilateral.

Classification
Microtia Weerda Classification

Grade 1: Smaller ear

Grade 2: Rudimental, malformed but some recognisable components

Grade 3: 'Peanut' ear: Small, deformed tissue often containing cartilage

Grade 4: Anotia

Clinical Presentation
Noticed at birth/newborn baby check.

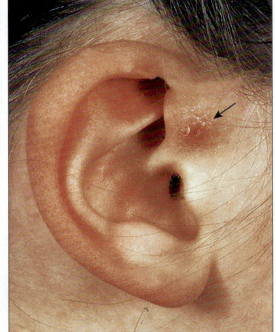

Figure 19.14 Infected preauricular sinus.

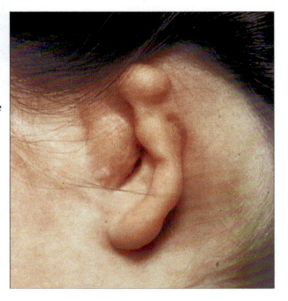

Figure 19.15 Microtia.

Treatment
Cosmesis: Autologous tissue reconstruction or by a bone-anchored prosthesis from 10 years. Hearing loss: Addressed with bone-conducting hearing aid from birth, which can be converted to a bone-anchored hearing aid from 5 years.

MIDDLE EAR ANOMALIES

Minor ossicular abnormalities to major deformities of the middle ear cleft associated with microtia and meatal atresia, and result in a conductive hearing loss.

Treatment

Results of attempted surgical correction for these major anomalies are poor. The treatment of choice is therefore amplification via conventional air-conduction hearing aids if the external auditory meatuses are present, or a bone-conduction hearing aid if they are not.

INNER EAR ANOMALIES

Anomalies of the cochlea, vestibule, semicircular canals, aqueducts and internal auditory meatus can occur in isolation or in combination with various syndromic and non-syndromic conditions.

Presentation

Severe bilateral sensorineural hearing loss, may be progressive.

Treatment

Audiological evaluation, appropriate amplification, speech and language therapy (SLT), support from a teacher of the deaf, and genetic counselling. Some are suitable for cochlear implantation, whereby the auditory nerve endings are electrically stimulated in response to sound.

RHINOSINUSITIS WITH OR WITHOUT NASAL POLYPS

Incidence

Incidence is 4% in childhood. Uncommon in children under the age of 10 years.

Classification

EPOS2020 Position Paper.
  Paediatric rhinosinusitis:
  Presence of two or more symptoms, one of which should be nasal blockage/obstruction/congestion or nasal discharge (anterior/posterior nasal drip) with or without facial pain/pressure, with or without cough. With either endoscopic signs of nasal polyps, and/or – mucopurulent discharge (primarily from middle meatus) and/ or oedema/mucosal obstruction (primarily in middle meatus) and/or CT changes (mucosal changes within the osteomeatal complex and/or sinuses).
  Paediatric Acute rhinosinusitis:
  Sudden onset of two or more of the symptoms:

- nasal blockage/obstruction/congestion

- discoloured nasal discharge

- cough (daytime and nighttime) for < 12 weeks

Symptom free intervals may occur if the problem is recurrent, with validation by telephone or interview. Questions on allergic symptoms (i.e. sneezing, watery rhinorrhoea, nasal itching, and itchy watery eyes) should be included.
  Paediatric Chronic rhinosinusitis (with or without nasal polyps):
  Presence of two or more symptoms one of which should be either nasal blockage/obstruction/congestion or nasal discharge (anterior/posterior nasal drip) with or without facial pain/pressure with or without cough for ≥ 12 weeks, with validation by telephone or interview.

Clinical Presentation

Nasal obstruction, discharge and anosmia and secondary sinusitis. Polyps are associated with conditions such as cystic fibrosis (Figure 19.16), Young syndrome, primary ciliary dyskinesia, Kartagener syndrome or immune deficiency syndromes.

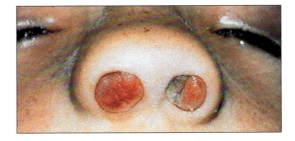

Figure 19.16 Cystic fibrosis: bilateral nasal polyps in a child.

Differential Diagnosis

Allergic and non-allergic rhinitis, olfactory loss and facial pain, nasal tumours, ANCA-associated vasculitis

Treatment

N. Saline. Intranasal steroids. Treat allergic rhinitis and GORD. Sweat test, RAST test, serum immunoglobulins including IgG subclasses and ciliary function tests may be useful. Consider adenoidectomy. CT Scan if surgery (Functional Endoscopic Sinus Surgery) is required.

Prognosis

High rate of recurrence and medical treatment must be continued postoperatively. Acute rhinosinusitis may be complicated by periorbital cellulitis (Figure 19.17), subperiosteal abscess (Figure 19.18), orbital abscess, cavernous sinus thrombosis, cerebral abscess and optic neuritis. Treatment of complications in children requires prompt referral to the paediatric otolaryngology team, CT scan of the sinuses and brain, ophthalmological and, if necessary, neurosurgical opinion.

NASAL MASS

The differential diagnosis of a nasal mass is as shown in Table 19.1.

NASAL GLIOMA AND MENINGOENCEPHALOCOELE

Incidence

Incidence is 1 in 20–40,000 births.

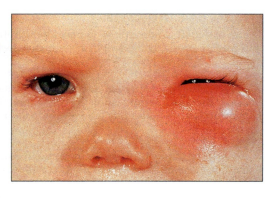

Figure 19.17 Periorbital cellulitis and subperiosteal abscess in a 9-month-old child.

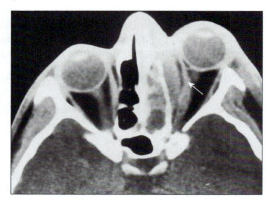

Figure 19.18 Periorbital cellulitis and subperiosteal abscess: axial CT scan of the child in Figure 19.17 demonstrating the subperiosteal abscess.

Classification

Nasal gliomas and meningoencephalocoeles are rare congenital nasal swellings resulting from herniation of cerebral tissue through the anterior skull base during fetal development. Nasal gliomas do not have an intracranial connection whereas meningoencephalocoeles maintain an intracranial connection.

Table 19.1: Differential Diagnosis of a Nasal Mass

Congenital	Acquired

• Glioma
• Meninogoencephalocoele
• Epidermoid cyst
• Dermoid cyst
• Chordoma
• Craniopharyngioma
• Thornwald cyst
	Inflammatory
	  • Abscess
	  • Polyp
	  • Antrochoanal polyp
	  • Mucocoele
	Benign
	  • Haemangioma
	  • Lymphangioma
	  • Lipoma
	  • Angiofibroma
	  • Neuroblastoma
	  • Neurofibroma
	  • Papilloma
	Malignant
	  • Lymphoma
	  • Rhabdomyosarcoma
	  • Thyroid carcinoma
	  • Nasopharyngeal carcinoma

Presentation

Rarely picked up on Antenatal scanning. Nasal obstruction, feeding difficulties and sometimes a visible mass in the nose (Figure 19.19). Due to its intracranial connection a meningoencephalocoele will increase in size with crying, straining or coughing and is pulsatile, unlike a glioma. Any polypoid mass within the nose should raise the suspicion of a possible intracranial connection.

Treatment

CT or MRI scan is mandatory. These lesions usually require complete excision via an endoscopic intranasal approach. Simple excision may lead to a CSF leak. A large skull base defect may need neurosurgical repair.

Prognosis

Excellent.

JUVENILE NASOPHARYNGEAL ANGIOFIBROMA

Incidence

Incidence is 1 in 15,000 males, peaking at 7–14 years of age.

Aetiology

A juvenile nasopharyngeal angiofibroma (JNA) is a benign vascular neoplasm that affects young males. It arises in the region of the sphenopalatine foramen and expands into the pterygopalatine fossa and nasopharynx.

Clinical Presentation

Epistaxis, progressive nasal obstruction, headaches and visual disturbance. Flexible Nasendoscopy (FNE) reveals a mass in the nasopharynx.

Treatment

A CT scan with contrast (Figure 19.20) or an MRI scan should be performed but avoid biopsy, as it may result in torrential haemorrhage. Preoperative embolisation, followed by surgical resection a few days later via an open approach (mid-facial degloving) or endoscopic approach. Very large lesions and recurrences can be treated with radiotherapy.

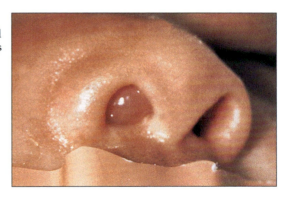

Figure 19.19 Nasal glioma in an infant.

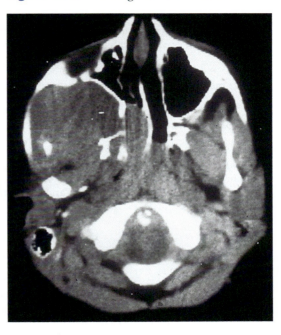

Figure 19.20 Axial CT scan of large right postnasal angiofibroma.

Prognosis

Excellent when there is total microscopic clearance of the tumour. Natural regression between 20–30 years old.

NASAL FOREIGN BODIES

Incidence

Nasal foreign bodies are common in 2–5-year-old children.

Clinical Presentation

Witnessed or history of unilateral, purulent, malodorous discharge or with nasal obstruction. Button batteries may cause rapid ulceration. Foreign bodies may be multiple and bilateral.

Differential Diagnosis

Rhinosinusitis, adenoiditis, sinonasal malignancy and unilateral choanal atresia.

Treatment

Retrieval using an angled hook, drawing the object from behind forwards under direct vision. The first attempt, under appropriate restraint, is generally the most successful because thereafter compliance is reduced. Inappropriate instrumentation may force the foreign body deeper into the nasal cavity or even into the lower airways. Clinical detection can be difficult. Rarely CT scan may be required to detect the foreign body, followed by examination under general anaesthesia.

CHOANAL ATRESIA

Incidence

Incidence is 1 in 8000 live births, Female:Male = 2:1. Unilateral:Bilateral = 2:1. Other congenital anomalies occur in over 50% of patients, and up to 30% may have CHARGE syndrome.

Aetiology

Congenital malformation, failure to develop a communication between the nasal cavity and the nasopharynx. It can be unilateral and more rarely, bilateral.

Classification

10% are membranous, the rest being bony or mixed bony/membranous.

Genetics

CHD7 gene causes CHARGE syndrome.

Clinical Presentation

Bilateral presents at birth as an emergency with respiratory distress, as neonates are obligate nasal breathers. Unilateral often presents later with nasal obstruction and unilateral mucopurulent discharge: there is absence of air flow, and inability to pass a size 8 French gauge nasal catheter beyond 5 cm into the nose.

Differential Diagnosis

Piriform aperture stenosis, mid-nasal stenosis, foreign body

Treatment

FNE, CT scan (Figure 19.21), remember to decongest and suction the nose prior to imaging. Examination of the postnasal space under general anaesthetic confirms the diagnosis. Neonates with bilateral choanal atresia will require a taped-in oral airway or intubation and orogastric feeding tube until surgical correction is undertaken, usually within the first week of life. Stenting may be required. Surgery for unilateral atresia is performed electively usually after the age of 2 years. Repair is undertaken via a transnasal approach under endoscopic control. Repeat dilatations are needed.

Prognosis

Excellent in almost all cases with normal growth, development and function of the nose. However multiple subsequent dilatations are often necessary.

TONSILLITIS (ACUTE, CHRONIC AND RECURRENT)

Incidence

Common for children to have at least two episodes of tonsillitis during childhood.

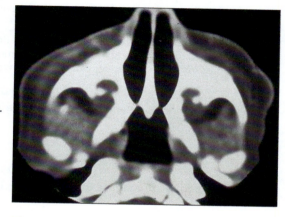

Figure 19.21 Bilateral choanal atresia: axial CT scan.

Aetiology

Viral due to the EBV, adenovirus or respiratory syncytial virus (RSV). Bacterial due to *Streptococcus pyogenes*, *Streptococcus pneumoniae*, *Staphylococcus aureus* or *Haemophilus influenzae*. Immunocompromised are more susceptible.

Clinical Presentation

Acute tonsillitis (Figure 19.22) is usually bilateral and presents with a sore throat, fever, abdominal pain, dysphagia, otalgia and tender cervical lymphadenopathy. Chronic tonsillitis is defined as lasting six weeks or more. Features associated with chronic tonsillitis include dysphagia, halitosis, tonsillar hypertrophy or fibrosis, debris-filled tonsillar crypts, persistent cervical lymphadenopathy and poor general health.

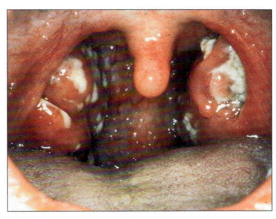

Figure 19.22 Acute follicular tonsillitis.

Differential Diagnosis

Toxoplasmosis, infectious mononucleosis

Treatment

Throat swabs are helpful in prolonged/resistant infections, when an unusual organism is suspected or in the immunocompromised. Full blood count, monospot and EBV-titres may be useful. Intravenous or oral penicillin for five days is the treatment of choice in acute infections (Clarithromycin in cases of penicillin sensitivity). Rehydration, antipyretic and analgesic therapy is required. Tonsillectomy is recommended for recurrent (SIGN guideline 117), chronic or complicated tonsillitis.

Prognosis

Most episodes are self-limiting. Complications include rheumatic fever, peritonsillar cellulitis or abscess, retropharyngeal or parapharyngeal abscess, septicaemia and upper airway obstruction.

PERITONSILLAR ABSCESS (QUINSY)

Aetiology

Unilateral collection of pus outside the capsule of the tonsil, following an acute or acute-onchronic infection.

Clinical Presentation

Unilateral sore throat, trismus, dysphagia.

Treatment

Incision and drainage, with intravenous antibiotics are needed; usually under general anaesthetic but needle aspiration under local anaesthesia may be sufficient in older patients. Recurrent quinsy requires tonsillectomy, ideally 4–6 weeks after the infection has resolved.

RETROPHARYNGEAL ABSCESS

Aetiology

Abscess arising in a retropharyngeal (prevertebral) lymph node, from which pus may track down inferiorly into the mediastinum. Causes include trauma secondary to a foreign body, tonsillitis, adenoiditis, cervical osteomyelitis or dental infection.

Clinical Presentation

Pyrexia, odynophagia, stiff neck and signs of upper airway obstruction are usual.

Treatment

CT scan, incision and drainage is performed under general anaesthesia with intravenous antibiotic cover.

OBSTRUCTIVE SLEEP APNOEA

Incidence

Incidence is etween 3–5% of children.

Aetiology

Hypertrophy of the lymphoid tissues of the Waldeyer ring (Figure 19.23). Retrognathia, macroglossia, midfacial hypoplasia and generalised hypotonia may also contribute.

Classification

Sleep-disordered breathing encompasses a spectrum ranging from snoring to obstructive sleep apnoea (OSA). OSA is the temporary cessation (apnoea) or reduction (hypopnoea) of airflow during sleep caused by an obstruction. OSA can be mild, moderate or severe depending upon the number of hyponoeas and apnoeas per hour.

Genetics

Associated with other conditions, e.g. Trisomy 21, Prader–Willi, Pierre Robin, Achondroplasia.

Clinical Presentation

Snoring, mouth breathing, a disturbed sleep pattern with frequent waking, witnessed episodes of respiratory obstruction, impaired growth and behavioural problems. In severe cases, sternal recession, pectus excavatum and ultimately cor pulmonale.

Treatment

Clinical diagnosis. Parental videos aid diagnosis. Polysomnography is required when history is unclear, patients have other diagnosis e.g. craniofacial abnormalities or if central sleep apnoea is suspected. Adenotonsillectomy cures most, but not necessarily those with other comorbidities. In these cases, other surgery (turbinoplasty, septoplasty, tongue base reduction), a nasopharyngeal airway and/or continuous positive airway pressure (CPAP) may be used in addition to adenotonsillectomy. Tracheostomy may be required in extreme cases.

DROOLING

Aetiology

Lack of oromotor control associated with a poor swallow reflex in children with cerebral palsy and other neurological conditions. Drooling is normal until 5 years old.

Clinical Presentation

Multiple changes of clothing or bibs, skin excoriation around the lips and chin. Bullying and affecting school.

Treatment

If posture is thought to contribute, physiotherapy can be beneficial. Speech and language therapy can improve lip closure, jaw elevation and tongue control. Anticholinergic drugs (hyoscine patches

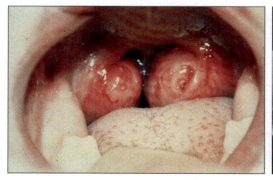
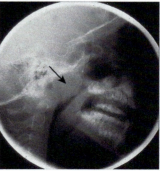

Figure 19.23 (Left): Tonsillar hypertrophy in a child with obstructive sleep apnoea. (Right): Lateral neck x-ray showing adenoidal hypertrophy.

or oral glycopyrrolate) reduce saliva production but are associated with side effects. Botulinum toxin injection offers temporary relief but needs repeating every few months and can cause dysphagia. Surgical options include submandibular duct ligation or transposition and submandibular gland excision with or without parotid duct ligation.

LARYNGOMALACIA

Incidence

Commonest cause of stridor in neonates and infants, accounting for 35–40% of cases.

Aetiology

May be partial or complete. Laxity of the immature laryngeal tissue allowing collapse of the supraglottic structures on inspiration, but the exact cause is unknown, associated with reflux.

Clinical Presentation

Stridor is inspiratory and variable. Onset is generally six weeks after birth and worse with effort (e.g. when feeding or crying). Difficulty with feeds, reflux and vomiting are common; failure to thrive occurs in severe cases. Other signs include tachypnoea, subcostal recession, tracheal tug and pectus excavatum.

Treatment

FNE or with a rigid laryngoscope, is necessary for all but the very mildest cases. Findings include long omega-shaped epiglottis, short aryepiglottic folds, redundant arytenoid mucosa and collapse of supraglottic tissues into the laryngeal introitus with inspiration are diagnostic. Mild laryngomalacia can be observed. Patients with failure to thrive can be treated with NG feeding or undergo endoscopic aryepiglottoplasty to trim the redundant supraglottic tissues. Treat reflux. SLT reviews are helpful.

Prognosis

Half will resolve in one year and 90% in two years.

SUBGLOTTIC STENOSIS

Classification

Cotton–Meyer grading: I: 0–50% endoscopic treatment; II: 51–70% endoscopic treatment; III: 71–99% resting stridor; IV: 100%.

Aetiology

Congenital causes: Elliptical, failure to re-canalise, prematurity.
Acquired causes: Circumferential trauma, GORD, high tracheostomy, infections, intubations.

Clinical Presentation

Stridor, failure to extubate, recurrent croup.

Treatment

Evaluate weight, voice, stridor and increased work of breathing. FNE. Conservative management for mild cases. Antibiotics if bacterial infection, steroids, adrenaline nebulisers, treat reflux if needed. MLB and endoscopic treatment (incision, dilatation, steroids, cricoid split). Open: Cricoid split, laryngotracheal reconstruction, cricotracheal resection, slide tracheoplasty, tracheostomy.

RECURRENT RESPIRATORY PAPILLOMATOSIS

Incidence

Incidence is 4 in 100,000 in children.

Aetiology

Human papilloma virus (HPV) Types 6 and 11 (Figure 19.24). Papillomas are benign exophytic proliferations of keratinised stratifed squamous respiratory epithelium. Can occur anywhere in the aerodigestive tract, but typically present in the larynx, especially the vocal cords.

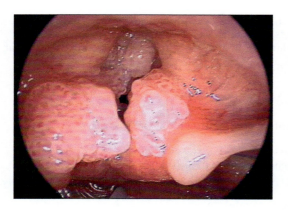

Figure 19.24 Endoscopic view of recurrent respiratory papillomatosis of the supraglottis and glottis.

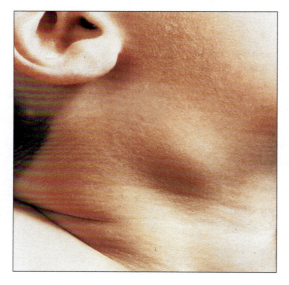

Figure 19.25 Second branchial arch cyst in an 8-year-old boy.

Clinical Presentation

Average presentation is 4 years old. Symptoms depend upon the location and severity of the disease, progressively hoarse voice, abnormal cry, stridor, respiratory distress and exercise intolerance. Younger children have a more aggressive clinical course. *HPV11* behaves more aggressively.

Treatment

Endoscopic examination. Biopsy is needed to confirm diagnosis and rule out malignant transformation. Biopsies should be performed yearly if disease continues. Typing of *HPV* using the polymerase chain reaction (PCR) helps direct prognosis discussions with the family. Aim of treatment is to maintain a good airway and adequate voice while awaiting spontaneous remission without causing long-term scarring of the larynx. This is achieved by 'debulking' the papillomas on a regular basis. Powered instruments ('microdebrider') have superseded CO_2 laser vaporisation as this causes less laryngeal scarring. Offer the Gardasil vaccination, rarely intralesional cidofovir, which remains controversial, but can be useful in florid disease. Tracheostomy is occasionally necessary but tends to cause tracheobronchial spread of papillomas and so should be avoided if possible.

Prognosis

No effective systemic or surgical treatment to eradicate HPV. The disease tends to remit after a number of years, but can progress to adulthood. Malignant transformation is rare.

BRANCHIAL SINUSES, FISTULAE AND CYSTS

Aetiology

Rare embryological anomalies that arise from incomplete fusion of the branchial arches, resulting in a sinus, cyst or fistula. Commonest is a second branchial cleft sinus or fistula, followed by first branchial cleft sinus or fistula and finally fourth branchial pouch sinus.

Clinical Presentation

First and second branchial cleft sinuses present with a congenital opening to the skin that intermittently discharges mucoid or mucopurulent fluid; occasionally, an abscess may develop. Branchial cysts usually lie deep to the anterior border of the sternomastoid at the junction of its upper and middle thirds (Figure 19.25). Fourth branchial pouch sinuses do not have an external opening and present with recurrent neck abscesses which may have undergone a number of incision and drainage procedures.

Treatment

Ultrasound shows size, position of a cyst and can show the pathway of a sinus or fistula. Sinogram or MRI scan can be performed. Fourth branchial pouch sinus require endoscopic examination of the piriform fossa, as surgical excision has been superseded by endoscopic ablation of the sinus opening in the piriform fossa. For first and second arch anomalies, surgical excision of the entire tract is curative.

PAEDIATRIC HEAD AND NECK MASSES

Incidence

Head and neck masses in children are common. Usually they represent, self-limiting reactive lymphadenopathy associated with upper respiratory tract infections. Congenital masses include thyroglossal duct cysts, dermoid cysts, branchial anomalies, haemangiomas and vascular malformations; 5% of paediatric malignancies arise in the head and neck region, the most common are lymphoma and sarcoma.

Treatment

Is the lump congenital or acquired, acute or chronic, rapid or slow growing, painful or painless, midline or lateral, solitary or multiple? Determine size; shape; smooth or irregular, solid or cystic; mobility; change in colour of the overlying skin; functional disability; and any other local or systemic features. Consideration of the above should lead to differential diagnosis. Ultrasound will give information regarding tissue density, size, location, depth and often diagnosis. CT and MRI scans can give additional information but require a general anaesthetic in small children. Serology, FBC, Mantoux test, thyroid function tests and chest x-ray may be required. An ENT opinion should be obtained as soon as possible. Fine needle aspiration cytology (FNA) is not often used in children; ultrasound guided core biopsy or open biopsy is preferable.

THYROGLOSSAL DUCTCYST

About 70% of congenital head and neck masses. Males = Females.

Aetiology

During development, the thyroid descends from the tongue at the foramen caecum into the lower neck. Tract usually disappears after descent, but remnant may persist anywhere along its course, enlarge and present as a cyst. The tract has an intimate relationship with the body of the hyoid bone.

Clinical Presentation

Usually presents in the first two decades of life as a solitary midline cystic neck swelling (Figure 19.26). Variable size. May become infected to form an abscess and discharge forming a sinus. The cyst lifts with protrusion of the tongue.

Treatment

Thyroid ultrasound to demonstrate the presence of normal thyroid tissue is mandatory – very rarely it may contain the only functioning thyroid tissue. Surgical excision is the treatment of choice because of the risk of infection and abscess formation, and rare possibility of malignancy arising in a thyroglossal cyst. An abscess requires incision and drainage, followed by excision of the cyst when the infection has resolved. Modified extended Sistrunk procedure removes the cyst, tract, body of the hyoid, and a core of tissue from thyroid isthmus to the foramen caecum at the tongue base.

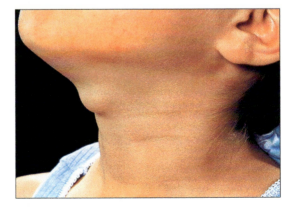

Figure 19.26 Thyroglossal duct cyst in a 7-year-old boy.

Prognosis

Excision of the cyst alone carries a recurrence rate of up to 50%. Wide excision using an extended Sistrunk procedure has a recurrence rate of less than 5%.

OROPHARYNGEAL, AIRWAY AND OESOPHAGEAL FOREIGN BODIES

Clinical Presentation

Any paediatric age groups. Small objects such as fish bones tend to lodge in the oropharynx, particularly tonsil, base of tongue and valleculae. Larger objects e.g. coins are typically found at the cricopharyngeal level. Older children may be able to localise a foreign body above the cricopharyngeus. Younger children present with drooling, dysphagia or irritability. Cough, wheeze, stridor, hoarseness, increased respiratory effort suggest a foreign body in the airway.

Treatment

A normal lateral neck x-ray or chest x-ray does not exclude a foreign body. The x-ray may demonstrate a radio-opaque foreign body (Figure 19.27), prevertebral soft tissue swelling, retropharyngeal or mediastinal air. CT may be helpful. Surgeons should have a low threshold for endoscopy to exclude an ingested foreign body. A spiking temperature suggests the possibility of complications such as a retropharyngeal abscess, perforated viscus, mediastinitis or septicaemia. If such a complication is suspected, the child should be placed nil-by-mouth, blood cultures obtained, high-dose IV antibiotics with anaerobic and gram-negative cover, and a contrast swallow or CT scan considered.

Bronchial foreign body may have a ball-valve effect, causing air trapping and hyperinflation of the affected lung. Inspiratory and expiratory chest x-rays may give clues as to the location of a foreign body and show hyperinflation, mediastinal shift (Figure 19.28) or atelectasis. However, there may be little to suggest the presence of a bronchial foreign body after the initial episode of coughing/choking. Bronchoscopy should be performed by an experienced surgical, anaesthetic and nursing team. Distal foreign bodies occasionally require flexible endoscopy and, very rarely, a thoracotomy may be required.

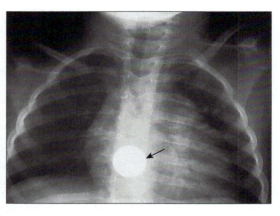

Figure 19.27 Chest x-ray demonstrating a radio-opaque body (coin).

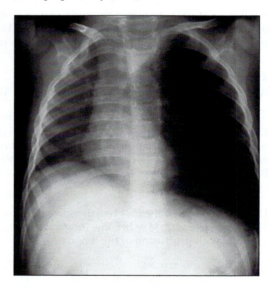

Figure 19.28 Hyperinflation of the left lung with mediastinal shift to the right due to air trapping by a foreign body in the left main bronchus.

20 Paediatric Plastic and Reconstructive Surgery

Neil Bulstrode, David Dunaway, Simon Eccles, Adrian Grobbelaar, Jonathan Leckenby, Loshan Kangesu, Paul Morris, Juling Ong, Patricia Rorison, Amir Sadri, Branavan Sivakumar and Gill Smith

INTRODUCTION

Plastic and reconstructive surgery covers a wide and varied set of sub specialties involving all parts of the body, including the head and neck, congenital hand and limb anomalies, as well as dermatological and soft tissue conditions (see also the chapter 'Dermatology'). The specialty is integral to many multidisciplinary teams and assists with the management and reconstruction of patients affected by trauma, malignancy and congenital deformity with the intention to improving function and form for patients, as well as their psychology.

There are several areas of plastic surgical practice that are beyond the scope of this chapter. The most common and important conditions are discussed and the reader is directed to further reading as appropriate.

HEAD AND NECK

Much of the work in paediatric plastic surgery centres on the head and neck. This includes the management of cleft lip and palate, craniofacial deformities, craniopagus conjoined twins, head and neck cancer, ear reconstruction, neurofibromatosis and other conditions. This requires collaborative working with other specialties including otolaryngology, neurosurgery, maxillofacial surgery, dental, orthodontics, audiology, speech and language, interventional and diagnostic radiology, psychology and others. The management centres on dealing with emergency situations and improving form and function. The input of psychologists is particularly important for these patients as issues will inevitably arise as a consequence of living with facial difference.

CLEFT LIP AND PALATE

Incidence

Cleft lip and/or palate (CLP) is the most common craniofacial deformity. In most cases it is a unilateral, but can be bilateral with varying levels of involvement of the structure from the lip to the back of the soft palate.

In the United Kingdom, the overall incidence is approximately 0.8 in 1000. In 2020 cleft palate alone (CP) was the most common of the four cleft types, representing 44.6% of all a known cleft types, followed by cleft lip (CL) (23.9%), unilateral cleft lip and palate (21.7%) and bilateral cleft lip and palate (9.8%). There is racial heterogeneity with rates higher in East Asians and lower among Afro-Caribbeans.

Aetiology

CLP results from a failure of fusion of the central (frontonasal) and lateral (maxillary) embryological processes that form the midface. The aetiology is largely unknown but likely multifactorial with environmental and genetic factors. There is only a 30% concordance rate among identical twins. Recognised environmental factors are maternal diabetes, smoking, alcohol and drugs (anticonvulsants, steroids). Folic acid supplementation plays a role in preventing CLP.

Classification

CLP can be unilateral or bilateral. In addition it can complete (involving all the lip/alveolus/palate) or incomplete (partial involvement of the lip/alveolus/palate). A microform (forme fruste) cleft lip is a form of incomplete cleft lip which is characterised by a vertical furrow or scar, vermillion notch, white roll imperfection, and varying degree of vertical lip shortness.

Genetics

No single gene has been identified as a cause for CLP. CP alone is genetically distinct from CLP. A parent affected by CLP has an approximately a 3–5% risk of having an affected child. The risk increases as increasing family individuals have CLP (e.g. the risk increases to 17% if there is one affected parent and sibling).

DOI: 10.1201/9781003175186-20

Clinical Presentation

Antenatal diagnosis represents the most common presentation (75–95%). In CP, the diagnosis is made at birth by direct visual inspect of the palate. In cases a CP is missed and is cause for feeding difficulty and failure to thrive. Rare variants of cleft palate such as submucous cleft palate will present with poor speech characterised by velopharyngeal incompetence.

Treatment

Cleft care is multidisciplinary with input dependent on the age of the child and needs.

Surgical repair is carried out at various time points. A cleft lip and hard palate are repaired in a thriving infant at approximately 3–4 months of age. A soft palate cleft is repaired between 6–9 months of age. The aim is to have a repaired soft palate before speech development to prevent development of compensatory speech characteristics. The alveolar cleft is repaired with bone graft during the period of mixed dentition when two-thirds of the canine root has developed, around age 8–10.

Prognosis

The overall prognosis is good. Up to 25% of patients will require secondary surgery either for complications such as fistula (10%) or the development of velopharyngeal incompetence due to poor soft palate lift or length. Patients with associated anomalies or syndromes have a poorer outcome.

CRANIOSYNOSTOSIS

Craniosynostosis (CS) is the premature fusion of the cranial sutures. The characteristic head shapes (trigonocephaly, scaphocephaly, brachycephaly and plagiocephaly) are the result of restricted growth perpendicular to the affected suture and the consequent overgrowth of the non-fused sutures.

Craniosynostosis affects 1 in 2250 live births and the aetiology is considered to include both genetic and environmental factors. For the vast majority of cases (80%) CS affects only a single suture (Figure 20.4) and no genetic cause is found.

When multiple sutures are involved, an identifiable genetic basis is more likely. This is particularly the case when the coronal sutures are affected.

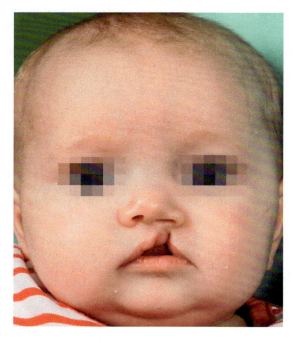

Figure 20.1 Left incomplete cleft of the lip and alveolus (gum).

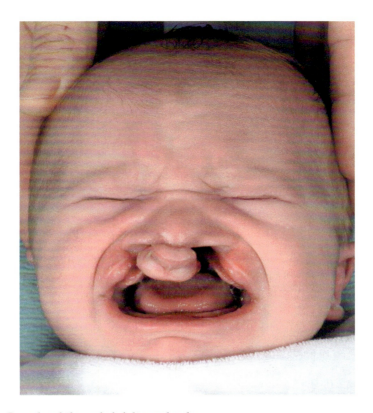

Figure 20.2   Complete bilateral cleft lip and palate.

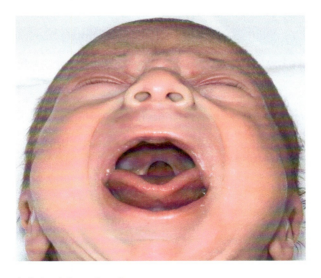

Figure 20.3   Isolated cleft of the soft palate.

Incidence

CS affects 1 in 2250 live births. The characteristic deformities of craniosynostosis result from restricted growth of the affected suture and the overgrowth of the non-fused sutures.

Metopic (1/2000, M > F)

Sagittal (1/4000, M > F)

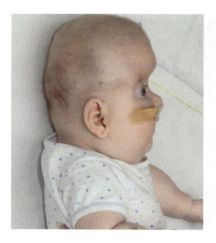

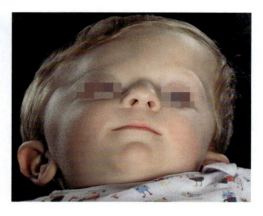

Figure 20.5 Plagiocephaly due to right unilateral single suture coronal synostosis. There is no threat to brain development.

Figure 20.4 Apert syndrome with multisuture or complex synostosis. There are risks to the airway, vision and increased intracranial pressure.

Unicoronal (1/8000, F > M)

Lambdoid (1/200,000, M = F)

A genetic cause is much less common and associated with coronal or multi-suture synostosis (MSS) (Figure 20.5).
   Muenke syndrome (*FGFR3*, 1 in 20,000)
   Crouzons (*FGFR2/3*, 1 in 25,000)
   Pfeiffers (*FGFR2*, 1 in 100,000)
   Aperts (1 in 100,000)

Aetiology

Craniosynostoses are 80% multifactorial and are associated with mechanical and genetic factors; 15% will have identifiable genetic mutations involving the *FGFR*, *TWIST*, *TCF12* and *ERF* genes. Craniosynostosis is not a key feature in the remaining 5% (e.g. hypophosphatemic rickets and vitamin D deficiency).

Pathogenesis

The foetal skull develops over the dura and is influenced by cellular signalling pathways and mechanical forces at specific regions to form sutures. These structures enable skull deformation during birth, rapid brain growth and provide protection to the brain. Craniosynostosis is the premature ossification of these sutures.

Classification

Craniosynostosis is classified by the affected suture and cause. Examples are:

1. Non-syndromic (multifactorial aetiology) sagittal craniosynostosis

2. *FGFR3* Muenke syndrome bicoronal craniosynostosis

3. MSS associated with hypo-phosphotaemic ricketts.

Clinical Presentation

Craniosynostosis usually presents at birth with progressive cranial deformity. Some will have additional problems (e.g. raised intracranial pressure (ICP)) particularly when more than one suture is involved (Tables 20.1 and Table 20.2).

Differential Diagnosis

Differential diagnoses for children with head shape and size anomalies are listed in Table 20.3.

Table 20.1: Functional Morbidities Associated with Craniosynostosis

Airway	Midnasal stenosis, maxillary retrusion	Multiple potential levels of airway obstruction
Orbital	Maxillary retrusion	Shallow orbits, exorbitism, globe subluxation, corneal exposure
Maxillary arch	Constricted maxillary arch, cleft in Apert's syndrome	Dental crowding, malocclusion
Aesthetics	Convex facial profile, orbital dystopias	Psychosocial
Neurodevelopmental	Cephalocranial disproportion, chiari malformation, hydrocephalus	Increased risk of seizures, developmental delay, autistic spectrum disorders
Extracranial features	Acne, acanthosis nigricans, cardiac anomalies, limb anomalies	

Table 20.2: Features of Craniosynostoses and Deformational Plagiocephaly.

Suture	Description	Features
Sagittal	Scaphocephaly	Frontal bossing, Sagittal ridge, occipital 'Bullett', low posterior vertex
Metopic	Trigonocephaly	Midline metopic ridge, Bitemporal narrowing, biparietal widening
Unicoronal	Anterior (synostotic) plagiocephaly	Ipsilateral brow retrusion, eye brow elevation and nasal root deviation. 'Harlequin sign' on plain AP skull x-ray
Bicoronal	Brachy turricephaly	Bilateral brow retrusion with bitemporal and brow widening. High wide frontal bossing.
Lambdoid	Posterior (synostotic) plagiocephaly	Ipsilateral posterior flattening, contralateral parietal bossing, ipsilateral mastoid bossing
Normal open cranial sutures	Posterior (deformational) plagiocephaly	Parallelogram shaped head, ipsilateral frontal bossing, ipsilateral anterior ear malposition. No nasal root deviation
Early multi-suture	Cloverleaf/Kleeblattschädel	Prominent central frontal bossing continuous with prominent anterior fontanelle, prominent temporal bulging, Hypertelorism, downslanting canthal angle, flat posteriorly
Late multi-suture	Microcephalic/ normocephalic	Normal head shape with lower head circumference for age. May have a bony prominence (Volcano) at site of anterior fontanelle

Table 20.3: Non-Craniosynostotic Differential Diagnoses

Metopic ridge	Normal head shape and bitemporal width, no hypotelorism. Ridge over metopic suture
Small/Closed anterior fontanelle	The anterior fontanelle closure is extremely variable (3 months to 3 years). Early closure in the absence of other features is not usually significant.
Large/persistent anterior fontanelle	A large fontanelle may be a feature of cleidocranial dysplasia.
Skull defects	Parietal foramina maybe features of genetic conditions (*MSX2*, *ALX4*) associated with CS
Microcephaly	A head circumference (HC) < 2 SD below the mean. Consider primary brain anomalies. If HC fails to increase with successive measurements this may reflect MSS
Macrocephaly	HC > 2 SD above the mean. Consider benign macrocrania of infancy, hydrocephalus, overgrowth conditions.

When there is diagnostic uncertainty, additional examinations (e.g. imaging, genetic testing) may be required.

Crouzon syndrome – multi-sutural cranosynostosis. Clinically normal hands and feet. midface retrusion. Significant risk of raised ICP.

Pfeiffer syndrome – bicoronal or cloverleaf phenotype. Broad radial deviation of the great toe and thumb. No cleft palate, midface retrusion.

Apert syndrome – bicoronal or cloverleaf phenotype, Complex complete syndactyly's. Cleft palate (70%), midface retrusion, hypertelorism

Genetic testing for syndromic Craniosynostosis:
Coronal or multiple sutures: *FGFR1, FGFR2, FGFR3, TCF12, TWIST* and *ERF*.
The midline sutures: *SMAD6*.

Treatment

Cranial vault surgery is generally performed for aesthetic reasons in the first two years of life. Vault expansion to address raised intracranial pressure may, however, be required at any time up to 10 years of age. In contrast, facial surgery is generally performed as late as possible to reduce the impact on facial growth and the need for repeated surgery. Surgery to address sight threatening exorbitism can be performed at any age to preserve vision.

The management of this heterogeneous group of challenging and rare conditions requires expert assessment and management by an experienced multidisciplinary team, which must continue throughout childhood and early life.

The age of the child, indication and deformity dictate the surgical technique used. Minimally invasive techniques (e.g. spring cranioplasty and endoscopic strip craniectomy and helmet [ESCR]) can be used before 5–6 months of age, whereas fronto-orbital, posterior and total vault remodelling are performed from 10–18 months.

Raised ICP develops insidiously and can lead to neurocognitive morbidity and vision loss. Regular ophthalmological testing (fundoscopy, electrophysiological testing, OCT) can reduce this risk. Posterior vault expansion is the mainstay of treatment for raised ICP.

Fronto-facial advancement surgery is used to alter appearance, improve the airway, correct occlusion and treat raised ICP in those with more complex presentations.

Prognosis

Most children with craniosynostosis have excellent aesthetic and functional outcomes. A higher level of care is required in children with syndromic CS to provide them with the best opportunities to lead independent lives.

CRANIOFACIAL MICROSOMIA

Craniofacial microsomia is a bilateral asymmetric craniofacial anomaly. It affects the first and second branchial arch structures and results in a correspondingly wide spectrum of functional and aesthetic morbidities. Mandibular hypoplasia, orbital dystopias, nerve palsies, microtia and soft tissue deficiencies of the face are characteristic of this condition. Grading systems are available to standardise assessment and guidelines are useful for management by an experienced multidisciplinary team. Extracranial manifestations are common, particularly in those with more severe craniofacial deformity. The prognosis for this condition is favourable for the majority of patients. More severely affected patients, however, often require functional interventions earlier in life and multiple staged reconstructions to address the various aspects of the deformity throughout childhood and adolescence.

Incidence

Craniofacial microsomia (CFM) is the second most common congenital craniofacial anomaly affecting between 1 in 3000 and 1 in 6000 live births.

Aetiology/Pathogenesis

The condition results in underdevelopment of the facial structures derived from the first and second branchial arches.

Classification

CFM has an extremely wide phenotypic presentation in both its severity and the facial structures involved. The use of a standardised assessment tools to grade the degree of orbital, mandibular, ear, nerve and soft tissue deformity is helpful for evaluation.

Genetics

CFM is sporadic in most cases with no genetic causes found.

Clinical Presentation

Diagnosis of craniofacial microsomia requires:

- Two major criteria
- One major and one minor
- Three+ minor criteria

Major criteria	Minor criteria
Mandibular hypoplasia	Facial soft tissue deficiency
Microtia	Pre-auricular skin tags
Orbital/facial bone hypoplasia	Macrostomia
Asymmetric facial movement (Cranial Nerve palsy)	Clefting
	Epibulbar dermoids
	Segmental anomalies of the spine

Over 50% of patients have extracranial manifestations[2] (CNS, cardiac, renal, and spinal anomalies) and are associated with a higher OMENS grade (Figures 20.6 and 20.7).

Functional and aesthetic problems reflect the spectrum of disease:

1. Tongue based upper airway obstruction secondary to micrognathia
2. Speech and feeding difficulties from skeletal deformity, clefts and nerve palsies
3. Hearing problems from anomalies of the inner, middle and external ear
4. Malocclusion due to asymmetric mandibular hypoplasia
5. Visual problems from orbital dystopia, rectus palsies, astigmatisms and epibulbar dermoids
6. Cranial and facial postural and skeletal asymmetry

Differential Diagnosis

Hemifacial atrophy, condylar growth arrest, hemifacial hypertrophy, vascular anomalies, proteus syndrome, condylar hyperplasia, deformational plagiocephaly, Unicoronal craniosynostosis, Treacher–Collins syndrome, Nager syndrome, Miller syndrome.

Treatment

Management is directed towards addressing functional problems, reducing secondary morbidities and is timed with growth. A management plan may include early interventions to address the airway, speech, vision and hearing. Appearance related interventions to address soft tissue asymmetry, occlusion and skeletal corrections are staged later in adolescence to achieve the stable clinical outcomes.

MDT management is essential. Airway support may be needed. Some patients require hearing aids and speech therapy. Soft tissue augmentation can be performed in stages throughout childhood, with autologous ear reconstruction performed from 9 years. Orthodontic and orthognathic surgery should be performed at the completion of facial growth to reduce the likelihood of relapse.

Prognosis

Long-term prognosis is generally good for patients with mild to moderate disease. More

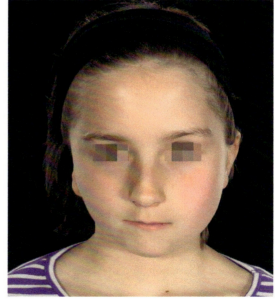

Figure 20.6 Right craniofacial microsomia with ear deformity.

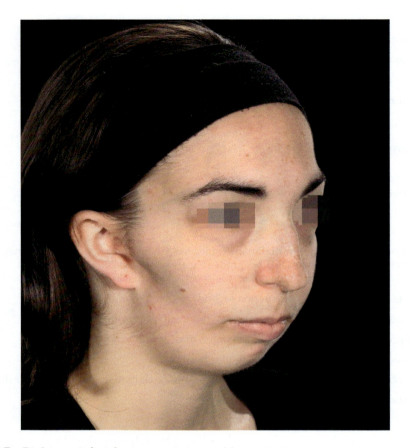

Figure 20.7 Right craniofacial microsomia in an older patient.

severely affected individuals will generally require earlier and multiple interventions to address functional morbidities and aesthetic asymmetries.

FACIAL PALSY

Incidence

Congenital facial paralysis accounts for 8–14% of all paediatric cases of facial paralysis. The incidence of facial paralysis in live births is 0.8–2.1 per 1000 births, and, of these, 88% are associated with a difficult labour.

Aetiology

Congenital (present at birth) facial paralysis is uncommon and is classified as traumatic or developmental, unilateral or bilateral, and complete or incomplete (paresis). Determining the aetiology is important because the prognosis and treatment differ depending on the underlying pathophysiology.

Clinical Presentation

Facial palsy may cause multiple problems for the newborn, such as difficulty with nursing and incomplete eye closure. If the paralysis does not resolve, it may affect the child's future speech, expressions of emotion, and mastication.

Diagnosis

An appropriate history and physical examination usually reveal the origin, but radiographic imaging and neuromuscular testing may be necessary for treatment planning.

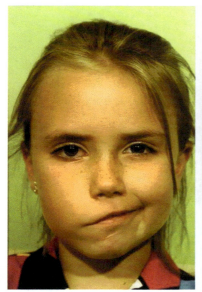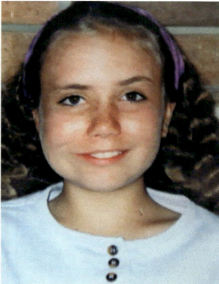

Figure 20.8   Patient with right sided facial palsy before and after two stage facial reanimation surgery with a cross facial nerve graft followed by a free pectoralis minor free flap. (Jonathan I. Leckenby and Adriaan O. Grobbelaar. Facial Reanimation Plastic Surgery: Principles and Practice, Chapter 22.)

An extended physical examination is needed to exclude other congenital malformations. Associated anomalies may include microtia, inner ear abnormalities, extraocular muscle paralysis, facial hypoplasia, other cranial nerve deficiencies, cleft palate, internal organ disorders, and extremity deformities. Bilateral facial paralysis is most commonly seen in children with Möbius syndrome.

Treatment

Treatment initially concentrates on protecting the cornea. Children generally require only the administration of artificial tears or taping of the eye at night. Small procedures like a platinum chain or tarsorrhaphy may be utilised to protect the eye if necessary. When indicated, formal reconstruction of the smile normally starts at the age of four years; the exact technique of reconstruction depends on the degree of the facial palsy and if the condition is unilateral or bilateral. Classically a two-stage reconstruction is performed, with the first operation the preparation of a new nerve cabled across the face from the healthy side to the non-functioning side. That is then normally followed by a transplanted muscle to replace the non-functioning facial muscles nine months later. In children with bilateral palsy another motor nerve must be utilised to power the new muscles transplanted into the face.

Prognosis

Depending on the degree of paralysis most patients can be improved with regard to both appearance and function.

MICROTIA AND EAR RECONSTRUCTION

Incidence

Microtia, or small ear, and atresia can be unilateral or bilateral (10% of cases) with an incidence of 1 in 6–8000 births. The condition affects the right side more than the left and can be involved in craniofacial microsomia and syndromes such as Goldenhar and Treacher–Collins.

Aetiology/Pathogenesis

The aetiology is unknown although the condition is associated with a family history of twinning. Early deficiency or embolism in the stapedial artery is one postulated cause.

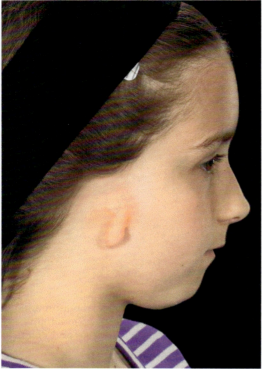

Figure 20.9   Patient with lobular microtia.

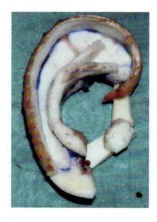

Figure 20.10   An ear framework carved and constructed from costal cartilage.

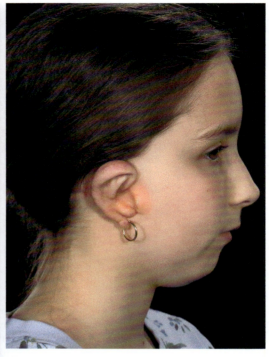

Figure 20.11   Same patient after two-stage surgery, placing the framework in a subcutaneous pocket and then creating the retro-auricular sulcus.

Clinical Presentation

Microtia is deficiency and deformity of the external ear and conductive hearing loss.

Diagnosis

Clinical examination by all relevant specialists including hearing assessment and renal ultrasound is advised.

Treatment

Treatment by a multidisciplinary team, involves audiology, surgeons (ENT, maxillofacial), orthodontists and psychology.

Hearing is the most important functional issue. Support is required for unilateral conductive hearing loss using either bone conduction and anchored hearing aids or implantable middle ear devices.

The options for ear reconstruction include no reconstruction. Surgical solutions are reconstruction with a staged carved rib cartilage framework placed in a subcutaneous pocket and, from nine years onwards, the use of a synthetic framework or a bone-anchored prosthesis.

Prognosis

The prognosis is excellent when treated by a dedicated multidisciplinary team. Patient reported outcome measures have shown good satisfaction with surgical intervention.

NEUROFIBROMATOSIS TYPE 1

Incidence

Neurofibromatosis Type 1 (NF1) is a multisystem condition, which occurs in 1 in 3000 live births. It is caused by and underlying abnormality in the gene coding for Neurofibromin, which transmitted as an autosomal dominant mutation, although there can be variable expression, resulting in a genetic mosaic. Spontanouse mutations also arise.

NF1 is transmitted on chromosome 17, and there are various subtypes which include Von Recklinghausen's disease. NF2 is transmitted on chromosome 22.

Aetiology

Tumour cells spread along multiple fascicles, causing diffuse thickening of peripheral nerves, mainly sensory nerves. NF1 is not limited by race or sex. It is however age specific, most signs are visible after birth, and the growth of individual lesions is highly variable.

Classification

There are no standardised classification systems, but Jackson (a craniofacial surgeon) attempted a classification of the craniofacial anomalies:

1. I – Mild (soft tissue only) plus seeing eye

2. II – Moderate (soft tissue and bone) plus seeing eye

3. III – Severe plus non-seeing eye

Other classifications are based on intracranial and cutaneous disease, and these lesions have been stratified with regard to the effect on the orbit, and to the various divisions of the trigeminal nerves that are affected.

Diagnosis

This requires a positive family history as there is autosomal dominant transmission as well as a high degree of suspicion.

Any two or more of the features below are also required:

1. Six or more *café* macules (> 0.5 cm in children or > 1.5 cm in adults)

2. Two or more cutaneous/subcutaneous neurofibromas or one plexiform neurofibroma

3. Axillary or groin freckling

4. Optic pathway gliomas

5. Two or more Lisch nodules (iris hamartomas seen on slit lamp)

6. Bony dysplasia (Sphenoid wing dysplasia, bowing of long bone +/– pseudarthrosis)

7. First-degree relative with NF1

NF1 should be differentiated from:

1. Autosomal dominant multiple *café au lait* patches

2. Schwannomatosis

3. Watson syndrome

4. Segmental/mosaic NF1

Clinical Features

Most children present with benign neurofibromas, but these have a 10% lifetime risk of malignant transformation; 33% of NF1 have plexiform neurofibromas, and of these 38% have head and neck tumours and 24% optic nerve gliomas. Other issues that may arise include:

■ Central nervous system gliomas

■ Sphenoid Wing dysplasia and/or buphthalmos

■ Additional problems:

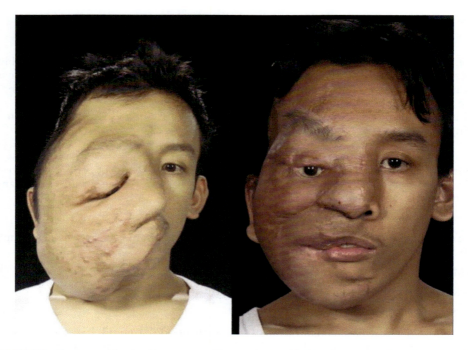

Figure 20.12 Patient with plexiform neurofibromatosis affecting the right side of the face before and after surgery.

- Learning difficulties (37%)
- Headaches (61%)
- Scoliosis (43%)
- Tibial Dysplasia (6%)
- Macrocephaly (63%)

Increased mortality is associated with:

- Malignant transformation
- Spontaneous haemorrhage causing hypovolaemic shock
- Airway compression and tracheostomy related complications
- Malignant peripheral nerve sheath tumours

Treatment

Management involves the surgical management of neurofibromas and plexiform neurofibromas by a specialist team. This must also include the monitoring of disease progression, including optic nerve gliomas.

Surgery can be successful in reducing the volume of plexiform neurofibromas and in children reducing the secondary impact on growth. Other medical teams will be involved including paediatric neurology, ophthalmology, and child and adolescent psychology, among others

Medical management involves the control of symptoms, including pain. More novel therapies have recently been trialled including the use of MEK inhibitors (mitogen-activated protein kinase inhibitor). This agent affects mutations along the MAPK/ERK pathway, and one such agent is Selumetinib. In trials this has been found to reduce the volume of plexiform NF1 and make them softer and less painful. BRAF inhibition may have a role in predicting outcome in plexiform size reduction.

Outcomes

Most NF1 patients lead normal lives. However, NF1 presents in many ways, and its outcome is often difficult to predict. The NF1 gene mutations can affect members of the same family in differing ways. Appearance and functional impairment are the main patient concerns, but one must also remember the increased risk of malignant transformation.

CONGENITAL HAND AND LIMB ANOMALIES

The incidence of upper limb anomalies in the United Kingdom is approximately 1 in 450 live births. Congenital hand differences arise from genetic or environmental influences on the foetus during development. Embryogenesis of the upper limb occurs between week four and eight of gestation and along three axes of development: proximo-distal, antero-posterior and dorso-ventral. The Oberg–Manske–Tonkin (OMT) classification, first proposed in 2010, is based on our current understanding of the aetiology, molecular genetics and developmental biology of congenital upper limb anomalies. Within this chapter we will provide an overview of examples within each of the three main themes of this classification; namely malformations – abnormal formation of a body part, deformities – an insult occurring after normal formation and dysplasias – abnormality in size, shape and organisation of cells within a tissue.

Malformations
Radial Longitudinal Deficiency (RLD)
Incidence
Overall incidence ranges from 1:30,000 to 1:100,000 live births.

Aetiology
Genetic and environmental factors such as thalidomide have been implicated in RLD.

Presentation
Typically patients present with a radially deviated and flexed wrist on a shortened forearm with a hypoplastic or absent thumb. Bayne and Klug categorised RLD into four types based on the amount of radius present. Type I is characterised by mild radial shortening. Cases with a hypoplastic (or 'miniature') radius are considered Type II, partial absence of the radius constitutes Type III, and total absence is Type IV. Associated conditions are common and can affect almost any organ system. These include blood dyscrasias such as Fanconi anaemia and Thrombocytopenia-absent radius, heart conditions such as Holt–Oram syndrome and multi-system disorders such as VACTERL association.

Example of radial longitudinal deficiency showing proximal hypoplasia, wrist deformity and thumb aplasia.

Differential Diagnosis
Underdevelopment of the radius can be established through clinical and radiographic examination of the upper limb. It is important to look for anomalies along the whole length of the upper limb and for associated conditions affecting other organ systems.

Treatment
The main aims of treatment in RLD are to create stable alignment of the hand and carpus on the forearm, maximise function and optimise growth potential. The soft tissue structures on the radial side of the wrist are short therefore treatment begins with a regime of stretching and splintage carried out by the parents under the guidance of a hand therapist. Subsequent surgical intervention depends on the severity of the deficiency and the child's overall functionality. In cases of severe hypoplasia, i.e. grades III and IV, the wrist deformity is usually addressed through initial soft tissue distraction by an external frame, followed by a wrist centralisation/radialisation procedure to create a stable ulno-carpal equilibrium or radial substitution procedure by free tissue transfer. Subsequently thumb reconstruction may be required and limb lengthening.

Prognosis
Outcomes of treatment vary according to the severity of the condition and stiffness of the digits. Soft tissue distraction in conjunction with centralisation/stabilisation procedures are effective in improving wrist position to optimise hand function and cosmesis. However regardless of treatment ulnar growth is compromised in the majority to around 50–60% of normal and upper limb strength is less than normal.

Deformations
Constriction Ring Sequence
Incidence

Constriction ring sequence (CRS) also referred to as amniotic band syndrome has a reported incidence of between 1:200 to 1:1500 live births.

Aetiology

The most widely accepted aetiology is an extrinsic theory of mechanical deformation of normally developed anatomy by amniotic strands.

Presentation

Multiple limbs are usually affected and associated musculoskeletal anomalies are commonly present. There is a predilection for the more distal extremities – in particular the longer central three digits and great toe. The severity of the deformity can vary significantly between affected limbs ranging from mild indentations to deep constrictions causing limb amputations. Distal digital autoamputations and fusions in the form of acrosyndactyly are also common.

Differential Diagnosis

CRS can be distinguished from other forms of intrinsic limb deficiency including transverse arrest and symbrachydactyly by the presence of rings elsewhere, acrosyndactyly, the more tapered shape of digital auto-amputations and a lack of more proximal hypoplasia.

Treatment

Early intervention is indicated in cases of acute vascular compromise, progressive lymphoedema and nerve compression. Release of acrosyndactyly can untether growth. More moderate constriction rings can be dealt with non-urgently. Some severe cases warrant more complex functional reconstruction through toe to hand transfers, skeletal lengthening and digital transpositions.

Prognosis

As with other congenital hand anomalies children adapt well but with growth further interventions may be required to preserve optimal function.

Dysplasias
Macrodactyly

Incidence

Macrodactyly has an estimated incidence of 1:50,000 live births.

Aetiology

Macrodactyly is deemed part of the PIK3CA related overgrowth spectrum of disorders (PROS).

Presentation

It can be isolated, involving a single digit or more generalised involving an entire extremity or other areas of the body. It may be associated with other conditions. Enlarged areas often correspond to the cutaneous distribution of specific nerves, i.e. nerve territory orientated macrodactyly (NTOM). Macrodactyly tends to follow two patterns of clinical progression – a static form where growth is commensurate with that of the child and a progressive form in which the growth is disproportionate.

Differential Diagnosis

Macrodactyly which tends to be more hamartomatous overgrowth should be distinguished from conditions such as pure vascular anomalies or single cell type tumours and malignancies.

Treatment

Management of these cases is challenging due to the extensive nature and relentless progression of the condition. The aims of treatment are to reduce bulk, maintain sensation and preserve joint motion whenever possible. Surgical options include epiphyseal ablation (epiphysiodesis), soft tissue debulking with or without skeletal reduction and sometimes amputation. Careful counseliing is crucial.

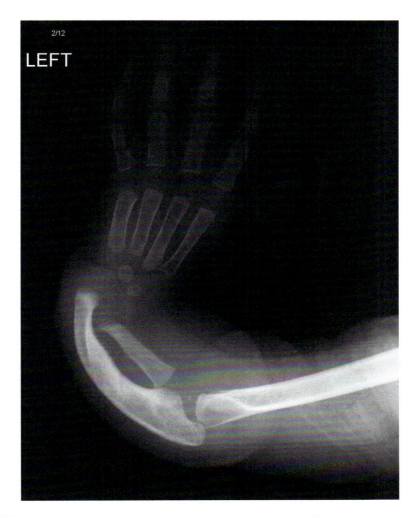

Figure 20.13 Image of child with radial longitudinal deficiency – demonstrating a short forearm, radial deviation at the wrist and an absent thumb.

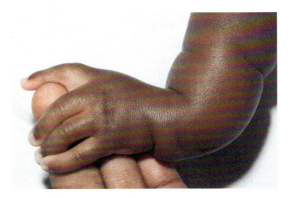

Figure 20.14 Radiograph of a child with Type II radial longitudinal deficiency.

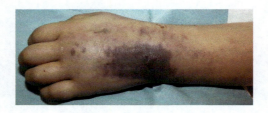

Figure 20.15   Early damage to the skin following extravasation.

Prognosis

Surgery can be complicated by problems of delayed healing but achieving a satisfactory result for the parents is particularly difficult. Control of more generalised and progressive overgrowth may need targeted medical therapy.

EXTRAVASATION INJURY

Incidence

An extravasation injury (EI) is an iatrogenic complication due to intravenous medication leaking into the tissues, leading to tissue necrosis and severe functional and aesthetic sequelae. This can occur in between 11 and 58% of hospitalised children. An extravasation injury occurs in 4.6% of failed intravascular devices.

Pathophysiology

Extravasation occurs if an intravascular cannula tip ends up outside of the vessel because of slippage or 'skewering' of the vessel on insertion leading to fluid being infiltrated into the surrounding tissues. Extravasation can also occur with incorrectly placed or dislodged intraosseous access.

The vast majority of extravasations are asymptomatic. Injury can be caused by either the volume or by the chemical properties of the substance extravasated.

Volume Effect

If a substantial amount of liquid is infiltrated, particularly in the limb, ischaemia and necrosis can occur. If the extravasation occurs beneath the deep fascia a compartment syndrome can develop.

Chemical Effect

The degree of tissue damage is related to the osmolality, pH and direct cytotoxicity. Vesicants such as chemotherapeutic agents are a particularly damaging and cause blisters and tissue necrosis. Other drugs leading to tissue damage include vancomycin, phenytoin, acyclovir, total parental nutrition, adrenaline, and dextrose with a concentration of more than 10%. All hospitals should have an agreed list of medication that requires active management to minimise this risk.

Clinical Presentation

A discreet swelling, skin colour changes (mottled, pale, increased capillary refill time), pain and difficulty flushing the IV cannula are common signs and symptoms. Skin necrosis and compartment syndrome are usually late signs.

Differential Diagnosis

Cellulitis or phlebitis at the cannulation site are common differential diagnoses.

Treatment

Early recognition and treatment are important in preventing tissue damage. Despite treatment, tissue damage may still occur but can be reduced.

Initially stop the infusion, attempt to aspirate as much of the solution as possible. Identify the agent, the volume and time has elapsed between the injury and identification.

Conservative management for non-vesicants is with limb elevation and regular assessment to monitor treatment.

Toxic substances (see above) must be diluted and washed out to limit tissue damage. This can be performed at the bedside. The 'Gault technique' utilises multiple small incisions made around the injury site and instilling saline and/or hyaluronidase.

Tissue necrosis may heal by secondary intention or require debridement and reconstruction with skin grafting to flap coverage.

Prognosis

Extravasation injuries are an emergency and early treatment can result in complete resolution or significant limitation of tissue damage. Early recognition and washout can prevent tissue necrosis and subsequent morbidity associated with functional loss and scarring.

REFERENCES

Extravasation Injuries
- Ghanem AM, Mansour A, Exton R, et al. Childhood extravasation injuries: Improved outcome following the introduction of hospital-wide guidelines. *J Plast Reconstr Aesthet Surg.* 2015 Apr;68(4):505–518.
- Gopalakrishnan PN, Goel N, Banerjee S. Saline irrigation for the management of skin extravasation injury in neonates. *Cochrane Database Syst Rev.* 2017;7(7):CD008404.
- Gault DT. Extravasation injuries. *Br J Plast Surg.* 1993;46(2):91–96.

Cleft Lip and Palatte
- Losee JE, Kirschner RE. *Comprehensive Cleft Care.* New York: McGraw-Hill Medical, ©2012.
- The Cleft Registry and Audit NEtwork (CRANE) Database. www.crane-database.org.uk

Craniosynostosis
- Mathijssen IMJ. Guideline for care of patients with the diagnoses of craniosynostosis. *J Craniofac Surg.* 2015;26: 1735–1807.
- O'Hara J., et al. Syndromic craniosynostosis: Complexities of clinical care. *Mol Syndromol.* 2019;10:83–97.

Craniofacial Microsomia
- Birgfeld CB, Luquetti DV, Gougoutas AJ, et al. A phenotypic assessment tool for craniofacial microsomia. *Plastic and Reconstructive Surgery J.* 2011;127(1):313–320.
- Horgan JE, Padwa BL, Labrie RA, et al. OMENS-Plus: Analysis of craniofacial and extracraniofacial anomalies in hemifacial microsomia. *The Cleft Palate-Craniofacial J.* 1995;32(5):405–412.
- Vento AR, LaBrie R, Mulliken JB. The OMENS classification of hemifacial microsomia. *The Cleft Palate Craniofacial J.* 1991;28(1):68–76.
- Renkema RW; and the ERN CRANIO Working Group on Craniofacial Microsomia. European guideline craniofacial microsomia. *J. Craniofacial Surgery.* 2020;31:2385–2484.

Microtia
- Cugno S, Bulstrode NW. Congenital ear anomalies. In Farhadieh, R., Bulstrode, N., Mehrara, B.J., and Cugno, S. (Eds), *Plastic Surgery: Principles and Practice.* Elsevier, 2021.

Hand Surgery
- Sivakumar B, Adamthwaite J, Smith P. Congenital hand surgery. In Farhadieh, R., Bulstrode, N., Mehrara, B.J., and Cugno, S. (Eds), *Plastic Surgery: Principles and Practice.* Elsevier, 2021.

21 Orthopaedics and Fractures

Deborah M Eastwood

Children change with growth: Their musculoskeletal system withstands and adapts to the applied forces over time. This process can be both 'painful and ungainly' causing parental concern. This chapter helps you identify what to worry about. Always plot the heights of the child and his/her parents on a growth chart.

Assess the presence/absence of the five Ss:

- Symmetry
- Stiffness
- Symptoms
- Skeletal dysplasias
- Systemic disorder

Symmetrical, asymptomatic problems in an otherwise normal child are not usually a concern.

NORMAL VARIATIONS OF GAIT AND POSTURE

Most 'odd walks' are simply normal variations. The foot progression angle is the angle the foot makes in relation to an imaginary straight line that the patient is walking (Figure 21.1).

Intoeing

An intoeing gait, arising from one of three sites, causes parental concern and childhood 'tripping' (Table 21.1).

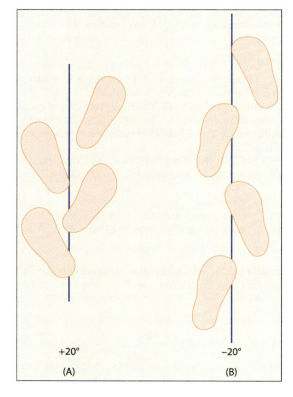

Figure 21.1 Foot progression angle demonstrating (A) extoeing and (B) intoeing gait patterns. the cause is identified on clinical examination. (From Williams *et al.* (eds), *Bailey and Love's Short Practice of Surgery*, CrC press 2013, with permission.)

DOI: 10.1201/9781003175186-21

Table 21.1: Intoeing

Cause	Age at presentation	Age at resolution	Treatment	Type
Metatarsus adductus (Figure 21.3)	Infant	2–3 years	Occasionally	Physiotherapy and/or casting
Internal tibial torsion	Toddler	4–6 years	Occasionally Very rarely	Gait education Tibial osteotomy
Femoral neck anteversion (Figure 21.2)	Child	8–11 years	Occasionally Very rarely	Gait education Femoral osteotomy

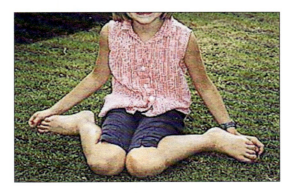

Figure 21.2 Child showing the 'w'-sitting posture characteristic of femoral neck anteversion.

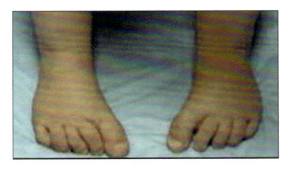

Figure 21.3 Metatarsus adductus – if the curved lateral border of the forefoot is correctible/flexible, by pushing on the medial border, no treatment is required; if it is stiff, then physiotherapy stretches and/or casting are implemented.

Extoeing

Extoeing is less common but may delay walking. The infant has an external rotation hip contracture; the older child, external tibial torsion when corrective tibial osteotomies may be required.

Tip-Toe Walking

This is part of the normal maturation of walking. A neurological abnormality must be excluded in bilateral cases and a dislocated hip or congenital anomaly creating a leg-length difference in unilateral cases (Figure 21.4).

Treatment

Spontaneous improvement is likely. Children may require physiotherapy or release of a contracted Achilles tendon.

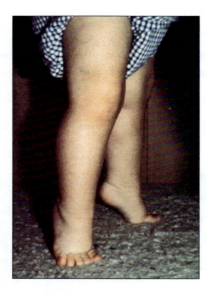

Figure 21.4 Child demonstrating a tip-toe gait; note that her knees are straight. A child with toe walking and flexed knees might have a neurological cause for the gait pattern.

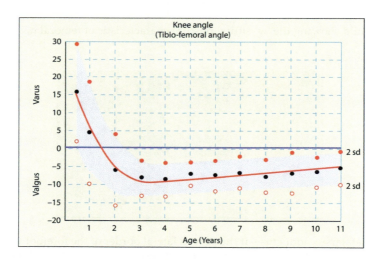

Figure 21.5 Graph depicting the change from genu varum to genu valgum to normal alignment during childhood years. (From Williams et al. (eds), *Bailey and Love's Short Practice of Surgery*, CrC press 2013, with permission.)

Bowlegs and Knock-Knees (Genu Varum and Genu Valgum)

Infant bow legs may become toddler knock knees, but by age 7–8 years alignment should be normal (Figure 21.5). When necessary, a standing leg alignment radiograph excludes a pathological cause and allows measurement of the deformity.

Treatment

For physiological deformities, spontaneous improvement is expected (unless bow legs/knock knees run in the family!). If the deformity is noted in later childhood and/or is progressive or asymmetrical an underlying cause should be identified. Treatment to improve alignment may be offered using guided growth techniques (Figures 21.6A and 21.6B).

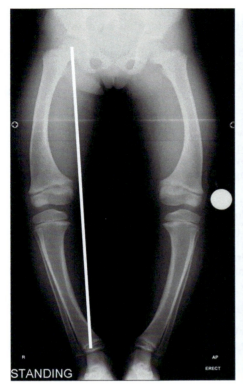
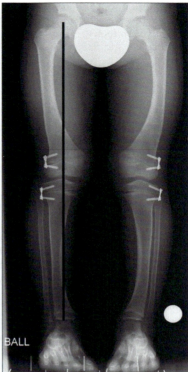

Figure 21.6 (A) AP leg alignment radiograph demonstrating bowlegs in a child with hypo-phosphataemic rickets. The mechanical axis links the centre of the hip to the centre of the ankle passing through the centre of the knee; on the right the line is abnormal lying outside the knee joint. (B) Same child as in 21.6A. Two plates have been inserted on the lateral aspect of the limb, spanning the growth plate and tethering growth on this side. Growth continues on the opposite side. With time (12m) the deformity corrects and the mechanical axis is normal

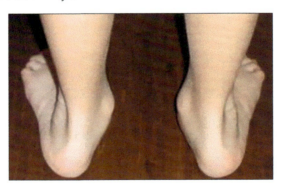

Figure 21.7 Flexible flat foot showing hindfoot valgus and the 'too many toes' sign when viewed from behind.

Flat Feet

All children under 3 years have fat, flat feet. Many children continue to have flat feet, associated with normal childhood joint laxity or conditions (such as trisomy 21) with excessive ligamentous laxity (Figure 21.7).

Flat feet are usually asymptomatic: they do *not* predispose the child to backache or arthritis in later life but cause parental concern. Most adults do *not* have flat feet although genetic factors (familial/racial) influence this; so spontaneous improvement is expected. The painless, flexible flat foot needs *no* treatment. Orthoses *do not* alter the natural history but can alleviate symptoms such as tired/achy calves or feet.

The symptomatic, rigid flat foot is usually due to a tarsal coalition or inflammation. Medical or surgical treatment may be required (Table 21.2 and Figure 21.8).

CONGENITAL AND DEVELOPMENTAL ABNORMALITIES OF THE LOWER LIMB

POSTURAL ABNORMALITIES (THE MOULDED BABY)

In utero, many babies are moulded and born with 'postural deformities': the foot lying in either calcaneovalgus (Figures 21.9A and 21.9B) or equinovarus. Torticollis and plagiocephaly (Figure 21.10) are common, as are asymmetric hip movements which may mimic a dislocated hip. Postural problems improve with time and/or stretching exercises.

CONGENITAL TALIPES EQUINOVARUS DEFORMITY ('THE CLUB FOOT')
Aetiology/Incidence

The foot with congenital talipes equinovarus (CTEV) points 'down and in' (Figure 21.11). It is present at birth and detectable on antenatal scans (but severity is difficult to judge).

Club feet may be postural, idiopathic, syndromic or neuromuscular in origin. For idiopathic feet, the incidence is 1–2 in 1000; 50–60% are bilateral and boys are more frequently affected. There is a small increased risk with a family history.

Treatment

- Idiopathic feet respond well to Ponseti treatment with weekly foot manipulations and above-knee plaster casts that sequentially correct the foot deformity (Table 21.3 and Figure 21.12).

Table 21.2: Differentiation between the Flexible and Rigid Foot

Type	Characteristics
Flexible	On tip-toe, the arch restores and the heel position corrects; subtalar joint movements are full and pain free
Rigid	On tip-toe, the arch fails to return; subtalar joint movements are restricted and often painful

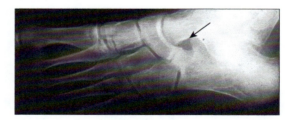

Figure 21.8 Oblique radiograph of the foot showing a calcaneonavicular coalition. the arrow points to the almost complete bony fusion where there should be a space.

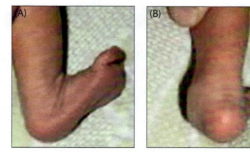

Figure 21.9 (A and B) an infant foot lying in a calcaneovalgus position.

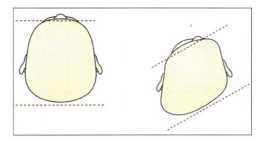

Figure 21.10   Line diagram of a plagiocephalic head secondary to intrauterine moulding.

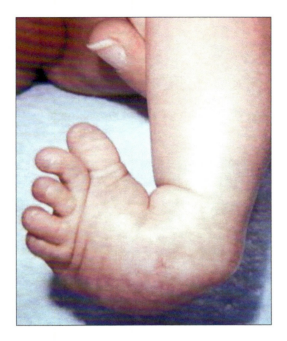

Figure 21.11   A club foot deformity: At birth the deformity was fixed.

Table 21.3:   Order of Deformity Correction with Ponseti Treatment

Description	Site of the deformity
Cavus	Pronation of the first ray
Adduction	Midfoot and forefoot
Varus	Subtalar joint
Equinus	Hindfoot

■ An Achilles tendon release performed in clinic is often required; 95% of idiopathic feet avoid a major surgical procedure. The child wears a system of 'boots and bars' at night and naptime until the age of 4–5 years (Figure 21.13).

Prognosis

■ Relapse is treated with further casting and/or a tibialis anterior tendon transfer. The affected foot is often smaller, the calf thinner and leg a little shorter.

■ Ponseti treatment of the non-idiopathic/syndromic club foot is not as effective but may lessen the extent of subsequent surgery.

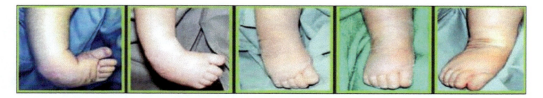

Figure 21.12 Photographs demonstrating correction of a club foot deformity after weekly castings.

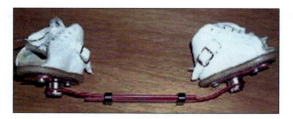

Figure 21.13 The 'boots and bars' worn for part of the day/night for the first four years of life to maintain correction.

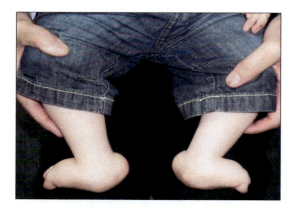

Figure 21.14 Bilateral congenital vertical talus deformities in a child with arthrogryposis: The feet have a 'rocker-bottom' appearance.

CONGENITAL VERTICAL TALUS

Aetiology/Incidence

- Congenital vertical talus (CVT) is much rarer than CTEV deformities. The child has a 'rocker-bottom foot': the foot may appear 'flat' with a bony lump (the talar head) where the arch should be; 50% are associated with other abnormalities and classified as syndromic feet (Figure 21.14).

Treatment

- A modified Ponseti technique manipulates the foot into position although overall the results are less successful than with a club foot and surgical treatment is often required.

DEVELOPMENTAL DYSPLASIA OF THE HIP

Aetiology/Incidence

Developmental dysplasia of the hip (DDH) describes a spectrum of hip pathology ranging from the irreducibly dislocated hip to one that is in joint but associated with a shallow ('dysplastic') acetabulum.

The incidence of neonatal instability may be as high as 20 cases per 1000 births, whereas the incidence of dislocated hips is about two cases per 1000 live births. Many hips unstable at birth stabilise spontaneously.

- The risk factors include:

  - Female

  - Breech position

  - Family history

All babies are examined at birth and at time points defined by the NIPE programme, to elicit signs of hip instability (Table 21.4 and Figure 21.15). Asymmetric thigh skin folds alone are not a risk factor; soft tissue 'clicks' are common and not considered worrying. It is important, however, to maintain a high index of suspicion as early detection is the key to successful treatment.

- If the examination is unclear and/or there are risk factors for DDH an ultrasound scan is necessary (Figure 21.16).

Treatment
Neonatal Presentation

- Dislocated and/or unstable joints must be reduced and held in joint by the simplest means possible. Treatment should be commenced between 2–6 weeks of age. A Pavlik harness (or similar splint) is worn for essentially 24 hours per day for a period of 6–8 weeks until the dysplasia resolves or the stability improves (Figure 21.17). If early treatment fails, the hip is treated as below as a 'late presenting' hip.

The orange lines define the bony aspects of the acetabulum and measure the alpha angle which should be more than 60°.

The orange circle outlines the cartilaginous femoral head which is lying outside the acetabulum. It should be positioned where the 'alpha' symbol is.

Late Presentation

Unfortunately, diagnosis is often delayed and the child presents with restricted hip movements or a limp. The clinical signs are:

- A leg-length difference (Galeazzi sign positive).

Table 21.4: Questions to Ask on a Neonatal Hip Examination

1. Is the hip dislocated?	If so, is it reducible?	Ortolani positive
	If not …	Ortolani negative
2. Is the hip dislocatable?	Does it sublux/dislocate?	Barlow positive
3. Is the hip clinically normal?	If so, are there risk factors requiring further investigations?	Ultrasound scan for diagnosis

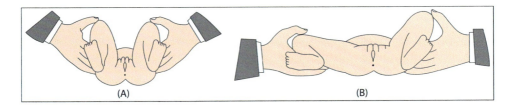

(A) (B)

Figure 21.15 Neonatal hip examination. (A) Line diagram of a child with hips and knees flexed to 90° about to undergo a neonatal hip examination; (B) limited abduction in flexion of the baby's left hip. Note the fingers on the lateral proximal thigh at the level of the greater trochanter. Once limitation of abduction has been identified, the examiner can use this finger to lift up on the trochanter to see if the hip will reduce (Ortolani test: positive if the hip reduces). The hips must be flexed to at least 90° before the hips are abducted: less flexion and the limitation of abduction is much less obvious.

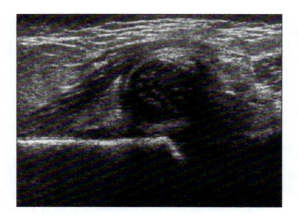

Figure 21.16   An ultrasound scan showing a femoral head lying outside the acetabulum (a dislocated hip); such a scan is *not* incompatible with a 'normal' clinical examination.

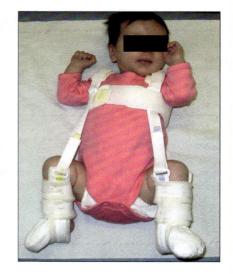

Figure 21.17   A baby wearing a Pavlik harness: The hips should be flexed to a right angle and the anterior straps should lie across the baby's thigh.

- The short leg lies in external rotation (Figure 21.18).

- Limited abduction in flexion; in unilateral cases a difference may be significant (Figure 21.19).

- Beware bilateral cases: the child waddles but the signs on examination are symmetrical and thus harder to identify.

- After 4–5 months, x-rays are the investigation of choice (Figures 21.20 and 21.21).

- The longer the hip has been 'out', the more aggressive the treatment.

- After walking age, an open reduction is usually required and with further delay femoral and/or pelvic osteotomies would be required.

- The more surgery that is needed, the less likely the child is to have an excellent outcome: early detection is therefore important. Long-term follow-up is required to monitor hip development and minimise the risks of degenerative change

LIMB LENGTH DISCREPANCIES
Aetiology/Clinical Presentation

- Limb length discrepancies (affecting upper or lower limbs) may be secondary to a wide variety of congenital and acquired causes and the 'surgical sieve' helps you consider all possibilities (Table 21.5).

- Congenital abnormalities are classified according to an internationally recognised system illustrated in Table 21.6.

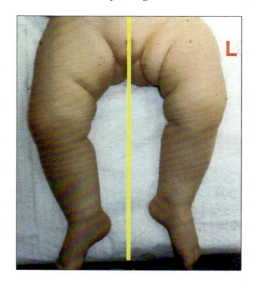

Figure 21.18   A child (under anaesthetic) demonstrating a short left leg, asymmetrical skin creases and a widened perineum suggestive of a dislocated left hip. The Galeazzi sign would have been positive on the left leg.

- A small difference causes no problems. It is possible to predict (via a downloaded 'app' or using standard graphs) what the discrepancy will be at skeletal maturity and if this is more than 2–2.5 cm, treatment is advised.

- The clinical discrepancy is measured by standing the child with a block under the foot on the shorter side to level the pelvis: the difference is 'checked' on a standing radiograph (Figure 21.22).

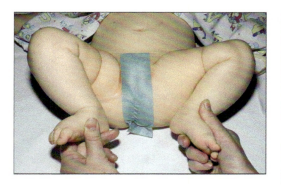

Figure 21.19 Clinical photo of a child (under anaesthetic – hence no fingers on the thighs) demonstrating limitation of abduction of the right hip.

Treatment

May involve the following options:

1. Controlling growth of the longer leg via an epiphyseodesis (growth plate 'fusion') (Figure 21.23).

2. Limb lengthening treatment with correction of associated deformity via application of an external fixator (Figure 21.24).

3. Operative shortening of the longer limb: Unusual.

4. Rarely, amputation and prosthetic limb use.

5. A combination of the first two approaches and the use of orthotic supports.

Treatment choice is multifactorial; determined by the function and comfort of the abnormal leg and a holistic assessment of the child.

FIBULA HEMIMELIA
Aetiology/Incidence

This is the most common major congenital lower limb deformity (1:20–30,000 live births) (Figure 21.25) It has characteristic features, that highlight this 'field defect' occurs during embryogenesis affecting the distal limb predominantly.

The diagnosis is made on clinical suspicion/examination and on plain radiographs.

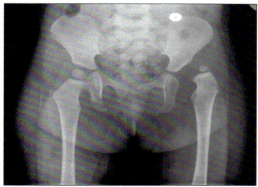

Figure 21.20 AP pelvic radiograph demonstrating a dislocated left hip representing a late presentation of DDH. The ossific nucleus (within the cartilaginous anlage) is smaller on the left than on the right, the proximal femur is laterally displaced and the bony acetabulum is abnormally shaped; the acetabular index is high).

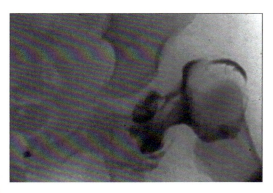

Figure 21.21 Arthrogram of the left hip: Dye has been injected into the joint to outline the dislocated cartilaginous femoral head.

Table 21.5: Congenital and Acquired Causes of Limb Length Discrepancy

Congenital	Acquired
Generalised, e.g. skeletal dysplasia	Traumatic
Localised: failure of formation of a limb	Infective
	Metabolic
	Neoplastic
	Vascular
	Inflammatory

Table 21.6: Congenital Leg-Length Discrepancies

Category	Description	Example
I	Failure of formation of parts • Transverse • Longitudinal	Congenital amputation Fibular hemimelia
II	Failure of differentiation	Vertebral body fusion; radioulnar synostosis
III	Duplication	Extra digits
IV	Overgrowth	Gigantism; macrodactyly
V	Undergrowth	
VI	Congenital constriction band syndrome	Often affects hands/feet with poor formation of the digits
VII	Generalised skeletal abnormalities	Skeletal dysplasia, e.g. achondroplasia

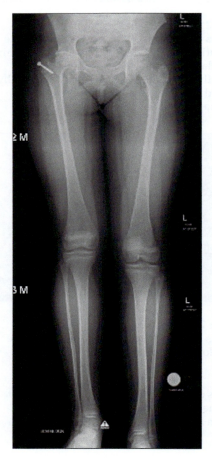

Figure 21.22 Standing ap limb length and alignment radiograph; the child has a short right leg secondary to poor development of the proximal femur following osteomyelitis as an infant. She is standing on a 3 cm block which levels her pelvis. She is awaiting an epiphyseodesis.

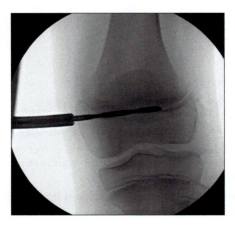

Figure 21.23 Left knee: Intra-operative radiograph demonstrating the technique of a 'drill epiphyseodesis' of the distal femoral physis. The drill bit must pass along the physis causing enough damage to stop it growing.

Treatment

■ For this and for all other limb deficiencies is guided by the principles outlined above for the management of a limb length discrepancy. The overall principle is to obtain a well-aligned limb of suitable length but with functioning, stable and comfortable joints. Surgery is associated with complications that may adversely affect outcome.

PROXIMAL FEMORAL FOCAL DEFICIENCY

■ Proximal femoral focal deficiency (PFFD) (Figures 21.26 and 21.27) is much less common (1 in 50,000 live births). Again the whole limb is affected but the features are more pronounced at hip level. Without a working hip joint, limb function will be poor.

CONGENITAL TIBIAL DEFICIENCY

■ This is the rarest lower limb congenital anomaly (1 in 1,000,000 live births). The foot may be normal but depending on the severity of the tibial deficiency there may be no functioning ankle or knee joint (Figure 21.28).

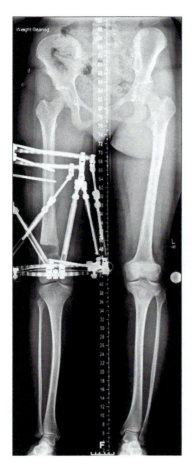

Figure 21.24 AP standing radiograph demonstrating leg length and alignment: The right femur has undergone an osteotomy with application of an external fixator to support the limb whilst the deformity is corrected and the femur lengthened.

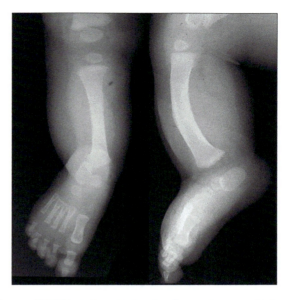

Figure 21.25 AP and lateral radiographs of a child with fibula hemimelia. There is no fibula present on the right lower leg but there are five toes.

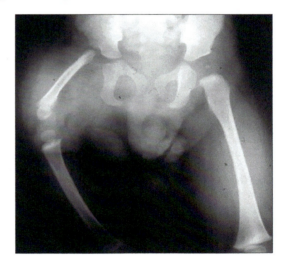

Figure 21.26 AP radiograph of both legs of a 6-month-old child showing an under-developed proximal femur on the right. The fibula is also absent. The whole of the right leg is the same length as the left thigh (femur). This is an example of proximal femoral focal deficiency.

Treatment

- If the proximal tibia and the quadriceps are present then a below-knee amputation may be possible; otherwise, the treatment of choice is a through-knee amputation and artificial limb fitting (Figure 21.29).

COMMON CONGENITAL TOE PROBLEMS
Curly Toes

- Medial deviation of the lesser toes is of no clinical significance but cosmetic concerns are common. The curly toes are treated easily by flexor tenotomy (Figure 21.30).

- Laterally deviated tips of the second/third toes are common and essentially asymptomatic.

- Over-riding toes (Figures 21.31 and 21.32) may rub on shoes.

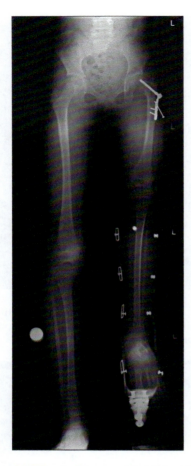

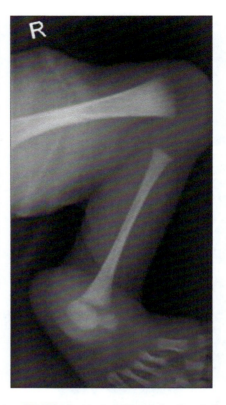

Figure 21.28 Lateral radiograph of an infant with an absent tibia: The fibula looks 'large' and may be mistaken for the tibia; the clue is the significant foot deformity and the fibula lies 'behind' the femur.

Figure 21.27 An 11-year-old child with proximal femoral focal deficiency who has undergone hip surgery to stabilise the joint and who wears an extension prosthesis; she has elected to keep her foot and she has refused limb lengthening surgery. (There is also a loose screw!)

Syndactyly (webbing) of the lesser toes is a cosmetic problem; separation can be considered but surgery is more extensive than patients realise.

Ingrowing toenails are a frequent cause of pain. Basic advice about nail care and footwear is usually all that is needed. If infections are troublesome, wedge excision of the lateral nail edge is necessary with phenolisation of the nail bed to prevent regrowth.

OTHER CONGENITAL/ACQUIRED LOWER LIMB PROBLEMS

BLOUNT DISEASE

In this condition there is disordered growth in the posteromedial tibial physis.

- The aetiology is unknown. The infantile form is common in those of Afro-Caribbean origin but the adolescent-onset disease affects all ethnic origins.

- Risk factors include early walking and obesity. The child presents with progressive bow leg deformity often with significant intoeing. There are classical radiographic features (Figure 21.33).

- Treatment is surgical (Figure 21.34).

- Guided growth techniques applied early in the pathological process reduce the need for extensive surgery (as seen in Figure 21.6B).

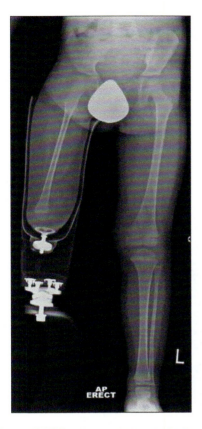

Figure 21.29 Same child as in 21.28 aged 4.5 years following a through-knee amputation. He is wearing his sport prosthetic limb.

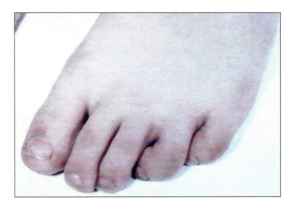

Figure 21.30 A clinical photograph of the forefoot of a young child with curly fourth and fifth toes.

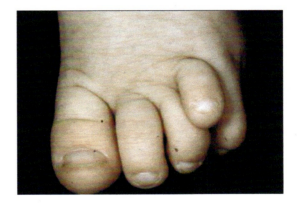

Figure 21.31 An 'over-riding' fourth toe is usually due to a short metatarsal, and often part of a syndrome.

CONGENITAL PSEUDARTHROSIS OF THE TIBIA

This rare condition presents clinically with an anterolateral bow (defined by where the apex of the bow is) of the tibia with or without a fracture (Figure 21.35). Classic radiographic changes are noted and 50% of cases are associated with neurofibromatosis. Once fractured the tibia is reluctant to heal and long-term orthotic treatment may be necessary, with surgery to obtain bony union and restore leg length.

POSTEROMEDIAL TIBIAL BOW

This may present as a calcaneovalgus foot deformity but the problem is in the tibia (apex of the deformity is posteromedial) (Figure 21.36). The deformity resolves with time but the child may be left with a short leg requiring surgery.

PES CAVUS (THE HIGH-ARCHED FOOT)

A high-arched foot suggests an underlying neurological abnormality, particularly with asymmetry and/or a progressive change in

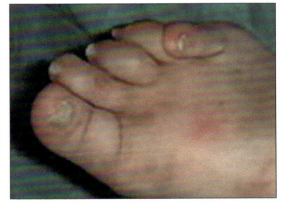

Figure 21.32 An over-riding fifth toe is due to a congenital malformation; surgical treatment is simple and reliable.

585

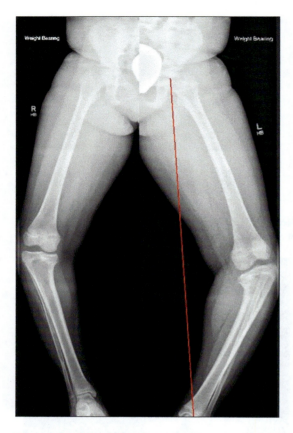

Figure 21.33 AP limb alignment view demonstrating bilateral severe bow legs secondary to Blount disease (note the mechanical axes): A condition caused by poor function of the posteromedial proximal tibial physis and epiphysis.

foot shape (Figure 21.37). Spina bifida, tethered cord syndrome and peripheral neuropathies should be considered. Investigations may involve spinal MR and/or neurophysiological testing.

Treatment includes:

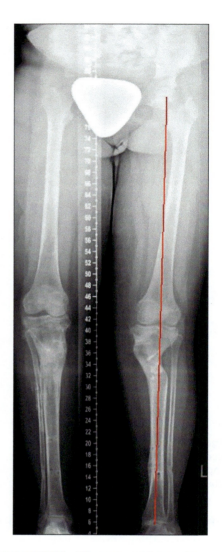

Figure 21.34 The same patient as in 21.33 following deformity correction using an external fixator; the left leg has a correct mechanical axis (despite the crooked tibia).

- Physiotherapy/orthotic supports: to prevent contractures whilst maintaining function and comfort.

- Surgical correction of deformity.

CLASSIC CAUSES OF LOWER LIMB PAIN

Growing Pains

These must be a diagnosis of exclusion but they are a legitimate cause of children's pain and parental distress. They are defined as:

- Pain lasting for > three months.

- Symptom-free intervals.

- Pain at the end of the day or that wakes the child at night; not necessarily joint-related.

- Symmetrical symptoms of equal severity which may alternate from limb to limb.

586

- Unilateral symptoms may require further investigation to exclude rarities such as tumours and infections.

- Treatment involves reassurance, explanation and conservative measures.

Knee Pain
Osgood–Schlatter Disease

- Tenderness and swelling are localised to one or both tibial apophyses.

- Pain is often asymmetrical, exacerbated by exercise and/or by prolonged periods of sitting with bent knees.

- Symptoms are frequently precipitated by growth or a minor injury.

- Conservative treatment consisting of relative rest, reassurance and analgesia is helpful.

Anterior Knee Pain Syndrome

- Symptoms of ill-defined pain around the front of the knee, with giving way and clicking, exacerbated by prolonged sitting or by activity, are often present in both knees of teenagers.

- Patellofemoral crepitus and discomfort on patellofemoral compression are present.

- Patella subluxation must be excluded.

Patellofemoral Subluxation

- Frequently presents in adolescent girls.

- Treatment is usually conservative with physiotherapy to strengthen the quadriceps muscle.

- It may be associated with ligamentous laxity.

- Surgical reconstruction is required in cases of persistent subluxation/dislocation (Figure 21.38).

Other conditions include:

- Osteochondritis dissecans.

- Discoid meniscus.

Foot Pain
Kohler Disease

- Presents with dorsal forefoot pain and swelling in young children.

- The radiological appearances (Figure 21.39) resolve spontaneously and without sequelae.

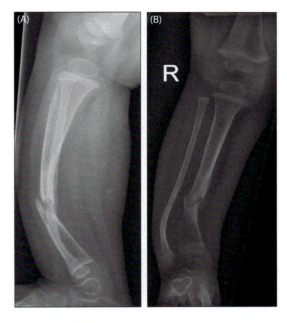

Figure 21.35 Lateral (A) and ap (B) radiographs of a child's right tibia/fibula showing a bowed tibia with an anterolateral apex: The diagnosis is tibial pseudarthrosis associated with neurofibromatosis.

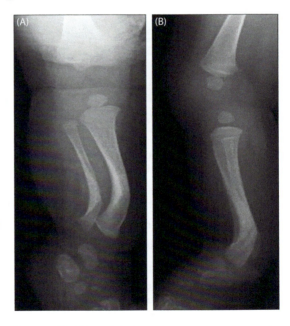

Figure 21.36 AP (A) and lateral (B) radiographs of a child's tibia/fibula showing a bowed tibia with a posteromedial apex; the bow usually straightens spontaneously but the leg is often slightly short.

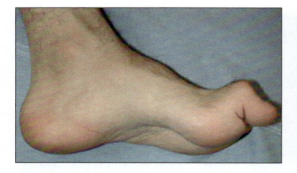

Figure 21.37 A lateral clinical photograph of a high-arched (cavus) foot with clawing of the great toe, often seen in adolescents; a neuropathic cause must be sought and excluded.

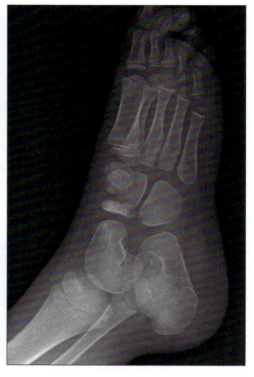

Figure 21.39 Oblique radiograph of the foot showing increased density in the navicular consistent with Kohler's disease.

Sever Disease
Enthesopathy of the calcaneal apophysis

- Presents with heel pain related to activity.
- Calf muscle tightness may be a contributing factor.

Freiberg Osteochondrosis

- Presents with forefoot pain.

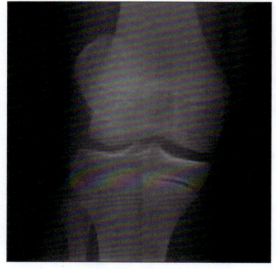

Figure 21.38 AP radiograph of the right knee showing the patella subluxed laterally.

- Avascular change in the second metatarsal head seen on x-ray.
- It may present as an incidental x-ray finding.
- If symptoms persist, bony spurs/fragments may need excision.

THE CHILD WITH A (PAINFUL) LIMP

Children may limp because of pain, weakness, deformity or to gain attention. The causes vary from sepsis to a spinal tumour and from a leg-length discrepancy to a shoe that rubs. It is essential to exclude serious pathology and identify rare but important cases of sepsis, Perthes disease and a slipped upper femoral epiphysis. Many conditions, such as sepsis and juvenile arthritis, can present at any age but certain hip conditions afflict particular age groups.

History

The following points will help distinguish these conditions:

- Symptom onset: sudden or gradual?
- Symptom duration.

- Concurrent events: recent viral infection, trauma, new shoes or sport?

- General health: is the child well or ill?

- Examination:

  - Must include all joints and soft tissues.

  - A brief neurological examination.

  - Measurement of leg length,

  - Pain on movement or on weight-bearing?

Investigations:

- AP *and* 'frog' lateral pelvic radiographs.

- Further imaging may be required.

BONE AND JOINT INFECTION (OSTEOMYELITIS AND SEPTIC ARTHRITIS)

The pathology of osteoarticular infection must be understood by any doctor involved in the care of children (Figures 21.40 and 21.41). Prompt, accurate diagnosis still saves lives and preserves joint function. The following comments refer to acute or acute-on-chronic infections.

- There is no substitute for regular assessment and continuity of care.

- Diagnosis is based on clinical assessment supported by haematological results.

- With a prompt diagnosis, radiographic features should be minimal (Figure 21.42).

- Management is guided by the site and severity of the infection and local hospital protocols but must adhere to certain principles:

- Intravenous antibiotics are required.

  - With an improvement in clinical and haematological parameters, intravenous therapy is changed to oral therapy.

- The affected limb must be rested.

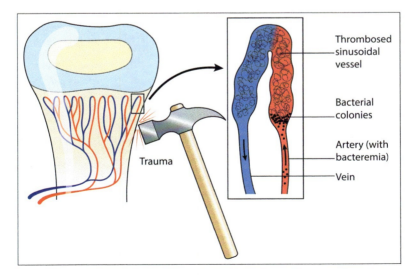

Figure 21.40 Diagram depicting the effects of minor trauma on the metaphysis of a long bone: The haematoma and thrombosis in the blood vessels allows passing bacteria to be 'trapped' in the region and encourages colonisation and the development of an osteomyelitis. (From Williams *et al.* (eds). *Bailey and Love's Short Practice of Surgery*, CRC Press, 2013, with permission.)

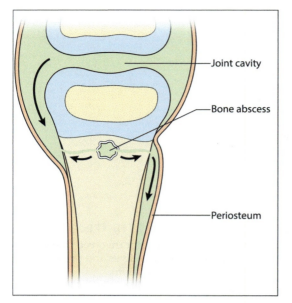

Figure 21.41 Diagrammatic representation of what might happen if an abscess forms within the metaphysis: pus may 'discharge' into the joint (secondary septic arthritis) or out through the cortical bone, lifting the periosteum and causing a subperiosteal abscess. (From Williams *et al.* (eds). *Bailey and Love's Short Practice of Surgery*, CrC press, 2013, with permission.)

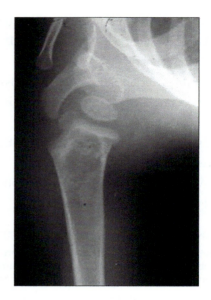

Figure 21.42 AP radiograph of a proximal humerus demonstrating a lytic area within the metaphysis compatible with infection. The child responded promptly to intravenous antibiotics: no surgery was required. It takes seven to ten days for changes to be seen on a plain radiograph.

- Appropriate analgesia must be prescribed.

- Pus in the joint, the soft tissues or in the bone requires surgical drainage.

TRANSIENT SYNOVITIS VERSUS SEPTIC ARTHRITIS

There is a qualitative difference between these conditions; transient synovitis remains a diagnosis of exclusion and should *not* be considered in a child < 2 years of age.

Four clinical predictors have been identified, to differentiate between septic arthritis and transient synovitis:

- History of fever.

- Non-weight bearing status.

- Erythrocyte sedimentation rate > 40 mm/h.

- White cell count > 12×10^9/l.

- With all four factors present, the probability of joint sepsis is > 90%.

  - C-reactive protein > 20 mg/l is a fifth predictive factor.

Ultrasound scans define the joint effusion (Figure 21.43).

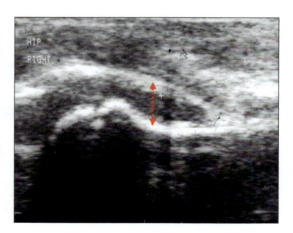

Figure 21.43 Ultrasound scan of the right proximal femur demonstrating a joint effusion. the red dotted line shows how far the fluid has displaced the capsule from the surface of the bone. (From Williams *et al.* (eds). *Bailey and Love's Short Practice of Surgery*, CRC Press, 2013, with permission.)

The solid black arrows point to the femoral head (epiphysis), the femoral neck (as it flares up to the metaphysis) and the capsule of the hip joint.

LEGG–CALVE–PERTHES DISEASE (OFTEN CALLED PERTHES DISEASE)

Perthes disease is characterised by avascular necrosis (AVN) of the femoral head leading to its collapse. As the blood supply returns, healing occurs but with deformity. The radiographic appearances are dramatic (Figure 21.44).

- Rare; affects boys predominantly.

- Presents between 4–8 years of age.

- Aetiology unknown, rarely bilateral.

Treatment aims to minimise femoral head deformity, reducing the risk of osteoarthritis.

- Non-surgical methods maximise the range of movement to maintain the femoral head shape.

- Surgical methods contain the vulnerable head within the acetabulum to protect against secondary deformity.

The prognosis is better in younger children and those with less involvement.

SLIPPED UPPER FEMORAL EPIPHYSIS
Aetiology/Incidence

In this important, rare (5 per 100,000) condition the femoral head (the epiphysis) slips off the neck (the metaphysis). A prompt diagnosis is associated with a significantly better prognosis; surgical treatment is essential.

Boys are more frequently affected and classically patients are overweight. Children often present with pain in/around their knee or non-specific symptoms of groin discomfort and an intermittent limp (externally rotated FPA).

Subtle radiographic changes may be more visible on a frog-lateral hip view than on the AP view: thus *both* must be requested.

Other conditions such as hypothyroidism and renal failure increase the risk of a slip. If the slip happens acutely, this is just like a fracture (Figure 21.45).

Treatment

A pin/screw is inserted up the femoral neck into the epiphysis to 'fix' the head onto the neck: the further the head has slipped off the neck, the more technically difficult this is (Figure 21.46).

More aggressive surgical procedures restore normal anatomy but the risks and benefits must be assessed carefully.

UPPER LIMB ABNORMALITIES

NEONATAL BRACHIAL PLEXOPATHY

Damage to the neonatal brachial plexus during delivery can occur in several high-risk situations:

- A large-for-dates baby and/or born to a diabetic mother.

- Abnormal intrauterine positions: a transverse lie or a breech presentation.

- A prolonged labour and/or a forceps delivery.

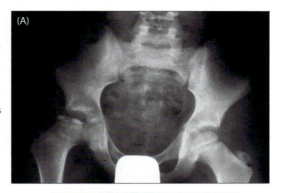

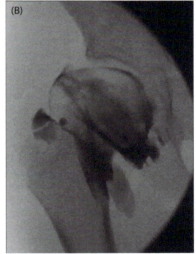

Figure 21.44 AP pelvic radiograph (A) showing right hip Perthes disease: The epiphysis appears to be in pieces; (B) an arthrogram outlines the cartilaginous head and confirms that this is still spherical.

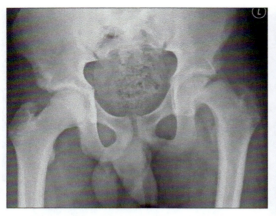

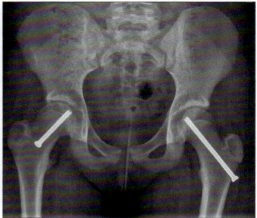

Figure 21.45 AP pelvic radiograph of an adolescent complaining of acute left groin pain. He is unable to walk and has essentially sustained a pathological fracture of his femoral neck but it is called an acute, severe slip of the upper femoral epiphysis.

Figure 21.46 AP pelvic radiograph of a patient with bilateral groin pain; both epiphyses had slipped, the left more than the right. Both were 'pinned *in-situ*' to stabilise the situation.

The child presents with a paralysed arm of variable severity and with the complete lesion there may also be a Horner syndrome. The diagnosis is initially clinical; other causes of a 'pseudo-paralysis' such as a clavicular fracture or shoulder join sepsis must be excluded.

Ideas on the timing of further investigation (neurophysiological testing and MRI) are changing and will be reflected in your local referral protocols.

All infants should receive physiotherapy to maintain a normal range of passive joint movement and prevent contractures.

TORTICOLLIS

The child presents with a 'cock-robin' head tilt due to a tight sternocleidomastoid muscle that pulls the affected side down and tilts the head round. The muscle may be torn during delivery especially if forceps were used; a 'tumour/swelling' is rarely found.

The tight muscle responds to physiotherapy-supervised stretching. Untreated, the head tilt leads to noticeable facial asymmetry. Surgical release is merited after the age

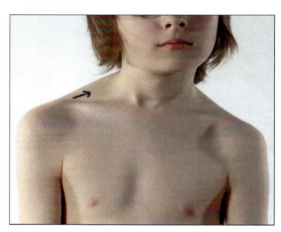

Figure 21.47 Clinical photograph of a child with a 'cock-robin' head posture secondary to a torticollis. This is thought to be secondary to a sternomastoid tumour, never more than a benign haematoma within the muscle. By this age, the muscle is contracted and unresponsive to physiotherapy.

of 18–24 months (Figure 21.47). A squint with diplopia may encourage a child to adopt the same posture but without muscle tightness.

Torticollis noted at birth may be due to a cervical spine abnormality and should be referred immediately. One that develops later acutely, often with pain, minor trauma and/or an upper respiratory tract infection must be assessed urgently for atlantoaxial rotatory instability.

CONGENITAL UPPER LIMB ANOMALIES

RADIAL CLUB HAND

- This longitudinal deficiency affects approximately 1 in 30,000 live births. Radial club hand is often associated with abnormalities of other systems:

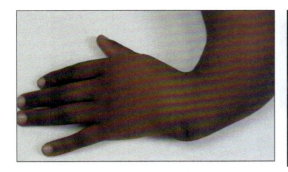

Figure 21.48 Clinical photograph of a child with TAR (Thrombocytopaenia Absent Radius) syndrome; the thumb appears normal.

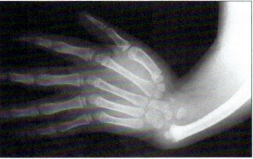

Figure 21.49 AP radiograph of the arm of the same child as in 21.48 showing an absent radius but well-developed thumb.

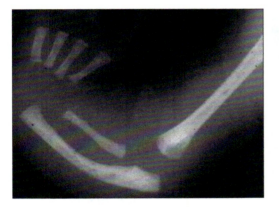

Figure 21.50 AP radiograph of a forearm of a child with Holt–Oram syndrome and a radial club hand; the radius is under-developed, the thumb is absent and there is significant deviation of the hand with respect to the forearm. (From Williams *et al.* (eds). *Bailey and Love's Short Practice of Surgery*, CRC press, 2013, with permission.)

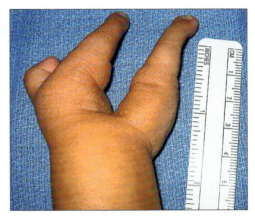

Figure 21.51 Clinical photograph of a cleft hand (ectrodactyly): In this case part of the ulnar club hand anomaly.

- TAR syndrome (Figures 21.48 and 21.49).
- Holt–Oram syndrome (Figure 21.50).
- Function may be surprisingly good.

Treatment options depend on the quality of the thumb (often poor) and whether or not the condition is bilateral:

- Physiotherapy and splinting are essential in early management.
- Surgery may help with wrist position and instability.
- Forearm lengthening and pollicisation of the index finger may be indicated.

ULNAR CLUB HAND

- Rare and often associated with other limb abnormalities (Figure 21.51).
- Surgical options include constructing a 'one bone forearm' and procedures to maximise function.

RADIOULNAR SYNOSTOSIS

In utero, failure of separation of the cartilage anlage results in a forearm with no pronation/supination movement (Figure 21.52). The hand on the end of the arm is effectively stuck in one position. The condition is often bilateral.

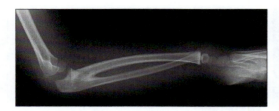

Figure 21.52 Lateral radiograph of a child's forearm: There is a proximal radioulnar synostosis and the radial head is dislocated. It is impossible to obtain a 'good' lateral view as the synostosis limits pronation/supination movement.

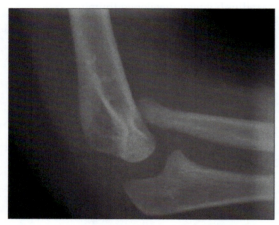

Figure 21.53 Lateral radiograph of the elbow showing a congenital anterior dislocation of the radial head: the proximal portion of the radius is malformed and the head deficient.

Careful functional assessment is required before treatment. Surgery exchanges one fixed position for another but it cannot restore movement: the fixed position of choice varies with hand dominance and cultural needs.

CONGENITAL DISLOCATION OF THE RADIAL HEAD

This may be associated with a radioulnar synostosis (Figure 21.52) or not (Figure 21.53); *if* pain and/or stiffness interfere with function, surgical excision can be considered later.

OTHER MINOR UPPER LIMB ABNORMALITIES

Trigger thumbs are common, often present from birth but not noticed until some months later. The tip of the thumb is held flexed: sometimes the child or their parent can straighten it but with active flexion the thumb gets stuck again. If the problem persists past 1 year of age, surgical release of the tight flexor tendon sheath pulley is curative (Figure 21.54).

Polydactyly of the hands or feet is one of the common, uncommon conditions. There is an association with other medical conditions such as renal disease or more widespread skeletal problems (Figure 21.55).

Pseudarthrosis of the clavicle is rare; it always affects the right side (except in dextrocardia) and presents from birth with a non-tender lump. It is often mistaken for a simple fracture but when it does not heal, the diagnosis is clear (Figure 21.56).

Symptoms are unusual in childhood but become more noticeable with time. Operative treatments reduce the 'fracture' and 'fix it' to encourage healing.

Sprengel shoulder is rare. The embryonic descent of the shoulder from the cranial end of the embryo fails, leaving the scapula in the root of the neck rather than on the posterior wall of the chest (Figures 21.57 and 21.58). Symptoms include difficulty with overhead movements. Cosmetic concerns are common; surgical repositioning of the scapula is possible.

EXAMPLES OF GENERALISED CONDITIONS AFFECTING THE MUSCULOSKELETAL SYSTEM

BENIGN JOINT HYPERMOBILITY SYNDROME

All children are lax jointed: this is normal. Joint laxity is maximal at birth, declining rapidly during childhood, less rapidly during the teens, and slowly during adult life.

Women are more lax jointed than men and there is significant ethnic variation. The clinical tests for joint laxity developed by Beighton

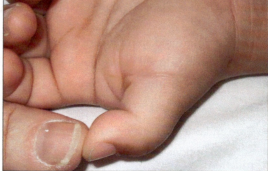

Figure 21.54 Clinical photograph of a trigger thumb: The thumb is flexed at the interphalangeal joint and cannot be straightened. Surgical release of a tendon pulleys solves the problem.

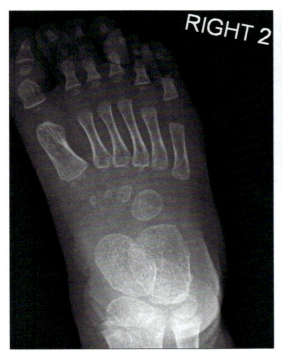

Figure 21.55 AP radiograph of a foot showing six well-formed digits: polydactyly is a common congenital anomaly.

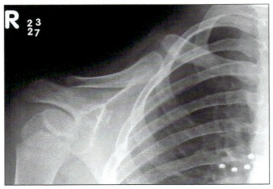

Figure 21.56 Radiograph showing a pseud-arthrosis of the clavicle. It was presented in late childhood and was of cosmetic concern only.

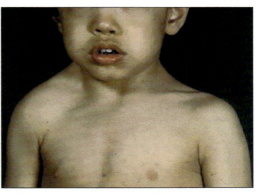

Figure 21.57 Clinical photograph of a child with a 'lump in the neck', which represents the failed embryological descent of the right scapula: a Sprengel shoulder.

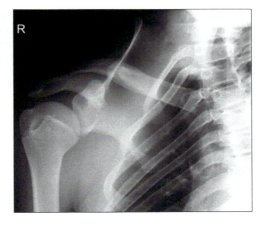

Figure 21.58 AP radiograph showing a high riding right scapula in keeping with a Sprengel shoulder.

are helpful. A child who scores five or more is hypermobile and may become symptomatic. Symptoms in children include joint and back pains, occasionally subluxations or frank dislocations, ligament, muscle and tendon injuries after mild trauma and fasciitis.

However, most children are asymptomatic and musicians (of all ages) with lax finger joints suffer less pain than their less flexible peers. Gymnasts/ballet dancers also have supple joints but in addition they have good muscle strength and co-ordination. Symptomatic children can be helped by experienced physiotherapists.

ARTHROGRYPOSIS

This descriptive term means stiff joints. Several hundred different causes have been established. A full neurological assessment is indicated as treatment and prognosis may be affected if an underlying cause can be identified.

The generalised form (arthrogryposis multiplex congenita) is much more disabling than the distal form (Figure 21.59). Some forms of arthrogryposis are genetic. The infant's joints have not moved *in utero* and the limbs are 'featureless', lacking skin creases and muscle bulk.

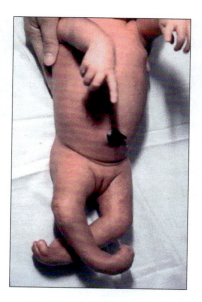

Figure 21.59 An infant with generalised joint contractures in keeping with a diagnosis of arthrogryposis multiplex congenita.

Physiotherapy and splinting are the mainstays of early treatment; some improvement in passive range of movement is common but active control may remain poor. Surgical options are available for specific problems but must be considered in the light of overall functional abilities.

NEUROMUSCULAR CONDITIONS WITH ORTHOPAEDIC CONCERNS

CEREBRAL PALSY

This results from a non-progressive injury to the developing brain and classically affects the motor cortex. Other areas may be affected: the larger the insult to the motor cortex, the greater the risk of associated damage. Although the damage is non-progressive, the musculoskeletal effects are progressive and variable depending on the tonal abnormality (spastic, hypotonic or dystonic).

Children are classified according to the GMFCS (Gross Motor Function Classification System) which predicts, with some accuracy, functional abilities as an adult. Physicians must remember that a child does not have to walk to function independently. There may be considerable differences in treatment aims for GMFCS I–III children compared to their non-walking GMFCS IV/V counterparts.

As with other neuromuscular conditions, orthopaedic care is small part of the multidisciplinary management plan. Treatment should prevent deformity and maximise function; orthopaedic surgery may be appropriate but in combination with physiotherapy and orthotic use. Treatment aims may include:

- Control of spinal deformity (Figure 21.60).

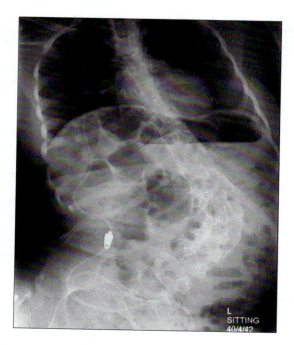

Figure 21.60 AP spinal radiograph in a child with total body involvement spastic cerebral palsy: There is a severe, spinal curve.

- Maintaining joint position.

- Control of muscle balance to prevent contractures.

Regular clinical and radiographic review identifies hips that are subluxing and which may benefit from surgical treatment (Figure 21.61).

SPINA BIFIDA

Worldwide, despite programmes of folate supplementation, antenatal screening and the possibility of termination of the pregnancy, many babies are born with spina bifida. There is a significant burden of childhood disability due to the sequelae of myelomeningocoeles.

The clinical picture is variable. Changes in neurological function raise the possibility of a tethered cord and/or Arnold–Chiari malformation and hydocephalus. Investigations include an ultrasound scan in infancy or a MRI later in childhood.

The child requires multidisciplinary management. Orthopaedic management is directed by the level of the lesion, associated problems including the intellectual impairment and the function achievable. Joints are often flaccid rather than contracted and splinting an insensate limb to provide joint stability is difficult. Immobilisation following surgery may lead to further disuse osteoporosis and pathological fractures in the recovery period (Figure 21.62).

THE SPINE

CONGENITAL DEFORMITIES

These problems are present at birth: they represent failures of formation (a hemivertebra) or of segmentation of vertebral bodies. The clinical result is usually scoliosis and treatment is based on the potential for curve progression. With kyphosis, progressive neurological deficit is common. Bracing is ineffective.

SCOLIOSIS

Aetiology/Incidence

- Scoliosis is a curvature of the spine in three dimensions: the 's' shape is visible on the x-ray but the rib hump concerns the patient and her mother (Figure 21.63). The aetiology may be idiopathic, neuromuscular, syndrome-related or congenital, and this, as well as age of onset, affects the natural history.

- Most curves are adolescent idiopathic scoliosis (AIS). It is most common in girls and there may be a family history. If the

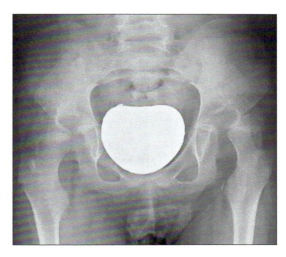

Figure 21.61 AP pelvic radiograph of a girl with spastic cerebral palsy, GMFCS level 4: Both hips are subluxed and painful, the femoral necks show significant valgus deformity (i.e. they are straight).

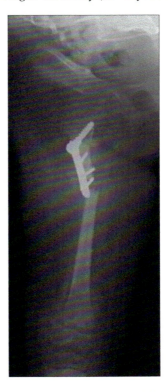

Figure 21.62 A child with spina bifida underwent an operative procedure to relocate his right hip; in the postoperative period he sustained two fractures, one proximally and one distally. Both healed with abundant callus but he was left with a stiff knee that severely limited his independent mobility.

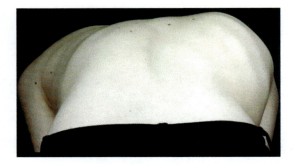

Figure 21.63 The Adams forward bend test highlights the rotational component of scoliosis and the 'rib hump' is obvious. (From Williams *et al.* (eds). *Bailey and Love's Short Practice of Surgery*, CRC press, 2013, with permission.)

curve starts in infancy or early childhood, the prognosis is worse as the spine has more time to grow and to curve (Figure 21.64). Curves are usually painfree; a painful scoliosis is a 'red flag' and requires investigation.

Treatment

This is dictated by the size of the curve and the risk of progression:

■ Curves with a Cobb angle < 25° are watched.

■ 25–45° curves are braced.

■ Curves > 45° and/or progressive may merit surgical treatment.

The standard treatment involves spinal fusion which limits further growth and lung development; if possible, surgery is delayed. More recently 'growing rods' have allowed earlier surgical intervention.

Aetiology influences treatment choice: neuromuscular curves have a different prognosis and hence management plan compared with idiopathic or congenital curves or those associated with osteogenesis.

SCHEUERMANN DISEASE (KYPHOSIS)

Kyphosis refers to the round-backed posture common to all thoracic spines; the normal kyphosis is 20–50°. Kyphotic curves in excess of this may be postural or structural (secondary to Scheuermann disease). This presents as a progressive curve in adolescence. The aetiology is unknown.

Treatment ranges from physiotherapy and bracing to surgery.

SPONDYLOLISTHESIS

Spondylolysis refers to a defect in the spinal vertebra which may be congenital or acquired (e.g. trauma). Spondylolisthesis occurs when the

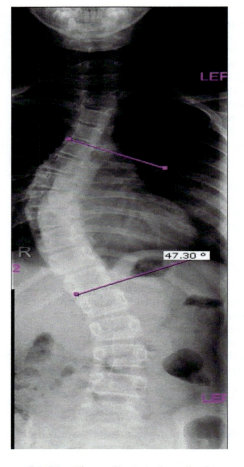

Figure 21.64 The scoliosis is described in terms of the apex of the curve: This lower thoracic curve, apex convex to the right, with a Cobb angle of 47° may warrant surgical treatment. (From Williams et al. (eds). *Bailey and Love's Short Practice of Surgery*, CRC press, 2013, with permission.)

upper vertebra slips forward on the lower. Mild slips are often asymptomatic and do not require treatment.

Treatment choice depends on the degree of slip and symptoms. Mechanical back pain may respond to conservative methods but the neurological involvement usually requires surgical intervention.

BACK PAIN

- Children should not suffer from back pain and thus if present there must be a worrying cause for it and pain is one of the 'red flag' signs for spinal pathology (Figure 21.65). However, back discomfort in the adolescent or prepubertal child is quite common and can be treated with advice regarding posture, physiotherapy and analgesic medication.

- Red flag symptoms and signs for spinal pathology include:

  - Systemic illness, fever or weight loss

  - Progressive neurological deficit

  - Unrelenting or night pain

  - Spinal deformity

In the presence of such signs/symptoms investigations to find the underlying cause must take place.

TRAUMA

Children have a reputation for bouncing rather than breaking when they fall and there are specific fracture patterns that only happen in the immature skeleton:

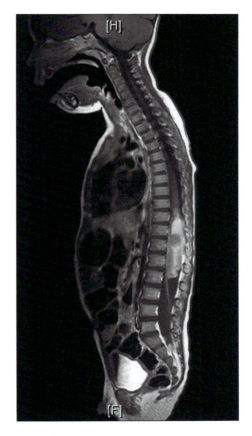

Figure 21.65 Lateral MRI demonstrating a large astrocytoma of the lower cord. The child presented with back pain that was waking him regularly from sleep. Night pain is a 'red flag' sign.

- Buckle fractures (Figure 21.66).

- Greenstick fractures (Figure 21.67).

- Injuries to the physis or growth plate (Figure 21.68).

- Children's ligaments are stronger than their bones so avulsion fractures are more common than ruptured ligaments in this age group.

- The growth plates may be mistaken for fractures so radiographs must be reviewed carefully and matched to the history and the physical signs. There will be tenderness at the site of a fracture.

Fractures in children heal rapidly and remodel with growth so some malalignment at the fracture site can be accepted:

- Deformity in the plane of movement of the adjacent joint will remodel if the child is still growing but rotational malalignment does not.

- Fractures involving the joint surface (intraarticular injuries) and/or the growth plate do not 'remodel' (Figure 21.69).

As with adults, basic principles must be adhered to and resuscitation ('save a life before a limb') is the key to good trauma management. It is always important to note the neurovascular status of

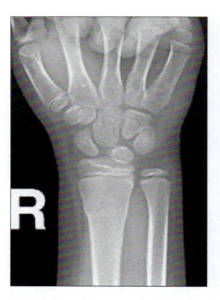

Figure 21.66 A child's AP wrist radiograph demonstrating a buckle fracture of the radial metaphysis: The fracture line is barely visible but the cortex is not completely smooth and is 'buckled'.

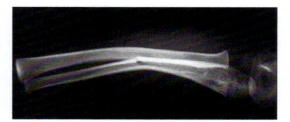

Figure 21.67 AP radiograph of the forearm demonstrating a greenstick fracture of the ulna. The bone is intact but may need to be broken to improve the deformity.

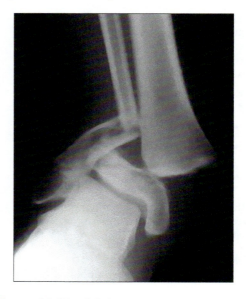

Figure 21.68 A Salter–Harris Type 2 distal tibial fracture with considerable displacement: The fracture must be reduced carefully without damage to the growth plate.

the limb distal to the injury and to care for any open wounds (Figure 21.70). Infection prevention is an essential part of any trauma protocol.

SPECIFIC PAEDIATRIC INJURIES

PHYSEAL INJURIES

These are classified according to the Salter–Harris system (Figure 21.71) based on:

- The severity of the injury to the physeal layer responsible for growth (see Figures 21.68, 21.69 and 21.70).

- Displacement at the articular surface (see Figure 21.69).

The physis is radiolucent on plain radiography and the extent of the injury must be gauged by looking at the displacement/position of the ossified metaphyseal and epiphyseal portions. Additional imaging techniques may help visualise the fracture fully.

Treatment

In general terms, the more severe the injury (SH Types III/IV) the more likely it is that an operative procedure will be required to reduce the physis and the joint surface and minimise future growth disturbance and joint damage.

PULLED ELBOW

In young children, it is easy to sublux the radial head when the child is pulled by the hand. The child cries and is then noted to have a limp arm with the elbow flexed and the forearm pronated.

Reduction is easy and often inadvertent with forearm supination leading to a click as the radial head relocates and movement improves. Normal function returns promptly. Recurrence is not unusual, but the children do grow out of this tendency.

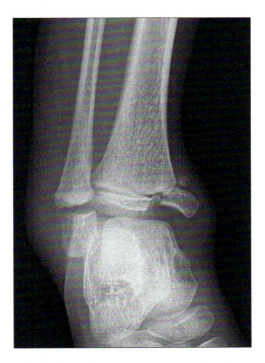

Figure 21.69 AP radiograph of the ankle demonstrating a significant physeal injury with disruption of the physis and the joint surface (Fibula SH Type 1, Medial malleolus SH Type IV).

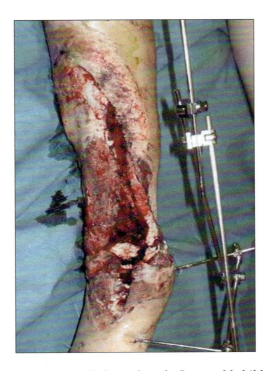

Figure 21.70 A major open injury to the lower leg of a 5-year-old child: ATLS principles ensured that the airway, breathing and circulation were managed in conjunction with the major soft tissue injury. Joint stiffness and physical damage are inevitable with this injury.

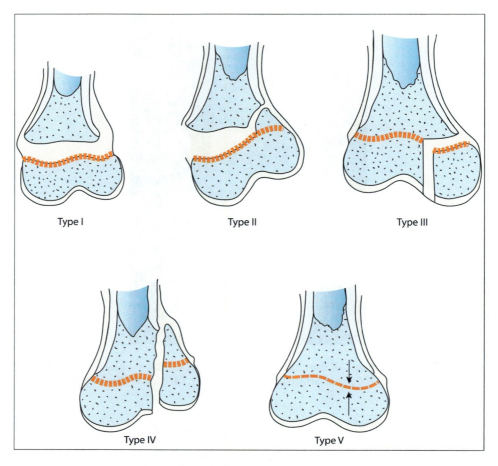

Figure 21.71 Salter–Harris classification of growth plate injuries. Type I: Shear through physeal plate; Type II: Partial shear through physeal plate and partial metaphyseal fracture (commonest injury) Type III: partial physeal separation with an intra-articular epiphyseal fracture; type IV: Plane passes from joint surface through physis and metaphysis; type V: Compression of the physis.

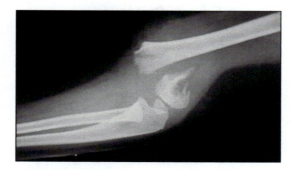

Figure 21.72 A lateral radiograph of a severely displaced supracondylar fracture of the humerus: The proximal fragment may have 'button-holed' through the biceps muscle and the brachial artery and/or the median nerve may become entrapped between the fracture fragments, either as a result of the injury or attempts to reduce the fracture.

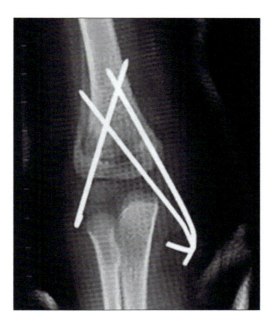

Figure 21.73 AP radiograph of a reduced and stabilised supracondylar fracture of the humerus. The arm is in plaster. the growth plate is not affected.

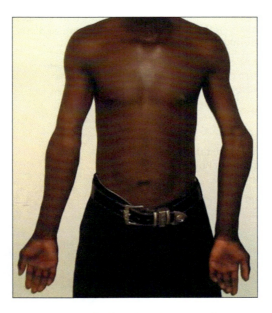

Figure 21.74 Cubitus varus is an unsightly deformity secondary to a poorly reduced fracture on the left arm. A corrective osteotomy is sometimes required.

FRACTURES AROUND THE ELBOW

Elbow fractures are common in childhood and associated with both acute problems such as neurovascular injury and compartment syndrome, as well as chronic deformity and malfunction.

Supracondylar Fractures of the Humerus

This the perhaps the potentially most serious injury. The Gartland classification 1–4 directs the need for closed reduction and pin insertion to stabilise the position (Figures 21.72 and 21.73). A careful neurovascular assessment of the hand must be made pre- and post-treatment and the following symptoms should raise the possibility of a compartment syndrome:

- Anxiety
- Analgesic requirement
- Agitation

Management of the pink but pulseless hand remains controversial but the orthopaedic team must be notified in all cases where the pulse is 'missing'.

A cubitus varus malunion deformity does not improve with time (Figure 21.74); it is noticeable and may cause symptoms. Surgical treatment can help.

Pitfalls Around Forearm Fractures

It is a basic tenet of orthopaedic management that an x-ray taken to look at an injury must include the joint above and the joint below, i.e. the whole bone. A failure to do so means the following injuries are all too frequently missed:

- Monteggia fracture: fracture of the ulna with radial head subluxation (Figure 21.75).
- Galeazzi fracture: Fracture of the radius with distal radioulnar subluxation.

Buckle Fractures

Torus or buckle fractures of the distal radius and/or ulna are common. They require little if any treatment:

- A wrist splints or a tubigrip bandage may be sufficient.
- Local hospital protocols may suggest that no follow-up of these fractures is required.

LOWER LIMB INJURIES

Fractures of the Proximal Femur

These are rare and usually due to high-velocity trauma (Figures 21.76).

AVN, malunion and growth arrest are feared complications. Urgent surgical management is required with screw or plate fixation.

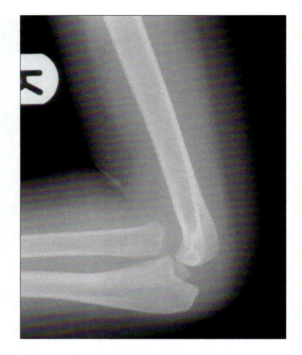

Figure 21.75 Lateral radiograph of a forearm injury, where no ulnar injury was seen and the radial head dislocation was 'missed': the ulnar injury was a greenstick fracture.

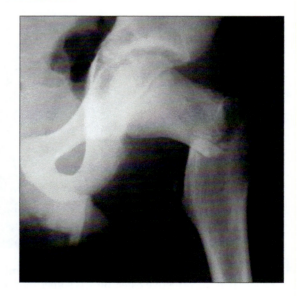

Figure 21.76 AP radiograph of a fractured neck of femur: in the elderly this is due to minor trauma, in a child a result of major trauma or in pathological bone.

An acute slipped capital femoral epiphysis should be treated similarly (see Figure 21.45).

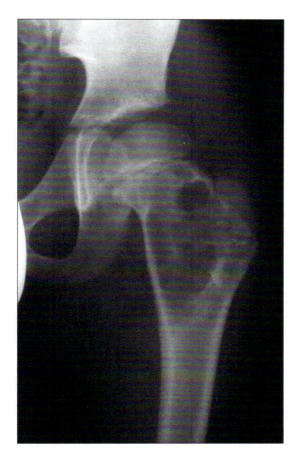

Figure 21.77 AP radiograph of the left proximal femur: there is a large bone cyst occupying most of the femoral neck. If this were to fracture, a poor outcome is likely thus it is wise to treat this cyst before it fractures.

Fractures of The Femoral Shaft

This is a common injury. Treatment depends on the age of the patient and the fracture site and methods include traction in the infant or child, flexible nails in the older child and standard adult techniques in the adolescent. Cast treatment is appropriate in selected cases. External fixation techniques may be required in open fractures or in the multiply injured patient.

Fractures of the Patella

The normal variant of a bipartite patella is frequently misdiagnosed as a fracture. Fractures should be tender to the touch and associated with some soft tissue swelling. Tendon avulsion fractures are associated with sporting injury or patients with neuromuscular disability.

Other Avulsion Injuries

■ Tibial spine avulsion injury (anterior cruciate ligament).

■ Injury to the tibial apophysis (patella tendon).

■ Avulsion of the hamstrings from the ischial tuberosity.

The avulsed bone fragment enlarges over time leading to radiographic features in the chronic injury that raise the possibility of a tumour. A careful interpretation of history, examination and x-ray and appropriate further imaging should clarify the issue.

Fractures of the Tibia/Fibula

One particular type of minimally displaced proximal tibial fracture is worthy of mention.

The **Cozen fracture** is an essentially undisplaced proximal metaphyseal fracture that is associated with the development of a knock-knee over the first 6–12 months after plaster cast removal. This represents a short-lived growth abnormality. Spontaneous improvement is usual but occasionally surgical treatment is required.

PATHOLOGICAL FRACTURES

A 'normal' fracture occurs as a result of an abnormal force applied to a normal bone. A pathological fracture occurs under two circumstances:

- When a normal force is applied to an abnormal bone.

- When an excessive force is applied to a normal bone in abnormal circumstances, such as may occur in cases of non-accidental injury.

Abnormal Bones

Pathological fractures through abnormal bone occur throughout childhood for a variety of causes:

- At birth, due for example, to osteogenesis imperfecta.

- In childhood, secondary to generalised poor bone density, for example, in neuromuscular conditions or fibrous dysplasia.

- In conditions of localised poor-quality bone formation, for example through simple bone cysts (Figure 21.77) or benign or malignant tumours.

Non-Accidental Injury

When excessive force is applied directly to a normal bone, fractures occur; the injury in a young child is often non-accidental. Such cases are more common than we would like to admit affecting children of all ages and from all walks of life. A high index of suspicion is required when the following features are associated with a fracture or soft tissue injury:

- Inappropriate and/or inconsistent history.

- Delay in presentation.

- Fracture in the non-walking child.

- Presence of multiple bruises of different ages (particularly in the non-walking child).

- There is no excuse for not examining any child fully and in cases of a poorly explained fracture, an examination to look for other injuries may save the life of the child. Child Protection Policies are an inherent part of NHS practice and you must be familiar with your local guidelines and referral protocols.

- Some injuries are 'classical' with a high specificity for non-accidental injury:

  - Fractures in children below walking age

  - Posterior rib fractures

  - Scapular fractures

  - Metaphyseal 'corner' fractures

  - Multiple fractures at different stages of healing

FURTHER READING

- Blom A, Warwick D, Whitehouse M, eds. *Apley and Solomon's System of Orthopaedics and Trauma.* 10th Edition. Productivity Press, 2017.
- Wenger DR, Pring ME, Pennock AT, et al. *Rang's Children's Fractures.* 4th Edition. Wolters Kluwer, 2018.

22 Urology

Naima Smeulders and Abraham Cherian

CONGENITAL URINARY FLOW ANOMALIES

Hydronephrosis

Definition

Hydronephrosis denotes dilatation of the urinary collecting system of the kidney – the pelvicaly-ceal system. Ureteronephrosis refers to dilatation of the ureter. The degree of dilatation is assessed on ultrasound by measuring the diameter of the renal pelvis at the renal parenchymal–pelvic junction in the anterior–posterior plane and that of the ureter behind the bladder. A diameter of ≤ 8 mm for the renal pelvis and < 5 mm for the ureter is deemed normal. Hydroureteronephrosis can result from impairment to the flow of urine or the retrograde reflux of urine.

Significance

In the past, the management of hydronephrosis was straightforward as children presented with symptoms, such as infection or pain, which warranted surgery. Today, antenatal ultrasound identifies a congenital anomaly of the urinary tract, primarily hydronephrosis, in 1 in 150 pregnancies. Long-term natural history studies have shown that dilatation often improves or resolves spontaneously; hydronephrosis does not equate with obstruction and the need for surgery.

Antenatal Hydronephrosis

In utero, hydronephrosis is defined as foetal renal pelvic diameter ≥ 5 mm in the second and ≥ 7 mm in the third trimester. When antenatal hydronephrosis is discovered, it is essential to confirm the diagnosis after birth (Figure 22.1). Knowledge of the prenatal evaluations during the progression of pregnancy forms the starting point of the assessment of the newborn, and should include the degree of unilateral or bilateral hydronephrosis, ureteric dilatation, renal size and parenchymal appearance, size of the foetal bladder and the amniotic fluid volume in relation to gestational age. Foetal urine production commences around the tenth week of pregnancy and accounts for the majority of amniotic fluid by the second trimester. The likelihood of significant postnatal pathology correlates to the severity of antenatal hydronephrosis.

Pelvi-Ureteric Junction Anomaly (PUJA)

Incidence

The incidence of pelvi-ureteric junction (PUJ) anomaly (PUJA) is 1 in 1500 live births, accounting for almost half of all antenatally diagnosed hydronephrosis. PUJA is bilateral in 10 to 20%; left to right ratio is 2:1 and male to female ratio is 2:1.

Aetiology/Clinical Presentation

The majority are primary and congenital in origin, although the problem may not become apparent until much later in life. The lack of an anatomical blockage combined with abnormal smooth muscle and neural arrangements at the PUJ have led to the concept of a 'functional obstruction' with impaired peristalsis of urine across the PUJ. While spontaneous improvement occurs in many, others will suffer progressive renal loss if left untreated.

Alternatively, or additionally, extrinsic compression of the PUJ by aberrant vessels crossing to the lower pole of the kidney can result in acute distension of the renal pelvis – typically intermittent – causing renal angle or loin pain accompanied by nausea and vomiting. Pyelonephritis/pyonephrosis, haematuria and hypertension are less common presentations.

Diagnosis

Serial imaging is pivotal in the assessment of PUJA. The diagnosis of PUJA can be suspected on ultrasound when this shows renal pelvic dilatation without ureteric dilatation and a normal urinary bladder (Figure 22.2). Diuretic renography with mercaptoacetyltriglycine (MAG3) is the

DOI: 10.1201/9781003175186-22

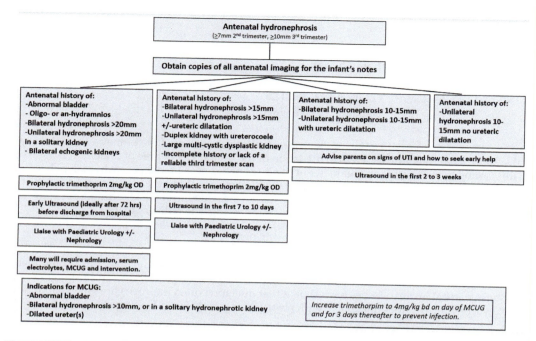

Figure 22.1   Flow diagram of assessment of newborn with antenatal hydronephrosis (adapted with permission from Smeulders N. and Paul A. hydronephrosis. In: Wilcox D, Godbole P, Coopper C [eds]. www.pediatricurologybook.com). MCUG – micturating cystourethrogram; UTI – urinary tract infection.

most popular functional imaging modality in PUJA today, providing information on differential renal clearance through the extraction of tracer from the blood as well as the excretion through the urinary tract by the disappearance of tracer (Figure 22.3). Assessment of drainage is controversial: while good drainage is easy to define, impaired drainage does not necessarily indicate obstruction. Instead this may reflect poor hydration, poor overall renal function, on-going filling of a capacious pelvicalyceal system, a full bladder or gravity – a further acquisition after change in posture and micturition is therefore essential. Even then, sequential renography documenting changes in differential function may be needed to identify those with obstruction, which is defined by Koff and Campbell as a restriction to urine flow, which if left untreated will cause progressive renal deterioration (Figure 22.4).

Treatment

The gold standard operation for PUJA is the Anderson–Hynes pyeloplasty, which allows excision of the fibrotic PUJ segment followed by a funnel-shaped tension-free anastomosis of the ureter to the renal pelvis, enabling dependent drainage. Success rates consistently exceed 95%, whether by an open or laparoscopic approach. Nephrectomy is recommended for those with gross dilatation in a very poorly functioning kidney in the presence of a normal contralateral kidney (Tables 22.1A and 22.1B).

Vesico-Ureteric Junction Anomaly (Megaureter)
Incidence/Classification

Congenital vesico-ureteric junction anomaly (VUJA) most frequently presents as a result of detection of the associated dilated ureter (primary megaureter), left to right ratio of 1.8:1, male to female ratio of 2:1. Ultrasound, micturating cystourethrogram (MCUG) and diuretic renography assessment allows VUJA and its megaureter to be classified into obstructed, refluxing, non-obstructed and non-refluxing, or both obstructed and refluxing. Co-existing anomalies occur in 16%, including PUJA, multi-cystic dysplastic kidney (MCDK), renal ectopia and agenesis. It is sometimes difficult to differentiate between a PUJA and VUJA or dual pathology, and an intra-operative contrast antegrade or retrograde pyelo-ureterogram may be required to clarify the anomaly (Figure 22.5).

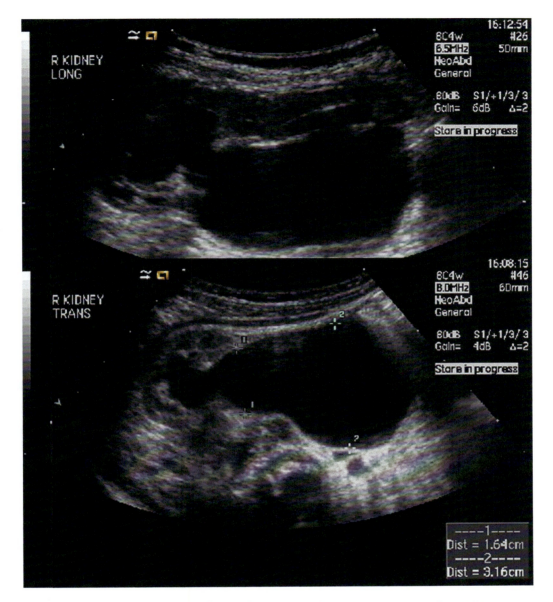

Figure 22.2 Ultrasound: longitudinal and transverse view of right hydronephrotic kidney. Distance 1 indicates the renal pelvic diameter in the anterior–posterior plane (AP pelvis) and distance 2 the extra-renal pelvic diameter.

Treatment

As spontaneous improvement is frequent, close observational management is recommended for the asymptomatic infant with stable or improving dilatation and differential function. Many advocate antibiotic prophylaxis, particularly for refluxing megaureters, and some also advise circumcision. Surgical intervention is indicated in 10–20% of primary megaureters for break-through febrile urinary tract infections (UTI), deteriorating function or dilatation. Ureteric reimplantation after excision of the stenotic VUJ segment, with or without ureteric tapering, previously the gold standard, is now reserved for those who fail endoscopic balloon dilatation or cutting balloon endo-ureterotomy with temporary placement of a JJ stent. For those with < 10% differential function, nephroureterectomy is advised.

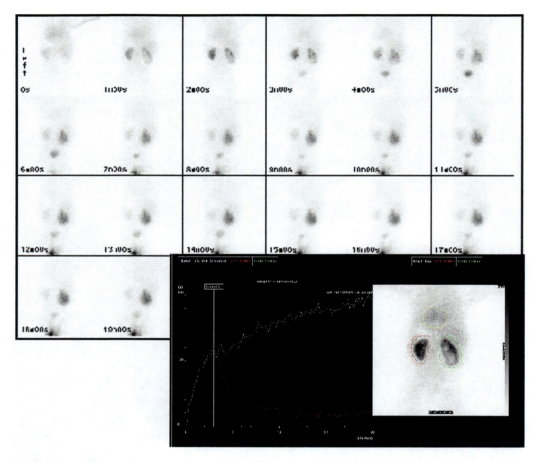

Figure 22.3 MAG3 renogram: Equal split differential function. While prompt drainage is observed from the left kidney, there is continuous accumulation of tracer in the hydronephrotic right kidney even after change in posture and micturition.

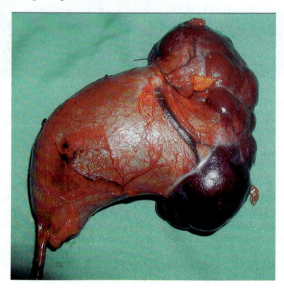

Figure 22.4 Pelvi-ureteric junction obstruction: gross pathology.

Table 22.1A: Indications for Close Observational Management of Unilateral PUJA

- Asymptomatic infant
- Stable or decreasing hydronephrosis on serial ultrasound
- Stable or improving differential renal function on MAG3

Table 22.1B: Indications for Surgery in PUJA

Absolute indications	Relative indications
	Recommendations for a 'prophylactic pyeloplasty' vary between units:
• Symptoms • Declining function • Increasing hydronephrosis (usually precedes renal deterioration)	• Hydronephrosis > 30 mm • Hydronephrosis > 20 mm with calyceal dilatation • Hydronephrosis (> 20 mm) in a solitary kidney or bilaterally • Intrarenal hydronephrosis (gross calyceal dilatation)

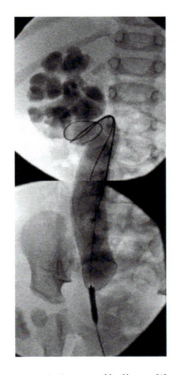

Figure 22.5   Intra-operative fluoroscopic image of balloon dilatation of right vesico-ureteric junction for the obstructive primary megaureter.

Vesico-Ureteric Reflux

Incidence/Clinical Presentation

The retrograde flow of urine from the bladder into the ureters either on bladder filling ('passive' vesico-ureteric reflux [VUR]) or on voiding ('active' VUR) accounts for approximately 25% of antenatally diagnosed hydronephrosis. More than 90% of those with antenatally detected reflux are male, whereas those presenting symptomatically with UTI are predominantly female. VUR may be intermittent. Its prevalence is 1–2% of the paediatric population overall, but 30% amongst those with UTI.

Aetiology

VUR may be secondary to urethral obstruction (e.g. posterior urethral valves), and neuropathic (e.g. spinal dysraphism, following pelvic surgery) or non-neurogenic bladder dysfunction (e.g. detrusor-sphincter dyssynergia). Where there is no underlying aetiology, VUR is described as primary. While this was previously thought to be purely the result of an abnormal VUJ, which is

Table 22.2: International Reflux Study Committee Classification

- Grade I – reflux into a non-dilated ureter
- Grade II – reflux into a non-dilated renal pelvis and calyces
- Grade III – mild/moderate dilatation of ureter, renal pelvis and calyces
- Grade IV – moderate tortuosity and dilatation of ureter, renal pelvis and calyces with obliteration of angle of fornices but papillary impressions maintained in most calyces
- Grade V – gross tortuosity and dilatation of ureter, renal pelvis and calyces with loss of papillary impressions in most calyces

often familial (34% of siblings and 50% of offspring), today VUR is recognised as part of a generalised abnormality of the urinary tract, including renal dysplasia and hypoplasia, bladder dysfunction and a possible predisposition to UTI.

Diagnosis

Micturating cystourethrogram (MCUG) is the gold standard and allows the severity of VUR to be graded (see Table 22.2). MCUG is an invasive investigation and prophylactic antibiotics must be increased to treatment dose for three days to reduce the risk of sepsis (Figure 22.6). For children who present symptomatically later in life, or to assess for VUR resolution, an indirect cystogram using MAG-3 renography can be obtained once a child has been potty-trained.

Renal dysplasia and scarring is best assessed by a DMSA isotope scan (Figure 22.7). Since the advent of routine antenatal ultrasound scanning it has become clear that about 60% of 'renal scars' in newborns ascertained to have VUR are the result of abnormal kidney development rather than secondary to infection.

Treatment

Spontaneous improvement is the norm, with persistent VUR more likely with higher grade, bilaterality, older age at presentation and renal dysplasia/scarring.

The goal of treatment is the prevention of renal injury, leading to hypertension and renal failure. The management of VUR continues to be debated. Previous randomised controlled studies found surgical correction of VUR to offer no advantage on renal outcome over antibiotic prophylaxis. Today, antibiotic prophylaxis is recommended only for Grade 3 VUR and above. No agreement exists on the role of circumcision, endoscopic injection and ureteric reimplantation. In contrast, the importance of optimising bladder and bowel function is beyond doubt and universally accepted.

Posterior Urethral Valves
Incidence/Clinical Presentation

A congenital membrane obstructing or partially obstructing the posterior urethra occurs in up to 1 in 4000 male births. Posterior urethral valves (PUV) accounts for almost 10% of antenatally diagnosed uropathies, and can affect the development of the entire urinary tract. An enlarged or thick-walled bladder, bilateral hydronephrosis with or without hyperechogenic renal parenchyma and oligo- or anhydramnios in a male foetus on antenatal ultrasound suggests PUV (Figure 22.8). Oligo- or anhydramnios can have secondary effects on pulmonary and limb development, culminating in Potter syndrome.

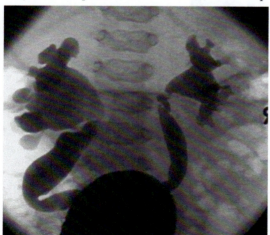

Figure 22.6   Bilateral vesico-ureteric reflux shown by a micturating cystourethrogram.

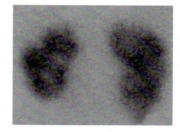

Figure 22.7   DMSA scan showing bilateral renal scarring in vesico-ureteric reflux.

Antenatal decompression by placement of a JJ stent between the foetal bladder and amniotic cavity may restore an adequate volume of amniotic fluid and hence lung maturation (Figure 22.9). So far, no benefit has been shown for renal and bladder outcomes from *in utero* vesicoamniotic shunting, which tends to be performed quite late, during the second half of pregnancy.

The newborn may show signs of chronic kidney disease (CKD), sepsis or pulmonary hypoplasia. While many boys with PUV are detected antenatally, others present in infancy (UTI/sepsis, dysuria, haematuria, CKD) or thereafter (incontinence). The quality of the urinary stream is misleading and voiding pressures in boys with PUV are as high as in normal male infants.

Ultrasound may show a dilated posterior urethra in addition to a thick-walled bladder (keyhole sign), upper tract dilatation and abnormal renal parenchymal morphology. MCUG is still the gold standard for diagnosis, although compared to cystourethroscopy its sensitivity is 80–90% (Figure 22.10).

Treatment/Prognosis

The three initial aims of treatment are to resuscitate the child in renal failure or sepsis, to drain the bladder and then to incise the PUV endoscopically. Subsequent management focuses on the long-term consequences of PUV for the urinary tract. CKD is present in 50% at the time of diagnosis. Four factors are associated with poor outcome in the long-run: presentation before the age of 1 year, bilateral VUR, proteinuria and daytime incontinence at the age of 5 years. Antenatal diagnosis carries a worse prognosis initially, with mortality or Stage V CKD in the first ten years of life predetermined by renal dysplasia and the severity of *in utero* obstruction. However, better renal function is observed in the second decade of life for antenatally detected PUV than for those presenting symptomatically later in childhood; preservation of renal function seems to benefit from early diagnosis and nephro-urological care. The association between poor renal outcome and urinary incontinence, present in 14–38% of boys with PUV, points to bladder dysfunction playing a major role in secondary renal damage. Indeed, the need for proactive management of the bladder in boys with PUV is well-established.

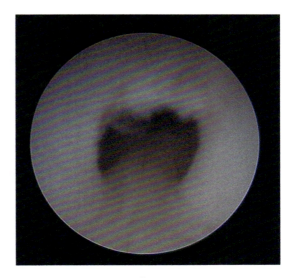

Figure 22.8 Endoscopic view of posterior urethral valve.

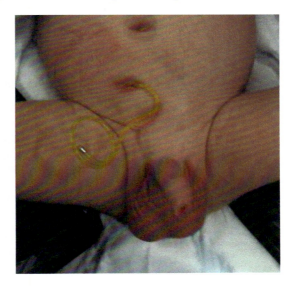

Figure 22.9 Newborn boy born with antenatally placed vesico-amniotic shunt *in situ*.

Multi-Cystic Dysplastic Kidney
Incidence/Aetiology

A faulty interaction between an abnormal ureteric bud and the metanephric mesenchyme during embryogenesis may result in a non-functioning kidney consisting of variable-sized cysts and an

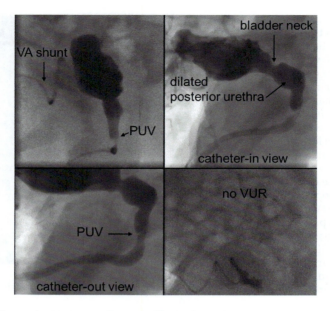

Figure 22.10 Micturating cystourethrogram. Note the trabeculated bladder, hypertrophied bladder neck and dilated posterior urethra above the posterior urethral valve (PUV). VA – vesico-amniotic; VUR – vesico-ureteric reflux.

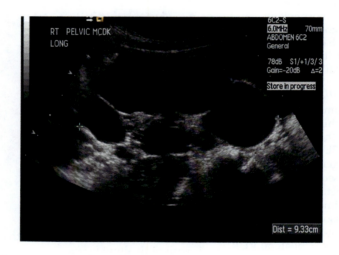

Figure 22.11 Multi-cystic dysplastic kidney: Typical ultrasound appearance. Note the absence of normal renal parenchyma.

atretic ureter (Figure 22.11). Today, the majority are detected antenatally, affecting 1 in 4000 live births. Contralateral anomalies, primarily PUJA and VUR, may be present in 20%.

Treatment

Serial ultrasounds have shown that these kidneys involute spontaneously: approximately one-third by 2 years of age, half by 5 years and two-thirds by 10 years. However, if the kidney fails to decrease in size or enlarges, nephrectomy is indicated (Figure 22.12). Although hypertension and malignant change have been reported, their incidence is similar to the normal population.

Renal Agenesis, Ectopia and Fusion

The apparent absence of a kidney on ultrasound may reflect a congenital deficiency (agenesis), involution of a MCDK or an ectopic location yet to be identified.

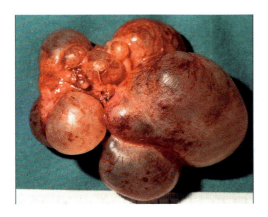

Figure 22.12 Multi-cystic dysplastic kidney: Gross specimen. No normal renal parenchyma can be seen.

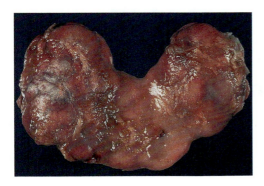

Figure 22.13 Horseshoe kidney.

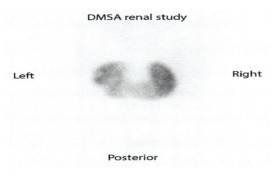

DMSA renal study

Left   Right

Posterior

Figure 22.14 DMSA isotope study of a horseshoe kidney.

Incidence

- Unilateral agenesis: 1 in 1000 to 1500 births, i.e. a solitary kidney; bilateral renal agenesis is incompatible with life (Potter syndrome).

- Horseshoe kidney: 1 in 400 to 1800 births; a fibrous band or renal tissue (isthmus) joins the two kidneys across the midline (by the lower poles in 95%).

- Simple ectopia: 1 in 1000 births, i.e. the kidney is placed on same side as its ureter (60% pelvic, rarely in the thorax, in 10% bilateral) (Figures 22.13 to 22.15).

- Crossed ectopia: 1 in 7000 births, i.e. the kidney lies on the opposite side to the insertion of its ureter into the bladder (usually left kidney crosses to the right, with fusion to the contralateral kidney in 85%).

Clinical Presentation/Diagnosis

Most are incidental findings on ultrasound imaging and may be part of multiple congenital anomalies such as the VACTERL association. Other urogenital abnormalities frequently coexist, for instance, contralateral VUR can be detected in one-third of unilateral renal agenesis, a PUJA occurs in 20% of horseshoe kidneys, and renal ectopia is associated with vaginal agenesis, bicornuate uterus or a contralateral ectopic ureter. Renal isotope imaging (DMSA) will reveal all functioning renal tissue. Occasionally, further clarification of the anatomy is required by magnetic resonance urography (MRU) or by intraoperative retrograde studies.

Treatment

Treatment is only required for clinically significant consequences, e.g. for VUR or PUJA.

Duplex Kidneys

Where a kidney has two parts (moeities) each with their own collecting system it is called a duplex kidney (Figure 22.16). In 60% the ureters join before their insertion into the bladder (incomplete duplex) and in the other 40% the two ureters enter the bladder separately (complete duplex). As a result of the way the ureters are incorporated into the bladder during development, the lower moiety ureter orifice lies above the upper moiety ureteric orifice (Mayer–Weigert Law). The terminal upper moiety ureter is prone to a cystic dilatation (ureterocoele).

Incidence/Clinical Presentation

Some degree of duplication is extremely common (approximately 1 in 100), bilaterally in 40%. Complete duplication occurs in 1 in 1000 and is bilateral in 25%. Where there is a family history the incidence increases to 1 in 12. Most duplications are an incidental finding. Others are

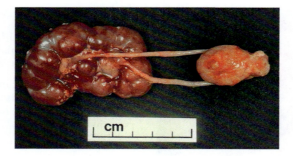

Figure 22.15 Fused kidneys with right and left moeity ureters draining to the bladder on their respective sides.

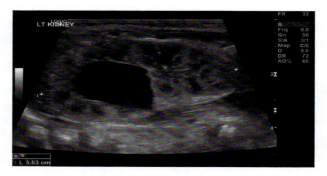

Figure 22.16 Ultrasound longitudinal image of left duplex kidney. Note the marked hydronephrosis of the upper moeity.

associated with hydronephrosis (Figure 22.16), and today, many of these are detected on antenatal ultrasound screening. An ureterocoele is seen in 1 in 5000. This may be obstructive to its associated moeity, and if very large the ureterocoele may prolapse into the bladder neck causing obstruction to the entire urinary tract. The lower moeity ureter is ectopic (high and lateral – where it is prone to VUR) in 1 in 2500 (40% of complete duplex systems). The upper moeity ureter is ectopic in 1 in 10,000 (10% of duplex systems). While in boys, the ectopia of the upper moeity ureter is always above the urinary sphincter, in girls the ectopia may be into the vagina causing dribble incontinence on top of a normal voiding pattern. As a general rule, the more ectopically a ureter inserts, the more dysplastic its associated renal moiety (Stephen hypothesis).

Diagnosis

On ultrasound, the only feature of an uncomplicated duplex kidney may be its greater renal length. Where there is hydronephrosis, this may preferentially affect one moiety of a complete duplex. Providing both moieties have functioning renal tissue, MAG-3 renography may show two distinct pelvicalyceal systems (Figure 22.17). A DMSA may be needed to clarify the degree of function in each renal moiety. An ureterocoele may be observed on ultrasound or it may show as a filling defect during the early filling phase of a MCUG (Figures 22.18 and 22.19). During the MCUG, contrast may reflux into the lower moiety pelvicalyceal system, which is orientated lateral and inferior – referred to as the 'drooping lily sign'. A MRU may be needed to demonstrate the very small poorly functioning upper moiety responsible for the dribble incontinence from its ectopic ureter, known as a 'cryptic upper moiety' (Figure 22.20).

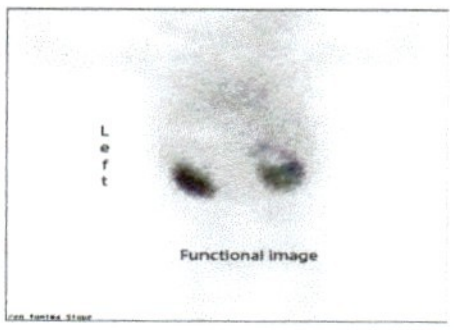

Treatment

No treatment is required in an asymptomatic child with a duplex system not complicated by obstruction, reflux or ectopia. No follow-up is needed for those without hydronephrosis. Endoscopic ureterocoele puncture may be needed to relieve obstruction to its

Figure 22.17 MAG-3 renogram demonstrating very poor function in the upper moeities of bilateral duplex kidneys.

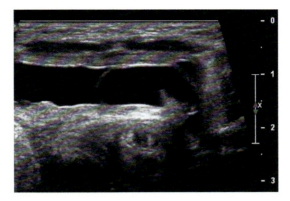

Figure 22.18 Ultrasound: longitudinal view of bladder demonstrating a large ureterocoele prolapsing through the bladder neck into the urethra.

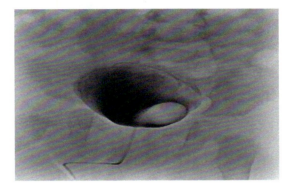

Figure 22.19 Micturating cystourethrogram: Early filling phase showing a large intravesical ureterocoele.

moiety or to the bladder outflow. Where intervention is indicated for VUR to the lower moiety or contralateral ureter, endoscopic injection may be attempted; similar success rates to simplex systems were noted in a recent meta-analysis (64% versus. 68%). As the distal upper and lower moiety ureters share a common blood supply, a combined mobilisation and reimplantation of both ureters is needed during intravesical ureteric reimplantation. Mobilisation of the upper moiety ureter / ureterocoele may leave a defect in the bladder neck that will require repair and risks bladder dysfunction. However, as the renal moieties of the most ectopic ureters typically are very poorly functioning, heminephrectomy allows extensive bladder surgery to be averted in most. For those with better function in both moieties, an anastomosis between the two moiety ureters or renal pelvises can similarly avoid extensive bladder dissection and is becoming increasingly popular.

INCONTINENCE
Development of Continence
In infancy, voiding occurs as a result of a reflex co-ordinated in the brainstem. With increasing age, bladder capacity increases and the frequency of voiding reduces. By around four years, voluntary inhibition of the voiding reflex has been attained.

Continence requires normal:

- mobility and brain function
- bladder capacity and compliance
- bladder sensation

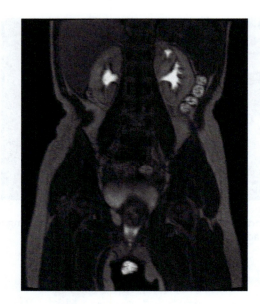

Figure 22.20 MRU demonstrating a 'cryptic' upper moiety for the left kidney. Its ectopic ureter insertion into the vagina is responsible for a dribbling incontinence on top a normal voiding pattern.

- voluntary detrusor contraction
- co-ordinated with sphincter control (competence and relaxation)

Aetiology

The key to tackling incontinence is to understand the aetiology, which frequently can be deduced from a careful history and examination followed by basic non-invasive assessments. Structural causes, such as the exstrophy–epispadias complex or an ectopic ureter, and neurogenic patholo-gies, for example, the spinal dysraphisms or secondary to anorectal anomalies, have to be differen-tiated from the far more common functional causes.

Exstrophy–Epispadias Complex
Incidence

Maldevelopment of the cloacal membrane and lower abdominal wall results in a spectrum rang-ing from epispadias (1 in 120,000), through vesical exstrophy (1 in 50,000) to cloacal exstrophy (1 in 300,000 live births).

Epispadias

Epispadias is the mildest form and generally seen in boys (Figures 22.21 and 22.22). The bladder is covered but the urethra opens on the dorsum of the penis. The penis is typically wide and short with dorsal curvature. In girls, the urethra is patulous and the clitoris bifid. In addition to recon-structing the genitalia, surgery for continence is required in the majority of patients as the defect extends through the sphincter and bladder neck.

Bladder Exstrophy

In this anomaly, the bladder opens onto the abdominal wall between split rectus abdominis muscles and separated pubic bones (pubic diastasis) continuing as an open urethral plate on the dorsum of the penis in the male and between divided clitori and labia minora in the female to the anterior edge of the vagina (Figure 22.23). The anus is anteriorly positioned (functionally normal) and the umbilicus is low-lying above the bladder plate. Inguinal herniae are a common association.

The surgical care of these babies has been centralised to a handful of institutions and each have developed their technique for closure of the bladder and abdominal wall, bladder neck repair as well as reconstruction of the penis.

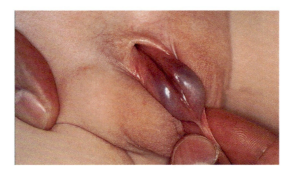

Figure 22.21   Epispadias without exstrophy.

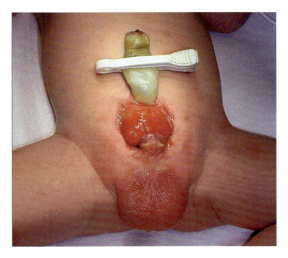

Figure 22.22   Classic bladder exstrophy with epispadias in a male.

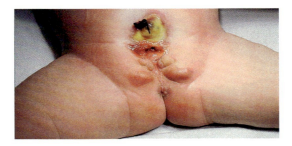

Figure 22.23   Classic bladder exstrophy in a female.

Cloacal Exstrophy

This is the most severe and rarest form of the exstrophy complex (Figure 22.24). Here, the bowel, usually at the ileocaecal valve, opens in the midline between two hemi-bladders, accompanied by diastasis of the pubis and a small epispadiac penis as well as an exomphalos into the cord. Other anomalies are frequent, such as spinal dysraphism (30%) and Arnold–Chiari malformation, lower limb (25%), renal and cardiac anomalies and a foreshortened intestine. Until 60 years ago, this condition was universally fatal, but since the 1980s survival has been over 90%.

In addition to the above surgery, hindgut reconstruction to a colostomy or ileostomy is required. Pelvic osteotomy is employed to help approximate the pubic diastasis (Figure 22.25) and support the closure.

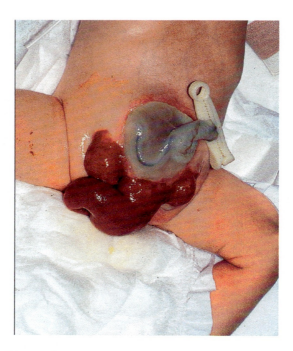

Figure 22.24 Cloacal exstrophy.

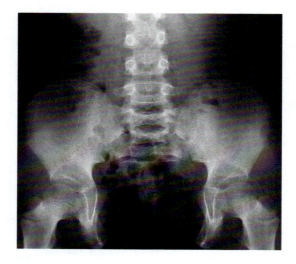

Figure 22.25 Widened symphysis pubis.

Cloacal Malformation
Definition

Cloacal malformation is a congenital anomaly of unknown cause, which occurs exclusively in females. In early foetal life, the urethra, vagina and anus fail to separate resulting in a common channel opening onto the perineum (Figure 22.26). Although classed under ano-rectal malformations this anomaly is more appropriately described as belonging to the spectrum of uro-rectal septum malformations; it is a spectrum of disorders and not a singular entity.

Incidence

Cloacal anomaly occurs 1 in 50,000 births.

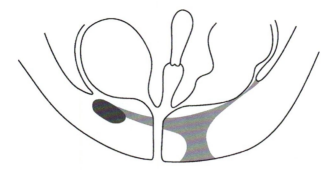

Figure 22.26   Classic long common channel cloaca.

Presentation

Antenatally, a cystic lesion within the foetal pelvis with or without upper urinary tract dilatation in a female, or obvious hydrometrocolpos should raise the possibility of a cloacal malformation. Counselling should include possible diagnoses, interventions both ante- and postnatally, centre for delivery, timing and modes of delivery. Differentials include vaginal atresia, imperforate hymen, urogenital sinus anomaly, cloacal malformation, ovarian cyst or duplication anomalies of the hindgut. Increasing size of the cyst, foetal ascites, anhydramnios or oligohydramnios, and urinary tract dilatation may require tapping of contents or placement of shunts.

After birth, the absence of an anal opening and instead the presence of a single perineal opening in a girl is a cloacal malformation until proved otherwise.

Clinical Features

Associated malformations occur in over 90%: 60% CKD (50% have renal failure at 5 years of age and up to 20% need kidney replacement therapy, such as dialysis or transplantation, before transition to young adult services), 60% spinal dysraphism, 60% cardiac anomalies and 20% have the appearance of genital ambiguity but their hormonal profiles are normal. A variety of subtypes are recognised: a broad categorisation involves the length of the common channel being short or long.

Management

For the best outcomes, an MDT co-ordinated holistic approach is essential. The immediate concerns are respiratory support, if there is pulmonary hypoplasia, and urinary tract drainage, if there is urinary tract obstruction. Stool diversion (colostomy) from the complex is essential to prevent contamination of the urinary tract and in preparation for definitive reconstruction. This is carried out within the first 48 hours of life. The next priorities are to establish feeding and conduct investigations to understand the anatomy, renal function and associated malformations.

Investigations include FBC, urea and electrolytes, Creatinine, ultrasound of the urinary tract and spine, MAG-3 renogram, genitogram/cystogram, distal loopogram, echocardiogram as well as an examination under GA and endoscopy through the common channel to provide details of the particular configuration of the anomaly. MRU can add further understanding to help guide reconstruction, which is usually performed between six and nine months of life, once the child is thriving (Figure 22.27). The goals of treatment are to restore anatomy and function. A variety of secondary procedures are required in later years in up to 50%. Psychological support is an essential component of care. Well-managed early life and transition to adult services is extremely important and has life-long consequences.

Neuropathic Bladder
Incidence/Aetiology

In most children, neuropathic voiding dysfunction is congenital: it must be assessed for in children with spinal dysraphism (1 in 2500) or anorectal anomalies. It is important to consider that this dysfunction can change typically at times of rapid growth such as in the first two years of life or in adolescence. Cord trauma or infarction, transverse myelitis, tumours or pelvic surgery may result in acquired neuropathic voiding dysfunction.

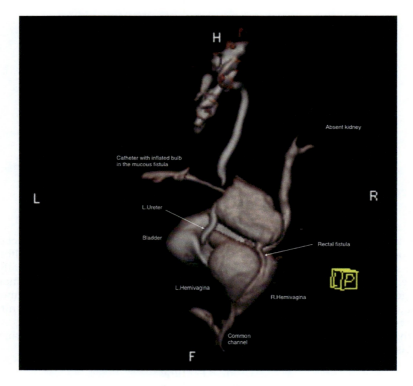

Figure 22.27 MRU reconstruction demonstrating the pelvicalyceal systems, ureters as well as the relation of the bladder, hemi-vaginas, the rectum and its fistula to the common channel.

Clinical Features/Diagnosis

Physical examination may reveal overt lower extremity neurological deficit and/or a hairy patch, dimple or skin tag on the spine may point to spina bifida occulta. Ultrasound will demonstrate upper tract hydronephrosis, bladder wall thickness and volume, and in children less than three months the terminal spinal cord. A plain film may show bony spinal abnormalities and constipation; however, for further details of spinal cord abnormalities MRI is required (Figure 22.28). Ultrasound is also used during non-invasive bladder function assessment to ascertain the voiding pattern and efficiency. Urodynamics assess the pressures within the urinary tract during bladder filling and emptying through a small catheter placed into the bladder. MCUG can provide further information during filling and voiding, including secondary VUR, and is combined with urodynamics (videourodynamics) after infancy. DMSA isotope scanning assesses the kidneys for renal damage.

Treatment

Regular careful assessment is essential to achieve the treatment aims:

■ preservation of renal function

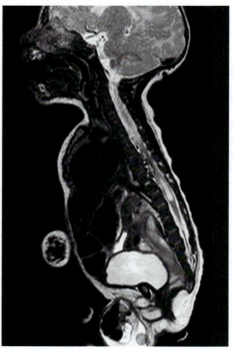

Figure 22.28 MRI: T2-weighted sagittal image. Note the hypoplastic spinal cord and segmental anomalies, as well as the large bladder.

Table 22.3: Management of Neuropathic Bladder

Proportion (%)	Bladder detrusor	Sphincter/ bladder neck	Pressures, i.e. risk to kidneys, continence	Management
7	Normal	Normal	Normal	Monitor for change
23	Hyporeflexic	Acontractile	Low pressure incontinence	Catheterisation for emptying; Surgery for continence
15	Hyporeflexic	Hypercontractile	Variable pressure	Regular catheterisation, may be continent without major surgery
11	Hyperreflexic	Acontractile	Variable pressure	incontinence Anticholinergics +/– catheterisation, surgery for continence +/– upper tracts
44	Hyperreflexic	Hyperreflexic	High pressure, high risk	Anticholinergics and regular catheterisation, may need vesicostomy/augmentation cystoplasty to protect kidneys

- continence

- sexual function.

Many require frequent bladder catheterisation and daily medication, and a proportion require major surgery to achieve these goals (Table 22.3).

Prognosis

With careful monitoring and high levels of compliance, renal damage can be minimised. Surgery for continence is required for a proportion, with subsequent life-long monitoring for side effects or late complications.

DISORDERS OF SEX DEVELOPMENT

Disorders of sex development (DSD) is a complex group of disorders with diverse pathophysiology that affect the internal and/ or external genitalia (Figure 22.29). Patients present in the newborn period with atypical genitalia or in adolescence with abnormal sexual development during puberty. Patients with DSD are best managed by a multidisciplinary team, and where this experience is not available referral to a regional DSD centre is mandatory. For further information on how to evaluate a new patient with DSD the reader is referred to the chapter 'Endocrinology'.

Hypospadias
Incidence/Clinical Presentation

Hypospadias occurs 1 in 300 live male births. This congenital abnormality is characterised by any combination of the following key features:

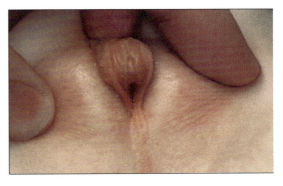

Figure 22.29   Ambiguous genitalia.

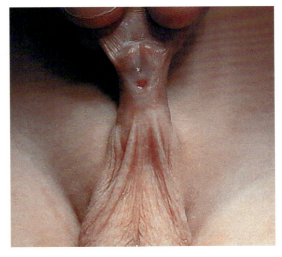

Figure 22.30   Distal hypospadias.

- A ventral urethral meatus abnormally positioned anywhere from the glans penis to the perineum (Figures 22.30 and Figure 22.31).

- Chordee forces the penis to point down to the scrotum when erect.

- A 'hooded' foreskin present only on the dorsal side.

623

It is important to distinguish an incompletely virilised hypospadiac penis from a virilised female or other DSD. This is facilitated by the palpation of the testes. Bilaterally descended testes point to a XY karyotype. However, if one or both testes are undescended or impalpable, DSD must be excluded.

Treatment

While for the most minor degree of hypospadias, no surgery or only excision of the hooded prepuce can be considered, the remainder are likely to require operative correction. The first step of surgery is the correction of the chordee, followed by urethroplasty and skin cover. Depending on the abnormality, the surgeon will advise either a single-stage or two-stage procedure using the prepuce as a graft for the urethroplasty. Therefore, parents must be counselled against circumcision of a newborn baby boy with hypospadias.

Prognosis

A cosmetically acceptable result should be attainable. However, complications are common: 5% meatal or urethral stenosis, 10–15% urethra–cutaneous fistula and 2–5% dehiscence of part of the repair. Voiding difficulties may become apparent only in adolescence.

Undescended Testis
Incidence

Testicular descent occurs during the fifth to seventh months of pregnancy, the left descending before the right. An undescended testis is observed in 1 in 50 to 100 term infants and in up to one-third of premature babies. Descent after birth does occur spontaneously but is rare after the first few months of life.

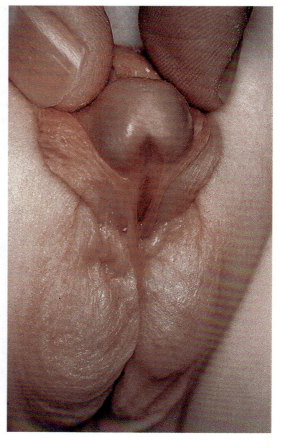

Figure 22.31 Penoscrotal hypospadias.

Clinical Presentation/Investigation/Classification

A careful history and examination allows the testis palpated outside the scrotum to be categorised into:

- An undescended testis: A testicle that is found in the line of its normal path of descent but outside the scrotum.

- An ectopic testis: A testicle that lies outside the normal path of descent, for instance, in the thigh or the perineum.

- An ascended testis: a previously normally descended testis that with growth has failed to retain its scrotal position.

- A retractile testis: A normal testis that on initial examination appears above the scrotum or in the inguinal canal but can be brought to the scrotum without tension once the cremasteric reflex has been overcome.

An impalpable testis requires further assessment under general anaesthesia. If the testis remains impalpable at this point, diagnostic laparoscopy will demonstrate one of three scenarios:

- The *vas deferens* and testicular vessels run to an intra-abdominal testis.

- The *vas deferens* and testicular vessels end blindly within the abdomen, pointing to testicular loss before the fifth month of pregnancy.

- The *vas deferens* and testicular vessels leave the abdomen through the deep inguinal ring. Subsequent groin exploration may reveal a testis within the groin or demonstrate the vas deferens and vessels to be blind-ending, presumably due to torsion or a vascular event during descent. This is known as the 'vanishing testis syndrome'.

Treatment

Retractile testes require no intervention. Orchidopexy is performed for palpable testes. If the testicular vessels to an intra-abdominal testis are short, the vessels may be stretched by securing the testis to the opposite side of the pelvis for several weeks, before routing the testis to the scrotum (Shehata technique). Alternatively, for a two-stage Fowler–Stephens

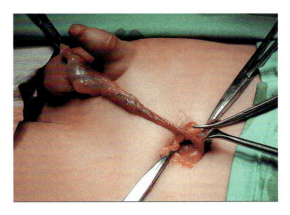

Figure 22.32 Undescended testis being brought down into the scrotum at surgery.

procedure, the testicular vessels are divided and, after a period to permit the collateral blood supply along the *vas deferens* to strengthen, the testis is mobilised on this second blood supply to the scrotum. Inguinal orchidopexy carries a 5% risk of testicular atrophy, and this increases to 10% for mobilisation of an intra-abdominal testis (Figure 22.32).

Prognosis

Surgery cannot reverse the maturational failure of the undescended testis but it can reduce the impact from further thermal injury. Historical data have documented normal semen analysis in 60% of men with unilateral and 25% of those with bilateral undescended testis, although paternity is achieved by up to 90% and 65%, respectively. Since then, the recommended age for orchidepexy has steadily decreased. So far, improved sperm counts and mobility as well as a reduced malignancy risk have been reported. The risk of malignancy is estimated to be two to three times that of the normal population for boys who had an orchidopexy before puberty. Monthly testicular self-examination should commence at puberty.

Acute Scrotum

Clinical Presentation

Sudden onset of scrotal pain, redness and/or erythema warrants emergency review in case of torsion of the testis, whose chance of viability reduces with each hour. In young children, the first symptoms are frequently atypical and non-specific, necessitating a high index of suspicion and scrotal examination in all boys presenting with abdominal pain or mere vomiting. The child must refrain from eating and drinking as emergency surgical exploration under general anaesthesia may be the only way to establish the diagnosis.

Differential Diagnosis

- Torsion of testis: can occur at any age but is more common after 10 years of age and affects 1 in 4000 males under the age of 25 years each year. A testis torted in the perinatal period is virtually never salvageable; however, the contralateral testis should undergo dartos pouch fixation to prevent contralateral torsion and loss of both testes.

- Torsion of hydatid of Morgagni: twisting of the appendage of the testis classically produces a tender dark spot above a non-tender testis; peak age of 11 years.

- Idiopathic scrotal oedema: careful examination will demonstrate the painless, salmon-pink oedema to extend beyond the confines of the scrotum. This condition is self-limiting; peak age 5 to 6 years.

- Epididymo-orchitis is uncommon in childhood and associated with urinary tract pathology and therefore requires a follow-up ultrasound scan of the urinary tract and pelvis.

- Incarcerated inguinal hernia (see the chapter 'Neonatal and General Paediatric Surgery').

- Trauma: rare.

■ Testicular tumour: although the vast majority of testicular tumours present as an assiduous painless mass, the sudden detection by a parent may result in an acute presentation (Figure 22.33).

Urolithiasis

Incidence

Over the last decades, the incidence of urinary tract stones in children has risen, particularly in adolescence, to as high as 1 in 5000 in some parts of the Western world. Marked geographical variation nevertheless persists: while very rare in Greenland and Japan, a 'stone belt' extends from the Balkans across Turkey, Pakistan and northern India. Overall, boys are twice as often affected as girls and tend to present at a younger age.

Aetiology

Unlike the adult population who have mostly idiopathic stones, most renal calculi in children are either infective, metabolic or are associated with an underlying anatomical abnormality. (Figure 22.34). Bladder stones are particularly prevalent in children with bladder augmentation (Figure 22.35).

The organisms most commonly associated with infective calculi are the urea splitting *Proteus* spp. and *Escherichia coli*. Today, a metabolic abnormality is detected in 44% of children with urolithiasis in the United Kingdom. Hypercalciuria (57%) is the most common metabolic abnormality, followed by cystinuria (23%), hyperoxaluria (17%), hyperuricosuria (2%) and unclassified hypercalcaemia (2%).

Clinical Presentation

Presenting features are macroscopic haematuria, UTI or abdominal pain; however, one in six children appear to be asymptomatic. Obstruction related to calculi may result in pyonephrosis, perinephric abscess, or progressive pyelonephritis and renal loss; emergency admission and relief of obstruction is required.

Imaging

Ultrasound is the first line modality. Where additional detail is needed, ultra-low dose CT scanners and protocols have made abdominal x-ray (AXR) and intravenous urography (IVU) obsolete. Functional imaging will detect renal

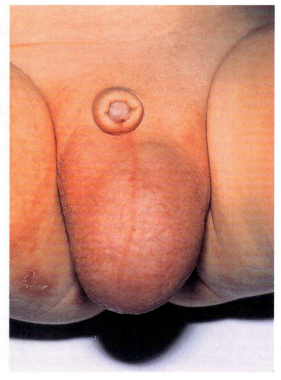

Figure 22.33 Scrotal mass caused by a tumour.

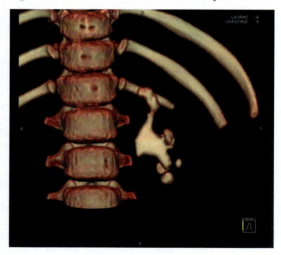

Figure 22.34 CT reconstruction of a left staghorn calculus.

damage resulting from the stone and diuretic renography may help identify underlying anatomical abnormalities, such as PUJA, VUJA or VUR.

Treatment

Once sepsis/infection has been controlled and obstruction relieved, the first aim of management is to clear all stones. Today, minimally invasive techniques are available even for the youngest of children and, as in adults, have largely replaced open surgery.

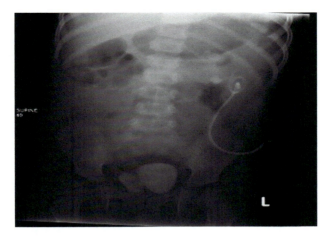

Figure 22.35 Plain abdominal radiograph showing two massive bladder stones and a staghorn left renal stone. A perinephric drain has been placed to drain a perinephric abscess.

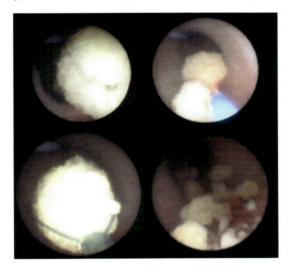

Figure 22.36 Intra-operative images of ureterorenoscopic laser stone disintegration and extraction.

- Extracorporal shock wave lithotripsy (ESWL) uses a shockwave generated outside the body and focused through the body tissues onto the stone to break the stone into smaller pieces, which can then be passed out of the body within the urine.

- Ureterorenoscopy (URS) employs tiny telescopes passed though the urethra and bladder to gain access to stones in the ureter and kidney (Figure 22.36).

- Percutaneous nephrolithotomy (PCNL) uses image guidance to gain keyhole access into the kidney. Stones are fragmented using a lithoclast and removed through the keyhole tract (Figure 22.37).

- Bladder stones can be removed by open or keyhole surgery (percutaneous cystolithotomy, PCCL) or cystoscopically.

As a result of the high incidence of underlying metabolic, anatomical or functional causes for stone formation, children are at significant risk of recurrent stone formation. Once stone clearance has been achieved, management moves on to the prevention of recurrence. A high fluid intake for urine solute dilution is essential for all. Other treatments will depend on underlying aetiologies.

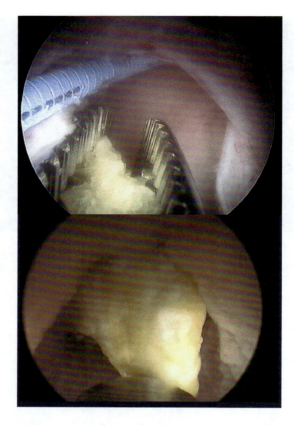

Figure 22.37 Intraoperative images of stone fragment extraction and lithoclast stone disintegration via the percutaneous nephrolithotomy tract.

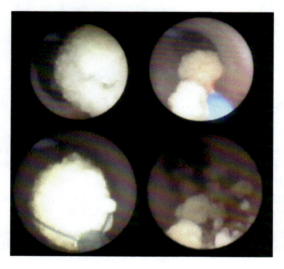

Figure 22.38 Intra-operative images of stone fragment extraction and lithoclast stone disintegration via the percutaneous nephrolithotomy tract.

NEOPLASIA

Childhood tumours of the urinary tract occur most commonly in the kidney (mostly Wilms tumour), the bladder-prostate (as rhabdomyosarcoma) or the testis/paratesticular. The reader is referred to the chapter 'Oncology' for further details. The uro-oncology surgeon has a major role in diagnosis/staging, stabilising children ahead of chemotherapy, surgical resection and function preservation/restoration.

FURTHER READING

- Wilcox DT, Thomas DFM (eds). *Essentials of Paediatric Urology*, 3rd edition. London: CRC Press, 2021.
- Wilcox D, Godbole P, Cooper C (eds). *Pediatric Urology Book*. http://www.pediatricurologybook .com.

23 Allergic Diseases

Ru-Xin Foong, Nandinee Patel, Adam T Fox and Stephan Strobel

INTRODUCTION

Allergic diseases describe disorders mediated by an exaggerated Th2 immune response to normally harmless environmental allergens. Prevalence rates have increased over time in low, middle and high income countries around the world. This is thought to be partly due to changes in environmental exposures and rapid urbanisation. Development of allergic diseases is the result of a complex interplay between genetic, epigenetic, and environmental factors during a vulnerable period.

Common terminology used in the field of allergy are defined in the glossary below.

ANAPHYLAXIS

Definition

Anaphylaxis is a systemic hypersensitivity reaction that is usually rapid in onset and may only rarely cause death if treated appropriately. Severe anaphylaxis is characterised by potentially life-threatening compromise in airway, breathing and/or circulation, and may occur without typical skin features or circulatory shock (WAO 2020)

Prevalence and Pathophysiology

The lifetime prevalence of IgE-mediated anaphylaxis is 0.3–5%.

Clinical Features

Allergic reactions where airway, breathing or circulatory signs occur are categorised as anaphylaxis. Speed of anaphylaxis onset can vary depending on amount of allergen exposure and route of exposure. Anaphylaxis can also be triggered by exercise with allergen exposure (exercise induced anaphylaxis) or without a known trigger (idiopathic anaphylaxis). Biphasic anaphylaxis (recurrence of anaphylaxis within 72 hours of the first reaction) occurs in approximately 5% of reactions, and patients should be informed of this possibility.

Diagnosis

Anaphylaxis is a clinical diagnosis and diagnostic criteria are published to support prompt diagnosis.

Treatment

Intramuscular adrenaline is the first line treatment for anaphylaxis. Delayed adrenaline administrated is noted to increase the risk for biphasic reactions and the need for additional treatment. In approximately 10% of anaphylaxis reactions, a single dose of adrenaline is insufficient to resolve the anaphylaxis. Current recommendations are for patients at risk of anaphylaxis to have access to at least two adrenaline autoinjector devices in the community.

Prognosis

In drug allergy fatality occurs in up to 0.51 per million people/year. In food allergy fatality occurs in up to 0.32 per million people years. Although the risk of fatality from anaphylaxis is rare, these represent potentially avoidable fatalities where prevention should be the goal.

FOOD ALLERGY

Food allergy and intolerance can be divided into IgE-mediated (immediate-onset symptoms) and non-IgE-mediated (delayed onset symptoms), depending on the underlying allergic mechanism. Adverse responses to food which are not mediated through an immune pathway are known as food intolerances and are not discussed further. Subtypes of adverse responses to food are shown in Figure 23.3.

DOI: 10.1201/9781003175186-23

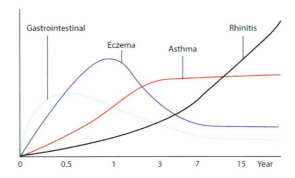

Figure 23.1 The Allergic March – Depiction of the point-prevalence of allergic diseases over time described as the allergic or atopic march.

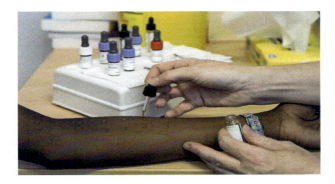

Figure 23.2 Skin prick testing.

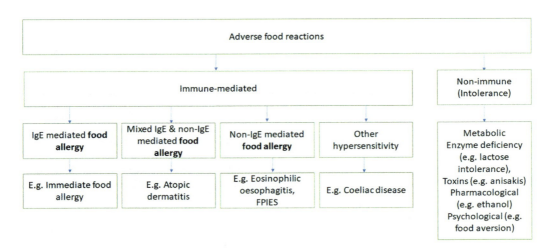

Figure 23.3 Classification of adverse reactions to food.

Prevalence

Around 1% of adults and 3–5% of children worldwide have food allergies; the prevalence may be even higher in the first year of life, estimated at 6–8% in Western countries. Whilst egg and cow's milk allergy are universally common causes of food allergy, the prevalence of additional food allergies varies, and is influenced by geographic location and distinctive dietary habits. The prevalence of peanut allergy in the United Kingdom has nearly doubled over the past decade, and now

Table 23.1: Common Terminology in Allergy

Hypersensitivity: A harmful, exaggerated immune response that has the potential to cause tissue damage.

Atopy: an inheritable pre-disposition to produce IgE antibodies towards harmless environmental allergens. The likelihood of developing allergic disease is only 13% if neither parent is atopic, this increases to 29% if one parent is atopic and 47% if both parents are atopic.

Sensitisation: The presence of IgE antibodies to an allergen(s). Antibodies may be detected within plasma or within tissues, bound to mast cells and basophils. Sensitisation may exist without the presence of clinical symptoms of allergy.

Allergen: an environmental antigen that has the capacity to generate an allergic immune response and binds to IgE antibodies.

Allergic reaction: The constellation of symptoms and signs occurring in an allergic individual following exposure to an allergen.

Allergy: The clinical expression, through reproducible symptoms, of an exaggerated immune response to usually innocuous environmental allergens.

The Allergic March: A term describing the natural history and sequential development of allergic phenotypes over time. This concept has now been superseded to a degree by the idea of single and multi-disease clusters over time **(Figure 23.1).**

Immediate allergy: IgE-mediated hypersensitivity, where clinical reactions typically occur within two hours of allergen exposure in a susceptible individual.

Delayed allergy: Description of a non-IgE-mediated (commonly cell-mediated) hypersensitivity, where clinical reactions typically occur mostly longer than two hours after allergen exposure in a susceptible individual.

Skin prick testing (SPT) (Figure 23.2): A rapid *in vivo* test performed in individuals suspected of having an IgE allergy. A standardised liquid extract of the allergen is placed on the skin and a lancet is used to prick the skin beneath. In sensitised individuals, tissue resident mast cells may be activated causing a localised wheal to develop around the puncture site. The size of the wheal predicts the likelihood of a clinical allergy but not reaction severity.

Intradermal testing: An *in vivo* test where a small volume of allergen is injected into the dermal layer and the skin assessed for evidence of local reaction after ~20 mins. It is more commonly used in testing for Type 1 drug allergies.

Patch testing: This *in vivo* test is performed by applying allergen under a seal to the skin (usually on the back) for an extended period and reviewing after 72 hour for any skin reaction. Sensitivity and specificity are unreliable and used mainly for contact (Type 4 hypersensiitvity).

Serum specific IgE testing: Serum is assessed for the presence of IgE antibodies to a whole allergen source (sensitisation). The sensitivity and specificity for clinical allergy varies greatly by allergen.

Component resolved diagnostics: Diagnostic approach that uses purified native or recombinant allergens to detect the sIgE antibodies response against the individual allergenic molecules 'components' in addition to whole allergens. Multiple 'components' have been identified. Over 16 components have been identified in peanut of which only a small number (~2) are used in clinical practice.

Oral food challenge (OFC): This is the gold standard procedure for diagnosing an IgE-mediated and delayed onset food allergy. Allergen is ingested in an incremental fashion in a supervised setting with observation in between doses for signs of an immediate or delayed reaction. If the food challenge is completed, and the top dose is ingested without symptoms, the food may then be re-introduced into the child's regular diet.

approximates 1.8%. An Australian study found a peanut allergy rate of 3% in children at 1 year of age. The prevalence reduces from infancy to young adults reflective of a substantial proportion of food allergy diagnoses self-resolving during childhood. Prevalence of self-reported food allergy can be up to ten times higher than challenge-proven allergy and reflects over-perception by patients and the importance of careful history and specialist assessment to make an accurate diagnosis. In specialist cohorts, approximately half of patients will avoid multiple food allergens.

IgE-MEDIATED FOOD ALLERGY

Pathophysiology

IgE-mediated food allergies develop due to the development of pathological T-helper Type 2 immune responses to innocuous food proteins (allergens) exposed to the body at key barrier sites (including the skin, gastrointestinal tract and lungs). This results in sensitisation (the production of allergen specific IgE antibodies which then bind to basophils, mast cells and eosinophils). On subsequent exposure to the same food allergen, specific allergen peptides are recognised by these specific IgE antibodies and activate the effector cells to release inflammatory mediators including histamine resulting in an immediate allergic reaction.

Clinical Features

Phenotypes of immediate food allergies can vary, and a few subtypes are described below. However, they are usually typified by allergic reaction symptoms which occur within two hours (usually within minutes) of exposure to the allergen. Multiple organ systems may be involved (generalised) or symptoms may occur only at the site of exposure (localised) and the severity of symptoms can vary but includes fatality secondary to anaphylaxis. Symptoms of an allergic reaction may include any of those listed in Table 23.2. Figure 23.4 shows an example of a child who has developed urticaria.

Primary Food Allergies

Primary food allergy can occur to any food. The prevalence of different food allergies varies across the globe. In the United Kingdom common food allergies include: hen's egg, cow's milk, wheat, peanut, tree nuts (e.g. cashew, walnut, hazelnut), sesame and fish. In the United Kingdom the following allergens must be labelled on pre-packaged goods: celery, cereals (including wheat and oats), crustacea, hen's egg, fish, lupin, cow's milk, mollusc (e.g. mussels), mustard, tree nuts, peanuts, sesame seeds, soybean, sulphites (which are chemical compounds that contain the sulphite ion which can cause respiratory and other symptoms). Patterns of co-allergy exist (walnut allergy is often co-associated with pecan allergy, and cashew with pistachio allergy). The amount of allergen ingestion required to trigger an allergic reaction will vary (in a normal distribution), e.g. one child may develop symptoms after exposure to a drop of milk whereas another only may react after ingestion of half a glass of milk. The trigger level and the reaction severity experienced may be affected by a host of 'co-factors': exercise, infection and other stress factors can all impact on the reaction. Phenotypes can also vary within a particular food or food group. In hen's egg allergy, over two-thirds of allergic individuals can tolerate baked egg without symptoms. In fish allergy in the United Kingdom, some forms may be tolerated (e.g. tinned tuna) as the major allergen (parvalbumin) is usually found within white muscle in fish.

Secondary Food Allergy – Pollen Food Allergy Syndrome

Patient's suffering from pollen food allergy syndrome have primary sensitisations to aeroallergens (e.g. birch pollen). Some fruits and vegetables will contain proteins (usually in their peel), with a similar structure to this pollen and therefore on ingestion of the raw fruit, the immune system

Table 23.2: Symptoms of an IgE-Mediated Allergic Reaction

Organ System	Symptoms
Skin	Urticaria, lip or face angioedema (Figure 23.3), erythema, pruritus
Oropharayngeal, ENT	Oral or throat pruritus, tongue angioedema, rhinitis, conjunctival injection, itchy eyes
Gastrointestinal	Abdominal pain, nausea, vomiting
Laryngeal	Hoarse voice, tight throat, throat lump sensation, painful throat, painful swallow
Respiratory	Wheezing, tight chest, difficulty breathing
Cardiovascular	Tachycardia, hypotension, pallor
Neurological	Reduced Glasgow Coma Scale, collapse, agitation

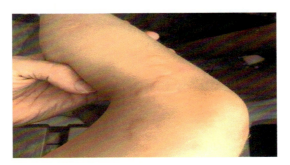

Figure 23.4 Clinical presentation of hives following exposure to a food allergen.

recognises these and triggers allergic symptoms. In these individuals who have developed cross-reactivity, ingestion of raw fruits containing cross-reactive allergens often results in local symptoms (e.g. oral allergy syndrome) but rarely causes systemic symptoms due to the labile nature of these allergens. Similarly, food processing (e.g. through cooking for the production of apple juice or apple pie) will result in denaturing of these labile allergens so they are 'unrecognisable' by the individuals and will not cause reactions. Onset of pollen food allergy usually occurs in older children, following a period of aeroallergen sensitisation.

Food-Dependant Exercise Induced Anaphylaxis

Foods allergic reactions can be affected by exercise acting as a 'co-factor'. Food-dependant exercise induced anaphylaxis exists where a food is usually tolerated but has the capacity to cause anaphylaxis, when the food is ingested close to or during exertion. Common food triggers include wheat (e.g. omega-5-gliadin) and shellfish. The clinical presentation can include cutaneous, respiratory, gastrointestinal, and cardiovascular symptoms that occur within ten minutes or up to four hours after the food has been. Most patients can tolerate the culprit food allergen and exercise independently. Conventional allergy tests (SPT and sIgE) may be helpful but it is primarily a clinical diagnosis. The diagnostic test is a modified exercise challenge under close medical supervision. The management for patients includes i.m. epinephrine injection as for normal anaphylaxis treatment. Once the culprit food has been identified, avoidance of any food triggers for at least four to six hours before exercise and one-hour post-exercise is recommended.

Diagnosis

Diagnosis is based on a combination of reaction history (e.g. swollen lips following peanut ingestion, see Figure 23.5), assessment of sensitisation based on SPT and/or serum IgE testing which gives a clinical likelihood of allergy. Table 23.3 provides some useful questions to consider when taking a food allergy focused history. Confirmation, if required, is by oral provocation challenge which remains the definitive diagnostic procedure.

Treatment

Currently management includes complete allergen avoidance and provision of medications for the management of accidental allergic reactions, alongside training for families on the prompt

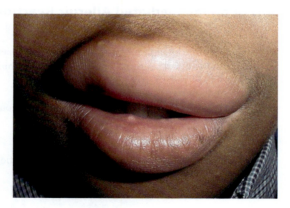

Figure 23.5 Lip angioedema in a 10-year-old boy following ingestion of cow's milk.

Table 23.3: Taking a Food Allergy History

Questions to ask when a food-allergic reaction is suspected:
1. What symptoms occurred as part of the reaction?
2. The ingredients and amounts of the food consumed (and route of exposure) prior to the reaction and preceding meal
3. Have those food been eaten and tolerated before this occasion? Have those foods been eaten and tolerated after this reaction?
4. Time interval between suspected food allergen ingestion and onset of symptoms
5. Other relevant factors (other active health conditions and health symptoms, current medications). Other contacts with similar symptoms. Previous history of similar symptoms.

recognition and response to reactions (see the section 'Anaphylaxis'). All paediatric patients with a diagnosis of IgE-mediated food allergy should be provided with a written allergy action plan. Dietetic review is helpful to provide comprehensive allergen avoidance advice (including potential sources of hidden allergen, e.g. peanut flour as a thickener in sauces), information on alternative sources of nutrients (e.g. calcium in a cow's milk allergic child) and assess adequate nutrition for growth (in a multiple food-allergic child). Interval specialist review is recommended for assessment of natural resolution of allergy. Nevertheless, there is a growing move towards more active management in an attempt to modify the disease trajectory to immune re-training using food immunotherapy protocols. Several phase 3 trials have reached completion and we are at the beginning of a new management strategy for paediatric food allergy. Food immunotherapy involves exposing the patient to a small amount of allergen which is gradually increased over time to achieve desensitisation (an increase in the amount of allergen the patient can ingest without reaction, which is dependent on regular exposure to the allergen).

With pollen food syndrome, strict food avoidance is not mandatory and patients often find a balance of inclusion of processed forms of the food. Additionally, unless any concerning factors are present, i.m. epinephrine is not usually prescribed.

Prognosis
Cow's milk, hen's egg and wheat allergy are common food allergies in infancy and are commonly outgrown in the first decade of life (e.g. wheat allergy has a two-third resolution rate by 12 years of age, egg allergy has more than 80% resolution by 3 years of age). Other food allergens demonstrate later onset (e.g. shellfish) or a more persistent profile e.g. peanut, tree nuts and shellfish (approximately 80% of peanut allergy will persist into adulthood).

Prevention
Many risk factors associated with the development of food allergy have been suggested. The strongest evidence for prevention in high-risk infants (significant early onset eczema) from developing allergies seems to be the early introduction of peanut and egg into the infant weaning diet from four to six months.

NON-IgE-MEDIATED FOOD ALLERGY
Pathophysiology
The mechanisms of development of non-IgE-mediated food allergies is less well understood. However, in eosinophilic gastrointestinal disease T-cells are implicated as the major cell in disease development and symptoms. These cell-mediated pathways explain the non-immediate nature of symptom presentation in these diagnoses.

Clinical Features and Treatment
The most common non-IgE-mediated-reactions tend to involve the gastrointestinal tract and these include cow's milk protein allergy (CMPA), food-protein induced enterocolitis (FPIES) and eosinophilic gastrointestinal diseases (EGID). Management is diagnosis dependent and discussed below.

Cow's Milk Protein Allergy
CMPA is one of the most common food allergies seen in young children with a peak often in the first year of life. Reactions may occur immediately (including anaphylaxis). Other delayed reactions are triggered 2–72 hours after ingestion of cow's milk protein or the picture may be more mixed. This reaction is seen in either formula or mixed-fed but less commonly in breast-fed (e.g. via maternal ingestion of cow's milk) infants. These infants can present with a wide range of symptoms including gastrointestinal reflux, vomiting, diarrhoea, blood and/or mucous in the stools, abdominal pain/discomfort, constipation, or faltering growth. Additionally, exacerbations in atopic eczema may be noted (Figure 23.6).

However, these are common symptoms in infancy and careful clinical assessment is required to avoid overdiagnosis. Allergy testing including SPT and specific cow's milk IgE are often negative in delayed responses, although they are positive in individuals with immediate symptoms. Diagnosis of delayed reactions is made via a detailed clinical history and a trial of cow's milk elimination diet for at least four weeks. In formula-fed infants the choice of extensively hydrolysed or amino acid formulas is based on severity of symptoms, evidence of impaired growth and age. In over 50% of patients cross-sensitisation will occur to soya protein and therefore soya milk as

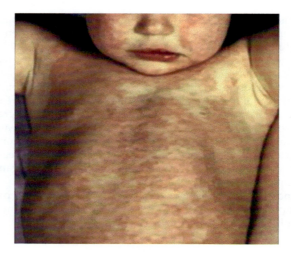

Figure 23.6 Atopic dermatitis exacerbation (with facial involvement and extensive erythema) noted in an 18-month toddler with cow's milk protein allergy.

milk replacement should also be avoided. Confirmation of diagnosis is by re-introduction and cow's milk proteins. Following diagnosis confirmation, cow's milk should continue to be avoided for at least six months with subsequent re-introduction attempted thereafter. In the EuroPrevall birth cohort of children with non-IgE-mediated cow's milk allergy, 100% of the children were tolerant to cow's milk within one year after diagnosis. Nevertheless, in reality a proportion of children will continue to have symptoms beyond 1 year of age and in these cases, switching to a plant-based calcium-enriched drink is the preferred option.

Food Protein Induced Enterocolitis (FPIES)

FPIES is a condition where two to four hours following exposure to an allergen, a child presents with profuse vomiting, diarrhoea and lethargy and hypothermia with hypotension occurring in about 15% of patients. The most common foods to cause FPIES vary by global region, In the United Kingdom, cow's milk and soya FPIES are common, whilst fish and crustacea are more common in Mediterranean countries and rice in the Far East. Patients are often initially misdiagnosed as having an acute infective illness (e.g. gastroenteritis or sepsis) which can result in a delay in their diagnosis. Diagnosis is clinical. The gold standard for diagnosing FPIES is by an oral food challenge which should be performed in a hospital setting due to the risk of hypotension and potential requirement of intravenous fluids. Management options for an acute reaction include intravenous fluids and ondansetron (a specific $5HT_3$-receptor antagonist which blocks $5HT_3$ receptors in the gastrointestinal tract), which, when given early may curtail a reaction. Once diagnosis is confirmed, allergen avoidance is recommended. Interval food challenges may be needed to assess if the patient has outgrown the allergy at the earliest by 18–24 months after the initial diagnosis. Infant FPIES is often outgrown by age 3–5 years.

Eosinophilic Gastrointestinal Disease (EGID)

EGID is a chronic immune mediated disease characterised by gastrointestinal symptoms and histologically by increased eosinophil-predominant inflammation (Figure 23.7).

EGID include a range of diseases that affect different parts of the gastrointestinal tract with tissue eosinophilia being a hallmark feature. They are classified according to their site, depth and severity of the inflammation seen in the gastrointestinal tract with the most common being eosinophilic oesophagitis (EoE), eosinophilic gastroenteritis and eosinophilic colitis. The pathogenesis is thought to be related to a hypersensitivity reaction that triggers the accumulation of eosinophils which release immunomodulatory cytokines that lead to local tissue damage. Children with EoE present with symptoms such as dysphagia, food bolus impaction, food aversion/refusal, reflux and/or growth failure. Families often report a child taking increasingly long to complete a meal (especially with foods like bread) and require large volumes of liquid during a meal, to assist with swallowing. Diagnosis is confirmed via endoscopy showing typical features (furrows and rings)

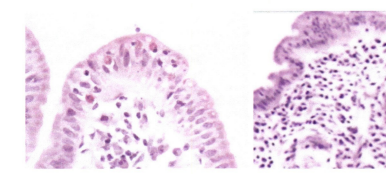

Figure 23.7 Eosinophilic infiltration in the mucosal epithelium in a duodenal biopsy in a child with Eosinophilic Gastrointestinal Disease (EGID).

and a multi-site biopsy displays more than 15 eosinophils per high power field. Treatment includes topical steroids (e.g. oral viscous budesonide) and/or an elimination diet of up to six common allergenic foods (i.e. cow's milk, soya, egg, wheat, peanut, fish) for at least four to six weeks. With symptom improvement, re-introduction of foods is important with repeated endoscopies to confirm histological improvement between introductions. In all cases of food elimination diets in the management of EGID, a multidisciplinary approach to care is important often including allergists, dieticians and gastroenterologists.

ATOPIC ECZEMA

Atopic eczema (atopic dermatitis) is a chronic inflammatory, pruritic skin condition that develops early in childhood and follows a remitting and relapsing course. It is often the first presentation of allergic disease in children. It is caused by a combination of genetic and environmental factors and may be exacerbated by many factors including infection, irritants and allergens in some individuals. It can occur in infants as young as 4 weeks of age and is a risk factor for the development of IgE-mediated food allergies.

Prevalence

The prevalence of atopic eczema has markedly increased in countries during the past three decades and affects 15 to 30% of children. Around 45% of atopic eczema begins within the first six months of life; 60% begin during the first year, and 85% begin before 5 years of age; 70% of these children have a spontaneous remission before adolescence.

Genetics and Pathophysiology

Familial genetic factors affect the skin barrier and the immune response including T-cell driven inflammation, are important in the underlying mechanism of eczema. Filaggrin (FLG) is an abundantly expressed protein in the outer layers of the epidermis and plays a crucial role in skin-barrier formation and protection against ultraviolet radiation. The gene for FLG is situated on chromosome 1q21 and carriers of FLG mutations are at significantly increased risk of developing atopic dermatitis, contact allergy, asthma and allergic rhinitis. Patients with atopic dermatitis who carry a FLG mutation appear to be predisposed to more severe, persistent forms of the disease and possibly to peanut allergy.

Clinical Features

Many differing phenotypes (e.g. follicular, erythrodermic) exist and the appearance of each can vary in different skin types. The clinical manifestations of atopic dermatitis vary with age. Eczema can occur in discrete patches or be diffuse over regions of the body. Common additional sites in infants include cheek involvement and seborrheic dermatitis of the scalp. In older children, facial exacerbations, particularly around the eyes, can occur and may be secondary to aeroallergen sensitisation.

Type IV hypersensitivity (contact dermatitis) can overlap with eczema, at any site. It is difficult to control eczema at specific sites (e.g. hands, eyelids and around piercings) The impact of itch symptoms should not be underestimated, as it can often disturb sleep, and affect a patient's quality of life.

Diagnosis

Diagnosis is clinical with hallmarks of itch and roughness of the skin on touch. Several validated scores (e.g. POEM, SCORAD) can be used to track the percentage of the body affected and flare severity over time, and thus the effectiveness of treatment. In troublesome infective flares, skin swabs for microbial culture assist in directing the focused use of antibiotics or antivirals. In severe or unremitting cases it is important to assess if any overlap immune syndromes may exist. (e.g. hyper IgE syndrome, ectodermal dysplasia, Wiskott–Aldrich syndrome) see the chapter 'Immunology'. Potential exacerbating factors may be detected through careful history.

Atopic eczema is a risk factor for the development of IgE-mediated food allergies in childhood (80% of food-allergic children will report a history of atopic eczema during infancy).

Food allergens: Children with early onset eczema (under 1 year) have a higher likelihood of food allergens contributing to the onset or persistence of exacerbations through a non-IgE-mediated mechanism (over 60% of infants with severe eczema starting under 3 months of age). Cow's milk, soya, hen's egg and wheat are common exacerbating factors in allergic patients. No validated, diagnostic test is available. If the history is suggestive, of this, a trial of allergen exclusion for three to four weeks may be tried followed by re-introduction. Improvement in eczema symptom control during exclusion with recurrence of symptoms on re-exposure would suggest food as a contributing factor. To avoid nutritional deficiencies, food exclusions should only be undertaken with the advice of an experienced professional. Screening for IgE sensitisations is usually unhelpful since atopic children often have raised total non-specific IgE sensitisations without clinical relevance.

Other foods (e.g. tomatoes, packaged meat), may cause erythema at eczema sites on ingestion as a non-allergic phenomenon, secondary to its histamine content.

Non-food allergens: If aeroallergens are suspected as an exacerbating factor in facial eczema (more common in older children), SPT or blood IgE testing may demonstrate IgE antibodies to specific aeroallergens (e.g. house-dust mite, cat dander, grass pollen) and specific allergen avoidance advised. Sensitisation to indoor airborne allergens often occurs earlier than sensitisation to pollen.

Treatment

The mainstay of eczema management is the use of topical agents: emollients, wet wrap treatment and anti-inflammatory agents (topical steroids or steroid-sparing calcineurin inhibitors) proportional to the severity eczema. Systemic immunosuppression (e.g. methotrexate) have been the traditional step-up treatment for difficult to control eczema. However, Dupilumab (an anti-IL4 and anti-IL13 monoclonal antibody) is now licenced for use and has been shown to reduce eczema severity and percentage skin surface area affected as well as reducing the itch. Multiple additional biologic agents are now explored (see the chapter 'Dermatology'). Optimisation of eczema management will aid restoration of epidermal barrier function and may reduce sensitivity to airborne or contact allergens.

ALLERGIC AIRWAYS DISEASE: Allergic Rhinitis, Rhinoconjunctivitis and Allergic Asthma: Aspects Related to Food Allergies

Allergic airways disease encompasses a variety of symptoms and conditions that affect the shared, connecting mucosal lining of the airways, from the nose to the lungs. The level of inflammation at each site will affect symptom control at the other sites. These diagnoses often exist together i.e. allergic rhinitis tends to be higher in patients with allergic asthma.

ALLERGIC ASTHMA

Prevalence

The incidence of asthma in childhood is about 10–15% with some European countries reaching rates of about 20%. Food allergies and asthma often co-exist with one another and share similar risk factors. It has been reported that 4–8% of asthmatic children have food allergies and approximately 50% of food-allergic children have asthma. UK data suggest a childhood diagnosis of food allergy is associated with an almost three-fold increase in a diagnosis of asthma in adulthood.

Genetics and Pathophysiology

Asthma arises from a complex interplay of genetic and environmental factors. Several phenotypes and endotypes exists under the umbrella diagnosis of asthma. In allergic asthma eosinophilia is often demonstrated and aeroallergen exposure has an impact on respiratory inflammation in sensitised individuals. Genome wide association studies demonstrate numerous loci with significant association with asthma, eczema and rhinitis as well as responsiveness to asthma treatments including biologics. Children with (poorly controlled) asthma and food allergies have a heightened risk of developing more severe clinical reactions on food exposure including anaphylaxis and are therefore at greater risk of fatal anaphylaxis. Around 75% of children with peanut allergy develop asthma.

All children with asthma and food allergies should have regular follow up for the management of their asthma and food allergies including access to emergency epinephrine autoinjectors.

Clinical Features and Diagnosis

A detailed description is provided in the chapter 'Respiratory Medicine'. We focus on key allergic aspects of asthma below. IgE-sensitisation to aeroallergens (commonly house-dust mite and cat dander from infancy and grass and tree pollens in childhood/adolescence) can contribute to airway inflammation in sensitised individuals. This may be suggested by a history of exacerbations on allergen exposure. Some aeroallergens (e.g. cat dander) can be potent at triggering wheeze with a degree of desensitisation (hypo-responsiveness) brought about by constant exposure. Removal of the allergen during holidays may exacerbate clinical sensitivity on return. Food allergies do not normally present with isolated or chronic respiratory symptoms.

Treatment

The mainstay of treatment for allergic asthma (inhaled corticosteroids and bronchodilators) is detailed further in the chapter 'Respiratory Medicine'. Anti-IgE monoclonal antibody treatment has been licenced as an add-on treatment in those with an allergic phenotype. Biologics targeting other aspects of the allergic pathway (e.g. Interleukin 4, 5, 13) are likely to become future licenced treatment options for children. There is emerging evidence to suggest that desensitisation of children with allergic rhinitis to grass or tree pollen may be less likely to progress to the development of asthma if they are desensitised to the causative pollen.

ALLERGIC RHINOCONJUNCTIVITIS

Prevalence

Up to 40% of the population are affected by allergic rhinoconjunctivitis at some point in their lives, with increasing prevalence with age. By 4 years of age approximately 20% show sensitisation to aeroallergens. The incidence of rhinitis peaks around 12–15 years of age. Although symptoms may worsen during the first few pollen seasons, they often stabilise and can disappear entirely over time in about 20% of children.

Genetics and Pathophysiology

Genetic backgrounds of atopy including family history, presence of early atopic eczema and/or food allergies can increase the risk of developing allergic rhinitis. Most reactions to seasonal allergens tend not to appear before the child is 2–3 years of age.

Clinical Features

Common symptoms include nasal symptoms and ocular symptoms (Figures 23.8A and 23.8B). Other hallmark clinical signs of children with severe rhinitis include the: 'allergic shiner' (a darkening of the lower eyelids due to suborbital oedema), 'allergic crease' (a transverse skin crease above the tip and below the bridge of the nose caused by constant rubbing) and 'allergic salute' (upward rubbing of the nose with the palm of the hand due to persistent itching and trying to open the nasal passages). A proportion of patients may exhibit isolated nasal symptoms in 'allergic rhinitis'.

Symptoms can disturb sleep, attention and can have significant adverse effects on a child's quality of life. Common triggers of seasonal symptoms include grass, tree and weed pollen (except in tropical regions where these may become perennial allergens) whereas perennial allergens include house-dust mite, animal dander and moulds).

Diagnosis

Clinical examination typically reveals prominent inferior turbinates and inflammation demonstrated by mucosal pallor and clear discharge. Rarely, sensitisation is not noted on SPT or blood IgE testing but local investigation (e.g. via conjunctival challenge or intranasal challenge) may only

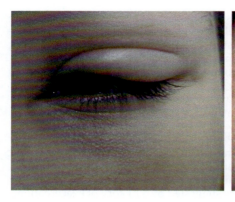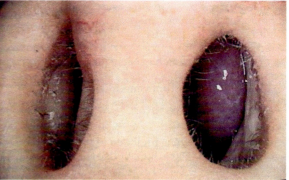

Figure 23.8 (A) Eyelid angioedema noted in a child with significant allergic rhinoconjunctivitis secondary to tree pollen sensitisation (B) inflamed inferior turbinate in left nostril obstructing airflow.

demonstrate the presence of local IgE. Validated scores exist for the assessment of disease severity and the impact of symptoms on daily activities, which can be used for the assessment of the effect of treatments. In early onset, or atypical presentations of rhinitis, alternative diagnoses must be eliminated first.

Treatment

The first line of treatment includes environmental allergen avoidance measures in combination with the use of non-sedating antihistamine on an as-required basis if symptoms are infrequent. For more persistent bothersome symptoms, intranasal corticosteroids provide the greatest effect on symptom control. Topical antihistamine eye drops may be used as an add-on treatment. For children who are on maximal therapy but still experience significant symptoms, sublingual and subcutaneous immunotherapies have been shown to be effective for grass, tree, and house-dust mite aeroallergens. Aeroallergen immunotherapy consists of a three-year treatment course where an individual is exposed to a small dose of a specific aeroallergen known to significantly contribute to symptoms. This is achieved on a regular basis via the sublingual route or subcutaneous route to desensitise their immune system to future allergen exposure.

DRUG ALLERGY

Prevalence

Drug hypersensitivity reactions represent adverse effects of drugs taken at a dose that is tolerated by normal subjects and which clinically resembles allergy. They are suspected in 3–15% of paediatric patients, although allergy is confirmed in only one-tenth of cases and are not discussed in detail at this stage.

Clinical Features

Drugs and under certain conditions, vaccines, can result in allergic reactions. Some of the more common medications that can cause drug reactions include: antibiotics, anti-hypertensives, anti-convulsants, local anaesthetics agents and general anaesthesic agents (i.e. neuromuscular receptor blocking agents, opioids). In Gel and Coombs Type I reactions, speed of onset of symptoms may be dependent on route of administration with intravenous administration usually causing symptoms within minutes of exposure (Figure 23.9).

In Gel and Coombs Type IV cutaneous hypersensitivity reactions, symptom onset may occur four to six weeks after commencement of dosing. It is for this reason that a detailed drug and symptom history should be made, as well as an assessment of other known tolerated drug classes and the likelihood of needing further treatments. Vaccine-related drug allergic reactions are uncommon, especially severe adverse reactions such as anaphylaxis. If reactions do occur, testing to vaccine constituents (e.g. gelatine, egg protein, cow's milk, preservatives (i.e. thimerosal, aluminium, phenoxyethanol), yeast, dextran, latex) should be considered. Allergic reactions to vaccines should be distinguished from other non-allergic adverse events secondary to vaccines (e.g.

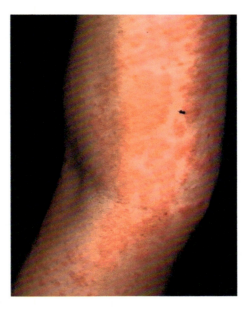

Figure 23.9 Urticaria appearing rapidly after ingestion of ceftriaxone in an adolescent being treated for pneumonia.

non-immune vasovagal events and immune [non-allergic] e.g. localised swelling and erythema or fever).

Diagnosis

In suspected allergy, the aim of investigation is to find suitable, safe alternative drugs or drug classes for future use. Where an allergy is unlikely, the purpose of testing is to de-label the assumed allergy. Depending on the pre-test likelihood of allergy, no further confirmatory testing may be required (e.g. anaphylaxis following intravenous penicillin use or drug reaction with eosinophilia and systemic symptom [DRESS] to ciprofloxacin). Depending on the reaction suspected, SPT, intradermal drug testing, basophil activation testing or lymphocyte transformation tests may be appropriate. Allergy testing can be highly predictive for some drugs (e.g. allergic reactions to neuromuscular blocking agents) as these drugs are the most common cause of allergic reactions during the onset of general anaesthesia.

Treatment and Prognosis

If a medication is required despite the presence of a Type 1 allergy, with no alternative agents available, rush drug desensitisation may be attempted. For intravenous medication this involves a staged process of slow exposure. Pre-medication to suppress allergic reactions may not consistently effective. Exposure would be repeated at each future drug administration if this was an interval dosing medication (e.g. three monthly ceftazidime for cystic fibrosis). This carries a high risk of systemic reactions and therefore should only be performed in specialist settings with access to intensive care support. Drug provocation tests can be performed for diagnostic clarity and de-labelling or to confirm safe alternatives. The natural history of drug allergies varies according to the underlying immunological mechanism. Penicillin allergies can be outgrown and individuals rarely becoming re-sensitised to it.

Antibiotic Allergy

Beta-lactam allergy is the most reported drug allergy (80–90% of reactions reported as cutaneous). Cutaneous presentations classically occur at the time of viral infections and so it can be very difficult to determine whether associated rashes (drug allergies usually present with cutaneous manifestations) arise from the index infection for which the antibiotic was prescribed or are due to the antibiotic or both. Therefore, clarification when the child is well can be helpful. Diagnostic tests are limited to specific serum IgE, SPT and/or intradermal tests or basophil activation testing which is restricted to research settings. The sensitivity and specificity of these tests are highly variable; sensitivities are generally low but specificities high. Often, if a side-chain reaction is implicated as the targeted allergen (e.g. amoxicillin allergy) penicillin may be tolerated and this should be assessed through oral drug provocation testing.

URTICARIA AND ANGIOEDEMA

Urticaria is an 'itchy' skin condition (also called hives or wheals) that can occur as an allergic manifestation, often, as the result of allergen exposure. Angioedema is the swelling of the skin at mucous membranes (e.g. lips, eyes). Chronic urticaria (CU) is a distinct condition in which urticaria occurs (unrelated to allergy) and persists for over six weeks. CU is rare in infancy and childhood affecting 0.1–3% of children.

Aetiology/Pathophysiology

CU is not an allergic condition, although allergies may co-exist (like in any other individual). The central effector cell is the dermal/mucosal mast cell, which on degranulation releases vasoactive mediators such as histamine, a major mediator of urticaria and angioedema. Most commonly, no known trigger is found for 'chronic spontaneous urticaria'. CU is sometimes associated with circulating 'auto-immune factors', i.e. the immune system wrongly targets skin cells (mast cells). This process results in the itchy skin and mucosal hives and swelling. These IgG autoantibodies can be detected and are usually present in 40–60% of cases; if present, their presence predicts a more prolonged disease course.

Clinical Presentation

CU presents as episodes of urticaria that persists beyond six weeks (Figure 23.10).

Angioedema is associated in 80% of cases. In children, the condition typically arises in otherwise healthy individuals, often with no known trigger or secondary to a preceding infective illness. Occasionally, autoimmune conditions (i.e. thyroid disease, coeliac disease, and vasculitis) are associated and may be suggested by history. A subset of patients may have symptoms triggered by a range of physical triggers (e.g. cold, heat, pressure, vibration, cholinergic activation) defined as chronic inducible urticaria. Overlap with vasculitic and rheumatological disorders presenting with urticaria and urticaria pigmentosa should be considered dependent on history and age of presentation.

Investigation

Investigation is based on suspected aetiology. Physical urticarias may be confirmed through a range of physical trigger testing (e.g. temperature test) and autoimmune screening may be indicated if history is suggestive. However, in self-limiting chronic spontaneous urticaria with angioedema, investigations are usually unhelpful.

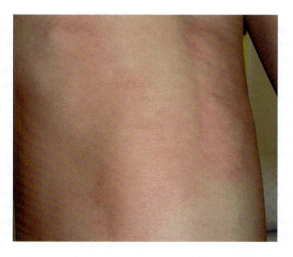

Figure 23.10 Patchy urticaria at the trunk with surrounding erythema in a child with chronic urticaria experiencing urticaria five days a week.

Treatment and Prognosis

High-dose non-sedating antihistamines are the first line treatment (up to a maximum of four times the daily dose). Anti-IgE monoclonal antibody has been licenced for the treatment of chronic, spontaneous urticaria but not inducible urticaria. Trials off therapy or weaning therapy are recommended at intervals to assess for spontaneous resolution. Resolution occurs in over two-thirds of patients within five years of onset.

FURTHER SUGGESTED READING

- Foong RX, Dantzer JA, Wood RA, et al. Improving diagnostic accuracy in food allergy. *J Allergy Clin Immunol Pract*. 2021;9(1):71–80. doi:10.1016/j.jaip.2020.09.037.
- Conrado AB, Patel N, Turner PJ. Global patterns in anaphylaxis due to specific foods: A systematic review. *J Allergy Clin Immunol*. 2021. doi:10.1016/j.jaci.2021.03.048.
- Tsuang A, Chan ES, Wang J. Food-induced anaphylaxis in infants: Can new evidence assist with implementation of food allergy prevention and treatment? *J Allergy Clin Immunol Pract*. 2021;9(1):57–69.
- Lopes JP, Sicherer S. Food allergy: Epidemiology, pathogenesis, diagnosis, prevention, and treatment. *Curr Opin Immunol*. 2020;66:57–64.
- Marrs T, Lack G, Fox AT, et al. The diagnosis and management of antibiotic allergy in children: Systematic review to inform a contemporary approach. *Arch Dis Child*. 2015;100(6):583–588.
- Cardona V, Ansotegui IJ, et al. World allergy organization anaphylaxis guidance 2020. *World Allergy Organ J*. 2020;13(10):100472. Published 2020 Oct 30. doi:10.1016/j.waojou.2020.100472.
- Sicherer SH, Sampson HA. Food allergy: A review and update on epidemiology, pathogenesis, diagnosis, prevention, and management. *J Allergy Clin Immunol*. 2018;141(1):41–58. doi:10.1016/j.jaci.2017.11.003.
- Sokolowska M, Eiwegger T, Ollert M, et al. EAACI statement on the diagnosis, management and prevention of severe allergic reactions to COVID-19 vaccines. *Allergy*. 2021;76:1629–1639. doi:10.1111/all.14739.
- Satitsuksanoa P, van de Veen W, Tan G, et al. Allergen-specific B cell responses in oral immunotherapy-induced desensitization, remission, and natural outgrowth in cow's milk allergy. *Allergy*. 2024;00:1–20. doi:10.1111/all.16220.

Index